Principles of total hip arthroplasty

Principles of
total hip arthroplasty

NAS SER EFTEKHAR, M.D., F.A.C.S.

Associate Clinical Professor of Orthopaedic
Surgery, College of Physicians and Surgeons,
Columbia University, New York;
Associate Attending Orthopaedic Surgeon and
Chief of Hip Service, New York Orthopaedic Hospital,
Columbia-Presbyterian Medical Center, New York;
Consulting Orthopaedic Surgeon, Valley Hospital,
Ridgewood, New Jersey

Illustrated by
ROBERT J. DEMAREST

Director of Medical Illustration,
College of Physicians and Surgeons,
Columbia University

with **841** illustrations

THE C. V. MOSBY COMPANY

Saint Louis   1978

The C. V. Mosby Company
11830 Westline Industrial Drive, St. Louis, Missouri 63141

Library of Congress Cataloging in Publication Data

Eftekhar, Nas S   1935-
    Principles of total hip arthroplasty.

    Bibliography: p.
    Includes index.
    1. Hip joint—Surgery.   2. Artificial hip joints.
3. Arthroplasty.   I. Title.
RD549.E37   617'.58   78-18471
ISBN 0-8016-1496-1

GW/U/B 9 8 7 6 5 4 3 2 1

To my teacher

SIR JOHN CHARNLEY

for his
contributions to orthopaedic surgery

Foreword

I am pleased to write a foreword for this monumental book, *Principles of Total Hip Arthroplasty,* written by one of my most dedicated and successful pupils. Dr. Nas Eftekhar came to me as a postgraduate student to study total hip replacement over eleven years ago and became so immersed in the subject that he doubled his originally proposed stay and evidently has never regretted this.

Eftekhar's book is appearing at a most opportune time; it is a reminder that results of consistently high quality, with a minimum of complications, are obtained only by concentrating on the minutiae of a surgical technique, provided always that the technique itself is well conceived. In this respect it is significant that although total hip replacement has now been "released" for general use for over a decade, many surgeons are still ready to change their methods for the most recent ideas and do this even though no fundamentally new principle may be involved and even though new hazards might lie ahead. This is the eternal hope for a magic method "which anyone can do."

The reader cannot fail to get the message so well put over by Eftekhar: that success depends on minute attention to originally planned detail. There is no place for mixing different techniques in the hope of getting a hybrid better than the root stock.

But let it not be thought that this foreword is merely complacent. No surgical technique can ever be 100 percent successful, though it is possible that some day total hip replacement might get very near this. We must openly face the weakest aspects of any well-tried technique in efforts to improve in specific directions. Only when we have come to the end of all efforts to improve on specific details will it become reasonable to abandon ten to fifteen years of past experience and submit large numbers of patients to totally new and untried principles.

Professor Sir John Charnley

Foreword

There has long been a need for a textbook on total hip replacements. Dr. Nas Eftekhar has filled this need. This book is accurately written and includes the history of hip arthroplasty, covering anatomical features, techniques, complications, and follow-up. Dr. Eftekhar has written in a lucid and readable manner. Being meticulous in accuracy, his illustrations are outstanding.

Dr. Eftekhar has limited his work and research to implant surgery and has made several important contributions to the philosophy as well as the biomechanics affecting total hip replacements in the human being. Probably one of the most important contributions is his discussion of the removal of the greater trochanter versus nonremoval. It should be of great interest to all surgeons who do extensive hip surgery. At no time does Dr. Eftekhar compromise in principle, and his very strong feelings shine through repeatedly in the text.

This book reflects the teacher. Dr. Eftekhar is a very positive, superb, and stimulating teacher both in the clinic and in the operating room. His approach is that of a scholar. I have no hesitancy in stating that this will become a classic text in total hip replacement and will be used by medical students, residents, and hip surgeons.

Dr. Nas Eftekhar is to be congratulated on spending endless hours to present such a fine work, which I believe to be the first comprehensive book on total hip replacement.

Frank E. Stinchfield

Preface

This text is directed toward the resident in training and the orthopaedic surgeon in practice. It is also intended to provide a reference for the surgeon who is already equipped with an adequate practical apprenticeship in hip surgery.

The title, *Principles of Total Hip Arthroplasty*, is intended to signify a logical basis for "reconstructive hip surgery" rather than to merely describe a method of *hip replacement by prosthesis*. On this ground the patient is treated and not the hip; the patient is considered first, and the hip is reconstructed by individualizing the clinical problem based on anatomical and pathological findings.

Because of the importance of preoperative and postoperative management, eight chapters (Parts two and three) are devoted to methods of evaluation and prophylactic measures with the hope of minimizing complications. Equal importance has been placed on the recognition of postoperative complications, which must be considered thoroughly when recommending elective surgery such as total hip arthroplasty (Part five). In this context, Chapter 8 was constructed to formulate some criteria for patient selection but not with the aim of establishing a "code of practice."

Because of the lack of adequate clinical information at this time, two recent developments are excluded from the text: (1) total hip replacement by the use of porous materials for biological ingrowth and (2) total hip replacement by articular resurfacing. As technology evolves and the long-term clinical findings of these procedures are evaluated, poor results are as likely to be caused by error in the selection of suitable candidates for surgery as by error in surgical technology itself.

This book is based on an unusual large-scale clinical experience. The clinical examples presented throughout the text are from patients I have seen, treated, or consulted, including some patients with prior treatment. No clinical situation is presented or exemplified that did not in fact occur. Good results obtained from total hip arthroplasty are cited throughout the text, but there are also failures that often can be traced to a common cause, that is, patient selection and/or surgical error in technique. It is my hope that this book will in some way help those who are interested in the medical and surgical management of suffering patients afflicted with and handicapped by hip disorders.

Owing to my good fortune and their generosity, a number of outstanding educators, colleagues, and friends graciously reviewed prepublication drafts of the chapters of this book and gave me their comments and constructive suggestions. The entire text was reviewed by Dr. Frank E. Stinchfield and Sir John Charnley. Chapters 3 and 4 were reviewed by Dr. C. Andrew L. Bassett; Chapters 5 and 9 by Dr. Ralph S. Blume and Dr. Leonard Brand; Chapter 3 by Dr. Vittorio Castelli, Dr. Jorge O. Galante, Dr. Austin D. Johnston, and Dr. Peter Walker; Chapter 7 by Dr. Stuart W. Cosgriff; Chapters 6 and 16 by Dr. Alexander Garcia and Dr. Phillip J. Nelson; the Introduction, "A Historical Note on the Development of Hip Arthroplasty," and Chapters 5 and 9 by Dr. Sawnie R. Gaston; Chapters 7 and 12 by Dr. Thomas Goss; Chapters 13 and 14 by Dr. Hugo A. Keim; Chapters 15 and 17 by Dr. Howard A. Kiernan and Dr. J. Drennan Lowell; and Chapters 1, 2, and 4 by Dr. Charles S. Neer II. It is with great pleasure that I thank them for their numerous kind remarks and corrections.

Since the dramatic beginning of the original work of Sir John Charnley, an incredible mass of information, at an almost explosive rate, continues to grow in this challenging field. With newer technology developing and unforeseen problems arising in clinical situations, innovative solutions are being sought. With this in mind, undoubtedly it will be required that this text be revised in the future.

N. S. Eftekhar

Acknowledgments

As in all endeavors in life, much help comes from others who contribute but usually are not visible on the scene to receive credit for their efforts.

Foremost among my colleagues I thank my teachers in orthopaedics: Thomas Hunter, F.R.C.S.; Douglas Freebody, F.R.C.S.; Professor Robert A. Robinson, M.D.; Professor Robert D. Ray, M.D., Ph.D.; and Professor Sir John Charnley. It is with great pleasure that I offer my sincere thanks to my teacher, Sir John Charnley, for the encouragement and support he has given me while writing this volume.

With warmest regards I wish to acknowledge my senior colleague, Frank E. Stinchfield, M.D., the former Chief of Orthopaedics at the New York Orthopaedic Hospital at Columbia-Presbyterian Medical Center, for his talent in surgery and his dedication to education and, above all, his devotion to patient care. He will be recorded in the history of surgery for founding two important societies: The Hip Society and The International Hip Society. For his unselfish dedication as an educator, for his guidance, and for his time, despite his enormous work load as president of the American College of Surgeons, in reading this manuscript and making many invaluable suggestions, comments, and constructive criticisms I am indebted.

Among the positive features of this book is the outstanding artwork by my friend Robert J. Demarest. It is my special privilege to thank him for his talent and patience during the long, tireless three years of work that he put into the preparation of the illustrations. He patiently watched, photographed, and sketched many operations and used much of his extra time in the rendering of the final product by his innovative transparent watercolor technique. He never compromised, he never began to illustrate before mastering the subject, and he never released a work that was not considered perfect. In addition, he supervised the entire artwork of the book by organizing the drawings and x-ray photographs included in the text. I thank him for his superior work. My thanks to Angela Icca LaValle for the graphic art. The photography is by Mr. Renald VonMuchow and Mr. Donald Garbera. Mr. Garbera's outstanding reproduction of radiographs and Mr. VonMuchow's photography of patients, specimens, and histology has added to the visual reproduction in this text. For their excellent work and cooperation I am grateful. Special thanks are due to Cintor Division of Codman & Shurtleff in the United States and Chas. F. Thackary, Ltd. in England for their permission to use the instruments illustrated in this text. My thanks also to Mr. Rudolph Gand for his innovative mind and the technical assistance he has given me in designing and manufacturing the special instruments used in surgery.

I owe a debt of gratitude to Mark G. Lazansky, M.D., and James Pugh, Ph.D., at the Hospital for Joint Diseases for the light and electron microscopy of cement specimens used in Chapter 4. My thanks to my colleague and associate in the Orthopaedic Research Laboratories, Mr. Robert J. Pawluk, who has been extremely helpful to me in my research work and has kindly permitted me to use illustrations of animal experimental work in Chapter 3.

The manuscripts were typed and retyped and

Acknowledgments

edited again and again by Ms. Kathleen (Keen) Bailey. For her talents, grammatical corrections, editing, and hard work, I am grateful. I am also appreciative of additional secretarial assistance by my office secretaries, Mrs. Harriet Miller and Ms. Carrie Wittreich, and part-time assistants, Ms. Maria Voyantes and Ms. Virginia Olsen.

I wish to express my appreciation to the orthopaedic nursing staff and physiotherapists for the excellent care given to the patients both on the floor and in the operating room. Without their dedication and care there would have been no success in surgery. The orthopaedic resident staff and fellows in hip surgery at the New York Orthopaedic Hospital have contributed a great deal to the material presented in this book. They

have assisted me in surgery and have supervised and given superb care to patients. My special thanks to them for their outstanding work. I am equally grateful to the orthopaedic attending staff at the New York Orthopaedic Hospital in asking my opinion in certain unusual cases and allowing me to include some of their cases and results in the studies that have been reported in this text.

I deeply appreciate the love and understanding of my wife, Barbara, and my children, Kimberly and Kirt, in sacrificing so much to allow me to complete this task. Without their support and encouragement this work could never have been finished.

xiv

Contents

Contents

xvii

Contents

Principles of total hip arthroplasty

A historical note on the development of hip arthroplasty

We must welcome the Future, remembering that soon it will be the Past; and we must respect the Past, remembering that once it was all that was humanly possible.

GEORGE SANTAYANA

The philosophies of one age have become the absurdities of the next, and the foolishness of yesterday has become the wisdom of tomorrow.

SIR WILLIAM OSLER

In science the credit goes to the man who convinces the world, not to the man to whom the idea first occurs.

SIR WILLIAM OSLER

Preserved skeletons show that osteoarthritis and rheumatoid disease have afflicted man since earliest times. Half a million years ago, Java man suffered from osteoarthritis of the hip.[20] While a complete citation of historical milestones in the development of surgery of the hip joint is beyond the scope of this book and can be found in other sources,[47] this section briefly explores the groundwork that led to the concept of a movable hip joint and the development of total hip replacement. The history of hip arthroplasty may be considered in five major steps: osteotomy arthroplasty, interpositioning arthroplasty, reconstructive arthroplasty, replacement arthroplasty, and total arthroplasty (bipolar replacement).

OSTEOTOMY ARTHROPLASTY

For centuries the problem of rendering an ankylosed hip mobile captured the imagination of surgeons. The first enterprising surgeon of record was John Rhea Barton of Lancaster, Pennsylvania, who performed an osteotomy on an ankylosed hip in 1826.[2] By intertrochanteric osteotomy, he devised an artificial joint that he manipulated 20 days after surgery to maintain

mobility. After 6 weeks the hip joint was mobile, and 3 months later the patient walked with a cane and had functional mobility at the site of the osteotomy. However, 6 years later the hip lost full range of motion. The patient died of pulmonary tuberculosis 10 years later, but it was said that he enjoyed a pain-free functional joint until his death[47] (Fig. 1, A).

In 1863 Sayre[42-44] reported an osteotomy for an ankylosed hip following resection of a bone fragment, which was a modification of Barton's operation.

INTERPOSITIONAL ARTHROPLASTY

A New York general surgeon named Carnochan used a wooden block between the surfaces of a resected neck of a mandible in 1840,[5] and Verneuil used soft tissue for interpositional arthroplasty in 1860, but it was Ollier's work in 1885[37] that created immense interest in this procedure. By that time, interpositioning materials such as muscle, fibrous tissue, celluloid, silver plates, rubber sheets, magnesium, zinc, and decalcified bone were being used. The interpositioning of these materials between the articulating surfaces was helpful in maintaining

1

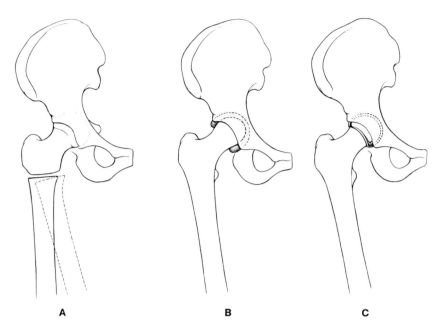

A   B   C

Fig. 1. A, Osteotomy arthroplasty as first performed by John Rhea Barton, who performed an osteotomy on an ankylosed hip in 1826 in order to maintain motion at osteotomy site. **B,** Example of interpositional arthroplasty performed by Ollier and others in 1885. Numerous interpositioning materials such as muscle, fibrous tissue, celluloid, silver plates, and rubber sheets were used. **C,** First formal Vitallium mold (cup) arthroplasty was performed by Smith-Petersen in 1937.

motion at the site of osteotomy and in preventing recurrence of bone growth. However, continuous motion usually led to ankylosis at the site of arthroplasty.

In the early 1900s Murphy,[35,36] Lexer,[24] and Payr[38] advocated the use of tensor fascia lata muscle for interpositioning arthroplasty, while at the same time Foedral found that pig's bladder was sufficiently strong to withstand the stress of weight bearing and intra-articular pressure. In 1919 Baer[1] popularized pig's-bladder arthroplasty at the Johns Hopkins Hospital.

Skin was used as an interpositioning material in the first decade of this century by Loewe[25] and later by Kallio.[23] During this same period, Sir Robert Jones[21] of Liverpool used gold foil to cover a reconstructed femoral head in femoral arthroplasty.

The popularity of interpositional arthroplasty eventually spread to Italy and Germany. In Italy, Putti[40] used every feasible material available in a large number of patients (Fig. 1, *B*).

In 1923 Smith-Petersen placed a glass mold in a patient's hip.[48-50] Although it proved too fragile, as did Pyrex and available plastics, the concept of a mold prosthesis had been born and

proved to be a major contribution in the development of hip arthroplasty. In 1937 Smith-Petersen at the suggestion of his dentist, John Cooke, used Vitallium, a cobalt-chromium alloy, as an interpositioning material.[50] This proved to be clinically successful, and the Smith-Petersen mold became a valuable tool in the armamentarium of the orthopaedic surgeon. Thus after half a century of other experimental work, it is Smith-Petersen who must be given credit for proving that the acetabulum will tolerate a foreign body performing a weight-bearing function (Fig. 1, *C*).

RECONSTRUCTIVE ARTHROPLASTY

Brackett[3] and Whitman[56,57] described the concept of arthroplasty of the hip joint via reconstruction of the upper femur (Fig. 2, *A*). Among others, Magnusen,[27] Colonna,[9] Luck,[26] and Wilson[59] modified these reconstructive procedures to suit each individual problem.

Sir Robert Jones[21] popularized a neck osteotomy known as Jones' pseudarthrosis (Fig. 2, *B*), and Girdlestone[11,12] used resection of the hip joint in order to maintain motion (Fig. 2, *C*). Charnley's central dislocation-stabilization oper-

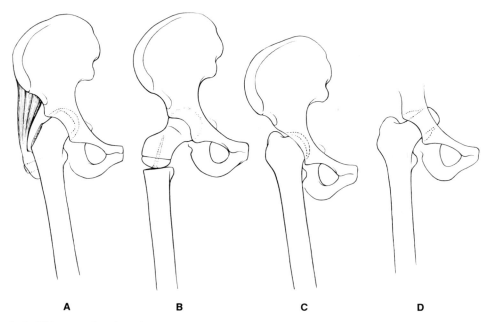

Fig. 2. A, Whitman arthroplasty by reconstruction of acetabulum and transfer of abductor muscles. **B,** Type of arthroplasty proposed by Jones using osteotomy of neck and retaining motion at site of osteotomy. **C,** Example of Girdlestone operation. Head and neck are resected and superior portion of acetabulum is removed. **D,** Charnley's central dislocation-stabilization operation proved a great value in certain patients by producing motion as well as mechanical improvement for hip.

ation proved of great value in creating a pain-free and stable hip during the pre-total-hip era,[6] (Fig. 2, *D*). In some patients this operation was the product of a failed arthrodesis procedure.

REPLACEMENT ARTHROPLASTY

Groves[15-17] in England used a prosthetic replacement of the femoral head in 1927 with limited success. It was made of ivory, never functioned well, and finally failed. Prior to this ivory prosthesis, Delbet[10] in France used a rubber prosthesis in 1919.

In 1940 Drs. Harold Bohlman and Austin Moore removed a tumor from the upper end of a femur and inserted the first metallic prosthesis. They published an original case report in the *Reporter of the Columbia Medical Society* in South Carolina in 1942 and in the *Journal of Bone and Joint Surgery* a year later.[33] This is the first known metallic replacement hemiarthroplasty.

The credit for the widespread use of the femoral head replacement belongs to the Judet brothers, who received much acclaim for their plastic (methyl methacrylate) prosthesis in 1948[22] (Fig. 3, *A*). However, breakage and loosening of the

prosthesis and absorption of bone often called for secondary intervention, and the celebrated original results eventually fell into disrepute. The Judet prosthesis was subsequently made of nylon and other synthetics that had become available. The Judets' contribution is significant because it proved that mechanical replacement of the hip utilizing plastic material can be tolerated in the human body with minimum tissue reaction.

In 1951 Peterson[39] devised a short-stemmed steel prosthesis, which was fixed to the femoral shaft by screws. Other innovations were Mac-Bride's "doorknob" and J. E. M. Thompson's "light-bulb" prostheses.[54]

Throughout the 1950s, more than 50 types of prostheses were introduced; the short-stem type was replaced by the intramedullary long-stem type, which gave more stability, and the non-metallic type was replaced by the metallic type, which provided greater durability. Numerous designs used here and abroad today share common features of the two types developed by F. R. Thompson[52,53] in 1950 (Fig. 3, *C*), and A. T. Moore[31] in 1952 (Fig. 3, *B*). The acetabular replacement by a fixed cup was introduced by

3

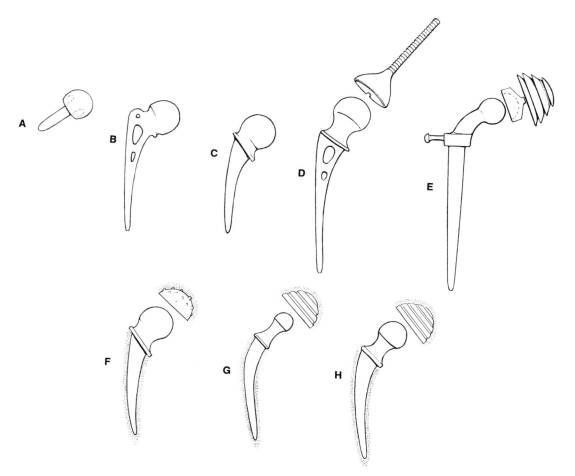

Fig. 3. Hemiarthroplasty prostheses. **A,** Acrylic Judet; **B,** self-locking Moore; **C,** Thompson. Total arthroplasty (bipolar) prosthesis. **D,** Ring; **E,** Sivash; **F,** McKee-Farrar; **G,** Charnley; **H,** Müller. NOTE: no cement was used in **D** and **E,** but acrylic cement was employed in **F, G,** and **H.**

Urist[55] and others. However, failure usually resulted from the bipolar nature of arthritis and the loosening of these devices.

TOTAL ARTHROPLASTY (BIPOLAR REPLACEMENT)

In English literature, as far as we can determine, total hip replacement was first introduced by Wiles[20,58] in 1938 at the Middlesex Hospital in London. He used stainless steel parts that fit into one another precisely. The acetabular component was anchored to a buttressed plate by screws, and the femoral component was secured to the neck of the femur by a bolt. He placed this total hip joint into six patients with severe rheumatoid arthritis but reported in 1950 that the procedure was not totally satisfactory. No other work was found recorded until 1951 when

Haboush[18] published his experiences with self-curing acrylic cement in total hip arthroplasty at the Hospital for Joint Diseases in New York City. In 1952 Haboush used a Vitallium prosthesis, but because he did not apply the principles of arthroplasty (equalization of forces) and because cement was used only for fitting and not for the transmission of the load, the results were poor. A similar prosthesis had been used in 1951 by McKee and Watson-Farrar,[30] who later used acrylic cement with improved results.

It is of historical interest to note that attempts at fixating a prosthesis date back to 1890 when Gluck,[13,14] in a lecture to the German Medical Society, discussed the use of bone glue or cement to fasten ivory devices.[45] At that time, cement was composed of colophony, pumice powder, and plaster of paris. It was apparently well tolerated and became walled off in the marrow cavity.[46]

McKee[28] states that he developed a series of models of total hip replacements, but these were not inserted into a human until 1951, when the first artificial lag-screw joint was introduced. From 1956 to 1960, he had a 54% success rate; revision was required mainly because of loss of fixation. His rate of success increased with the use of methyl methacrylate introduced by Charnley[29] (Fig. 3, *F*).

After trying a number of prostheses, Müller[34] developed a plastic acetabular cup with a 32-mm. chromium-cobalt-molybdenum femoral head, which he has used extensively in his clinic since 1966 (Fig. 3, *H*). Peter Ring[41] began his clinical experience with total joint replacement by metallic components (metal against metal) without cement in 1964 (Fig. 3, *D*). It was somewhat parallel to the work of Russian surgeons who originally developed a metal-to-metal "single unit" prosthesis but subsequently used an interpositioning high-density polyethylene surface (Fig. 3, *E*).

Since the original work by the British surgeons, numerous other devices of metal against metal and metal against plastic have been introduced in the United States and abroad. As most of these are in the experimental stage, the future will reveal their merits and shortcomings.

From 1952 to 1957, Wiltse and his associates[60] conducted entensive experiments with acrylic cement, and Henrichson and his associates[19] experimented on pigs to test tissue reaction to acrylic cement. Since then, many laboratory experiments have been undertaken to determine the safety and mechanical properties of cement and its biological compatibility in humans.

Dr. Frank E. Stinchfield of New York must be recognized as one of the most outstanding of those orthopaedic surgeons who have contributed to the advancement and better understanding of problems related to surgery of the hip joint. His scientific contributions in mold arthroplasty, femoral head replacement, and most recently, total hip arthroplasty span years of detailed studies. Under the leadership of Dr. Stinchfield, American surgeons anticipated the extraordinary demand by the public for total hip joint arthroplasty and established The Hip Society in 1968. The express primary purpose of The Hip Society is to study improvements, benefits, risks, and long-term clinical results of opera-

tions such as total hip arthroplasty. In addition to founding The Hip Society in the United States, Dr. Stinchfield has also been instrumental in establishing The International Hip Society for the advancement and better understanding of problems related to surgery of the hip joint throughout the world.

CHARNLEY'S CONTRIBUTIONS TO MODERN SURGERY OF THE HIP

In 1958 John Charnley first reported his clinical experiences with the replacement of a human joint using steel femoral components and Teflon. In 1960 he described fixation of the components with acrylic. In November of 1962, the acetabular component was replaced by a more wear-resistant plastic, high-density polyethylene (Fig. 3, *G*).

Charnley's development of low-friction arthroplasty (LFA) and the introduction of self-curing acrylic cement represent the most significant developments in orthopaedic surgery of this century. His work from 1954 to 1974 is best described in his own account of the evolution of LFA at his clinic at Wrightington Hospital.[8] In this paper, presented at the College of Physicians and Surgeons of Columbia University at the time he received the honorary Lasker Award in recognition of his achievement, Professor Charnley divides his work into six basic phases of development.

Basic research into the lubrication of normal animal joints

Squeaking in an artificial joint indicates friction at the site, which does not occur naturally in joints. Charnley observed this in 1954 and began to investigate the phenomenon of lubrication that produces low friction, but the only direct experimental work he found was by Dr. E. Shirley Jones, who had reported a very low friction coefficient of 0.02 in animal joints, based on work with a homemade contraption duplicating joint action. Dr. Jones concluded that lack of friction was due to hydrodynamic lubrication; that is, in a ball-bearing situation, fluid enters the zone of contact and lubricates it. Charnley further speculated that oscillation on load bearing prevents this hydrodynamic action; he decided that synovial fluid could not be the crucial factor contributing to low friction in normal joints, as cartilage remained smooth even after it was wiped clean. He concluded that "boundary"

5

lubrication was a specific feature of intra-articular cartilage and responsible for low frictional resistance. He then assumed that a material such as polytetrafluoroethylene (Polytef),* which was self-lubricating, would be an appropriate substitute for the damaged cartilage and proceeded to use it with excellent temporary results.

The use of polytetrafluoroethylene (PTFE) or Polytef Teflon

In the first Polytef arthroplasty, both sliding surfaces were made of Polytef replacements for the damaged articular cartilage. Early results were "phenomenal," but after 12 months there was evidence of failure and mechanical loosening. The stump of the neck of the femur lost its blood supply and became necrotic; the assumption that nothing would stick to Polytef was proved false by the accumulation of a brown sticky material on the sliding surfaces, which prevented sliding and caused movement and wear between the plastic socket and the bone of the acetabulum.

Low-friction arthroplasty as a principle

From this failure, Charnley learned the significance of the principles of LFA: Not only must low frictional resistance be maintained within a joint, but the turning force (torque) transmitted from the metal femoral head to the socket must be resisted for a successful arthroplasty. Since torque is the product of frictional force and the length of the lever on which it acts, and since the frictional force between metal and plastic surfaces is constant for a given load, torque could be decreased only by reducing the diameter of the prosthetic head. Likewise, the frictional force and resistance (turning of the plastic socket in the acetabulum) can be augmented by using a socket with a thick wall, thereby increasing the outside diameter of the socket.

Charnley then began to work with a smaller diameter metal head and more efficient bonding of implants to bone.

Bonding of implant to living bone by quick-setting acrylic cement

Because "the points of direct contact between an implant and bone" that produce a tight fit are "points where the bone would absorb and

---

*Nonproprietary name and trademarks of drug: Polytef—PTFE paste for injection and Teflon.

leave the implant inadequately supported," Charnley felt that small amounts of acrylic cement used only as an adjuvant to a tight mechanical fit was a mistake. He therefore tried making the implant a loose fit, with acrylic used not as an adhesive but as a "grout," and found that this bold and generous use of cement improved the chance for fixation by a factor of 200.[7]

Introduction of high-density polyethylene

After the failure of Polytef, a salesman approached Charnley with a new product, high-density polyethylene, which he rejected, discouraged. However, one of his assistants decided to test it. It proved remarkably wear resistant, and although it lacked Polytef's self-lubricating property, it was capable of being lubricated by synovial fluid. This was a most fortunate coincidence, and after 5 years of testing, it proved to be a highly valuable material for the construction of artificial joints. The first high-density acetabular prosthesis was inserted in a human hip joint in November 1962.

Attempt to identify the cause of failures

Chemical rejection of the cement was first suspected as the cause of the 10% failure rate in total hip replacement surgery. The 90% success rate justified the continuation of the procedure but called for further investigation into the problem.

A clean-air operating room was designed, and with its use there were immediate dramatic results. Complications were reduced by more than half, and the concensus was that failure was largely caused by bacterial infection.

Although the clean-air idea is still not universally accepted, Charnely's statistics and the preceding facts attest to its validity.

Charnley's contribution to the understanding of total hip replacement is indeed a milestone in orthopaedic surgery. Much of the work presented here is based on his biomechanical concepts, which have influenced many surgeons and bioengineers throughout the world. His teachings and his work have been the mainspring of inspiration in the writing of this volume.

SUMMARY OF ESSENTIALS

■ The history of arthroplasty of the hip may be considered in five major historical phases: osteotomy arthroplasty, interpositional arthroplasty, reconstructive arthroplasty, replacement arthroplasty, and total arthroplasty.

- The history of arthroplasty begins with John Rhea Barton of Lancaster, Pennsylvania, who performed an osteotomy on an ankylosed hip in 1826 and maintained motion at the site by manipulation following osteotomy.
- Many surgeons in Europe and the United States attempted interpositioning arthroplasty at the turn of the century by placing a variety of materials between the articulating surfaces of the hip joint. An arthroplasty of this type performed by Smith-Petersen in 1923 led to the clinical success of cup arthroplasty, and he must be credited with proving that the acetabulum could tolerate a foreign body performing a weight-bearing function as a method for arthroplasty.
- Around the turn of the century, many surgeons used reconstructive procedures involving the acetabulum and the upper femur with the hope of formation of pseudarthrosis. Brackett, Whitman, Magnusen, Colonna, Jones, Girdlestone, and others are responsible for the development of arthroplasty of the hip without any formal interpositioning material.
- The Judet brothers' contribution was significant because it proved that mechanical replacement of the hip can be tolerated, a concept subsequently refined by Frederick Thompson of New York and Austin Moore of South Carolina.
- The concept of total hip arthroplasty is credited to many surgeons, with Wiles, Haboush, McKee, and Charnley among the early pioneers in the field. It must be recognized, however, that Charnley's major contribution to the understanding of total hip replacement, a milestone in the history of orthopaedic surgery, includes the introduction and popularization of acrylic cement for fixation and high-density polyethylene plastic as bearing material of the socket. Charnley's work has had a worldwide influence on many surgeons and engineers who are today working to identify the inherent problems in total joint replacement and to improve existing methods and materials.

REFERENCES

1. Baer, W. S.: Arthroplasty with the aid of animal membrane, Am. J. Orthop. Surg. **16:**1-29; 94-115; 171-199; 1919.
2. Barton, J. R.: On the treatment of ankylosis by the formation of artificial joints, North Am. Med. Surg. J. **3:**279-292, 1827.
3. Brackett, E. G.: Fractured neck of the femur—operation of transplantation of the femoral head to trochanter, Boston Med. Surg. J. **192:**1118-1120, 1925.
4. Bohlman, H. R.: Replacement reconstruction of the hip, Am. J. Surg. **84:**268-278, 1952.
5. Carnochan, J. M.: Archives of Medicine **284,** 1860. Cited in Thompson, F. R.: An essay on the development of arthroplasty of the hip, Clin. Orthop. **44:**79-82, 1966.
6. Charnley, J.: Compression arthrodesis, including central dislocation as a principle in hip surgery, Edinburgh and London, 1953, E & S Livingstone, pp. 242-255.
7. Charnley, J.: A biomechanical analysis of the use of cement to anchor the femoral head prosthesis, J. Bone Joint Surg. **47B:**354-363, 1965.
8. Charnley, J.: Total hip replacement, J.A.M.A. **230:**1025-1028, 1974.
9. Colonna, P. C.: A new type of reconstruction operation for old ununited fracture of the neck of the femur, J. Bone Joint Surg. **17:**110-122, 1935.
10. Delbet, P.: Résultat éloigné d'un vissage pour fracture transcervicale du fémur, Bull. Mém. Soc. Chir. Paris **45:**434, 1919.
11. Girdlestone, G. R.: Arthrodesis and other operations for tuberculosis of the hip. In Girdlestone, G. R., editor: The Robert Jones birthday volume, Cambridge, Mass., 1928, Oxford University Press.
12. Girdlestone, G. R., Watson-Jones, R., Stamm, T., and Pridie, K. H.: Discussion on the treatment of unilateral osteoarthritis of the hip, Proc. R. Soc. Med. **38:**363-368, 1945.
13. Gluck, T.: Autoplastik; transplantation; Implantation von Fremdkörpern. Berl. Klin. Wochenschr. **27:**421-427, 1890.
14. Gluck, T.: Referat über die durch das moderne chirurgische Experiment gewonnenen positiven Resultate, betreffend die Naht und den Ersatz von Defecten höherer Gewebe, Sowie über die Verwerthung resorbirbarer und lebendiger Tampons in der Chirurgie, Arch. Klin. Chir. (Berl.) **41:**187-239, 1891.
15. Groves, E. W. H.: Arthroplasty, Br. J. Surg. **11:** 234-250, 1923.
16. Groves, E. W. H.: Some contributions to the reconstructive surgery of the hip, Br. J. Surg. **14:** 486-517, 1927.
17. Groves, E. W. H.: Surgical treatment of osteoarthritis of the hip, Br. Med. J. **1:**3-5, 1933.
18. Haboush, E. J.: A new operation for arthroplasty of the hip based on biomechanics, photoelasticity, fast-setting dental acrylic, and other considerations, Bull. Hosp. Joint Dis. **14:**242-277, 1953.
19. Henrichsen, E., Jansen, K., and Krogh-Poulsen, W.: Experimental investigation of the tissue reaction to acrylic plastics, Acta Orthop. Scand. **22:** 141-145, 1953.
20. Jayson, M., editor: Total hip replacement, Philadelphia, 1971, J. B. Lippincott Co., p. 11.
21. Jones, R., editor: Orthopaedic surgery of injuries, London, 1921, Frowde, 2 vols.

22. Judet, J., and Judet, R.: The use of an artificial femoral head for arthroplasty of the hip joint, J. Bone Joint Surg. **32B:**166-173, 1950.
23. Kallio, K. E.: Arthroplastia cutanea. Proceedings of the Nordisk Ortopedisk Forenings Twenty-eighth Assembly in Helsinki, June, 1956, Acta. Orthop. Scand. **26:**327, 1957.
24. Lexer, E.: Über Gelenktransplantation, Med. Klin. Berlin **4:**817-820, 1908.
25. Loewe, O.: Über Hautimplantation an Stelle der freien Faszienplastik, Munch. Med. Wochenschr. **60:**1320, 1913.
26. Luck, J. V.: A reconstruction operation for pseudarthrosis and resorption of the neck of the femur, J. Iowa Med. Soc. **28:**620-622, 1938.
27. Magnuson, P. B.: The repair of ununited fracture of the neck of the femur, J.A.M.A. **98:**1791-1794, 1932.
28. McKee, G. K.: Artificial hip joint, J. Bone Joint Surg. **33B:**465, 1951.
29. McKee, G. K.: Development of total prosthetic replacement of the hip, Clin. Orthop. **72:**85-103, 1970.
30. McKee, G. K., and Watson-Farrar, J.: Replacement of arthritic hips by the McKee-Farrar prosthesis, J. Bone Joint Surg. **48B:**245-259, 1966.
31. Moore, A. T.: Metal hip joint—new self-locking Vitallium prosthesis, South. Med. J. **45:**1015-1019, 1952.
32. Moore, A. T.: The self-locking metal hip prosthesis, J. Bone Joint Surg. **39A:**811-827, 1957.
33. Moore, A. T., and Bohlman, H. R.: Metal hip joint—a case report. J. Bone Joint Surg. **25:**688-692, 1943.
34. Müller, M. E.: Die Huftnahen Femurosteotomien, Stuttgart, 1957, Georg Thieme Verlag.
35. Murphy, J. B.: Ankylosis: arthroplasty—clinical and experimental, J.A.M.A. **44:**1573-1582; 1671-1678; 1749-1766; 1905.
36. Murphy, J. B.: Arthroplasty, Ann. Surg. **57:**593-647, 1913.
37. Ollier, L. X. E. L.: Traité des résection et des operations conservatrices qu'on peut practiquer sur le systeme osseus, Paris, 1885, Masson et cie, Editeurs.
38. Payr, E.: Blütige Mobilisierung versteifter Gelenke, Zentrabl. Chir. **37:**1227, 1910.
39. Peterson, L. T.: The use of a metallic femoral head, J. Bone Joint Surg. **33A:**65-75, 1951.
40. Putti, V.: Arthroplasty, J. Orthop. Surg. **3:**421-430, 1921.
41. Ring, P. A.: Complete replacement arthroplasty of the hip by the Ring prosthesis, J. Bone Joint Surg. **50B:**720-731, 1968.
42. Sayre, L. A.: A new method for artificial hip joint in bony ankylosis—two cases. Trans. Med. Soc. N.Y. pp. 111-127, 1863. Cited in Shands, A. R.: Historical milestones in the development of modern surgery of the hip joint. In Tronzo, R. G., editor: The surgery of the hip joint, Philadelphia, 1973, Lea & Febiger, pp. 1-26.
43. Sayre, L. A.: Exsection of the head of the femur and removal of the upper rim of the acetabulum for morbus coxarius, N.Y. State J. Med. **14:**70-82, 1855.
44. Sayre, L. A.: Exsection of the head of the femur for morbus coxarius, Med. Record N.Y. **6:**281, 1871-1872.
45. Scales, J. T.: Acrylic bone cement—bond or plug? J. Bone Joint Surg. **50B:**698-700, 1968.
46. Scales, J. T., and Lowe, S. A.: Some factors influencing bone and joint replacements. In Jayson M., editor: Total hip replacement, London, 1971, Sector Publications Ltd., pp. 103-126.
47. Shands, A. R.: Historical milestones in the development of modern surgery of the hip joint. In Tronzo, R. G., editor: The surgery of the hip joint, Philadelphia, 1973, Lea & Febiger, pp. 1-26.
48. Smith-Petersen, M. N.: A new supra-articular subperiosteal approach to the hip joint, Am. J. Orthop. Surg. **15:**592-595, 1917.
49. Smith-Petersen, M. N.: Arthroplasty of the hip, a new method, J. Bone Joint Surg. **21:**269-288, 1939.
50. Smith-Petersen, M. N.: Evolution of mould arthroplasty of the hip joint, J. Bone Joint Surg. **30B:**59-75, 1948.
51. Thompson, F. R.: Vitallium intramedullary hip prosthesis—preliminary report, N.Y. State J. Med. **52:**3011-3020, 1952.
52. Thompson, F. R.: Two and a half years' experience with a Vitallium intramedullary hip prosthesis, J. Bone Joint Surg. **36A:**489-502, 1954.
53. Thompson, F. R.: An essay on the development of arthroplasty of the hip, Clin. Orthop. **44:**73-82, 1966.
54. Thompson, J. E. M.: A prosthesis for the femoral head: a preliminary report, J. Bone Joint Surg. **34:**175-182, 1952.
55. Urist, M.: Hip arthroplasty, Baltimore, 1965, The Williams & Wilkins Co.
56. Whitman, R.: A new treatment for fracture of the neck of the femur, Med. Rec. **65:**441-447, 1904.
57. Whitman, R.: The reconstruction operation for ununited fracture of the neck of the femur, Surg. Gynecol. Obstet. **32:**479-486, 1921.
58. Wiles, P. W.: The surgery of the osteoarthritic hip, Br. J. Surg. **45:**488-497, 1958.
59. Wilson, P. D.: Trochanteric arthroplasty in the treatment of ununited fractures of the neck of the femur, J. Bone Joint Surg. **29:**313-327, 1947.
60. Wiltse, L. L., Hall, R. H., and Stenehjem, J. C.: Experimental studies regarding the possible use of self-curing acrylic in orthopaedic surgery, J. Bone Joint Surg. **39A:**961-972, 1957.

PART ONE

BASIC SCIENCE

CHAPTER 1

Applied surgical anatomy of the hip

There is but little room for inexactness in the field of
surgery; a deviation of even a centimeter or two from the
correct approach may change success into disaster.

LORD BROCK

This chapter describes only those anatomical
features relevant to hip surgery. Information
given here will be referred to in subsequent
chapters (Chapters 2 and 12 to 14). It is intended
as a brief review of applied anatomy, thus many
anatomical details unrelated to hip replacement
have been omitted. The interested reader is referred to standard texts in anatomy.[2,5-9]

GROSS ANATOMY AND SURGICAL APPLICATION
Pelvis

The two coxal or hip bones, also known as
innominate bones, articulate firmly with the
sacrum and with each other at the pubis symphysis; with the sacrum and coccyx they form
the bony skeleton of the pelvis. The coxae are
tightly bound together with the sacrum and
coccyx by ligaments, forming the "pelvic ring."
The walls of the pelvis are padded with muscles
and other structures from within and without,
so that the living pelvis is very different from a
bony specimen. Therefore orientation of the
pelvis on the operating table could be somewhat
altered by the position of the soft tissue about the
hip. For example, when a patient is supine on
the operating table and severe bilateral flexion
deformity is present, a forward tilt of the pelvis
results, which can best be determined by the
presence and amount of compensatory lumbar
lordosis. Attention to the bony landmarks of the
pelvis and thigh, by observing the surface anatomy, will assist in the proper placement of the
incision at surgery (Fig. 1-1).

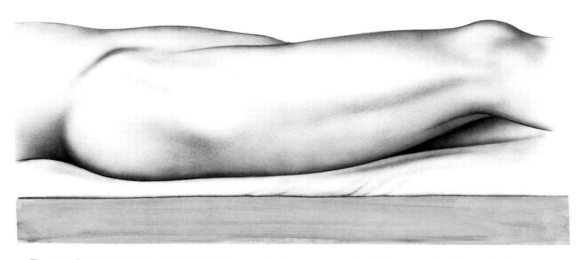

Fig. 1-1. Surface anatomy of hip and thigh as patient lies on operating table. Important landmarks include
anterosuperior spine, crest of ilium, greater trochanter, and iliotibial track. NOTE: concavity behind greater trochanter, denoting site of greater trochanter. Also observe prominent tensor fascia femoris and depression
between gluteus medius and tensor fascia femoris muscle. These surface landmarks should assist in proper
placement of skin incision at surgery.

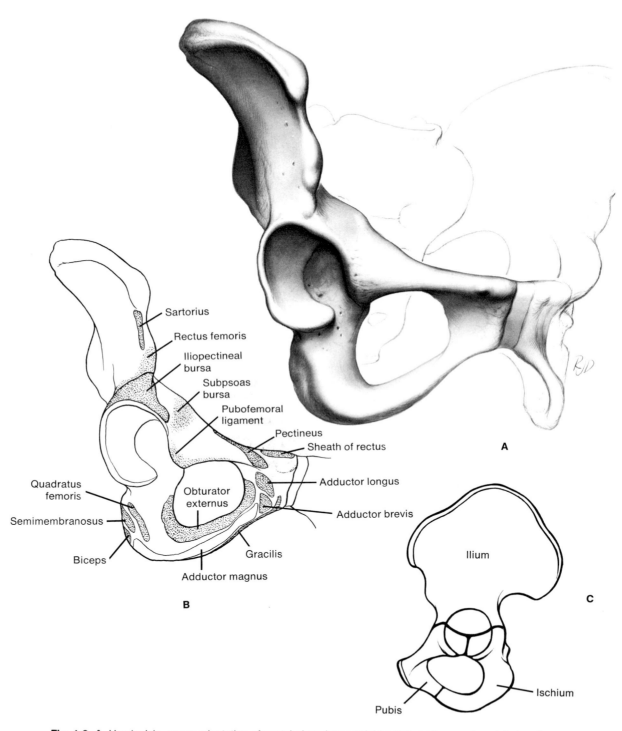

Sartorius

Rectus femoris

Iliopectineal bursa

Subpsoas bursa

Pubofemoral ligament

Pectineus

Sheath of rectus

Quadratus femoris

Semimembranosus

Biceps

Obturator externus

Adductor longus

Adductor brevis

Gracilis

Adductor magnus

Ilium

Ischium

Pubis

A

B

C

Fig. 1-2. A, Hemipelvis. NOTE: orientation of acetabulum, intracotyloid notch, and zone of acetabulum (acetabular fossa). **B,** Site of insertion (dotted area) and origin of muscular attachments about hip joint. **C,** Formation of hemipelvis.

The ilium, pubis, and ischium all contribute to the formation of the acetabulum, which faces not only outward but also somewhat downward and anterior. A mental visualization of the acetabular orientation is essential when directing the reamers for preparation of the acetabulum. The weight-bearing upper and posterior walls of the acetabulum are especially heavy, whereas the inferior wall is less substantial at the site of the acetabular notch (Fig. 1-2, *A*). The formation of the hemipelvis is of interest (Fig. 1-2, *C*). The iliac and ischial segments are massive and provide major support for muscular attachment and formation of the acetabulum (Fig. 1-2, *B*). The pubic bone (anteriorly) contributes to a lesser degree to the acetabulum. When preparing the acetabulum for the cup, one must strive to obtain the maximum fixation from the best available bone, namely, the iliac (superiorly) and the ischium (posteriorly). Although the inferior wall is absent in normal conditions, in protrusion or osteoarthritis a wall may be formed by fusion of opposing osteophytes extending beyond the intracotyloid notch. This wall may be used as a supporting structure for fixation of cement to the acetabulum.

The acetabular notch leads into the "acetabular fossa," a rough area at the center of the articulating portion of the acetabulum; it is the thinnest portion of the floor and a zone that may transilluminate on a dry specimen since the inner and outer tables of cortical bone are fused at this site without interpositioned cancellous bone (Fig. 1-3). It is of paramount importance to avoid deepening the socket beyond this zone or breaking through this area; this could lead to failure of fixation of cement and a complete medial migration of the prosthetic device. It is a fortunate coincidence that in most osteoarthritic hips, especially in congenital dysplasia, marked thickening of the floor has taken place, which allows further deepening at this level. This is usually evidenced by radiological "teardrop" widening on anteroposterior views of the pelvis (Fig. 1-4).

Ilium. The ilium is the component of the coxa that can be felt by the examiner's hand approximately 4 to 6 cm. inferior to the rib cage. It is somewhat fan-shaped with the hinge of the fan at the acetabular level. The margin of the fan extends from the anterior to the posterior border, with the iliac crest between them, thus separat-

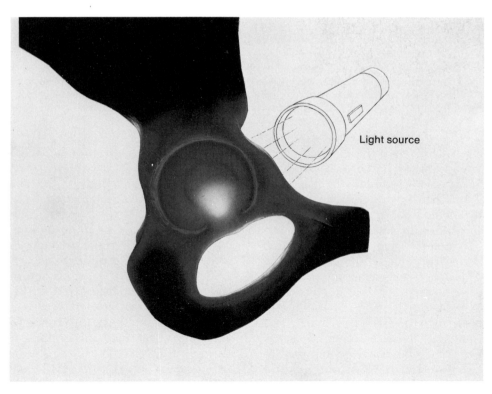

Fig. 1-3. Acetabular fossa may transilluminate on a dry bony specimen.

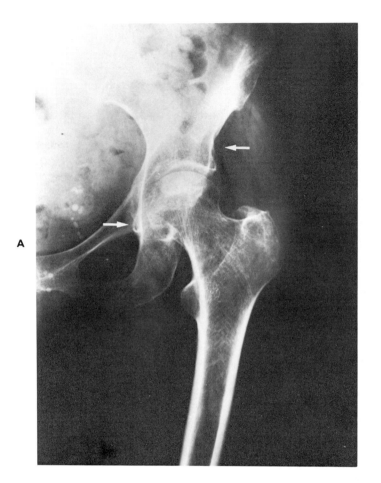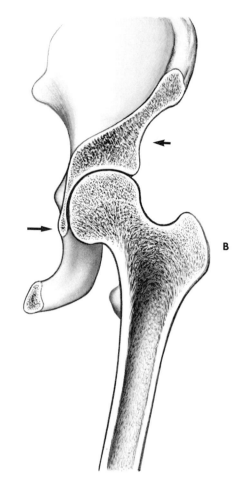

Fig. 1-4. Frontal view of hip joint. **A,** Anteroposterior representation of normal hip joint. Arrows indicate "teardrop" and cancellous zone of weight-bearing portion of acetabulum. **B,** Cross-sectional view of hip in frontal plane at site of "teardrop" illustrates "teardrop" representation and thinnest segment of acetabular floor. Top arrow also indicates superior weight-bearing cancellous zone of hip at level of acetabular roof.

ing the abdominal wall from the gluteal region. The hollow area between the rib cage and the crest allow the surgeon to palpate the iliac crest for the level of the pelvis, even through a draped surgical field. The anterior end of the iliac crest ends in an important landmark, the "anterosuperior spine," which gives origin to the inguinal ligament and may be palpated through the surgical draping. It is best done with both hands of *one* examiner at surgery. The two spines denote the transaxis of the pelvis. The acetabular cup is fixed in reference to this line (see Chapter 12).

A second landmark is an external lip that is prominent 5 to 7 cm. above and behind the anterosuperior spine and is known as the "tubercle of the crest." These landmarks should be considered as points of reference for (1) position of

the patient on the operating table, (2) placement of the incision, (3) trochanteric position, and (4) measurements of length of the extremity and orientation of the acetabular component. A fixed abduction or adduction may alter their locations in reference to the axis of the body, a major point to be remembered in the orientation of the acetabular cup guide at positioning.

The muscles of the lateral and posterior abdominal walls and fascia lata of the thigh are attached to the iliac crest and can be conveniently detached from their insertions to make the ilium accessible for bone grafting if necessary during hip replacement. Surgical draping must not make the iliac crest (from the anterosuperior spine to its posterosuperior spine) inaccessible.

The bony pelvis gives the appearance of hav-

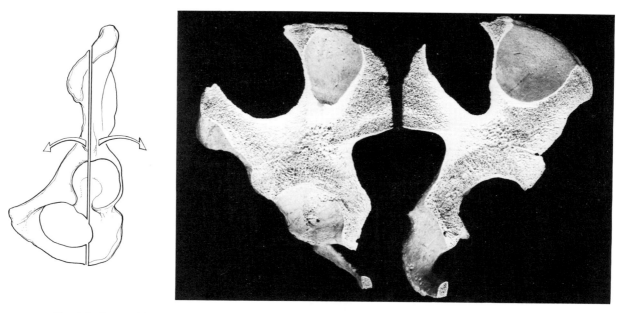

Fig. 1-5. Bony pelvis gives appearance of having been twisted on itself at site of acetabulum. Two planes cut each other nearly at right angles. Upper one roughly corresponds to ilium, and lower one corresponds to ischium and pubis. Photograph illustrates cancellous portions of ilium when pelvis is sectioned in plane of wing of ilium (drawing).

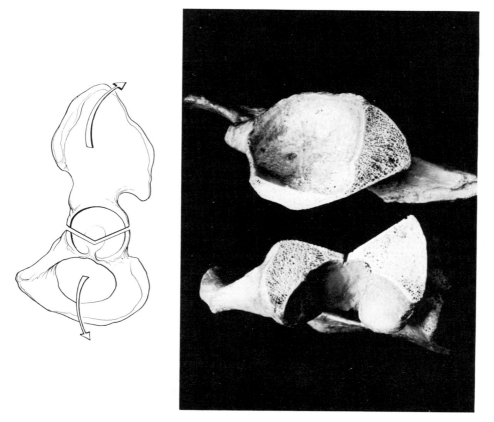

Fig. 1-6. Same as Fig. 1-5, but sectioned pelvis perpendicular to axis of ischium and pubis reveals segment of cancellous bone in regions of pubis and ischium. NOTE: posterior segment of ilium is also substantial and rich in cancellous bone. Drawing illustrates plane of sectioning of pelvis.

15

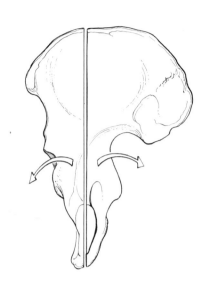 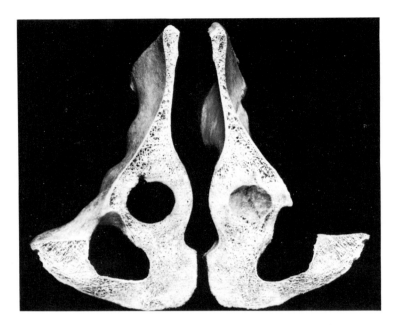

Fig. 1-7. Same as Figs. 1-5 and 1-6, but section of pelvis through ischium and pubis is perpendicular to plane of ilium. Photograph illustrates best available bone for fixation of total prosthesis, principally in region of ischium and ilium. Drawing illustrates plane of section of ilium used for photograph.

ing been twisted on itself at the site of the acetabulum (Figs. 1-5 to 1-7). Therefore the two planes cut each other nearly at right angles, the upper one roughly corresponding with the ilium and the lower one corresponding with the ischium and pubis. This is an important consideration in the orientation of the pelvis on the operating table; it also explains the lack of availability of bone in the iliac region despite the anteroposterior view of the radiographs of the pelvis that give a deceptive representation of a flat "iliac fan" as an excellent bony stalk in this region (Figs. 1-5 to 1-7).

The ilium with its wide gluteal surface is completely covered by glutei and only in a dissected bone specimen is it marked by anterior, posterior, and inferior gluteal lines (Fig. 1-8). The whole crest of the ilium extends between the anterosuperior and posterosuperior iliac spines. The "anterior gluteal line" marks the posterosuperior border of the margin of the gluteus minimus and the anteroinferior border of the origin of the gluteus medius. The posterior gluteal line separates the origin of the gluteus maximus from the medius. The inferior gluteal line is the inferior boundary of the origin of the gluteus minimus. The inner surface of the wing of the ilium is the iliac fossa; on its posterior por-

tion is the articular surface for the sacrum. Below the anteroinferior spine is an ill-defined notch, the "iliopubic eminence," which marks the junction of ilium and pubis. This landmark is a guide for the insertion of a pointed retractor, that is, Hohmann retractor, to visualize the anterior portion of the acetabulum at the junction of the ilium and the pubis (Figs. 2-2 and 2-10; see also Chapter 12). Below the posteroinferior spine is the deep greater sciatic notch, which may be conveniently palpated through the inner wall of the pelvis by subperiosteal dissection or following exploration of the sciatic nerve in the buttock. For example, with injury to the sciatic nerve following fracture dislocation of the hip joint requiring decompression of the sciatic nerve, the sciatic notch may be reached conveniently by palpating along the sciatic nerve to the point of its exit from the notch. Near the anterior border of the sciatic notch at the base of the wall of the acetabulum is another rounded thickness that marks the junction of the ilium and ischium.

Ischium. The ischium is the most massive contributing element of the posterior acetabular wall; it has facets on its posterolateral aspect for the origin of the hamstring muscles. Above this area is the lesser sciatic notch, which is

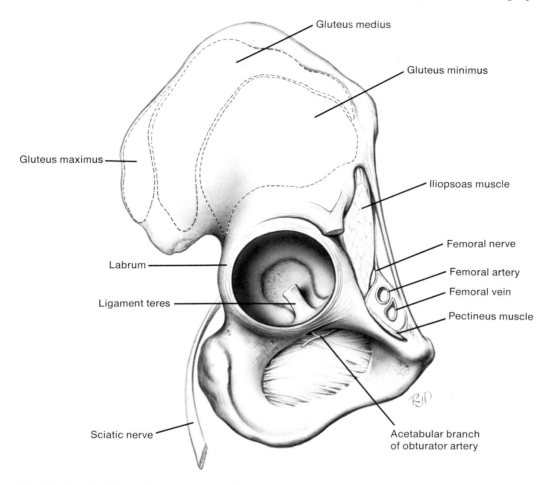

Gluteus medius

Gluteus minimus

Gluteus maximus

Iliopsoas muscle

Femoral nerve

Labrum

Femoral artery

Femoral vein

Ligament teres

Pectineus muscle

Sciatic nerve

Acetabular branch
of obturator artery

Fig. 1-8. Site of origin of gluteal muscles on ilium is indicated. Relationship of sciatic nerve to acetabulum, acetabular branch of obturator artery, femoral artery and vein, femoral nerve, and iliopsoas in relation to acetabulum should be noted. Acetabular floor is marked by horseshoe articulating zone and acetabular fossa. Ligamentum teres and its synovial folding are supplied by acetabular branch of obturator artery.

separated from the greater sciatic notch by a projecting sharp spike known as the ischial spine. In front of the ischium lies the body of the pubis. The ischium and the pubis jointly form the obturator foramen, bounded below by the "ischiopubic ramus" and the inferior ramus of the pubis projecting backward from the pubic bone. It is essential to assess the orientation of the body of the ischium with the bone of the pubis so that anchoring holes for cement fixation are created in the body of the ischium and not in the ilioischial junction or near the obturator foramen, a common error. (See Chapter 12.)

Pubis. This area is less developed in size than the ilium and ischium. The pubic body articulates at the symphysis with the pubic bone of the other side. Its superior ramus runs above

the obturator foramen to form part of the acetabular wall, and its inferior ramus curves inferiorly and posteriorly to fuse with the ischium. The direction and size of the pubis must be appreciated on a dry bony specimen and compared with its radiological magnification to ascertain its orientation, thus avoiding extensive preparation and removal of bone for anchorage at surgery (Figs. 1-2 and 1-8). (See Chapter 17.) The pubis, which anteriorly forms the boundary of the obturator foramen and inferiorly the ischiopubic ramus, gives origin to the adductor muscles (Fig. 1-2). The upper end of the symphysis pubis at the angle with the crest gives attachment to the rectus abdominis and terminates laterally in the prominent point of the "pubic tubercle," to which the inguinal ligament is at-

17

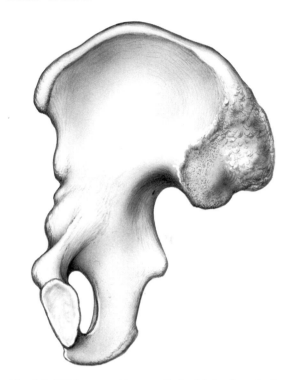

Fig. 1-9. Middle zone of inner wall of pelvis is of greatest concern because it comprises floor of acetabulum and is thinnest segment of pelvis. It is mainly covered by iliacus muscle.

tached. Lateral to this the superior ramus extends to the "iliopubic eminence" where it joins the ilium. Its inferior border gives attachment to the "pubofemoral ligament" of the hip joint and overhangs the obturator foramen. From the pubic tubercle, the pectineal line runs along the superior ramus to the "iliopectineal eminence." The pubic tubercle gives origin to the reinforcing capsular ligament—the pubofemoral ligament of the hip joint.

Inner wall. From the inner side of the pelvis, three contributing areas may be recognized.[1]

1. In the back and upper portion of each coxa, an articular surface shaped like an ear is termed the auricular surface; above and behind each auricular surface is a rough tuberosity for the strong interosseous sacroiliac ligament. Behind this area is the expanded posterior part of the crest for the erector spinae muscle. This area is of no interest to us in replacement surgery unless it has been invaded in previous surgery or disease.

2. The second area, however, is of greater concern: The ventral surface of the ilium, which is slightly concave and forms the bony iliac fossa, gives origin to and is covered by the iliacus muscle. It should be recognized that the ventral surface of the ilium is completely covered by the iliacus muscle, thus all neurovascular structures are well cushioned within the pelvis. Yet it is thin and may be easily penetrated if an attempt is made to structure an acetabulum at that level, for example, at the site of a pseudoacetabulum of a congenital dislocation of the hip (Figs. 1-9 and 1-10).

3. The third part, the lower portion, is comprised of the obturator foramen, which is covered by the obturator internus, which also arises from the periphery of this segment. Entry to the obturator foramen from the outside by deep dissection often leads to damage of the obturator vessels and bleeding, which may be a nuisance to control. Flow of excess cement in this region may cause obturator nerve palsy. The main trunk of the obturator nerve is closely applied to the iliopubic segment of the pelvis prior to entry to the thigh via the obturator foramen. (See Chapter 17.)

Acetabulum

Because of the importance of the acetabulum, knowledge of some details of this territory is essential. Over two fifths of the acetabulum is contributed by the ischium, less than two-fifths by the ilium, and only one-fifth by the pubis (Figs. 1-5 to 1-7). The so-called triradiate cartilage, which is responsible for the formation of the acetabulum (Fig. 1-2, C), develops from a variable number of small ossifying centers joined at the floor of the acetabulum and known as os acetabuli.[9] However, there is an ultimate fusion of these centers, making a unified floor. The nonarticulating surface, known as the "acetabular fossa" or the "pulvinar," contains some fibrofatty tissue (haversian fat pad) and opens below toward the obturator foramen at the acetabular notch (Fig. 1-8). At surgery this area is best exposed by traction on the stump of the ligamentum teres and curettage at its base; more conveniently, it may be excised by an electric knife to minimize bleeding. The acetabular fossa indicates the innermost and thinnest (transilluminating) zone of the floor. The surgeon should be warned of the danger of further deepening toward the midline in this area. The notch is bridged by the "transverse ligament," a tendinous structure continuous with the fibrocarti-

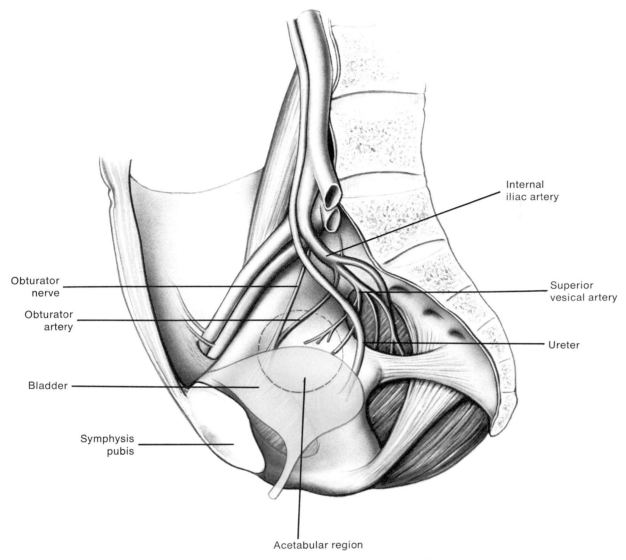

Internal
iliac artery

Obturator
nerve

Obturator
artery

Superior
vesical artery

Ureter

Bladder

Symphysis
pubis

Acetabular region

Fig. 1-10. Bony and ligamentous walls of pelvis minor are shown. Corresponding zone of acetabular floor is traced (circle) in background. Position of ureter and bladder in relation to acetabular floor is identified. Obturator nerve and artery and vein traversing behind iliopubic segment and small branches of superior vesical artery are shown. It is fortunate anatomical coincidence that no major vital structure is present immediately adjacent to bone of inner wall of acetabulum (circled). Note position of common iliac artery and vein in relation to lesser bony pelvis.

laginous acetabular labrum, which in turn is attached to the whole periphery of the mouth of the acetabulum (Fig. 1-8). The transverse ligament may be excised, but an incision at a line perpendicular to its fibers allows adequate entry to the bottom of the notch, where maximum exposure is needed. Incision may be anterior or posterior, but should be close to the bone. It is under the transverse ligament that vascular structures pass through the notch to enter the

ligamentum teres into the femoral head (Fig. 1-8).

On careful examination of the "articular lunate" surface of the acetabulum, the pubic articulating surface is distinct from the surface of the iliac segment, which is also marked on the rim by a small notch (Fig. 1-2). This is a common site for the iliopectineal bursa to communicate with the hip joint. The distinction is helpful in order to appreciate the dividing zones of the

19

acetabulum contributed by the ilium and pubis. The state of the acetabular cartilage of the iliac segment is best visualized when pin retractors are inserted to retract the superior capsule of the joint. (See Chapter 12.) The fibrocartilaginous acetabular labrum is attached to the bony rim within the capsule of the joint, adding to the depth of the cavity. At times it is quite hypertrophic and might be taken for the true bony periphery, leading to inadequate deepening. Its routine excision is required to provide visualization of the rim. Exposure of the bony rim is perhaps the most important step in preparation of the acetabulum and appreciation of the relationship of the bony masses and their articulating surfaces. When the prosthetic cup is inserted, a crescent is formed between the cup and the acetabulum, which is best packed with cement only after a full visualization.

In protrusio acetabuli the medial wall is often expanded and thin toward the midline. The very thin cortical bone should be carefully preserved at surgery. When a membranous defect is present, it may be reinforced by bone, graft, or wire mesh. (See Chapter 13.) In protrusion the acetabulum is barrel-shaped with a narrow opening, as if the acetabulum has been blown out like a balloon.

As the result of disease, such as protrusio acetabuli or rheumatoid disease, the acetabulum may be markedly distorted, with an altered relationship to the osseous and soft tissue of the pelvis. For example, in protrusio acetabuli, the floor of the acetabulum is extremely thin and

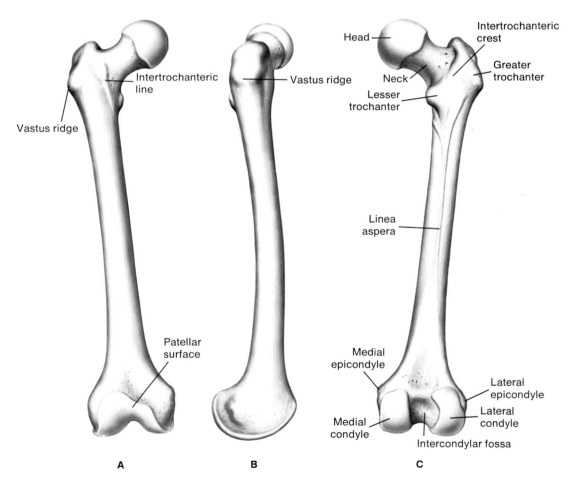

Fig. 1-11. A, Anterior view; **B,** lateral view; and **C,** posterior view. Upper femur consists of head, neck, and trochanters. Prominent greater trochanter at base (vastus ridge), lesser trochanter, and bony landmarks are helpful in orientation of osteotomy of greater trochanter as well as orientation of femoral component of prosthesis.

occasionally membranous, expanded toward the midline; the entrance of the cavity is narrowed like a barrel top, requiring expansion at the rim.

Femur

The femur is the longest bone of the skeleton and articulates with the hip bone above and the tibia below; it carries the patella in front of it. The femur consists of a shaft that is directed downward medially and slightly forward (Fig. 1-11). Its general curvatures, the details of its ends, and the complex angles of the upper femur must be fully understood in the normal as well as the pathological states. The shaft of the femur twists on itself (femoral torsion or anteversion). The patella in front of the femur provides an important landmark, a reference point when the

limb is positioned for orientation of the reamers during preparation as well as for insertion of the prosthesis. Therefore the patella should not be excessively hidden in the free leg drape.

The upper end of the femur consists of the head, neck, and the trochanters (Fig. 1-12).

Head and neck. The head has a separate epiphysis; the epiphyseal line practically, but not absolutely, corresponds with the edge of the articular surface.[1] A prolongation of the cartilage covering the surface of the front of the neck, which extends onto the bony ridge, is frequently found running along the upper front part of the neck. This ridge is called the eminence of the neck. The articular extension underlies the iliopsoas tendon if there is a large bursa opening, otherwise it seems to support the inner part of

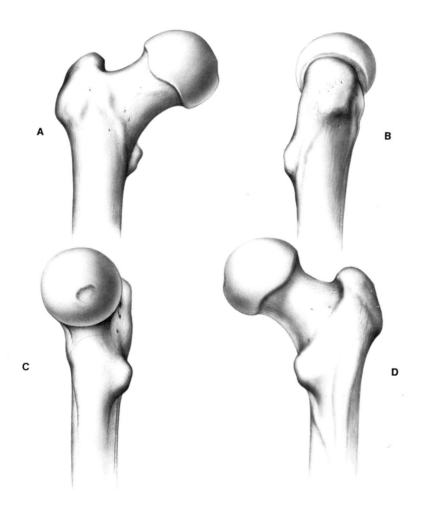

Fig. 1-12. A, Upper femur in frontal view; **B,** lateral view; **C,** lateral view with head in front; **D,** posterior view.

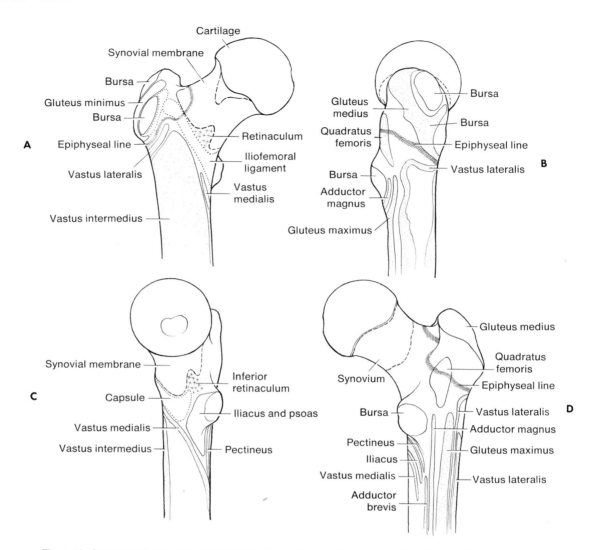

Fig. 1-13. Corresponding to bony landmarks in Fig. 1-12, site of major muscular attachment, capsular attachment, synovial folding attachments, and major ligaments and bursa are illustrated. **A,** Frontal view, **B,** lateral view; **C,** lateral view from front; and **D,** posterior view. (Outline of synovial capsular muscular and ligamentous structure was adopted from Breathnach, A. S., editor: Frazer's anatomy of the human skeleton, ed. 6, Boston, 1965, Little, Brown & Co.)

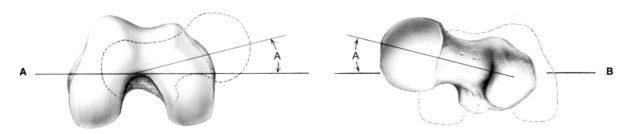

Fig. 1-14. Neck shaft angle both in anteroposterior and lateral planes must be considered prior to and during surgery. Excessively anteverted neck is common. **A,** Represents anteversion as femur is viewed from femoral condyles. **B,** Illustrates anteversion as femur is viewed from top of neck of femur.

the iliofemoral ligament. The head of the femur, larger in the male than in the female, forms two thirds of a sphere. (The sphericity of the head has been debated in the past.) The size and shape of the femoral head determines the size and shape of the acetabulum. Thus a small head removed at surgery is suggestive of a small acetabulum, a misshapen head (that is, flattened) denotes a misshapen acetabulum, and so on. The position and size of the fovea varies; one or two small foramina, which represent the entry site of a branch of the obturator artery (the ligamentum teres artery) and the vein, are sometimes seen. These are often absent in an arthritic hip. The synovial funnel that surrounds these vessels is attached in the depressed margin of the fovea and is terminated at the margin of cartilage covering the head. Numerous vascular foramina originate from the synovial membrane, which covers the entire anterior surface of this bone extending toward the head.

These typical anatomical characteristics are not present in an arthritic hip, in which the head and neck junction is often distorted by osteophytes; therefore the site for amputation at the femoral neck and the opening of the neck may not be clearly identifiable. The posterior aspect of the neck is usually smooth, and the line of reflection of the synovium is about halfway up the neck, continued up from the turned-up lower end of the intertrochanteric line. The obturator externus, obturator internus, and gemelli are closely applied to the upper neck of the femur and the quadratus femoris, posteriorly and inferiorly. The close relationship of these muscles should be appreciated when mobilization of the upper femur is necessary, requiring disinsertion of these muscles from the upper femur by maximum internal rotation of the limb, thereby facilitating their detachment (Figs. 1-12 and 1-13). The neck shaft angle both in the anteroposterior and lateral planes must be considered prior to and during surgery (Figs. 1-11 and 1-14). An excessively anteverted neck in a congenital dislocation of the hip or a displaced osteotomy at the neck shaft angle calls for special preparation of the upper femur. In a variety of conditions the neck length may be shortened and might require a careful evaluation prior to osteotomy to prevent further shortening. Displaced osteotomies or malunion of neck fractures in particular must be carefully evaluated, not only in relation to varus/valgus angles but to rotational

deformity as well. (See Chapters 13 and 14.)

Greater trochanter. The term "greater trochanter" is applied to the mass of bone that stands up at the base of the neck and gives attachment to the gluteal muscles. In situations like coxa vara or "sunken prosthesis" (for example, Moore self-locking prosthesis) the trochanter appears substantial in size since it "stays proud" (projected) in reference to the remainder of the shaft. It normally consists of the whole body at the base of the neck including the femoral tubercle at the top of the intertrochanteric line, the so-called upper aspect of the neck. The gluteus minimus bursa occupies the anterior smooth surface, and the piriformis inserts along the whole length of the upper crest of the trochanter, while the obturator internus and gemelli are inserted medial to and in front of it on the slope of the trochanter. On the lateral surface of the trochanter there is a well-marked oblique ridge for the insertion of the gluteus medius, which occupies the whole breadth of the ridge. Above the oblique ridge, the trochanter is completely covered by the gluteus medius insertion and its intervening bursa. The widened base of the neck is marked anteriorly by a roughened ridge of bone known as the "intertrochanteric line" and posteriorly by the "intertrochanteric crest," the prominent ridge between the two trochanters (Figs. 1-11 and 1-12). An understanding of the complex shape of the trochanter is important at the time of its removal and reattachment in total hip surgery.

On the lateral surface and at the base of the trochanter is the "vastus lateralis ridge." This landmark at the base of the greater trochanter is best palpated by placing a finger or thumb against the shaft of the femur over the vastus lateralis and moving upward to appreciate its projection while the vastus lateralis is still undetached from the shaft of the femur. The vastus ridge may be partially covered by a trochanteric bursa and is often best recognized following its removal. The ridge will identify the level of removal of the trochanter; it is also an eminence that is used for interlocking of the trochanter at the reattachment stage. The trochanter proximal to the ridge is the site of the tendinous insertion of the gluteus medius (Fig. 1-13). The intertrochanteric line marks the attachment site of the iliofemoral ligament. The strong lateral limb of the ligament goes to the tubercle at the upper end of the line (Fig. 1-15). The medial

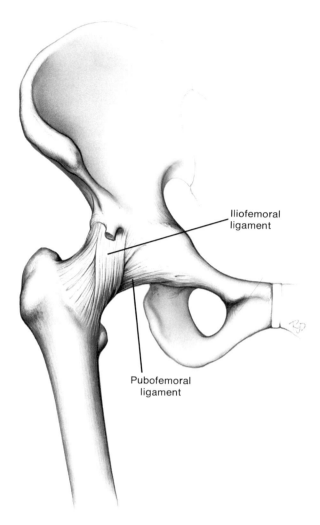

Iliofemoral
ligament

Pubofemoral
ligament

Fig. 1-15. Intertrochanter line marks attachment site of iliofemoral ligament. Strong lateral limb of ligament goes to
tubercle at upper end of line, medial band proceeds to lower
end of line. Capsular reinforcing ligaments provide anterior
stability for hip joint.

band proceeds to the lower end of this line with
its intermediate band, which goes to the thinner
portion of the line in between.[1] The interval between this line and the lesser trochanter offers
insertion to the muscular fibers of the iliacus.
The inner wall of the greater trochanter above
the neck is best identified following an opening
in the capsule. Recession of the digital fossa
toward the posterolateral aspect and the posterior ridge of the trochanter must be noted. The
posterior crest is further extended medially as
far as the lesser trochanter. This asymmetry
and the direction of the fossa hamper passing
of the clamp from the front to recover the saw-

band when its direction is not observed. If the
limb is fixed in external rotation owing to arthritis, the tip of the clamp naturally enters the
fossa, piercing the capsule posteriorly but superficial to the trochanteric crest.

Lesser trochanter. The lesser trochanter presents two surfaces: a posterior smooth surface
related to a bursa at the upper border of the adductor magnus and a rough medial area giving
insertion to the psoas major. This insertion is
continued down on the shaft to just below the
trochanter and above the ridge of the linea as-
pera femoris, which continues the intertrochanteric line over the medial aspect of the bone to
its posterior surface. The tendon's muscular
insertions can be detached from the lesser trochanter to free the upper femur. It is a safe surgical dissection when the disinsertion is done
next to the bone of the lesser trochanter, and it
should be performed from the front, with the
extremity in external rotation. As stated, the
posterior surface is completely free of tendinous
insertions and muscle attachments, but it is
covered by a well-formed bursa separating it
from the adductor magnus. At the site of the
lesser trochanter deep within the shaft, the femur is strengthened by a bony bar or column
visible at sections extending into the neck and
known as the calcar femorale.[3] The relationship
of the calcar femorale and the lesser trochanter
is observed at surgery following removal of the
greater trochanter when the leg is maximally
adducted. The lesser trochanter forms an additional landmark to the transcondylar line of the
knee joint, which should be observed in the
preparation of the femoral canal. It is particularly important in cases of excessive anteversion
of the femoral neck. The psoas tendon and the
iliacus muscle may be removed from the lesser
trochanter to mobilize the upper femur in difficult pathological situations. It must be noted,
however, that beyond this level no other soft
tissue structure keeps the femur attached to the
pelvis, and careless hyperadduction can cause
severe damage to the soft tissue of the medial
thigh. The lesser trochanter is an excellent point
of reference on x-ray films of the hip, indicating
the degree of hip rotation at the time radiographs
were obtained. A prominent lesser trochanter
indicates an externally rotated hip joint, whereas
the greater trochanter appears less prominent
than usual because the rotation causes its apparent "overlapping" by the femur head.

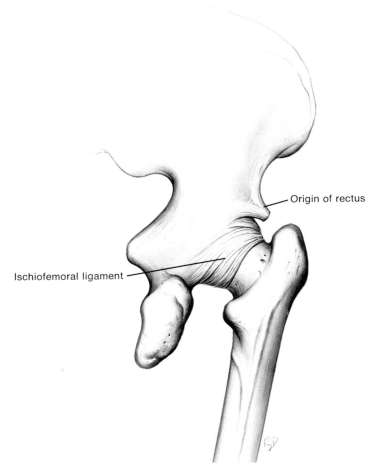

Origin of rectus

Ischiofemoral ligament

Fig. 1-16. Orbicular ligament may hinder dislocation of femoral head at surgery. This structure is best released at junction of ilium and ischium at posterior segment of acetabulum to allow head to escape from depth of acetabulum. Fibers of ischiofemoral ligament are closely applied to femoral head, thus retaining head of femur in socket.

Assembled hip joint

The hip is a simple ball-and-socket joint in which the spherical head of the femur fits closely in a deep bony cavity reinforced by strong ligaments and muscle tension. There has been much controversy in the past about the sphericity and the fit of the femur in the acetabulum and its true weight-bearing area. In pathological conditions the bony acetabulum is generally expanded and enlarged by arthritis and often deepened by osteophytes, especially in the superior and posterior portions. While this can be favorable in the replacement of arthritic hips, it is disadvantageous in the fracture of a normal acetabulum; that is, most of these neck fractures require replacement with an extremely small-sized prosthesis. In pathological conditions it is generally defective anteriorly as in most cases of osteoarthritis. The acetabulum is deepened by the fibrocartilaginous labrum attached to its rim; transverse fibers constituting the acetabular ligament bridge the gap formed by the acetabular notch and act as retaining structures for the head of the femur within the bony acetabulum. At the time of dislocation for replacement, it should be remembered that the constricting fibrocartilaginous labrum should be incised along with the posterior capsule to allow the head to escape from the depth of the acetabulum. (Additionally, a suction or vacuum effect at surgery may prevent the head from dislocating.) Whether the orbicular ligament or band of the capsule derives some of its fibers from the deep tendons of the gluteal muscula-

25

ture or from the reflected head of the rectus is only of academic interest. However, at times the hypertrophied "orbicular ligament" may hinder dislocation of the femur head at surgery. This structure is best released at the level of the junction of the ilium and ischium at the posterosuperior segment of the acetabulum. At the lower part of the neck many of these fibers pass into the inferior retinaculum, which closely surrounds the bone, and are closely applied to the femoral head, helping to retain the head of the femur in the socket (Figs. 1-8 and 1-16).

The Y-shaped ligament of the hip joint capsule (Bigelow's ligament) reaches the trochanteric line between a tubercle at its upper end and the medial side of the shaft (Fig. 1-15). The posterior and slightly medial aspect of the trochanter is marked by a vertical ridge known as the quadrate tubercle for the insertion of the quadratus femoris, which covers the bone medially to its insertion. The quadratus femoris attaches to the intertrochanteric crest. The crest is a part of the trochanteric mass removed (along with this muscle insertion) with a large size trochanter at surgery. Therefore it is not surprising to find that, despite removal of the trochanter from the femur, it assumes a position posterior to the acetabulum when the external rotators are contracted.

Reinforcing capsular ligaments of the hip joint

Reinforcing capsular ligaments of the hip provide stability for the joint and should be preserved at surgery. Anterior dislocation can be prevented by keeping the fibers tautly extended. The longitudinal fibers that cover the articular zone in front of the hip joint extend in a vertical plane from the anterior margin of the hip bone to the intertrochanteric line of the femur. The fibers attached to the anteroinferior spine are thicker than their counterpart fibers attached to the upper pubic ramus. Both of these ligaments reinforce the anterior capsule in a Y-shaped manner and are known collectively as the Bigelow's ligament. The direction and orientation of the contributing iliofemoral and pubofemoral fibers provide stability in maximum external rotation and extension, and the fibers are both tightened when the upright position is assumed. At surgery, an incision made along the midline of the neck of the femur generally divides the two portions of this ligament without severing

either. By preserving both components, the upper portion remains intact and attached to the capsule of the joint and the trochanter, while the inferior portion remains with the inferior capsule. Incision below the neck level preserves both divisions. These ligaments are proportionately shorter in women because of the greater obliquity of the female pelvis and the convexity of the female lumbar spine. They are better seen at surgery when the para-articular and precapsular fat is removed and blood vessels traversing this zone are transected.

The "ligamentum teres" has little significance in regard to hip replacement surgery except that, when present, it may make dislocation of the hip more difficult. But it is usually avulsed from the head and retained within the acetabulum at the position of maximum adduction. This ligament has a weaker synovial attachment to the head of the femur than the acetabular fossa and occasionally contains small vessels that bleed after dislocation. Remnants of the ligamentum teres are removed from the acetabular floor prior to preparation of the acetabulum in order to appreciate the depths of the pulvinar (acetabular fossa). The flattened base of the ligamentum teres is attached by two bands, one into each side of the acetabular notch, and one small strip between the two bands that blends with the transverse ligament (Fig. 1-8).[1] Therefore either part of the ligamentum teres base or the base in combination with the transverse ligament may be excised to allow access to the inferior portion of the acetabulum and the notch and to provide visualization of the fossa for deepening of the acetabulum. It should be remembered that the ligamentum teres is relaxed when the hip is in a semiflexed and abducted position and is taut when the hip is adducted. It is for this reason that firm adduction at dislocation allows for easy detachment from its insertion. Generally this ligament is absent in advanced rheumatoid and osteoarthritic hips.

Capsule of the hip joint

The capsule of the hip joint is a strong and dense fibrous structure. It attaches above the margin of the acetabulum 5 or 6 mm. beyond the labrum and should not be disturbed when the labrum is excised from within the capsular cavity. In front of the outer margin of the labrum, opposite the acetabular notch and further down, the capsule attaches to the transverse acetabular ligament and to the edge of the obturator foramen. On the neck in front it attaches to the trochanteric line above, to the base of the neck behind, and to the neck about 1 cm. above the trochanteric crest and below to the lower part of the neck close to the lesser trochanter (Fig. 1-13). The capsule is particularly thickened in the case of osteoarthritis and constitutes an especially heavy fibrous structure in the superior and inferior portions of the neck. It is shortened posteriorly in severe external rotation deformity and anteriorly when severe adduction deformity prevails. It may become expanded if the head has migrated cephalad. In a completely congenitally dislocated hip, the capsule may be divided into two separate segments connected by an isthmus (hourglass type). The capsule should not be disturbed if the exposure of the hip joint is complete, since it enhances the stability of the hip following replacement, and in toto resection will cause undesirable bleeding. On the other hand, if the trochanter is not removed, as in the anterior approach, a complete capsulectomy is a necessity for exposure prior to dislocation of the hip joint. From the front of the neck, retinacular fibers containing blood vessels enter the bone from the capsule at many points. The capsule of the joint is very thin posteriorly. Two sets of circular and longitudinal fibers reinforce it. The longitudinal fibers have

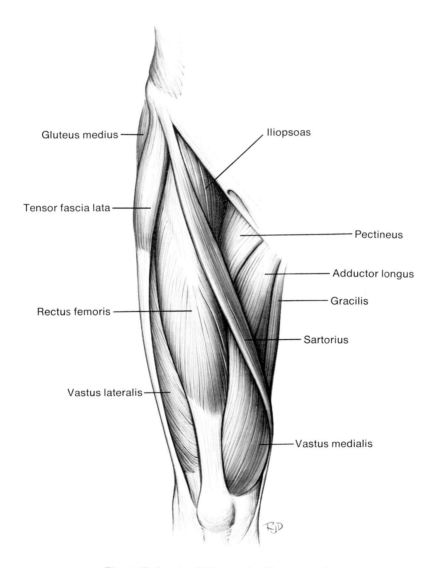

Fig. 1-17. Anterior thigh muscles (flexor group).

27

Basic science

been described previously; however, the circular fibers of the "zona orbicularis" are deep, forming a collar around the neck of the femur. These fibers only attach to the capsule, not to the bone. In addition to the longitudinal and circular ligaments, the "ischiofemoral ligament" reinforces the capsule. It has a spiral appearance on the back of the joint from its attachment to the ischium below and behind the acetabulum, and it directs upwards and laterally over the back of the neck of the femur. Some of its fibers are continuous with those of the "zona orbicularis," while others are fixed to the greater trochanter anteriorly and lead to the iliofemoral ligament.[2] This intricate system of reinforcing ligaments

substantiates the complexity of the capsule of the joint as a stabilizing mechanism of the hip that should not be disturbed unnecessarily if severe preexisting deformity of the hip is not present at surgery. Perhaps it is because of the efficiency of this design that a newly formed capsule after hip replacement does not usually give a full range of flexion.

Muscles about the hip joint

A gross anatomical representation of the muscles of the hip is illustrated in Figs. 1-17 to 1-19. The origins of the muscles and their attachments are shown in Figs. 1-2 and 1-17 to 1-19. The hip joint is covered by muscles on all sides,

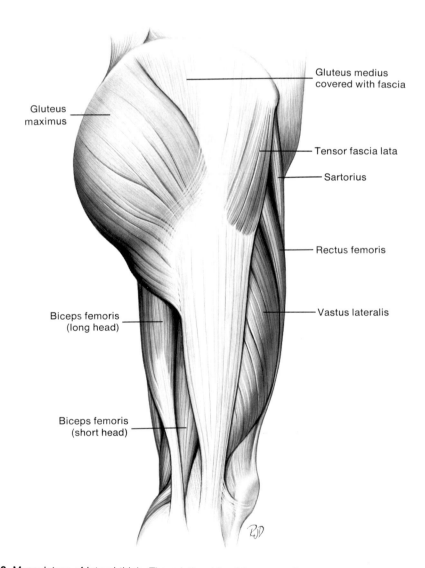

Fig. 1-18. Musculature of lateral thigh. The relationship of three muscles constituting the "pelvic deltoid."[4]

anteriorly by the lateral fibers of the pectineus, and lateral to the pectineus, the tendon of the psoas major with the iliacus on its lateral side. The femoral artery is on the psoas tendon, and the femoral nerve lies deep in the groove between the tendon and the iliacus (Fig. 1-8). More laterally, the straight head of the rectus femoris crosses the hip joint, and at the lateral border the deep layer of the iliotibial tract blends with the fibrous capsule. Superiorly, the reflected head of the rectus and the gluteus minimus covers the lateral part. Inferiorly, the lateral fibers of the pectineus lie on the capsule as they incline backwards; more posteriorly, the obturator externus crosses obliquely to gain the poste-

rior aspect of the hip joint. Posteriorly, the capsule is covered with the tendons of the obturator externus, which separate it from the quadratus femoris. The latter is accompanied by the ascending branch of the medial circumflex artery. Above the tendon of the obturator internus, the two gemelli are in contact with the joint and are separated from the piriformis by the sciatic nerve (Fig. 1-19). The nerve to the quadratus femoris lies deep to the obturator internus tendon and descends on the most medial part of the capsule. The piriformis crosses the uppermost part of the posterior surface of the articular capsule. When the trochanter is removed intra-articularly and the posterosuperior capsule and piriformis ten-

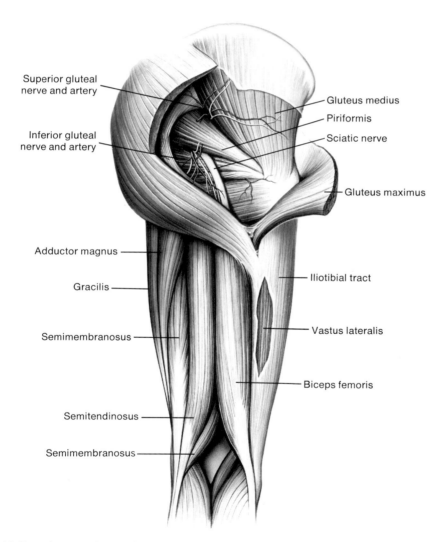

Fig. 1-19. Posterior musculature of thigh and buttock. Gluteus maximus has partially been removed to show deeper layers, which include short rotators, and position of sciatic nerve, superior and inferior gluteal nerves, and arteries; piriformis is "key" muscle.[4]

29

Table 1-1. Summary of functional anatomy of hip muscles

Function	Muscle	Nerve supply
I. Flexors		
A. Primary flexors	Iliopsoas	Nerve to iliopsoas
	Pectineus	Femoral or obturator
	Tensor fascia femoris	Superior gluteal
	Adductor brevis	Obturator
	Sartorius	Femoral
B. Secondary flexors	Adductor longus	Obturator
	Adductor magnus	Obturator
	Gracilis (anterior fibers)	Obturator
	Gluteus medius	Superior gluteal
	Gluteus minimus	Superior gluteal
II. Extensors		
A. Primary extensors	Gluteus maximus	Inferior gluteal
	Adductor magnus (posterior fibers)	Tibial
B. Secondary extensors	Semimembranosus	Tibial
	Semitendinosus	Tibial
	Biceps femoris	Tibial
	Gluteus medius	Superior gluteal
	Gluteus minimus	Superior gluteal
	Piriformis	Nerve to piriformis (L_4-S_2)
III. Adductors		
A. Primary adductors	Adductor brevis	Obturator
	Adductor longus	Obturator
	Adductor magnus	Obturator and tibial
	Gluteus maximus	Inferior gluteal
B. Secondary adductors	Pectineus	Femoral or obturator
	Gracilis	Obturator
	Obturator externus	Obturator
	Iliopsoas	Nerve to iliopsoas
	Hamstrings	Tibial
IV. Abductors		
A. Primary abductors	Gluteus medius	Superior gluteal
	Gluteus minimus	Superior gluteal
B. Secondary abductors	Tensor fascia femoris	Superior gluteal
	Piriformis	Nerve to piriformis
	Sartorius	Femoral
V. Internal rotators		
A. Primary internal rotators	Gluteus medius	Superior gluteal
	Gluteus minimus	Superior gluteal
	Tensor fascia femoris	Superior gluteal
B. Secondary internal rotators	Adductor magnus (posterior part)	Tibial
	Semitendinosus	Tibial
	Semimembranosus	Tibial
VI. External rotators		
A. Primary external rotators	Gluteus maximus	Inferior gluteal
	Piriformis	Nerve to piriformis
	Obturator externus	Obturator
	Obturator internus	Nerve to obturator
	Superior gemellus	Superior gemellus
	Inferior gemellus	Nerve to inferior gemellus and quadratus femoris
	Quadratus femoris	
	Adductor brevis	Obturator
	Adductor longus	Obturator
	Adductor magnus (anterior part)	Obturator
	Pectineus	Femoral or obturator
B. Secondary external rotators	Gluteus medius	Superior gluteal
	Gluteus minimus	Superior gluteal
	Sartorius	Femoral
	Iliopsoas	Nerve to iliopsoas
	Biceps femoris	Tibial

don are incised, brisk arterial bleeding at the site of division is a constant anatomical feature.

To the hip surgeon, knowledge of the origin and insertion of all muscles contributing to the movement of the hip is essential. For brevity, the functional anatomy and the sources of innervation of the hip muscles are presented in Table 1-1. For details of muscular origins and insertions, the reader is referred to standard anatomy texts.[2,5,6,8,9]

Seven noteworthy musculatures with their tendons traverse the hip joint in the back. From above downward they are: the posterior border of the gluteus medius, the piriformis, the gemellus superior, the tendon of the obturator internus, the gemellus inferior, the quadratus femoris, and the adductor magnus. The vertical muscles, the hamstrings, if seen at all, are located very close to the ischium. The description of the superficial structures of the hip (pelvic deltoid) by Henry[4] is of special interest. The "key muscle" in this region of the hip is the piriformis; at its upper edge one can identify the superior gluteal artery and nerve, and at its inferior bor-

der the most superficial structure to emerge is the inferior gluteal nerve. Along the postero-medial edge is the great sciatic nerve.[4] At surgery, when the external rotators are released (for example, the piriformis, detached from its insertion to the greater trochanter, and the quadratus femoris, detached from its femoral attachment close to the bone), it should be noted that the sciatic nerve is located halfway between the posterior border of the ischial portion of the acetabulum (Fig. 1-19).

Arteries and nerves

Major nerves and vessels in the hip region supply local structures as well as the lower extremity with blood and innervation. In the posterior aspect these structures include the sciatic nerve, posterior femoral cutaneous nerve, superior gluteal nerve and vessels, inferior gluteal nerve and vessels, and the nerves to the short rotators and articular branches. Anterior structures include the femoral cutaneous nerve branches, the obturator cutaneous nerve, the lateral femoral cutaneous nerve, and the femoral

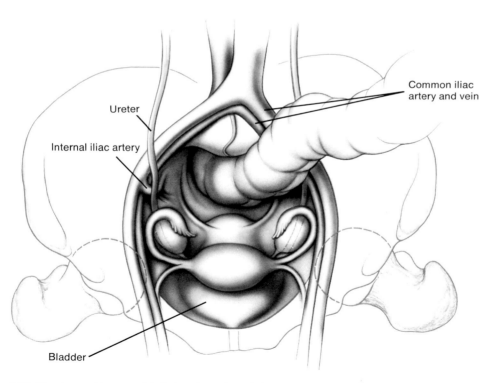

Fig. 1-20. Structures of lesser pelvis in female and proximity of its content to floor of acetabulum are shown. Distended bladder and ureter are closest viscera in addition to internal iliac artery and vein in region of hip joint.

31

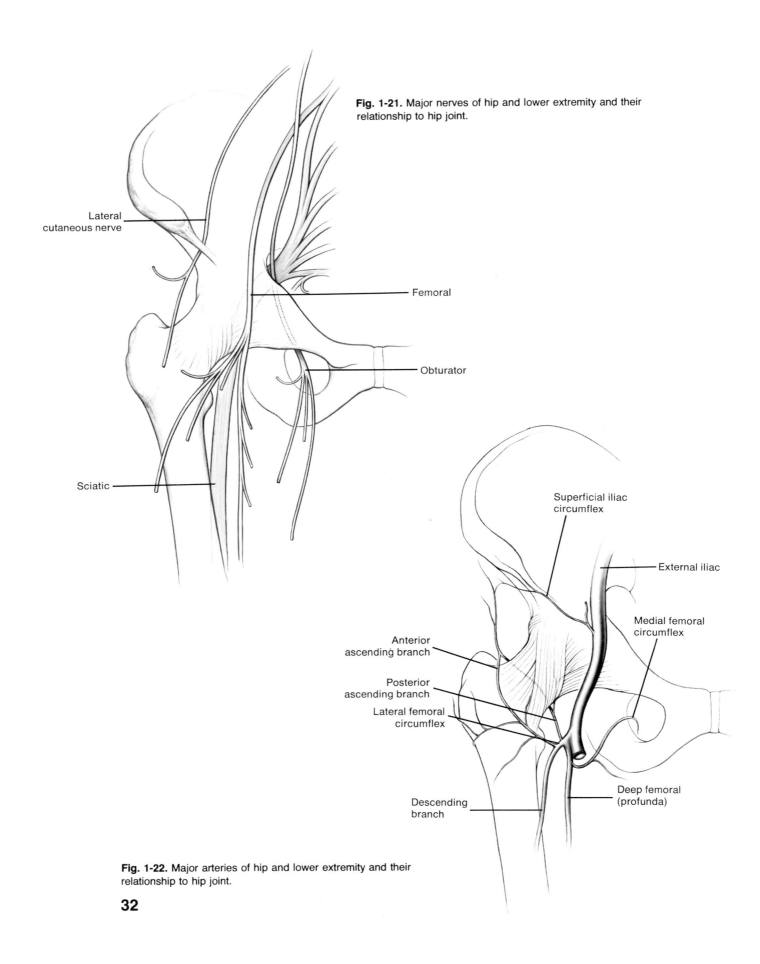

Fig. 1-21. Major nerves of hip and lower extremity and their relationship to hip joint.

Lateral cutaneous nerve

Femoral

Obturator

Sciatic

Superficial iliac circumflex

External iliac

Anterior ascending branch

Medial femoral circumflex

Posterior ascending branch

Lateral femoral circumflex

Descending branch

Deep femoral (profunda)

Fig. 1-22. Major arteries of hip and lower extremity and their relationship to hip joint.

32

nerve (cutaneous branches, articular branches, and muscular branches). Femoral vessels include the profunda (the largest branch) and femoral circumflex vessels, medial and lateral—both commonly a branch of the profunda.

The origin, distribution, and location of the major nerves and arteries of the hip joint are illustrated in Figs. 1-8, 1-10, and 1-19 to 1-22. The femoral nerves at the anterior rim of the acetabulum are the most vulnerable in the area, especially when this wall is defective as in congenital dysplasia. (See Chapter 13.) The sciatic nerve may be injured if the posterior wall is defective, that is, during a conversion of a difficult hip problem. Good exposure of the back of the pelvis and complete visualization of the nerve at this level ensures its safety if a bone grafting to the back of the acetabulum is planned. As stated, the obturator nerve may be injured during excessive preparation of the pubic segment of the acetabulum by anchor holes entering the obturator foramen or the iliopubic ramus and flow of cement into this area. In establishing the 'anchor holes,' location of these nerves must be borne in mind lest damage is caused by deep penetration of the cement. The relationship of the common iliac and femoral artery and veins to the wall of the pelvis is illustrated in an inlet view of the pelvis in Fig. 1-20. Inadvertent penetration of the pelvis may cause serious damage to these major vessels or viscera such as the bladder.

SUMMARY OF ESSENTIALS

- Knowledge of the gross anatomy of the hip is of paramount importance for the surgical approach and technique in relation to orientation and insertion of prosthetic components. The surgeon performing total hip replacement must study a bony skeleton and review anatomy in detail on a bony cadaveric specimen, dissecting the hip with particular attention to the neurovascular structures of the hip. A simulated hip replacement on a cadaveric specimen will expand the surgeon's comprehension of the gross anatomy of the pelvis and hip and may well prevent future surgical complications.
- The ilium, pubis, and ischium contribute to the formation of the acetabulum, which faces outward and somewhat downward anteriorly. In addition to structure, knowledge of the anatomical orientation of the acetabulum and pelvis is important. The weight-bearing upper and posterior walls of the acetabulum are especially heavy, whereas the

anterior wall is usually less developed. The inferior wall is less substantial at the site of the acetabular notch opening into the obturator foramen.

- The "acetabular fossa," a rough area located at the center of the articulating portion of the acetabulum, is the thinnest portion of the floor of the acetabulum. At this site the inner and outer tables of the pelvic bone are fused without interpositioned cancellous bone. This zone comprises the thinnest possible area beyond which damage may be rendered if deepening of the acetabulum is performed. In osteoarthritic hips (especially in congenital dysplasia) this area is thickened, and further deepening of the socket is possible here. This level corresponds with the radiological "teardrop" on an anteroposterior radiograph of the pelvis.
- The bony pelvis appears to have been twisted on itself at the site of the acetabulum, creating two planes at right angles to each other. The upper portion roughly corresponds to the ilium, and the lower corresponds to the ischium and pubis. This is an important consideration when observing the anteroposterior radiographs of the pelvis, which generally show the pelvis somewhat in a frontal plane and the ischium and pubis in a more sagittal plane. This deceptive x-ray representation of a flat "iliac fan" should be kept in mind when preparing the acetabulum. The three-dimensional configuration should also be kept in mind when orientation of the patient's pelvis on the operating table is being done.
- The greater sciatic notch may be conveniently reached both through the inner wall of the pelvis by subperiosteal dissection or from the outside by exploring the sciatic nerve in the buttocks.
- It should be recognized that the ilium and ischium are the major contributors to the formation of the acetabulum. The direction and the small size of the pubis must be appreciated on a dry bony specimen to avoid extensive damage at surgery. The anterior aspect of the pelvis is especially vulnerable at the zone of the pubic contribution to the acetabulum.
- Because the ilium and ischium each provide two fifths of the acetabulum and the remaining one-fifth is contributed by the pubis, the pubis particularly needs to be protected during the preparation of the acetabulum.
- The acetabular fossa containing fibrofatty tissue must be regarded as the key in identifying the depth of the floor at that level. By removal of the soft tissue from the fossa, the true depth of the socket may be appreciated. Preparation of the rim of the acetabulum involves heavy retraction of the capsule superiorly and anteriorly in addition to exposing the acetabular notch.
- The best access to the upper femur is by maximum adduction of the hip while observing the relation-

ship of the transcondylar line, patella, and lesser trochanter.

■ The size and shape of the acetabulum as represented by the size and shape of the head is a guide to the anatomical size of the socket selected at surgery and the amount of bone to be removed in order to accommodate the new socket.

■ Successful detachment and reattachment of the greater trochanter include appraisal of its size, shape, and location in relation to the shaft, the neck of the femur, the intertrochanteric line, the intertrochanteric crest, the tip, the digital fossa, the vastus lateralis ridge, and the quadratus femoris tubercle.

■ The lesser trochanter provides a reference guide for preparation of the upper femur and also denotes the medial muscular structures and the level of the calcar femorale. Both the lesser and greater trochanter denote degrees of anteversion or retroversion of the upper femur, but the best reference in this regard is the transcondylar line of the femur.

■ The capsule of the hip joint is preserved in some techniques of total hip arthroplasty, and with its reinforcing ligament, it can augment the stability of the hip joint. The capsular attachment to the periphery of the acetabulum provides an excellent support for retractors to aid visualization during surgery.

■ The key anatomical landmarks and their relationship to vital structures must be kept in mind for a safe surgical approach.

■ The anatomical discussion presented in this chapter is intended to apply to total hip arthroplasty. Specifics are thus limited to the replacement surgery, and the reader is advised to consult standard texts for detailed anatomy of the hip joint.

REFERENCES

1. Breathnach, A. S., editor: Frazer's anatomy of the human skeleton, ed. 6, Boston, 1965, Little, Brown & Co.
2. Grant, J. C.: Grant's atlas of anatomy, ed. 5, Baltimore, 1962, The Williams & Wilkins Co.
3. Harty, M.: The calcar femorale and the femorale neck, J. Bone Joint Surg. **39A:**625-630, 1957.
4. Henry, A. K.: Extensile exposure, ed. 2, Baltimore, 1957, The Williams & Wilkins Co.
5. Hollinshead, W. H.: Anatomy for surgeons, vol. 3: The back and limbs, New York, 1958, Harper & Row, Publishers, Inc.
6. Last, R. J.: Anatomy, regional and applied, ed. 2, Boston, 1959, Little, Brown & Co.
7. Lockhart, R. D., Hamilton, G. F., and Fyfe, F. W.: Anatomy of the human body, Philadelphia, 1959, J. B. Lippincott Co.
8. Romanes, G. J., editor: Cunningham's textbook of anatomy, ed. 11, London, 1972, Oxford University Press, Inc.
9. Warwick, R., and Williams, P. L., editors: Gray's anatomy, ed. 35 (British), Philadelphia, 1973, W. B. Saunders Co.

CHAPTER 2

Surgical approaches to the hip

A mind that understands principles will work out the methods.

HUGH OWEN THOMAS

. . . if the right instruments are used and if some points of technique during the operation are carefully considered, you will be soon able to do 80% to 90% of T.H.R.'s without removal of the greater trochanter. The operation is much easier and quicker.

M. MÜLLER

The most gentle way of retracting the gluteus medius and minimus is by detaching the greater trochanter. In a heavy muscled patient a considerable volume of gluteus medius lies anterior to the greater trochanter. How much of this muscle remains active after anterior exposure without detaching trochanter is unknown. To the damage that retraction may inflict on the gluteal muscles may be added to the danger of damaging the nerve supply of the tensor fasciae femoris.

J. CHARNLEY

During the past century numerous surgical approaches to the hip have been described, each of which claimed some advantage in the performance of certain surgical procedures. It is beyond the scope of this text to describe all these approaches, their usefulness, or their disadvantages.

Total hip arthroplasty requires greater exposure than most other hip procedures for complete access to the acetabulum and the upper femur. A complete fascial and muscular release should be considered a prerequisite to the correction of all existing fixed deformities. A knowledge of all alternative approaches to the hip is necessary in order to understand the anatomical basis for each, and each must be critically considered for its merits and disadvantages. All aspects of science are not crystallized, and the technology of total hip replacement is in the stage of evolution. Because a prosthesis and procedure (surgical approach) are interrelated, it is reasonable to suggest each prosthetic design should be used with the approach proposed by its originator.

When new approaches are recommended or modified, certain merits may be claimed for the approach itself while disregarding its disadvantages when applied to total hip replacement procedure. Few of these new approaches are truly original; many are either modifications or rediscoveries of approaches already in use. For a comprehensive discussion of this topic the reader is referred to surgical texts.[1,5-7,18,30]

A shortened operative time and reduction of blood loss are of concern to most surgeons in order to minimize morbidity. Likewise, early recovery during the postoperative course as related to surgical technique is a feature that must be considered. Whenever possible, the hip should be approached without detachment of muscular insertions, since detachment prolongs recovery time and increases morbidity. So the advantages of any approach must be contrasted with significant disadvantages such as restricted exposure leading to soft tissue damage from heavy retraction or technical errors as malpositioning or compromise fixation of the components and inadequate correction of the deformities. These

35

disadvantages are particularly critical when there is a severe anatomical distortion or scarring from previous operations.

An important consideration in any surgical approach to the hip joint is the positioning of the patient on the operating table, best ascertained when "landmarks" such as both anterosuperior spines and the greater trochanter can be palpated through the draping for orientation. For example, in the original technique of McKee and Müller, as well as that of Charnley, the patient remains in the supine position. This facilitates the positioning of the components in reference to the pelvis. However, many surgeons have modified these techniques by placing the patient in a variety of other positions ranging from semiprone to lateral decubitus and, at times, tilted a few degrees by elevating the operating side with a sandbag. Regardless of the surgical approach used, if the surgeon disregards the position of the patient on the table, the positioning of the components may be compromised.

Many surgical approaches to the hip have been described for specific operations, but familiarity of the surgeon with each approach does not necessarily mean it is suitable for total hip replacement. For example, Moore's "southern exposure" was designed for the insertion of the Moore self-locking prosthesis,[43,44] and while it is quite sufficient for this purpose, it is quite inadequate for total hip arthroplasty. This technique produces a deep wound without access to the stump of the femur or the acetabulum; deformity corrections may be difficult, particularly if extensive capsular release and mobilization of the upper femur are necessary.

Because more exposure is required for unrestricted access to the soft tissue and bone in total hip arthroplasty, the incision must be made with the patient's position and postoperative care in mind. It must also be versatile so that additional exposure of deep anatomical planes can be obtained if difficulties are encountered during the operation. It must be away from the perineum to avoid contamination and pressure on the suture line during recovery. And to spare operative time, it must not be excessively complicated, involving tedious dissection of neurovascular structures or violation of viable tissue.

COMMON SURGICAL APPROACHES TO THE HIP

Approaches commonly used in hip surgery are categorized according to anatomical planes of exposure as follows: anterior, anterolateral, lateral (transtrochanteric), posterior, posterolateral, and medial.

Anterior approaches

Despite extensive utilization in Smith-Petersen cup arthroplasty in the United States and Europe, the anterior approach has not gained popularity in total hip replacement because extensive time and intervention with muscle attachments are usually required to provide a complete exposure. Further, as with most anterior approaches, the Smith-Petersen approach requires extensive detachment of tendinous insertions and retraction of muscle, with potential damage to vital structures such as the femoral nerve and artery. Disturbance of the lateral cutaneous nerve of the thigh, with resultant numbness and "meralgia paresthetica," is another common complication. However, a limited anterior approach using only a segment of the Smith-Petersen approach is quite suitable for procedures such as biopsy. Common anterior approaches were described and popularized by Smith-Petersen[4,55,56] Heuter-Schade,[58] Fahey,[24] Luck,[37] and Jergenson and Abbott.[32]

Anterolateral approaches

The anterolateral approach without trochanteric osteotomy was popularized for total hip replacement by G. Kenneth McKee[40] and Maurice Müller.[47] Originally described by Watson-Jones,[62] this approach is versatile and provides good exposure of the neck of the femur and hip joint. The incision begins 1 inch distal and 1 inch posterior to the anterosuperior iliac spine, curves distally and laterally to the tip of the greater trochanter, and extends toward the lateral surface of the femoral shaft to 2 inches distal to the base of the trochanter (Fig. 2-1). The nerve to the tensor fascia femoris is found at the interval between the gluteus medius and tensor fascia femoris, which may inadvertently be damaged in exposing the capsule of the joint (Fig. 2-2).

To allow anterior dislocation of the femoral head, a complete capsulectomy is then performed, including the fibers of the reflected head of the rectus femoris (anteriorly) and the vastus lateralis (inferiorly) (Fig. 2-3). Dislocation at times is possible after complete capsulectomy and removal of osteophytes as well. The head is dislocated by traction, external rotation, and adduction, and the neck is cut at the desired

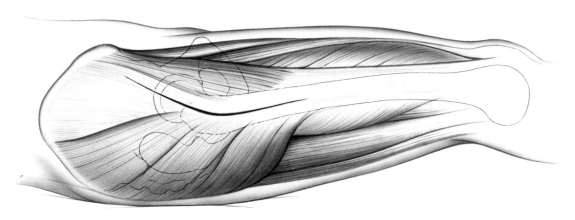

Fig. 2-1. Anterolateral exposure of Watson-Jones. Patient is positioned on operating table in supine position.

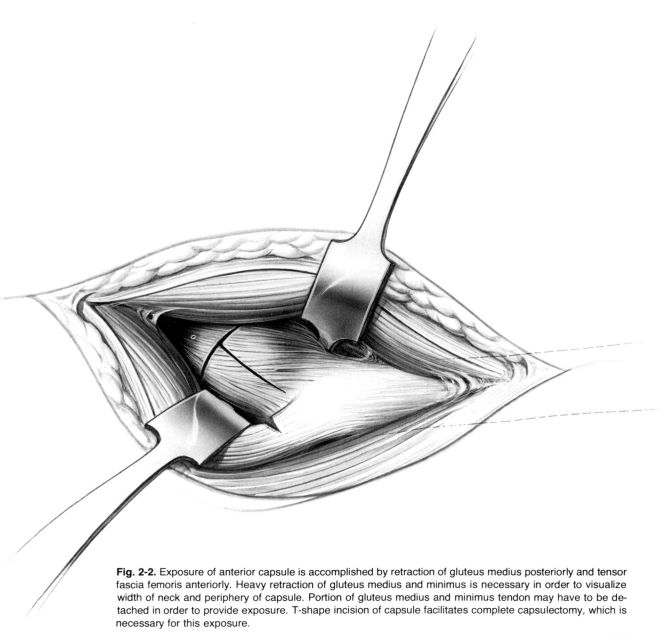

Fig. 2-2. Exposure of anterior capsule is accomplished by retraction of gluteus medius posteriorly and tensor fascia femoris anteriorly. Heavy retraction of gluteus medius and minimus is necessary in order to visualize width of neck and periphery of capsule. Portion of gluteus medius and minimus tendon may have to be detached in order to provide exposure. T-shape incision of capsule facilitates complete capsulectomy, which is necessary for this exposure.

37

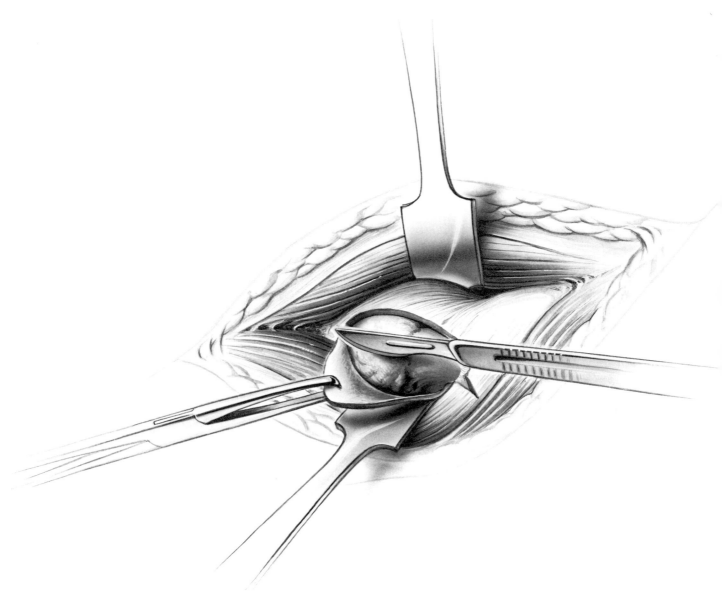

Fig. 2-3. Complete capsulectomy is essential in order to visualize head and periphery of acetabulum. Leg is positioned somewhat in external rotation.

level with a Gigli or oscillating saw (Fig. 2-4). The head is removed in a retrograde fashion, and exposure of the acetabulum is then completed with the aid of Hohmann-type retractors (placed anteriorly, posteriorly, and occasionally one inferiorly) (Fig. 2-5). Preparation of the acetabulum is completed with special reamers and cementing of the acetabular component according to the technique described in Chapter 12.

With this approach, division of the short external rotators may be done by placing the limb in external rotation; in particular, the piriformis should be placed under tension, pulled forward on a bone hook, and cut with a knife. During preparation of the medullary canal, a wide retractor with narrow points is placed under the greater trochanter to lift the femur forward, and the glutei are protected by a second small retractor, while the third retractor is hooked under the psoas muscle. Insertion of broaches should provide anteversion of no more than 10 degrees. The transcondylar axis of the knee serves as a reference (Fig. 2-6). To expose the opening of

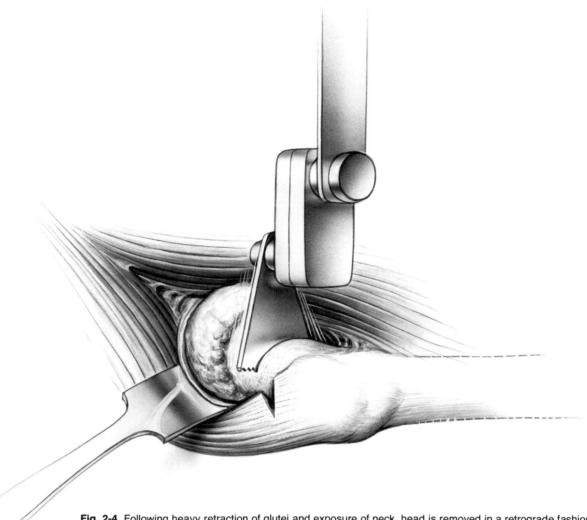

Fig. 2-4. Following heavy retraction of glutei and exposure of neck, head is removed in a retrograde fashion following osteotomy of neck.

the neck of the femur, considerable external rotation is necessary. To improve access, a portion of the gluteal tendon may be detached from the trochanter. Müller has emphasized the proper insertion of Hohmann retractors for better exposure in conjunction with this approach.[47] Figs. 2-2, 2-3, and 2-5 demonstrate the site of application of these retractors during the exposure of the hip.

For further details of the Müller and McKee techniques for total hip arthroplasty, the reader is referred to articles by these authors.[40,47] Figs. 2-1 and 2-4 illustrate the exposure of the hip joint through the anterior approach without removing the greater trochanter (Watson-Jones approach and Müller technique).

Lateral approaches (transtrochanteric)

No approach can be considered truly lateral unless the greater trochanter is removed or abductor tendons are disinserted or removed from it.[9,17] For this reason, distinction is made between the lateral and the anterolateral or posterolateral approaches. The lateral approach as originally described by Ollier in 1881 was made with a U-shaped skin incision at the trochanteric level.[18] This approach, which included trochanteric osteotomy, has been modified by many surgeons. Murphy, for instance, added a longitudinal extension at the midpoint ("goblet" incision).[18] Charnley has remained faithful to this surgical approach, using a straight midline incision. He used it for central stabilization and

39

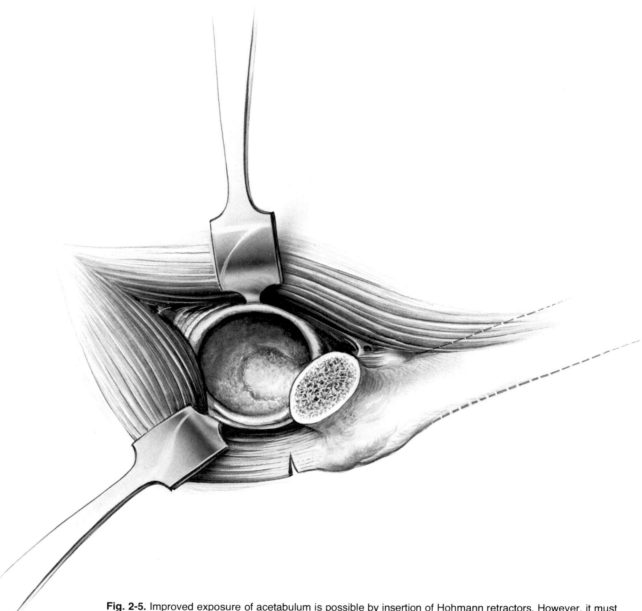

Fig. 2-5. Improved exposure of acetabulum is possible by insertion of Hohmann retractors. However, it must be recognized that heavy retraction of gluteal muscles is necessary since bulk of gluteus medius and minimus are further anterior on pelvis and greater trochanter.

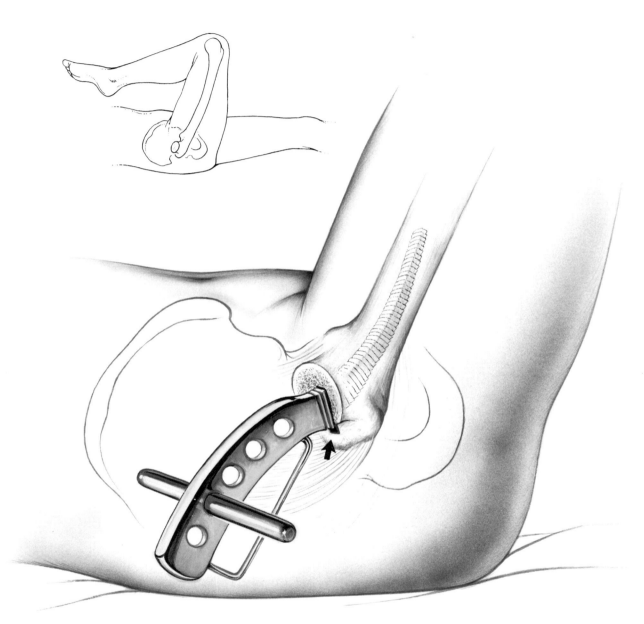

Fig. 2-6. Insertion of broaches in appropriate attitude is not feasible with anterior approach unless hip is maximally adducted, flexed, and externally rotated. This position is dangerous because of possibility of fracture of femur in osteoporotic person. Transcondylar axis of knee serves as reference for orientation of broaches and prosthesis. NOTE: valgus orientation of prosthesis is only possible if broaches are inserted as such to encroach onto greater trochanteric bed (arrow). In doing so fibers of gluteus medius and its tendon may be damaged.

central dislocation arthrodesis of the hip joint. We have used a modified oblique incision and, like Brady, find that it further improves exposure.[8] Aufranc and Stinchfield used this approach extensively in their work with mold arthroplasty.[4] In describing this approach, Harris,[28,29] recommended it for operations requiring extensive exposure.

I believe that a lateral approach is the most suitable in total hip arthroplasty; it is more physiologically sound when the greater trochanter is detached and subsequently reattached firmly to the lateral aspect of the shaft. While it provides wide exposure both anteriorly and posteriorly, there is no interference with neurovascular structures of the hip, and muscle fibers are spared from damage by avoidance of heavy retraction. It is particularly suitable for total hip replacement because it permits correction of deforming soft tissue structures where difficult anatomical situations are present and it permits restoration of tension and functional capacity of the abductor mechanism when the muscle fiber length is restored after transfer of the greater trochanter. Good visualization of the anterior and posterior aspects of the hip during dislocation is obtained, with a full view of the entire acetabulum following dislocation.

Following removal of the greater trochanter, the interval between the tensor fascia femoris medially and the anterior border of the gluteus medius and minimus laterally can be entered, but the nerve to the tensor fascia femoris may be spared. The capsule of the joint is incised but may be excised if absolutely necessary. A complete capsulectomy is not needed in order to obtain access to the acetabulum. Posteriorly, this approach permits detachment of the short rotators from the upper femur and the piriformis tendon from the greater trochanter as needed. Troublesome bleeding of the posterior shaft following detachment of short rotators can readily be controlled. With this exposure, potential damage to the sciatic nerve and the femoral nerve and artery is literally nonexistent. The details of this surgical approach, as used in total hip replacement can be found in Chapter 12.

Posterior approaches

As with anterior and lateral approaches to the hip, several posterior approaches have been described within the past century. There are numerous modifications of the posterior approach involving the skin incision and deeper incision, each with its limitations and advantages.* The posterior approach was first advised by von Langenbeck in 1874.[61] Kocher modified his approach, as described by Dumont in 1887.[1] Procedures described by MacFarland and Osborne, Zahradnicek, and Moore are basically alterations of the original incision and Kocher's approach, later further modified by Gibson.[25-27] Other posterior approaches were devised by Ober,[50] Osborne,[51] Caldwell,[10] Henry,[30] and Horowitz.[31] Gibson's modification of the posterior approach was described in 1949,[25] and then further modified by Marcy and Fletcher.[42] I have found this approach and exposure of the hip without removal of the greater trochanter helpful in partial replacement such as insertion of a femoral head prosthesis.[20]

Perhaps the most popular approach is Moore's "southern exposure,"[43,44] used extensively throughout the world in prosthetic replacement of the femoral head. Its advantages include relative ease and adequate exposure for insertion of a noncemented prosthesis. In this approach, the incision is begun approximately 4 inches distal to the posterosuperior iliac spine and is extended distally and laterally parallel with the fibers of the gluteus maximus to the posterior margin of the greater trochanter. It is then directed distally 4 or 5 inches parallel with the femoral shaft. In this approach the sciatic nerve is exposed and must be protected; it is not suitable for total hip replacement because of its depth without easy access to the upper femur.

Posterolateral approaches

Horowitz in 1952[31] and Marcy and Fletcher in 1954[42] described their modifications of Gibson's approach. These modifications constitute a posterolateral approach to the hip joint. I[19] have used this modified[42] approach extensively and find it the most suitable approach for adequate exposure and access to the acetabulum. It is a useful approach for the insertion of a femoral head prosthesis, and if total hip replacement is to be performed without removal of the greater trochanter, it is superior to the anterolateral approach of Watson-Jones as advocated by Müller and McKee. Its advantages include less forceful retraction of the glutei and better access

---

*See references 6, 25-27, 39, 42, and 43.

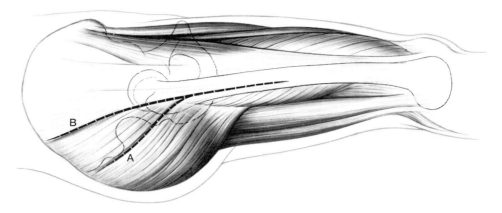

Fig. 2-7. Perhaps most popular approach for insertion of femoral head prosthesis is Moore's "southern exposure," *A.* In this approach incision is begun approximately 4 inches distal to posterosuperior iliac spine and is extended distally and laterally parallel with fibers of gluteus maximus to posterior margin of greater trochanter. It is then directed distally 4 or 5 inches with femoral shaft. This incision is not suitable for total hip replacement. Preferred incision is modified Gibson in that proximal limb of incision is aimed toward posterosuperior iliac spine, *B,* posterolateral approach (see text).

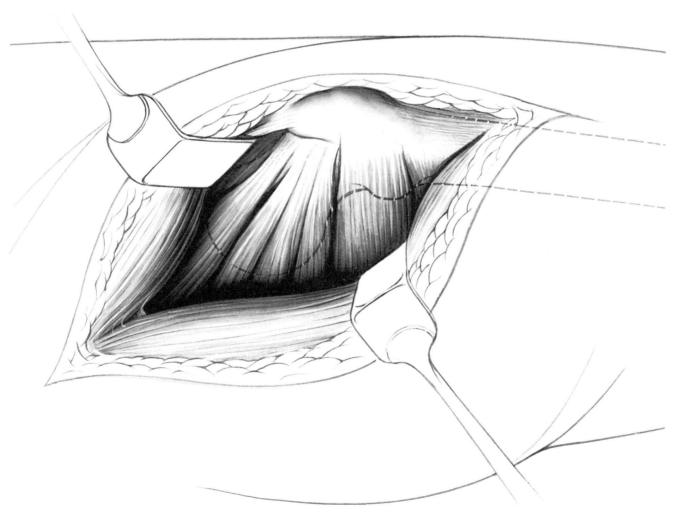

Fig. 2-8. Modified Gibson exposure (see text).

43

to the upper end of the femur in a bloodless field.

As in the other posterior approaches, for example, Moore's southern exposure, the patient must be placed in the lateral decubitus position (Fig. 2-13). However, the incision is made further laterally than in Moore's southern exposure (toward the posterosuperior instead of the posteroinferior iliac spine), eliminating the possibility of contamination of the incision and of the patient lying on the incision. In this exposure there is no need to visualize the sciatic nerve, since the incision is located just behind the femoral shaft and the dividing muscle interval between the posterior border of the gluteus medius and the upper border of the fibers of the gluteus maximus. There is no vascular structure along the approach line and no dis-

turbance to any muscular attachments. Yet, in an obese patient who might require further exposure, one third of the posterior attachment of the gluteus medius tendon may be excised for easy retraction and then simply resutured.

Unlike the southern exposure, in this approach the acetabulum is readily accessible, obviating the need for retracting the huge bulk of gluteus maximus muscle fibers. The skin incision begins three fingers anterior to the posterosuperior spine and progresses to the greater trochanter and the second limb then extends distally along the femur for approximately 6 inches (Fig. 2-7). The fascia and gluteofemoral bursa are incised in line with the skin incision, and the interval between the posterior border of the gluteus medius and the anterior border of the gluteus maximus is then

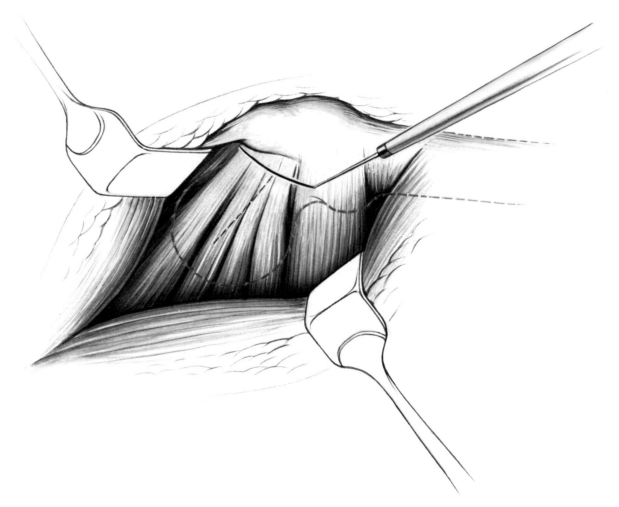

Fig. 2-9. By using diathermy knife, short rotators are detached from posterior aspects of femoral neck and greater trochanter.

entered (Fig. 2-8). The short rotators are then placed under tension by maximally rotating the limb internally. As much of the short rotators should now be detached as necessary to provide access to the whole width of the neck through the capsule (Fig. 2-9). The capsule is incised or excised as indicated to provide maximum exposure preserving the anterior part but excising as much from the posterior and inferior segments as necessary to allow dislocation by internal rotation of the hip. With excision of the capsule and placement of Hohmann retractors (anteriorly, posteriorly, and inferiorly), the acetabular exposure is complete and adequate (Fig. 2-10). The head of the femur may then be osteotomized, either in situ and removed in a retrograde manner, or removed with a Gigli saw following dislocation of the hip joint by maxi-

mum internal rotation (Fig. 2-11). Figs. 2-7 to 2-13 demonstrate the details of this approach. Details of the acetabulum preparation and insertion of the components are similar to those described for total hip replacement with tro-

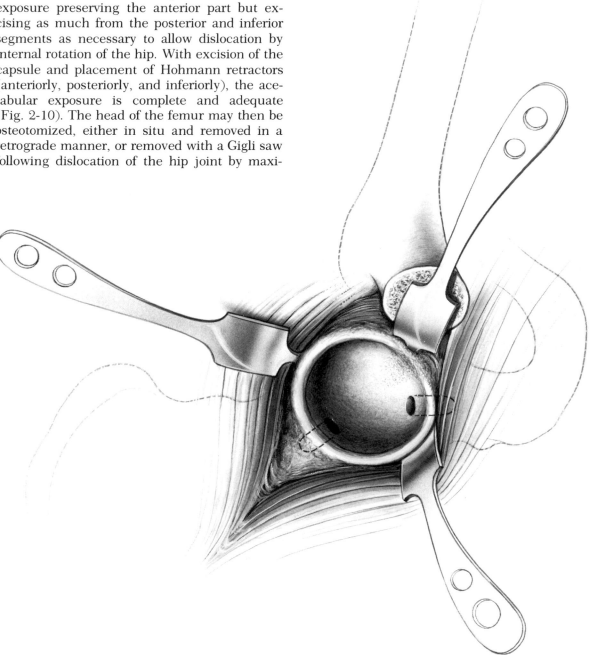

Fig. 2-10. Exposure of acetabulum with this approach is excellent. No heavy retraction of glutei is necessary. Use of Hohmann retractors facilitates complete exposure of acetabulum. NOTE: sciatic nerve need not be exposed or protected during operation (see text).

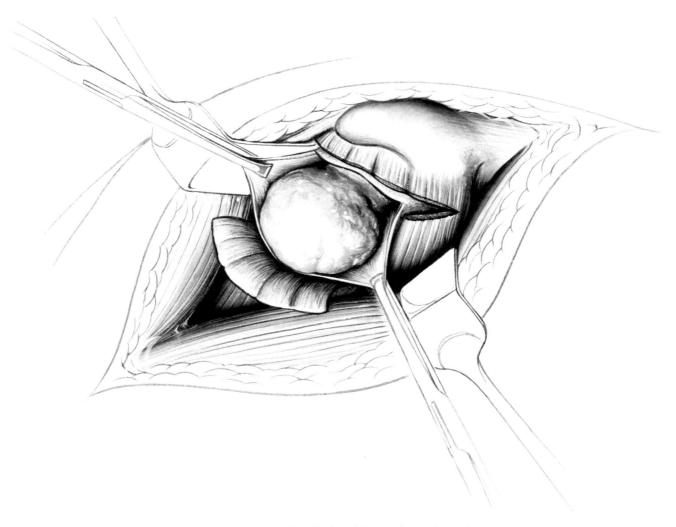

Fig. 2-11. Capsule is incised and retracted, head is then dislocated by maximum internal rotation of hip positioned in flexion.

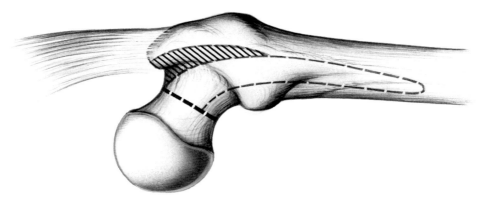

Fig. 2-12. Preparation of femur is similar to that of anterolateral approach but less damage to gluteal muscles is experienced during preparation of femoral canal. Note segment of bone to be removed from greater trochanteric area in order to allow valgus orientation for broach (shaded area).

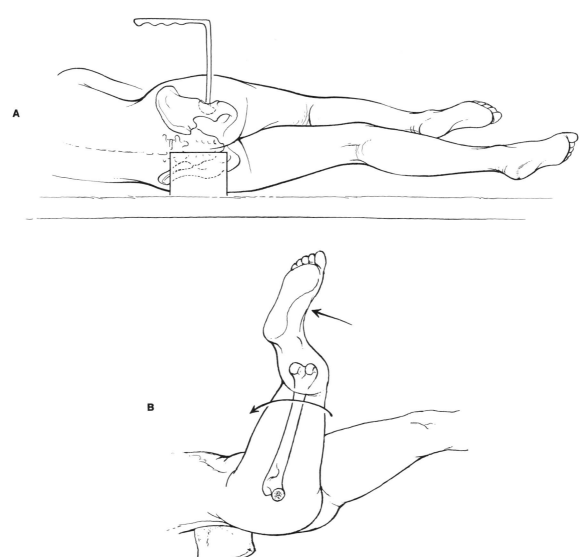

Fig. 2-13. A, Position of patient on operating table must be absolutely secured in order to make orientation of acetabular component possible with any degree of accuracy. **B,** During preparation of femoral canal, maximum internal rotation of lower extremity is necessary in order to produce access to upper end of femur.

chanteric osteotomy. Preparation of the upper femur is possible by maximum internal rotation of femur. The trochanteric bed must be entered in order to provide valgus orientation (Fig. 2-12). Fig. 2-13 illustrates the positioning of patient and orientation of the acetabulum and femur.

Medial approaches

Medial approaches to the hip joint are not suitable for performing total hip replacement,[21,38] as they provide only limited exposure of the proximal femur and the lesser trochanter. Approaches to the medial aspect of the hip may have a place in congenital dislocation hip surgery and in myotomy and neurectomy in the region of the adductors.

SUMMARY OF APPROACHES TO THE HIP AND AN ANALOGY

I compare the hip joint to a "house," and consider the various approaches to it: a main gate at the center, a second "walkway" at the front, and another in the back. The main entrance or gateway is the largest (the trochanter) and gives

47

the best and easiest access. The other routes, front and back, also allow entrance but are limited if greater traffic demand is placed on them. The "front walkway" (anterolateral approach) is situated between the tensor fascia femoris (anteriorly) and gluteus medius (posteriorly), the "back walkway" (posterolateral approach) is formed between the gluteus medius anteriorly and the upper border of the gluteus maximus posteriorly. With this analogy, one can readily see that "grand entrances" and major events are best arranged through the main gateway (by lifting up the greater trochanter and thus opening the main gateway), and less important events can take place via the secondary routes. If the main events are staged through the smaller entrances, there is reduced effect and efficiency, with unavoidable objects blocking the way and damage to the walkways.

For effective surgery, one can theoretically consider all three "possible approaches," but the "main gateway" is the most logical and effective course to follow.

CONTROVERSY OF THE TRANSTROCHANTERIC APPROACH

This aspect of total hip replacement technique remains controversial,* encompassing three schools of thought:

- Recommendation of routine trochanteric osteotomy in all cases
- Advocation of removal only in difficult anatomical situations
- Recommendation of total arthroplasty without trochanteric osteotomy

While controversy over the need for routine osteotomy of the greater trochanter continues, I believe this approach is indispensable in difficult anatomical situations and revision surgery. When adopted as a routine technique by surgeons who devote their careers to the surgery of the hip joint, the advantages are obvious and rewarding. In theory, osteotomy and transfer of the greater trochanter improve the mechanical situation of the hip and increase stability against dislocation. Based on personal clinical and teaching experience, I believe that the abductor muscle is better protected because it remains undamaged when the greater trochanter is removed. Certainly, a less experienced surgeon will have a greater margin of safety with the re-

moval of the trochanter. This is particularly true when he is confronted with an unexpectedly difficult anatomical situation at surgery, but he is also less confined when fixed deformity and severe contractures are present. Considering the mechanical analysis of the lever arm system, the functional load on the prosthetic joint is reduced, and this also may reduce socket wear, fatigue failure of the components, and cement fixation. These claimed features will be validated only when well-documented results of arthroplasty without trochanteric removal become available. (See Chapter 3.)

Disadvantages attributed to trochanteric osteotomy include increased blood loss and operative time, delayed postoperative ambulation, nonunion, symptomatic nonunion, rupture of wires (used for fixation of greater trochanter), painful bursitis, and dislocations resulting from separation of the trochanter.[2,22,23,47] These are rare, however (see Chapter 17), and must be balanced against the advantages, real and theoretical (Table 2-1). Complications of trochanteric osteotomy can be kept to a minimum only when the surgeon masters the technique by routine experience.

Table 2-1. Advantages and disadvantages of trochanteric osteotomy

Theoretical and practical advantages	Theoretical and practical criticism
Wide and extensive exposure	Increased operating time
Improved mechanics of the hip	Handling of the trochanter at surgery
Protection of anatomical structures	Delayed weight bearing postoperatively
Correction of fixed deformity	Increased blood loss
Ease of dislocation at operation	Trochanteric bursitis
Ease of preparation of acetabulum and femur	Trochanteric nonunion
Ease of insertion of components	Painful nonunion
Improved cement fixation technique	Breakages of wire and migration
Improved stability following surgery	
Improved quality of clinical results	
Low incidence of mechanical failure	

*See references 34-36, 41, 52, 54, 57, 59, and 60.

The criticism that osteotomy necessitates increased operating time and greater blood loss requires further study under controlled conditions for clarification. The criticism may be valid for surgeons who perform trochanteric osteotomy only in cases of technical difficulty in which extra time and blood loss would be routinely encountered regardless of the technique.

The question remains whether the greater trochanter should be osteotomized routinely or only in difficult cases. Routine osteotomy of the greater trochanter provides the surgeon with a unique experience in its handling, proper removal, and reattachment; with familiarity and practice, his efficiency increases. During surgery, therefore, the time spent removing and reattaching the trochanter will be regained because ease of exposure and better access facilitate proper surgical implantation of the prosthesis. Therefore regular use of osteotomy by the experienced surgeon reduces the number of technical complications in handling the greater trochanter. This experience is not gained if the surgeon osteotomizes the trochanter only occasionally, that is in difficult cases. In these surgical situations trochanteric complications are increased, and it is in these cases in particular that a good reattachment is of paramount importance for stability. Facileness gained from previous trochanteric experience will increase the probability of a straightforward, uncomplicated operation requiring minimum time and effort and ending with good results. Moreover, it is not always feasible to predict the difficulty or ease of a case by x-ray films and clinical examination prior to surgery and thus plan whether the trochanter should be removed or not.

It is often stated that rehabilitation is slow, and the patient must remain in bed for a longer period of time when the greater trochanter is removed. This is simply untrue. Rehabilitation following low-friction arthroplasty with routine osteotomy of the greater trochanter is not restricted because of the surgery on the trochanter. In the first 48 to 72 hours the patient is unable to move out of bed because of general recovery from surgery. When the trochanter has been well attached, there should be no difference in postoperative management and rehabilitation of these patients than with those operated without osteotomy of the greater trochanter.

Müller,[48] one of the proponents of surgery without osteotomy of the greater trochanter, believes that adequate instrumentation and an incision adequate for the exposure of the acetabular cavity and femoral neck produce results as good as those of osteotomy in more than 90% of primary operations. He believes that osteotomy is required in only about 10% of all cases where it will diminish the risk of breakage of the femoral shaft in severe osteoporotic or obese patients or when ankylosis is present. Müller has stated that the only reason he sees for osteotomy of the greater trochanter in any case is that after osteotomy it is easier to push the prosthesis down the femoral shaft into the correct valgus position, giving a better headward expansion of the cement and thus a better bond between bone and cement. The wires and screws fixing the greater trochanter also may supplement the cement fixation.

RATIONALE FOR ROUTINE TROCHANTERIC OSTEOTOMY

The rationale for routine trochanteric osteotomy may be considered within the framework of the three major areas: (1) biomechanical theory, (2) technical aspects, and (3) restoration of function.

Biomechanical theory

The biomechanical advantages of trochanteric osteotomy include:
- Reduction of socket load (wear and loosening)
- Reduction of stem load (loosening and fatigue fracture)
- Improved abductor power (excellence of gait)

Pauwels has analyzed the biomechanical principles of the moments of force on the hip joint, and Rydels practically related the load on the joint to muscular function based on analysis of the level arm systems.[3,11,13,14,16,53]

In theory, reducing the socket load may be accomplished by medial displacement of the socket or lateral displacement of the abductor mechanism (Fig. 3-12) or both. An elongation of the neck of the femoral prosthesis might have the same result, but with limited effect. A limp after total hip replacement may be a "sparing" phenomenon adopted by the patient. It may create a "disadvantageous ratio of leverage" in the hip, with excessive compensatory muscle forces

49

unnecessarily loading the implant. Loading the socket to such an extreme that the abductors do not function to their full capacity might cause future problems, even though short-term results are considered successful.

Equalization of the moments of the lever arms on the hip results in a reduction of the socket load, thus theoretically prolonging survival of the fixation. On the same theoretical basis, wear that is the function of both load and velocity can be minimized.[11,13,15] (See Chapter 3.)

Excess load on the socket may be detrimental and may cause eventual loosening of the prosthesis. This is borne out by statistical data suggesting an extremely low incidence of loosening in Charnley's low-friction arthroplasty as opposed to other types of prostheses.[3,12,15,45,46,49]

Lateral displacement of the greater trochanter is the only means of lever arm equalization when the floor of the acetabulum cannot be deepened because of anatomical restrictions. When medial displacement and the greater trochanteric transfer are both possible, it is advantageous to use the latter for equalization of the lever arms in young patients in order to avoid excessive damage to the floor of the acetabulum by deepening. Unfortunately, because of the multifactor sources of mechanical failure, the theoretical advantages outlined cannot be proved on clinical documentation alone. However, good judgment indicates the advisability of taking advantage of "all possible and theoretical" features that might be of long-term value.

Documentation of these theoretical values in regard to wear and loosening is not possible for the following reasons.

1. Unfortunately, no documentation of long-term results is available using a 22-mm. prosthetic head without detachment of the greater trochanter.

2. Degrees of deepening of the socket and lateral displacement cannot be independently evaluated in Charnley's operation.

3. Uncontrollable factors such as the patient's degree of activity and batch variations of plastics make comparison impossible.

4. Surgical technique, bone stock, bone pathology, and so on are almost never comparable in all situations.

5. No comparable data are available from total hip replacement procedures in which trochanteric osteotomy was not performed, but early clinical results are said to have been satisfactory,

nor is there any statistical data on the use of a large femoral head prosthesis without routine trochanteric osteotomy.[15]

Technical aspects

Exposure of the acetabulum. Good exposure of the acetabulum may be provided in some cases without trochanteric osteotomy. This is particularly true with a posterolateral technique (modified from Gibson) and the use of Hohmann retractors (Fig. 2-10). On the other hand, with Müller's technique, the anterior fibers of the gluteus medius often need detachment from the anterior aspect of the greater trochanter, in addition to forceful retraction of the anterior fibers necessary to expose the acetabulum. This is particularly true in large, muscular men (Fig. 2-2). As the hip becomes stiffer and severe contractures develop, anterior or posterior approaches become less satisfactory, and more force is necessary to expose the hip joint or dislocate the head.

With removal of the greater trochanter, however, a direct visualization is possible without a face-on view of the socket as if a "lid is off a tin." When the self-retaining retractors are in place and the limb is in maximum adduction with 30 to 40 degrees flexion across the opposite thigh allowing direct access to the acetabulum, its depth is better exposed and deficiencies of the rim or walls or osteophytes are revealed. Heavy retraction of the glutei in muscular or obese patients is obviated. Without trochanteric osteotomy, when unexpected difficulties are encountered, the surgeon may be forced to release the adductor tendons segment by segment from their insertions onto the femur without any formal planning for their subsequent reattachment. By removing the greater trochanter, the surgeon is formally making plans for its subsequent reattachment.

The most convenient utilization of pin retractors for exposure of the acetabulum when the trochanter is removed can be achieved by placing them intracapsularly and retracting the abductor system with its attached capsule cephalad; with the trochanter attached and the muscle intact, this is not feasible (see Chapter 12). Exposure without osteotomy is especially difficult in protrusion of the acetabulum in cases of rheumatoid disease, a sunken femoral prosthesis, or a small acetabulum. Overhanging ectopic bone or osteophytes cause difficulty in dislocation and prevent the surgeon from reaching the true depth of the acetabulum with instruments.

If the arthrotomy is done according to Charnley's technique by placing a cholecystectomy clamp inside the capsule and properly utilizing the Gigli saw, the major portion of the antero-superior, superior, and posteroinferior capsule is incised and remains with the abductor system (Fig. 12-16). In this case, no formal capsulectomy is necessary to provide exposure, and a complete capsulectomy adds to the operating time and blood loss.

Dislocation of the hip. With the greater trochanter removed, dislocation usually takes place with ease by maximum adduction of the hip following complete capsular incision at the posterior aspect. In this way the head of the femur emerges through the lateral aspect of the hip, and forceful external rotation, which often causes fracture of the femoral shaft, is avoided. Following dislocation, the shaft further displaces itself distally from the acetabular site, thus giving maximum access to the cavity (Fig. 12-27). Dislocation following osteotomy requires minimal manipulation of the shaft, a vital issue when severe osteoporosis or weakening of the femur is present as the result of a previously inserted nail and plates or a prosthesis. (See Chapter 14.) Dislocation is particularly difficult when the head of the femur has sunken into the pelvis and protrusio acetabuli is present. (See Chapter 13.)

Exposure of the stump of the upper femur. One of the most important technical aspects of total hip replacement is proper orientation of the femoral component in the femur, which must be done without perforation or damage to the upper shaft during preparation. Without release of the abductors (osteotomized trochanter), the hip cannot be fully adducted with delivery of the upper femur into the wound. It is at this point that the femoral broaches are often misdirected and perforate the shaft of the femur. The importance of valgus orientation of the stem and failure of the stem owing to varus placement cannot be overemphasized (Fig. 12-33). In order to visualize the alignment of the femur, it is often necessary to direct the tip of the prosthesis toward the center of the knee and somewhat medial to it. This is only possible when the hip can be fully adducted across the opposite thigh with the patient in the supine position (Fig. 12-34).

Reaming of the medullary canal. We emphasize the importance of removing the loose cancellous bone in the calcar region for better cement support in the valgus positioning of the prosthesis. It is best to ream the femur while it is in a full valgus position. The tapered reamers are aligned with the center of the knee joint but in valgus inclination. This obviously cannot be done without damage to the abductor muscles if one aims the reamer at the femur's medial cortex when entering the opening at the top. In fact, much cancellous bone must be removed from inside the trochanter cut surface and the entire top of the neck of the femur has to be gouged out to the trochanteric level in order to provide entrance in a valgus orientation (Fig. 12-33). With the trochanter and the abductors undetached, valgus alignment is impeded by the muscular mass. Slow insertion of the femoral component accompanied by repeated ramming of the cement into the medial zone between the bone of the calcar and prosthesis can be best facilitated following removal of the greater trochanter.

Insertion of cement into the upper femur. For cement insertion, the limb should be in maximum adduction and the knee supported by the second assistant, since only with a direct line of access to the femur can pressure be exerted onto the cement mass (Fig. 12-42). Injection of cement into the endosteal bone is possible only with forceful thumb pressure (double thumb pressure technique). The T-shaped top of the femur following removal of the trochanter permits access to use this technique (Fig. 12-33). A delicate and uncontrolled "stuffing" of the cement causes lamellation and blood admixture when the exposure and access to the top of the femur are restricted.

Ability to mobilize the upper femur. Following detachment of the greater trochanter, as the extremity is adducted, the contracted anterior and posterior capsule can be removed (in cases with long-standing fixed deformity or heterotopic bone formation in the medial aspect of the femur). At times, because of previous operations, the upper femur must be detached from the wall of the pelvis in order to provide space between the upper end of the femur and the pelvic wall. This is especially needed in mobilizing an ankylosed or arthrodesed hip, which can safely be accomplished by this maneuver (Fig. 14-2). Similarly, in cases of "upriding" femur (interrupted

Shenton's line on x-ray film) or pseudarthrosis, a complete mobilization provides length and space, which otherwise would have to be compensated for by shortening the neck of the femur. Nowhere is the need for mobilization of the upper femur better exemplified than in the case of a frankly congenital dislocation of the hip in which the medial upper femur is bound tightly against the wall of the pelvis, requiring resection of the soft tissue in order to lower the level of the hip joint (Fig. 13-5). In this way, often as a benefit of the maneuver, considerable length is obtained.

Removal of a previous prosthesis. An intramedullary femoral head prosthesis (cemented or noncemented) requires removal prior to replacement. In revising a total hip arthroplasty, its removal is routinely required, regardless of the presence or absence of loosening in the femoral portion. Following osteotomy of the greater trochanter, it is possible to enter the curve of the upper portion of the prosthesis and gain access to the stem or the bones of fenestration of the Moore self-locking prosthesis. An attempt to remove the prosthesis without removing the trochanter may lead to fracture of the femur. After osteotomy, the bed of the trochanter is the logical site to enter, using a reciprocating saw (Fig. 14-8). A complete mobilization of the upper femur facilitates direct access to the medial aspect of the prosthesis, which allows placement of the chisel over the medial neck of the prosthesis for extraction (Fig. 14-9).

Preservation of the capsule of the hip joint. A complete capsulectomy is an additional surgical maneuver involving increased blood loss and time waste. In low-friction arthroplasty experiences, relief from pain has not been correlated with the extent of capsular removal, and since the capsule also is an important stabilizing element, it normally should not be sacrificed unless mobilization of the femur by extensive release is needed to compensate for deformity. Its preservation may also be necessary for stability following replacement surgery. With a lateral approach, it is possible to preserve the inferior part of the capsule as well as the anterior portion. The anterior capsule with its reinforcing Y-shaped ligament prevents anterior dislocation by external rotation during the immediate postoperative course. The test of stability of the hip as related to the capsule may be appreciated when an attempt at dislocation is made prior to

reattachment of the greater trochanter. Often considerable force is necessary to pull the two components apart when both the anterior and inferior capsule have been preserved. Preservation further prevents inadvertent excessive elongation of the neck of the femur and resultant lengthening of the extremity.

Resection of ectopic bone. When heterotopic bone formation leads to ankylosis and its removal is indicated (see Chapter 16), the transtrochanteric approach is invaluable. Complete access to the front and back of the joint, as well as the region of adductors, without excess trauma to the abductor muscles is achieved by this route (Fig. 16-23). After detachment of the trochanter and removal of the femoral component, complete access to the back of the femur and the joint is possible without damage to the sciatic nerve. In most cases revision of the femoral component is necessary because its removal facilitates access to the area of heterotopic bone.

Safety of glutei and nerve to tensor fascia femoris. As stated previously, damage to the abductor system is often unavoidable when these muscles are well developed and the anterior segment is considerably hypertrophied. Paradoxically, very athletic men with a well-developed abductor system are more prone to injury of their hypertrophied muscles than are frail, elderly patients. With the anterior approach, heavy retraction (despite partial release of the abductor tendon from the trochanter) may be necessary for visualization of the acetabulum and may damage the anterior fibers of the glutei. At times, the nerve supply to the tensor fascia femoris may also be in jeopardy. Since it is an important abductor muscle and an important stabilizing element, damage to its nerve supply must be avoided. Further, considerable muscle damage may be incurred when lever-type retractors are applied to expose the acetabulum.

Charnley has advocated removal of the greater trochanter with a broad strap of lateral capsule, performed by passing a Gigli saw through the joint to detach the trochanter. Then when the greater trochanter is advanced, appropriate tension is applied to the superior capsule to provide stability for the hip joint. He has emphasized this technique because excessive advancement of the abductor mechanism is needless and may even endanger the function of the muscle. Undoubtedly, good results can be achieved despite damage to the tensor fascia femoris muscle or its nerve. (This is demonstrated in male patients by palpation of this muscle.) However, the burden of this muscle's function must subsequently be placed on the gluteal system (gluteus medius and minimus). The opposite experience to the preceding is the hypertrophied tensor (contracted iliotibial tract) from paralysis of the gluteus medius seen in poliomyelitis as occurs in postpolio paralysis. The most gentle way of retracting the gluteus medius is by removal of the greater trochanter with the lateral capsule to expose the joint (see Chapter 12) and placement of a retractor along the supporting capsule. This will preserve the muscle fibers and protect the nerve to the fascia femoris at the interval between this muscle and the gluteus medius. From clinical observation it is not clear how much of this muscle can be damaged irreparably without interfering with satisfactory function, but routine detachment of the greater trochanter will ensure safety of the abductor mechanism.

Stability of the hip and muscle tension. When the greater trochanter is preserved and a complete capsulectomy is performed, the neck may be overly lengthened, with excessive stretch imposed on certain groups of hip muscles. On the other hand, in a severely deformed hip following the resection of a contracted capsule, adequate balance of the abductor group against the flexors, adductors, and extensors might not be accomplished. For example, when the adduction deformity is corrected and the extremity assumes abduction, the abductor system may be excessively lax. By removing the greater trochanter and capsular strut after the extremity is placed in optimal abduction on the operating table, the greater trochanter assumes its appropriate position and can then be fixed onto the lateral aspect of the shaft. It is also important to note that following medial displacement of the central rotation of the hip by deepening of the socket, additional laxity of the abductor mechanism is produced, which can be retightened at the distal attachment of the abductors (Fig. 14-5). It may be argued that a prosthesis with extra neck length will provide the same effect, but this will place excessive bending stress on the femoral component and may induce fracture of the stem or loosening of the cement in the shaft. Further, using an extra neck length prosthesis for elongation entails unnecessary lengthening of the extremity. Therefore a balance must be made

between the leg length and the muscle tension about the hip.

Resistance against dislocation. A stable hip is guaranteed by using the preoperative radiographical template, accurate placement of the level of the socket, correct level of osteotomy of the neck, avoidance of stretching or tearing of the inferoanterior capsule, and retaining the capsular strut following reattachment of the greater trochanter. The low incidence of dislocation following Charnley's low-friction arthroplasty constitutes impressive statistical data to this end (see Chapter 17). This lateral approach allows good assessment of the level of the socket at insertion. Transfer of the trochanter further augments the stability of the hip. While it is quite possible to provide stability in most cases without severe deformity, it cannot always be achieved in hips with severe deformity or scarified tissue from previous surgery. It is in these cases that stability can be augmented by distal transfer of the greater trochanter. (See Chapter 14.)

Correction of fixed deformity. Severe fixed deformity of the hip requires special attention during total hip replacement. Good exposure is difficult, and the contracted capsule and muscles require additional release. Direct visualization of the short external rotators (for example, piriformis, obturator internus, gemelli, and obturator externus) will be facilitated by removal of the greater trochanter, particularly needed when a strong fixed flexion deformity is present. This can be accomplished safely without risking damage to the sciatic nerve, which is a real danger in the anterior approach without removal of the trochanter. With complete access to the upper end of the femur the following structures may be released as necessary: iliopsoas, rectus femoris, vastus lateralis, and all short rotators. It can be projected that improved function of the abductor system and hip reduction helps in converting a positive Trendelenburg's test to a negative one and prevents recurrence of fixed adduction deformity.

Failed previous surgery. There is universal agreement (even among surgeons who prefer not to remove the greater trochanter) that trochanteric osteotomy should be done in cases of failed previous surgery or an anatomically distorted hip for which complete exposure and mobilization are required. Included in this group are "upriding" pseudarthrosis, failed osteotomy, failed femoral prosthesis with proximal and distal migration, and malformations secondary to previous total hip replacements (see Chapter 14). It is mandatory to remove the trochanter in attempts to revise a cemented femoral stem by rechannelization.

Restoration of function

As stated previously, a severely deformed hip can only be restructured with complete mobilization of the upper femur. In this way the hip joint is mechanically improved, aiming at full functional activity with an intact abductor mechanism (including the gluteus medius and minimus and the tensor fascia femoris). The fascial and muscular structure of the thigh can be compared to a sleeve that incorporates the iliotibial tract as well as muscular septa of the thigh. Although these structures are somewhat inelastic beyond a given point of traction, nevertheless they function only when the length of the musculature has been placed with the appropriate tension and orientation. Therefore the degrees of advancement of the trochanter may be varied according to the demands in each technical situation. For example, the capsule and abductor muscles are heavily contracted in a high-riding nonunion of the neck of the femur with marked displacement or a failed pseudarthrosis. If the trochanter is not removed in cases of severe deformity, it is impossible to restore the good general alignment necessary for functional abductors.

A good example of the need for reorientation is a case of severe osteoarthritis of the hip with hyperproductive osteoarthrosis and fixed flexion, adduction, and external rotation deformity (Fig. 13-35). In this situation the head and the acetabulum may be eroded superiorly and the hip subluxed outwardly. As a general rule, the greater trochanter is rotated externally and its posterior border is almost at the posterior lip of the acetabulum, with the gluteus medius and minimus in a disadvantageous position for their function as abductors. When the abductor function is impaired in this way (usually accompanied by contracted adductors and external rotators) without correction of existing deformities, the mechanical disadvantage of the abductor-adductor ratio balances and the function of the abductors remains impaired. Therefore it does not suffice to resurface the joint without removing the mechanical impairment of the hip joint

mechanism. Neither factor (deepening of the acetabulum nor lateral displacement of the greater trochanter) might appear substantial on the radiographs, but a combination of the two may result in a substantial improvement (see Chapter 3). This may reduce the demand on a long-standing weakened and atrophied abductor muscle. In experiences with cup arthroplasty, Johnston and Larson[33] found that shifting the central rotation of the hip medially and the greater trochanter laterally proportionally increased the frequency of negative Trendelenburg's tests. If these principles are applied to total hip replacement, a more accurate term would be "total hip reconstructive arthroplasty." In summary, on the basis of the foregoing, the removal of the trochanter in performing total hip replacement is not purely the surgeon's option. It is an essential and intricate part of the procedure to ensure short- and long-term success of total hip arthroplasty. For a statistical analysis of greater trochanteric complications see Chapter 17.

SUMMARY OF ESSENTIALS

- Full knowledge of all alternative surgical approaches to the hip and evaluation of the advantages and pitfalls of each equip the surgeon to choose the most suitable approach for total hip replacement.
- The best approach for any extensive surgery, including total hip replacement, is one that provides maximum exposure with minimum soft tissue damage. The positioning of the patient at surgery is an intricate part of surgical exposure; the position must allow optimum orientation for insertion of the cement and the prosthesis.
- Of the many surgical approaches described in the past, the anterolateral, lateral, and posterolateral approaches are most suitable for performing total hip replacement. The anterior, posterior, and medial approaches to the hip provide inadequate exposure of the upper femur and the acetabulum for this surgery.
- The anterolateral approach (without trochanteric osteotomy, that is, Watson-Jones exposure of the hip as used by McKee and Müller) and the posterolateral approach (modification of Gibson's approach without removal of the greater trochanter) both may provide adequate exposure of the acetabulum in a hip with no deformity and a good range of motion. However, access to the upper femur is somewhat limited, and its preparation and the insertion of cement are difficult to accomplish. Orientation of the femoral stem prosthesis may be in jeopardy when these approaches are used. With

severe anatomical distortion (for example, fixed adduction and flexion deformity) or in revision of failed previous operations, these approaches are inadequate and fraught with increased morbidity and risk of damage to the abductor muscles and nerves to the tensor fascia femoris.

- The transtrochanteric approach provides extensive exposure and protects the anatomical integrity of the hip structures. This approach provides access to the front and back of the hip joint, including the greater trochanter, and requires no muscle release other than removal of the abductors. This approach is considered physiologically sound when the greater trochanter is subsequently firmly reattached to the lateral aspect of the femoral shaft. It spares heavy retraction of the abductor muscles (therefore especially suitable for muscular individuals) and allows good exposure and access to the top end of the femur for proper insertion of the cement and orientation of the prosthesis.

- Included in the many advantages of a transtrochanteric approach to the hip are a wide and extensive exposure, protection of anatomical structures, correction of fixed deformities, ease of dislocation at operation, ease of preparation of the acetabulum, ease of insertion of components, improved cement fixation technique, improved stability following surgery, and above all, improved quality of the long-term clinical results.

- There are several theoretical and practical criticisms of the transtrochanteric approach. They include increased operating time, handling of the trochanter at surgery, delayed weight bearing postoperatively, increased blood loss, trochanteric bursitis, trochanteric nonunion, and breakage of wire and proximal migration of the trochanter. These criticisms are valid for the surgeon who is not fully acquainted with problems of the trochanter and who uses this approach only occasionally in his surgical experience. Choice of a surgical approach must be made within the context of total hip reconstructive arthroplasty (as opposed to simple replacement of the articular surfaces). Therefore the surgical approach must provide the opportunity to remove all deformity and balance the forces about the hip following reconstruction. Long-term success of arthroplasty depends entirely on excellence of surgical technique, and a good surgical exposure paves the way for good technique. Together they constitute an essential and intricate procedure, parallel in importance with the selection of patients and the choice of prosthesis.

REFERENCES

1. Acton, R. K.: Surgical approaches to the hip. In Tronzo, R. G., editor: Surgery of the hip joint, Philadelphia, 1973, Lea & Febiger, pp. 79-103.
2. Amstutz, H. E.: Complication for hip replacement, Clin. Orthop. **72:**123-137, 1970.
3. Andersson, G. B., Freeman, M. A. R., and Swanson, S. A. V.: Loosening of the cemented acetabular cup in total hip replacement, J. Bone Joint Surg. **54B:**590-599, 1972.
4. Aufranc, O. E.: Constructive surgery of the hip, St. Louis, 1962, The C. V. Mosby Co.
5. Bankes, S. W., and Laufman, H.: An atlas of surgical exposures of the extremities, Philadelphia, 1968, W. B. Saunders Co.
6. Bost, F. C., Schottstadet, E. R., and Larsen, L. J.: Surgical approaches to the hip joint. In American Academy of Orthopaedic Surgeons: Instructional course lectures, vol. 11, Ann Arbor, 1954, J. W. Edwards.
7. Brackett, E. G.: Study of the different approaches to the hip joint, Bost. Med. Surg. J. **CLXVI:**235-242, 1912.
8. Brady, L. P.: Lateral oblique incision for the Charnley low-friction arthroplasty, Clin. Orthop. **118:**7-9, 1976.
9. Burwell, H., and Scott, D.: A lateral intramuscular approach to the hip joint, J. Bone Joint Surg. **36B:**104-108, 1954.
10. Caldwell, J. A.: Subtrochanteric fractures of the femur, Am. J. Surg. **59:**370-382, 1943.
11. Charnley, J. C.: Comparison of dynamic frictional torque in different total hip implants by a pendulum method, Internal Publication No. 35, Centre for Hip Surgery, Wrightington Hospital, England.
12. Charnley, J. C.: Total hip replacement by low friction arthroplasty, Clin. Orthop. **72:**7-21, 1970.
13. Charnley, J. C.: Comparison of the lever systems in the low-friction arthroplasty and the McKee-Farrar arthroplasty. Internal Publications, Centre for Hip Surgery, Wrightington Hospital, England, September, 1971.
14. Charnley, J. C.: The rationale of low friction arthroplasty. In The Hip Society: The Hip, Proceedings of the first open scientific meeting of The Hip Society, St. Louis, 1973, The C. V. Mosby Co., pp. 92-100.
15. Charnley, J. C., and Cupic, Z.: The nine and ten year results of the low-friction arthroplasty of the hip, Clin. Orthop. **95:**9-25, 1973.
16. Charnley, J. C., and Ferreira, A.: Transplantation of the greater trochanter in arthroplasty of the hip, J. Bone Joint Surg. **46B:**191-197, 1964.
17. Colonna, P. C.: The trochanteric reconstruction operation for ununited fractures of the upper end of the femur, J. Bone Joint Surg. **42B:**5-10, 1960.
18. Crenshaw, A. M.: Campbell's operative orthopaedics, ed. 4, St. Louis, 1963, The C. V. Mosby Co.
19. Eftekhar, N. S.: Status of femoral head replacement, Part I, Orthop. Rev. **2:**19-23, 1973.

20. Eftekhar, N. S.: Status of femoral head replacement, Part II, Orthop. Rev. **2:**23-30, 1973.
21. Etienne, E., LaPeyrie, M., and Campo, A.: The route of internal access to the hip joint, Int. Abst. Surg. **84:**275, 1947.
22. Evanski, P. M., Waugh, T. R., and Orofino, C. F.: Total hip replacement with the Charnley prosthesis, Clin. Orthop. **95:**69-72, 1973.
23. Evarts, C. M., et al.: Total hip joint arthroplasty, J. Bone Joint Surg. **54A:**1562, 1972.
24. Fahey, J. J.: Surgical Approaches to bones and joints, Surg. Clin. North Am. **29:**65-76, 1949.
25. Gibson, A.: Vitalium-cup arthroplasty of the hip joint, J. Bone Joint Surg. **31A:**861-868, 1949.
26. Gibson, A.: Posterior exposure of the hip joint, J. Bone Joint Surg. **32B:**183-186, 1950.
27. Gibson, A.: The Posterolateral approach to the hip joint. In American Academy of Orthopaedic Surgeons Instructional course lectures, vol. 10, Ann Arbor, 1953, J. W. Edwards.
28. Harris, W. J.: A new lateral approach to the hip joint, J. Bone Joint Surg. **49A:**891-898, 1967.
29. Harris, W. H.: Extensive exposure of the hip joint, Clin. Orthop. **91:**58-62, 1973.
30. Henry, A. K.: Extensile exposure, Edinburgh, 1960, E. & S. Livingstone.
31. Horowitz, T.: The lateral approach in the surgical management of the basilar neck, intertrochanteric and subtrochanteric fractures of the femur, Surg. Gynecol. Obstet. **95:**40, 1952.
32. Jergenson, F., and Abbott, L. C.: A comprehensive exposure of the hip joint, J. Bone Joint Surg. **36A:**798-808, 1955.
33. Johnston, R. C., and Larson, C. B.: Biomechanics of cup arthroplasty, Clin. Orthop. **66:**56-69, 1969.
34. Lazansky, M. G.: Complications in total hip replacement with the Charnley technic, Clin. Orthop. **72:**40-45, 1970.
35. Lazansky, M. G.: Total replacement arthroplasty of the hip: the Charnley low friction technique, J. Bone Joint Surg. **52A:**834, 1970.
36. Lazansky, M. G.: Trochanteric osteotomy in total hip replacement. In The Hip Society: The Hip, Proceedings of the second open scientific meeting of The Hip Society, St. Louis, 1974, The C. V. Mosby Co., pp. 237-247.
37. Luck, J. V.: A transverse anterior approach to the hip, J. Bone Joint Surg. **37A:**534-536, 1955.
38. Ludloff, K.: The open reduction of the congenital hip dislocation and anterior incision, Am. J. Orthop. Surg. **10:**438-454, 1913.
39. McFarland, B., and Osborne, G.: Approach to the hip, J. Bone Joint Surg. **36B:**364-367, 1954.
40. McKee, G. K.: Development of total prosthetic replacement of the hip, Clin. Orthop. **72:**85-103, 1970.
41. McKee, G. K., and Watson-Farrar, J.: Replacement of arthritic hips by the McKee-Farrar prosthesis, J. Bone Joint Surg. **48B:**245-259, 1966.
42. Marcy, G. H., and Fletcher, R. S.: Modification of the posterolateral approach to the hip for insertion of femoral head prosthesis, J. Bone Joint Surg. **36A:**142-143, 1954.
43. Moore, A. T.: The Moore self-locking Vitallium prosthesis in fresh femoral neck fractures. In American Academy of Orthopaedic Surgeons Instructional course lectures, vol. 16, St. Louis, 1959, The C. V. Mosby Co.
44. Moore, A. T.: The self-locking metal hip prosthesis, J. Bone Joint Surg. **39A:**811-827, 1957.
45. Morris, J. B.: The McKee-Farrar and Charnley total hip replacement arthroplasty, J. Bone Joint Surg. **50B:**680, 1968.
46. Morris, J. B., and Nicholson, O. R.: Total prosthetic replacement of the hip joint, Clin. Orthop. **72:**33-35, 1970.
47. Müller, M. E.: Total hip prostheses, Clin. Orthop. **72:**46-68, 1970.
48. Müller, M. E.: Osteotomy of the greater trochanter, total hip replacement without trochanteric osteotomy. In The Hip Society: The Hip, Proceedings of the second open scientific meeting of The Hip Society, St. Louis, 1974, The C. V. Mosby Co., pp. 231-237.
49. Nicholson, O. R.: Total hip replacement: an evaluation of the results and technics, Clin. Orthop. **95:**217-223, 1973.
50. Ober, F. R.: Posterior arthrotomy of the hip joint, J.A.M.A. **83:**1500-1502, 1924.
51. Osborne, R. P.: The approach to the hip joint; a critical review and suggested new route, Br. J. Surg. **18:**49-52, 1930.
52. Parker, H. G., et al.: Comparison of immediate and later results of total hip replacements with and without trochanteric osteotomy. Paper presented at American Orthopaedic Association Meeting, San Francisco, June, 1974.
53. Rydell, N. W.: Forces acting on the femoral-head prosthesis: a study on strain gauge supplied prostheses in living persons, Acta Orthop. Scand. [37:Suppl.] **88:**1-132, 1966.
54. Sledge, C. B.: Discussion controversey in total hip replacement, osteotomy of the greater trochanter. In The Hip Society: The Hip, Proceedings of the second scientific meeting of The Hip Society, St. Louis, 1974, The C. V. Mosby Co., pp. 247-250.
55. Smith-Petersen, M. N.: Treatment of malum coxae senalis, old slipped upper femoral epiphysis, intrapelvic protrusion of the acetabulum, and coxa plana by means of acetabuloplasty, J. Bone Joint Surg. **18:**869-880, 1936.
56. Smith-Petersen, M. N.: Approach to and exposure of the hip joint for mold arthroplasty, J. Bone Joint Surg. **31A:**40-46, 1949.

57. Stinchfield, F. E., Henry, H., Eftekhar, N. S., and White, E. S.: Total hip replacement. In Ahstrom, J. P., Jr., editor: Current practice in orthopaedic surgery, vol. 5, St. Louis, 1973, The C. V. Mosby Co., pp. 135-157.

58. Sutherland, R., and Rowe, M. J., Jr.: Simplified surgical approach to the hip, Arch. Surg. **48:** 144-145, 1944.

59. Thompson, R. C., and Culver, J. E.: The role of trochanteric osteotomy in total hip replacement, Clin. Orthop. **106:**102-106, 1975.

60. Volz, R. G., and Mayer, D. M.: The predictive factors necessitating trochanteric osteotomy in total hip replacement, Orthop. Rev. **5:**23-25, 1976.

61. vonLangenbeck, B.: Vorstellung cines Falles von geheilter Enterotomie, Verhandl. d. Deutsch. Gesellsch. f. Chir. **7:**40-46, 1878.

62. Watson-Jones, R.: Fractures of the neck of the femur, Br. J. Surg. **23:**787-808, 1936.

CHAPTER 3

Biomechanics and biomaterials

"Don't throw away the cane."
WALTER P. BLOUNT

In this chapter the interrelationship of materials and mechanical aspects of the artificial hip joint will be discussed, covering the following areas: biomaterials and compatibility; forces about the hip; frictional force; fixation elements and methods; design of reconstruction (operation); prosthesis design features; wear, friction, and lubrication; and mode of failure of total hip prosthesis.

Concepts concerning biomaterials and biomechanics for artificial hip joints are rapidly changing. New developments are based on investigations in biomechanical laboratories and the correlation of these findings with clinical problems as long-term results of hip replacement operations become available. Work is in progress in many areas, but, even now, some years will elapse before laboratory investigation of a specific situation can be verified by observations in clinical practice.

Orthopaedic surgeons are concerned with treatment of areas of the body (after prosthetic structures are applied) that are in continuous movement. Unlike stationary devices that are used in fracture fixation, these devices are expected to perform a mechanical function of life-long duration by transmission of load and translation of motion.

Structures and mechanical functions are usually constructed to serve for a specific length of time, termed the "design life" by engineers. It is possible as an engineering exercise to calculate the magnitude of stresses (applied loads and mechanical properties of materials) and to conceptualize a design with expected behavior. However, it is not realistic to apply such a model to human function and the body environment expecting behavior comparable to calculated laboratory performances. On this premise, laboratory work has its limitations and can only be used as a guide or for verification of some aspects of clinical application.

In a young patient the magnitude of forces generated in the hip joint from various activities is incredibly difficult to estimate. Examples of extreme conditions are: contact sports, jumping, and running. The average load applied to the head of the femur in the stance phase of normal walking (heel strike of a 77-kg. person walking 0.9 m./sec.) may be around 100 kg./force. In walking 1 mile the dynamic intermittent load may increase to as much as four or five times the body weight. If the hip is loaded about 1,000 times, in the course of 1 year the bearing may be loaded as many as 1 to 2.5 million times. If we consider that the total hip joint may be required to perform for 50 years, this obviously surpasses most limits of engineering "design life"*—even barring the hostile environment of the body and the unusual physical demands made (that is, athletic performances). To produce such a prosthesis will be the greatest orthopaedic and engineering challenge in development yet to be faced by the surgeon and engineer.

BIOMATERIALS AND COMPATIBILITY

From earliest times, surgeons have tried to replace missing or deformed parts of the body. Crutches were among the early ameliorative attempts used by the most primitive men, and as technology grew, more sophisticated appliances were developed. A golden nose is said to have been worn by Tycho Brahe (400 years ago) to hide a cavity he had acquired in a tavern fight!

Efforts to replace tissues in the body were reported throughout early literature with occasional accounts of successful results, principally with metals. Early appliances—such as gold skull plates and segments of bone—have been documented, but it was not until this century that metallurgists developed alloys that were sufficiently mechanically stable and chemically

---

*Under ideal lubricating conditions some ball bearings may last 10^9 to 10^{10} cycles.

inert to be used for dependable insertion. After more than half a century of development, the orthopaedic surgeon is now able to use metal safely and predictably for repair and replacement surgery.

Because the development of implantable polymers (plastics) is relatively recent, the issue of their complete prosthetic acceptability has not been fully resolved. Some of these plastics have remained implanted in thousands of humans for as long as 20 years and have been well tolerated, but the question of long-term reactivity to them remains unanswered. Questions surrounding short-term results, applicability of animal test results to humans, and future degradation of plastics after 30 or 40 years are all facets of the larger issue that concerns the orthopaedic surgeon. Even though it has been suggested that the average cell life span in man and the rat are comparable, there are other factors present that do not allow exclusion of the idea that these materials may become harmful to the body over an extended period of time.

Electrolytic action in the body usually makes the use of dissimilar metals (alloys) for the two surfaces of a joint impossible; one exception is chromium and cobalt alloys, which have been used in combination for a total hip prosthesis (McKee-Farrar total hip prosthesis). In order that a metal-against-metal prosthesis withstand incumbent stresses (such as in the hip joint), it must have a large diameter head to permit flow of a lubricating film of fluid between the mating parts.

A simple ball-and-socket bearing (metal against plastic) exposed to tissue fluid is most effective, provided that (1) the plastic is wear resistant and (2) any particulate matter released as the result of wear will not cause tissue reaction in the body. Since the latter presents the most serious problems, the design and choice of materials should be aimed toward inertness of the wear by-product and tissue tolerance. In vivo research should be directed toward the selection of biocompatible materials for the bearing joints. Employing any new materials clinically must be done judiciously. For example, in experiences with Teflon (PTFE) for socket material, the procedure was limited to individuals with extreme disability for whom there was no alternate method of treatment at that time (prior to 1962). (Teflon already had a good reputation for its inertness in the body.)

The total joint prosthesis is a complex engineering product; it must be problem free to perform a "lifetime service" without failure. The material should be adequately fatigue resistant in order to withstand weight-bearing stresses. Wear must be minimal, and the level of frictional resistance reduced to a minimum in order to protect the fixation (bond) from excess stress. It should also withstand corrosion and degradation in the hostile environment of the body; further, the weight-bearing element must be capable of attenuating the forces (absorb energy), be compliant, and above all, must have local and remote biological compatibility. Only then can we safely apply it to young patients without future concern.

Metals as bearing materials

Metals used in the body may fail from breakage or corrosion. Attempts to identify problems related to new metals used in orthopaedic surgery have led to a body of knowledge and standards that will continuously be revised on the basis of new studies and findings.* Metals commonly used for bearings include: stainless steel, chromium-cobalt-molybdenum, and titanium alloy.

Stainless steel

Impurities in stainless steel prostheses may initiate corrosion leading to failure of the implant; they can act as stress concentrators and, along with corrosion, may result in fatigue fracture.[74] Two often found inclusions are magnesium sulfide and chromium oxide. A standard composition for stainless steel used in surgical implants taken from ASTM standard specifications X138 and F139 is shown in Tables 3-1 and 3-2.[46,104] In the United States these standards are set by the F4 Committee on Surgical Implants. The steel used in the United States by manufacturers of implants is known as AISI-316L. A similar steel, known as EN58J, is used in England; this steel is susceptible to galvanic corrosions, especially in environments such as salt solutions. (See p. 63, "Fatigue Failure of Metal.") (See Tables 3-1 to 3-3.)

Chromium alloys

Just as iron can be made into alloys of steel, cobalt can be made into alloys that will resist corrosion and improve its physical properties.

*See references 37, 38, 68, 74, 92, 102, 109, and 122.

Table 3-1. Mechanical properties of metallic alloys (ASTM)*

Properties	Stainless steel ASTM F55, F56 Wrought	Co-Cr ASTM F75 Cast	Co-Cr ASTM F90 Wrought
Hardness	RB 85-95	Rc 25-34	RB98
Hardness (cold work)	Rc 30	—	Rc65
Ultimate tensile strength	80,000 p.s.i.	95-105,000	130,000
Ultimate tensile strength (cold work)	140,000	—	250,000
0.2% (yield strength)	35,000	65,000	55,000
0.2% (cold work)	115,000	—	190,000
Max strain	55%	8%	50%
Max strain (cold work)	22%	—	10%
Modulus: E	29×10^6 p.s.i.	36×10^6	35×10^6

Properties	Stainless steel ASTM A296 Cast	Titanium (pure) ASTM F67 Cast/wrought	Titanium 6A1-4V alloy ASTM F136 Cast/Wrought
Hardness	RB70-85	RB100	Depends on surface treatment
Ultimate tensile strength	70,000 p.s.i.	90,000	125-130,000
0.2% yield strength	30,000 p.s.i.	80,000	115-120,000
Max strain	30%	18%	10%
Modulus: E	28×10^6	15×10^6	16×10^6

*ASTM = American Society For Testing and Materials.
From Dumbleton, J. H., and Black, J.: An introduction to orthopedic materials, Springfield, Ill., 1975, Charles C Thomas, Publishers.

(See Tables 3-1 to 3-3, ASTM standard composition and mechanical properties for cast cobalt[46,104]-chromium-molybdenum [Co-Cr-Mo] alloy for surgical implants.) This alloy is commonly used as cast material (Austenal Laboratories).* Tissue reaction to long-term implantation of chromium-cobalt-molybdenum (Co-Cr-Mo) is minimal, although it does occur.[37,38] Microscopically, the tissue around the implants is generally free of excessive fibrous tissue, and the cellular reaction is usually slightly less than that which is seen around stainless steel implants. Small black particles have been observed in the phagocytes near chromium-cobalt-molybdenum (Co-Cr-Mo) implants, and spectral chemical analysis of adjacent tissue in both animals and plants has revealed ions of all three metals.[74]

Titanium alloys

Titanium (Ti-6Al-4Va) alloys have been used in orthopaedic surgery for cup arthroplasty prosthesis, plate and screws, and other hardware. (Tables 3-1 to 3-3 show a standard composition for titanium.[46,104]) It has been suggested that the tissue reaction to titanium is minimal in the absence of wear; when wear occurs, rapid oxida-

*Vitallium is a trademark of Homedica, Inc., Rutherford, N.J.

tion of the particles may be expected with the formation of highly stable titanium salts. Spectral chemical analyses of tissue adjacent to implants have always demonstrated the presence of titanium in the tissues, even without severe tissue reaction.[74]

Tissue reaction to implants

Biological compatibility is a *conditio sine qua non* for any material to be developed or used for prosthetic devices. According to Clarke, a "bland" or biologically inert material is one "which does not destroy the vitality of adjoining tissues, which provokes no inflammatory response beyond that occasioned by the trauma accompanying the insertion and by its presence as a physical and nonvital structure, and which does not impede the process of fibrous or osteogenic repair."[36] In addition to its chemical makeup, the physical form of the material may determine the "tissue response" that must also be considered.[95,102,103] Teflon is a classic example in this regard; it causes no reaction when used in bulk in the body (that is, sheet form), but considerable tissue reaction is usually engendered by small particles. In experimental conditions most plastics will produce tumors in rats (also true

Table 3-2. Comparison of mechanical properties of materials used in total hip replacement in clinical and experimental work

Material	Type and condition	Ultimate tensile strength MN/m.²	Tensile yield stress MN/m.²	Young's modulus GN/m.²	Elongation at fracture (%)	Compressive strength MN/m.²	Vickers hardness MN/m.²	Fatigue strength (10^8 cycles) MN/m.²
Stainless steel	316, 316L annealed	520-620	250-330	200	75-36		1,400-1,800	245-300
Cobalt–chromium alloy	Cast	650-750	440-570	200	8		3,000-4,000	235-275
Titanium, pure	Annealed	550-620	480-510	100	15-20		2,400	250-280
Stainless steel	316, 316L cold worked	1,000-1,500	770-1,370	200	8		3,200	300
Cobalt–chromium alloy	'Wrought' cold worked	1,000-1,700	500-1,300	230	9		4,500	480
Cobalt–nickel alloy	MP 35 N hot-forged	850-1,200	650-1,000	230	35-55		3,000-4,000	540-600
Titanium alloy	6 A1, 4V annealed	930	825	100	10-15		3,500	400-440
Aluminium oxide ceramic	Al_2O_3	270	—	350	0	4,000	20,000	NA
Polyethylene	High molecular weight, RCH 1,000	43	22	0.5	450	20		NA
Polyamide	Nylon 66	85	NA	3	40-80	NA		NA
Polyacetal	Delrin	70	NA	3	75	NA		NA
Polyester	Polyethylene tere-phthalate	80	NA	NA	100-300	NA		NA
Polymethyl methacrylate	Bone cement	25	NA	2	5	80		<14
Cortical bone		80-160	NA	20	1-3	130-280	200-300	30

Vickers hardness is measured using a pyramidal indenter. The results have the dimensions of stress and are usually expressed as kilograms force per square millimetre but are here expressed as meganewtons per square metre for ease of comparison with the other properties. (Expressed in kgf./mm.², the numerical values would be approximately one tenth of those in the Table.)

Strengths and stresses are given in meganewtons per square metre (that is, 10^6 newtons per square metre), abbreviated to MN/m.².

Young's modulus has the dimensions of stress and is given in giganewtons per square metre (that is, 10^9 newtons per square metre), abbreviated to GN/m.².

The compressive strengths of metals and alloys are not given because they are not usually measured separately, being roughly equal to the respective ultimate tensile strengths.

The tensile yield stress of aluminium oxide ceramic is not given because this is a brittle material and does not yield.

'NA' in a space means that information is not available.

The hardnesses of plastics are not readily measured by indentation methods; the values obtained by the methods which are used are equivalent to values in the range 50-200 MN/m.².

The properties given in this Table, and throughout the book, are expressed in units of the Système International (SI). The following are the units chiefly used.

Mass: the kilogram (kg.), equal to 1,000 grams or 2.2 pounds.
Force: the newton (N), equal to 0.225 pounds force.
Length: the metre (m.), equal to 39.36 inches.
the millimetre (mm.), 10^{-3} metre.
the micrometre (μm.), 10^{-6} metre, equal to 39.36 microinches.
Stress: newtons per square metre (N/m.²) or, more usually, 10^6 newtons per square metre (meganewtons per square metre, MN/m.²).

From Swanson, S. A. V., and Freeman, M. A. R., editors: The scientific basis of joint replacement, New York, 1977, John Wiley & Sons, Inc.

Table 3-3. Standard compositions of surgical implant alloys

Composition (weight %)	Stainless steel ASTM F55 or F56 Wrought	Co-Cr ASTM F75 Cast	Co-Cr ASTM F90 (Vitallium) Wrought
Tungston	—	—	14-16
Cobalt	—	Bal (57.4-65)	Bal (46-53)
Chromium	17-20	27-30	19-21
Nickel	10-17	2.5 max	9-11
Molybdenum	2-4	5-7	—
Iron	Bal (59-70)	0.75 max	3.0 max
Carbon	0.03 max	0.35 max	0.05-0.15
Manganese	2.00 max	1.0 max	2.0 max
Phosphorus	0.03 max	—	—
Sulfur	0.03 max	—	—
Silicon	0.75 max	1.00 max	1.00 max

Composition (weight %)	Stainless steel ASTM A296 Cast	Titanium (pure) ASTM F67 Cast/wrought	Titanium 6A1-4V alloy ASTM F136 Cast/wrought
Cobalt	—	—	—
Chromium	16-18	—	—
Nickel	10-14	—	—
Molybdenum	2-3	—	—
Iron	Bal (62-72)	0.5 max	0.25 max
Aluminum	—	—	5.5-6.5
Vanadium	—	—	3.5-4.5
Titanium	—	Bal (99+)	Bal (88.5-92)
Carbon	0.06 max	0.10 max	0.08 max
Manganese	2.00 max	—	—
Phosphorus	0.045 max	—	—
Sulfur	0.030 max	—	—
Silicon	1.0 max	—	—
Oxygen	—	0.45 max	0.13 max

Trade name	Type	Manufacturer
Alivium	Co-Cr	Zimmer, Orthopedic Ltd., London, England
CoCroMo	Co-Cr	Orthopedic Equipment Company, Bourbon, Indiana
Francobal	Co-Cr	S.A. Benoist Girard & Cie, Heronville, France
Orthochrome	Co-Cr	DePuy, Warsaw, Indiana
Protosul	Co-Cr	Protek & Sulzer, Indiana
Tivanium	Ti-6A1-4V	Zimmer USA, Warsaw, Indiana
Vinertia	Co-Cr	Deloro Surgical Ltd., Stratton St. Margaret, England
Vitallium	Co-Cr	Howmedica, Rutherford, New Jersey
Zimaloy	Co-Cr	Zimmer USA, Warsaw, Indiana

From Dumbleton, J. H., and Black, J.: An introduction to orthopedic materials, Springfield, Ill., 1975, Charles C Thomas, Publisher.

for debris derived from the cobalt-chromium alloy).

Attempts have been made to establish a quantitative method for tissue response to particles of foreign material (or even autogenous bone dust) in which the frequency (concentration of particles per field, rated 0 to 4) is noted and an average is derived by examining many fields.[8,77] The inflammatory response, likewise, is classified as acute, subacute, or chronic—based on the predominant cell type present. Obviously, particles that cause tissue reactions, which are progressive by nature, are of particular concern, along with rare debris particles capable of producing remote reactions via the regional lymphatic system and the reticuloendothelial system.

Corrosion and fatigue

As stated before, when two dissimilar metals are electrically coupled with each other, they undergo galvanic corrosion owing to the flow of current stimulated by their differing electrical potentials. This corrosion may also occur when two identical electrodes are in contact with solutions of different electrolytic composition. The types of metal corrosion occurring in the body include:

1. Uniform corrosion—in which the attack affects the entire surface and undergoes corrosion
2. Pitting corrosion—which is indicative of a local attack resulting in the formation of deep and shallow cavities (pits)
3. Intergranular corrosion—which occurs at the metal's grain boundaries and which may be deep and rapid
4. Cracking—which is usually caused by tensile stresses causing fatigue fracture and exposing the interior of the metal to a corrosive environment; common in implants involving fracture fixation

In general, reactions to metals relate not only to the ionic behavior in a biological situation (the body environment) but also to the size, shape, movement, and other physical parameters of the implant itself.[96]

Types of tissue reaction

Tissue reactions to metallic implants may be classified into four general types.

Injury reaction. Injury reaction occurs at the time of the implantation of metal and includes damage to the bone and soft tissue as the result of drilling, reaming, and so on. This type of reaction naturally involves a local tissue repair reaction,[42,43] accompanied by phagocytosis in the form of acute and, subsequently, subacute inflammatory cells as well as osteoclastic activities to remove the necrotic bone.

Repair reaction. Repair reaction takes place as manifested by the healing of soft tissue and the formation of new bone as well as the replacement or removal of dead bone. Usually plump, active fibroblasts and macrophages are concentrated in the implant area, which is also rich in capillaries. This phenomenon is characteristically caused by the specialization of immature perivascular mesenchymal cells and monocytes for the removal of dead bone and the formation of new bone. In the initial phase young fiber bone is formed, and this tissue is gradually converted to mechanically sound lamellar bone. Whether bone or fibrous tissue will be formed in any given situation during the multiphases of repair depends largely on the local properties (physical and chemical) at the site of repair.

Corrosion reaction. The third type of reaction is corrosion reaction, which is characterized by redox reaction occurring at the interface between the metal (electrode) and the tissue fluids. For example, metals such as cobalt and nickel are mutagenic in cell cultures, while others are inert. The tissue response to metallic corrosion has been described by many authors; there is an electrochemical reaction adjacent to the metals that causes an inflammatory response to corrosion, leading to cell infiltration and fibrous tissue formation about the implant.[37,75] Bone reaction to this type of corrosion consists of osteolysis and osteoclasis leading to loosening of the implant and formation of reactive bone in an attempt to encapsulate the implant. This reaction is very similar to that which is seen in osteomyelitis.

Metal particle reaction. Metal particle reaction is the fourth type of reaction. Vitallium (cobalt-chromium-molybdenum alloy) has been recommended because of its electrochemical inertness and its minimal tendency to self-welding.[119] This alloy has been used for internal fixation devices for over 40 years. Although an increased concentration of metal ions around the implants was demonstrated by Ferguson,[50] it did not occur with chromium and cobalt in a static situation. When the alloy was used as a bearing joint component, the elements were released, found in the bloodstream, and excreted in the urine.[40] It was also demonstrated that these alloy particles would partially dissolve when incubated in horse serum. Although hypersensitivity to cobalt, chrome, and nickel is well documented,[9,91] Evans and his associates[49] were the first to draw attention to metal toxicity after total hip arthroplasty. McKee[81] and others have reported the cause of "early failures" of the McKee prosthesis as a nonspecific inflammatory response in the absence of infection. In analyzing seven patients with failed McKee-Farrar total hip replacements, Jones and associates[72] found that six of these patients were cobalt positive—but nickel and

63

chrome negative on skin patch testing. Macroscopic and histological necrosis of bone, muscle, and joint capsule around the prosthesis was found in five patients whose hips were explored. Severe bone resorption, pathological fracture of the acetabulum, and loosening or dislocations were observed. Increased cobalt concentrations in the urine and in a variety of tissues were also reported.[54]

Reports indicate that Vitallium alloy prosthetic components (metal against metal) provide excellent wear resistance under operating conditions, with a volumetric wear less than that of metal-to-plastic bearings.[113] But because of high "frictional torque" and the problems of loosening, tissue reaction, and remote accumulation of debris, it is probable that metal-to-metal prostheses will eventually be phased out and replaced by metal against high-density polyethylene. The most accepted metals—coupled with high-density polyethylene—are Vitallium alloy, 316.L stainless steel, titanium 6, aluminum 4 vanadium alloy. Galante found that the wear of ultra-high molecular weight polyethylene in sliding contact with titanium alloy was enormously greater than that generated by Vitallium alloy.[56-58] At a contact stress of only 238 to 277 p.s.i., the wear rate of titanium was 15×10^{-9} mm./mm. as compared to 1×10^{-9} mm./mm. with Vitallium; at higher contact stresses, wear rate was even greater. Also, the titanium specimens were severely scored after those tests (although contact was only with polyethylene, which became filled with a black powder); it appears that the passive oxide film covering the titanium surface was weakened by the sliding motion of the two materials. It should be noted that the conditions of wear testing may have influenced the results. In a more recent work Galante and coworkers have shown that the wear resistance of titanium can be considerably improved by appropriately manipulating the passivation layer by either chemical or thermal techniques. Those recent experiments regard titanium at least as good as Vitallium as tested in the laboratory—obviously the crucial experiments probably would have to be in vivo.[55]

Polymers as bearing materials

As with metals, the inertness of plastics is of concern in design and performance. Polymers used as bearing materials have opened an important new area in material selection in total joint replacement.[6,11] Ideally, after implantation a polymer should not deteriorate from attack by the body fluids nor from its own chemical changes. This material should not generate a foreign body reaction leading to formation of granulation tissue or hypersensitivity. It should be capable of withstanding stress without structural changes in order to provide strength for enduring service. It must be easily produced and manufactured and inexpensive, and the method of sterilization must be easy, practical, and economical. Finally, the quality control methods must be standardized to assure a uniform performance.

Most of the plastics implanted in the body have provoked sarcomas when implanted in rats and mice. Heuper advanced the idea that the chemical nature of the implant, not its shape, is what offends,[69] but the authoritative work of Oppenheimer and Oppenheimer[85] and Oppenheimer, Oppenheimer, and Stout[86] in 1952 demonstrated that sarcomas are caused primarily by the size and shape of the implant. Concerning implantation of carcinogenic material in animals, however, it must be noted that a direct correlation between animal experimentation and human experiences has never been established. It is of special interest (and a striking fact) that in spite of extensive implantation of plastics in the human body no benign or malignant tumors have ever been reported as having been caused by these synthetic materials; nor have any malignant or benign tumors ever developed in tissues that were in direct physical contact with surgically implanted synthetic organic materials at any location. Actually, there are very few examples in the literature concerning tumors in relation to implanted material in any animal phylogenetically above mice or rats. Clinical reports of tumors—presumably the result of inserted metals in the human body—are scarce,[67,80,98] and all have failed to demonstrate a direct relationship between the implanted metals and cancer in humans. Of special interest is the study of Hoopes et al. in 1967,[67] reporting a survey covering some 40,000 cases of breast augmentation with a variety of materials: they found only six cases of cancer in these augmentations, which on detailed study revealed no relationship between the implanted materials and cancer. Others have also attempted research to document the carcinogenicity of implanted materials in higher animals with notable failure.

Teflon for bearing

Extensive surgical experience with Teflon has shown that this material is chemically inert; it was greatly surprising to find, however, that severe bone absorption and destruction resulted when it was used for sockets in total hip replacement. Most of the 344 Teflon sockets inserted (1958 to 1962)[26] had to be revised, not because of excessive wear (2 to 3 years following surgery), but because of severe bone damage (acetabulum, calcar of femur, and trochanteric region). On examination of failed Teflon total hips, a porridgelike material was often observed. Cavities were often created at the interface between bone and cement, as if the wear products had been pumped into the osseous tissue, thus producing mechanical erosion. Charnley observed that, once the source of granulating Teflon particles was eliminated, the destructive process stopped (as evidenced by the presence of inspissated calcific Teflon granuloma). The mechanical erosion in the acetabulum (caused by Teflon) was also frequently observed in the upper femur when the stem had become loose, allowing entry of debris into clefts formed between the cement and bone. Teflon reactions were usually typified by multinucleated giant cells (often more than 100 nuclei) often within the vicinity of relatively large-sized birefringent particles. Iliac and aortic lymph nodes, as one might anticipate, contained giant cells and plastic material, but it is of special interest that, strangely enough, particles of Teflon within the lymph nodes were not birefringent.[15,26]

High-density polyethylene

Present-day experiences with total hip replacement based on postmortem studies and re-exploration of joints (both in personal experience and in literature) are favorable both regarding the mechanical properties (Table 3-4) and the biocompatibility of high-density polyethylene against chromium-cobalt or stainless steel—although it is not possible to say that tissue reaction will not occur from debris accumulated over a very long period of time.

Reoperation on patients reveals a quite benign appearance of high-density polyethylene against metal articular surfaces. Gross and histological sections reveal minimum to moderate inflammatory foreign body reaction (Fig. 3-1). Granulated particles of plastic mixed with organic materials (yellowish pink in color) are present, and macrophages are filled with highly refractile granules visible by polarized light (Fig. 3-2). The lymphatic drainage of the joint carries particles of plastic to the regional nodes. However, no lymphadenopathy has been seen in patients where high-density polyethylene was used, nor has lymphadenitis been reported in patients who have now gone beyond 10 years with high-density polyethylene.[26]

Reaction to PMMA

Histological evaluation of both animal and human bone and cement has been extensively reported by several authors.* Charnley reported in detail the histological findings of human specimens (37 calcar and 26 acetabulum) following death from natural causes; all specimens studied had a successful total hip replacement. The average time after operation was 7.3 years, the longest period 13 years, and there were 13 patients over 9 years after operation. It was emphasized that all of these cases were 100% successful arthroplasties. This is very important to note and is an essential feature in the proper interpretation of cement in contact with living tissue.[26,117] In available literature, considerable confusion has occurred when the studies of loose and infected prostheses have been reported along with successful cement-fixed implants.[35] Consequently, it is important to consider the histology of bone and cement contact in the absence of infection in two separate situations: (1) state of rigidity, that is, successful arthroplasty, and (2) state of looseness, that is, failure.

Table 3-4. Mechanical properties of ultramolecular weight high-density polyethylene

Property	UHMWPE
Elongation (percent)	400-500
Yield strength (1,000 p.s.i.)	3.1-5.5
Tensile strength (1,000 p.s.i.)	6.4
Compressive strength (1,000 p.s.i.)	2.7-3.6
Tensile modulus (10^5 p.s.i.)	0.6-1.8
Density	0.94-0.965

From Dumbleton, J. H., and Black, J.: An introduction to orthopedic materials, Springfield, Ill., 1975, Charles C Thomas, Publisher.

*See references 8, 26, 27, 33, 35, 66, and 117.

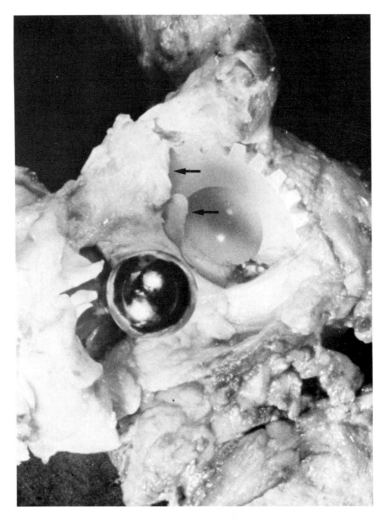

Fig. 3-1. Examination of postmortem specimens of total hip prostheses using high-density polyethylene against stainless steel has shown minimum tissue reaction. Gross specimen (postmortem) is removed 7 years and 3 months following successful low-friction arthroplasty. NOTE: marked capsular thickening as evidence of capsular repair (top arrow). At certain points thickness reaches more than 1 cm. Only evidence of gross histological tissue reaction was evidence of two small proliferative synovial-type reactions at inferior portion of joint (bottom arrow). Prosthetic components were rigidly fixed to bone by cement.

THE STATE OF RIGIDLY FIXED CEMENT
Gross appearance

Close contact between cement and bone is easily recognized when closely observing a horizontal or vertical cross-section of the femur or the acetabular region. Sometimes a layer of fibrous tissue is seen (by the naked eye) at the cement-bone junction, especially at the areas of cancellous bone in the acetabular region. On the other hand, this state almost never exists at the interface between cement and femur. At times, however, under low-power magnification, it appears that the cement is in direct contact with the bone, but there is a normal amount of fat cells close to the surface of the cement. The molding of the cement injected into the cancellous bone can be appreciated following careful removal of the cement from the bone. Three important histological features of the gross specimens are to be noted.

1. Negative impressions of the cement's forcible injection into the bone (through a mold of the interior surface of the bone)

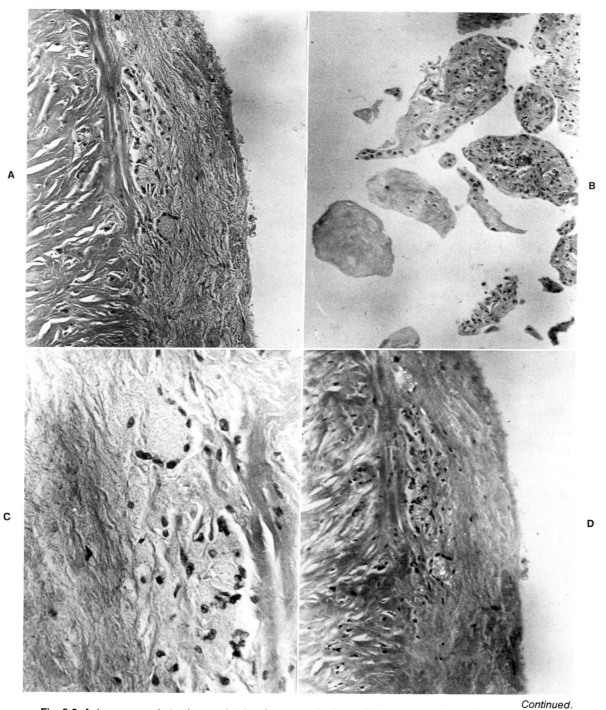

Continued.

Fig. 3-2. A, Low-power photomicrograph taken from capsular lining of joint showing giant cell reaction. Same patient as Fig. 3-1. **B,** Photomicrograph of portion of synovial lining. Tissue obtained from same specimen showing small but frequent giant cell reaction. **C,** High-power photomicrograph of giant cells presumably containing particles of high-density polyethylene. **D** to **F,** Similar to **A** to **C** but under polarized light. NOTE: double refractile material (HDP) within giant cells, evidence of wear particles of high-density polyethylene.

67

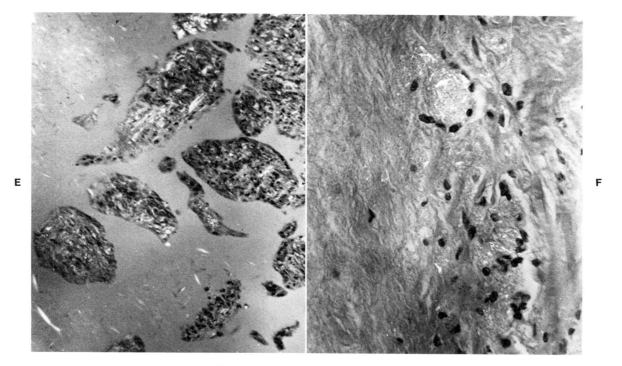

Fig. 3-2, cont'd. For legend see p. 67.

indicates that the bone is in contact with the cement.

2. Fibrous tissue with no preferred orientation interposed between bone and cement indicates the absence of contact, thus suggesting possible loosening or inadequate "pressure injection." It also may suggest areas of bone absorption and replacement by fibrous tissue.

3. Smooth surface areas of highly organized fibrous tissue or fibrocartilage suggest possible soft tissue contact, and load transmission zones.

Microscopy

To recognize the histology of cement-tissue contact areas one must be aware of the microscopic structure of acrylic cement itself when in contact with the tissue.

The polymer powder consists of spheres ranging from 38 to 80 μ. Because undecalcified sections are not satisfactory and for the purpose of detailed examination, the cement is usually dissolved out. The impressions left by the granules can easily be recognized as evidence of contact between the cement and the tissue (Fig. 3-3, *B*).

The postoperative tissue damage begins at surgery and leads to bone necrosis at the site of cement insertion. This is related to metaphyseal and intramedullary interference by the trauma of broaching,[17,106,107,110] and cell death by monomer[101,117,118] or heat of polymerization.[17,121] Therefore it is not unusual to find segmental or zonal necrosis in the trochanteric shaft or calcar region of the femur at a later stage. One frequently observes hemispherical cement impressions in direct contact with bone trabeculi containing living osteocytes (right up to its surface).

Interface. Within the first 2 or 3 weeks after insertion of the cement, a coagulum of connective tissue is visible (interposed between cement and bone). The repair is manifested by local hyperemia, migration of lipophages, and ingrowth of capillaries and fibroblasts. As time progresses, the interface tissue becomes more organized, with four types of contact between cement and bone generally observable for up to a year:

1. Direct contact points without recognizable cellular interpositioning
2. Areolar soft tissue—up to 300 μ in thickness in contact with the cement

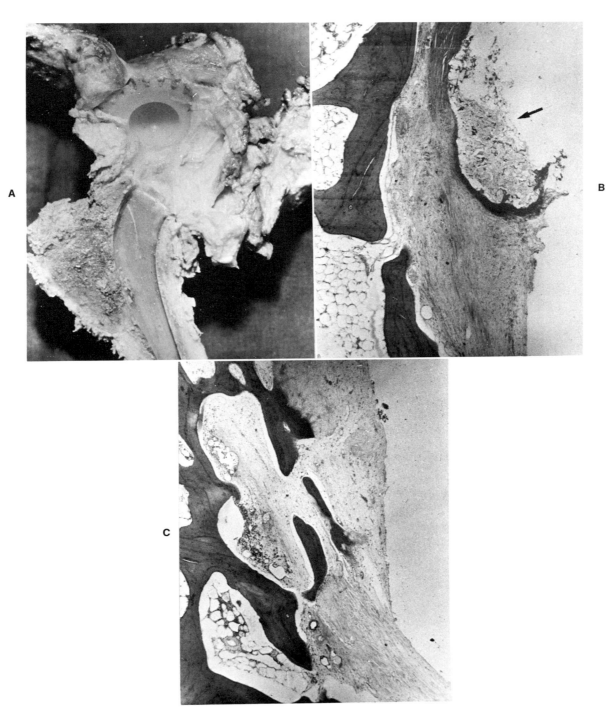

Fig. 3-3. A, Same specimen as shown in Fig. 3-1 but following removal of femoral component. Prosthesis was absolutely rigidly fixed in bone. There was no gross fibrous lining between metal and cement, but whitish fibrinoid-like material was smeared throughout length of prosthesis. There was smooth lining of interface between cement and bone without evidence of cavitation or cystic changes. **B** and **C,** Two areas of bone in contact with cement and interposed by fibrous tissue. Fibrous tissue is highly organized and in certain areas suggestive of fibrocartilage containing only occasional giant cells. NOTE: cement contact, **B,** with fibrocartilage and impressions of cement spheres within fibrocartilaginous layer. Portion of cement in this specimen had not been fully dissolved out of specimen (arrow). Healthy marrow is noted.

3. A thin layer of dense, fibrous tissue in contact with the cement
4. Weight-bearing zones of fibrocartilage in contact with the cement

In some areas both fibrous tissue and fibrocartilage are observed in the interface between bone and cement. When near the bone, fibrocartilage often demonstrates progressive conversion to bone. It is possible that these changes are metaplastic in nature, that is, the metaplasia of fibrous tissue into fibrocartilage may be the result of mechanical pressure, accompanied by progressive ossification of the deeper parts where there is direct contact between the fibrocartilage and old bone. Remarkable variation in the thickness of fibrous tissue is observed from one field to another in the same specimen.

Giant cells, usually indicative of foreign body reaction, are seen sporadically at the surface of fibrous tissue in direct contact with cement. Unlike the acetabulum, this membrane is usually not identifiable in the femur by gross examination. The fibers are oriented parallel to the surface of the cement. The permanent cement bed is established within 2 years, with fewer giant cells present with the passage of time; it is suggested that they are prevalent from 2 to 5 years following implantation.[17] The presence and frequency of giant cells is not particularly alarming as they are often insulated from underlying bone by a layer of fibrous tissue, which generally contains elongated nuclei lying parallel to the bone surface. Giant cells are usually found in areas of thick fibrous tissue in the non-weight-bearing areas (noncontact zones). There are rarely inflammatory cells; the frequent lodging of cement particles in the cytoplasm of the giant cells has been demonstrated.

Femur. Transmission of the load between cement and bone appears to take place at isolated points but mainly through the fibrocartilage. It may be that the fibrocartilage is metaplastic from original loose, fibrous tissue, which, as it responds to mechanical pressure, progresses with time into fully developed fibrocartilage capable of transmitting the load. Ossification frequently extends to this fibrocartilage area from underlying bone.

Occasional death of bone is also evident with osteoclastic activities; however, in some regions new osteoid is also formed and osteoblastic activities are often simultaneously present.

Bone appears to be remodelled in some areas, whereas in other zones new bone may be bridging two segments of dead bone (osteoblastic activity). These findings are not necessarily associated with failure, that is, loosening and so on. Necrotic bone is at times remodeled or reinforced by new bone. Replacement of the necrotic bone is usually completed within 2 years. Bone remodelling at the area adjacent to the cement is commonly observed in older specimens.

From the foregoing it must be recognized that this permanent cement bed (implant bed) of fibrous tissue is nonproliferative and has no detrimental effect on fixation. Rather, it is beneficial because of its antifretting effect (Fig. 3-3).[14] It is essential to recognize that macrophages and giant cells on the surface of cement remain permanently inactive if a perfect mechanical fixation is achieved. Conversely, if movement is present, these macrophages and giant cells are provoked, frequently resulting in loosening. Therefore, if the cement was slightly loose at the end of an operation, it will become completely loose as the result of motion. This, in itself, emphasizes the importance of a "perfect cement technique."

It is now clear that a fibrous layer containing giant cells is usually predominantly present in non-weight-bearing zones of endosteal surface of bone. But, here again, this layer of fibrous tissue is nonproliferative and rarely exceeds 50 to 100 μ in thickness; normal fat cells are usually observed adjacent to it. The thick layer of fibrous tissue as seen at the interface in most experimental work must be related to the lack of rigid fixation of the cement in these experiments. It is felt that the failure to achieve fixation in experimental animals as the result of pressure injection of cement is responsible for the formation of a thick fibrous layer. The macrophages and giant cells in the layer remain at a stable population permanently if a perfect mechanical fixation is achieved; however, with movement (if fixation fails) the cells are more provoked, forming granulomatous-type tissue.

In our laboratories[73] in order to characterize histologically the nature of the interface, three sets of experiments were conducted using 11 (7.7 to 13 kg. weight) adult beagles. Specifically the objective was to study the effects of monomer leaching and heat liberated from curing methacrylate plugs in situ. Separation of the two effects was accomplished in three group experiments: (1) plugs were cured and leached of monomer prior to plug implantation, thus the absence of heat and monomer. (2) Plugs were cured but not leached, thus the absence of heat only. (3) Plugs were implanted 4 minutes after the initiation of cement mixing, thus the presence of heat and monomer.

This experiment, which was designed to study the histological morphology of the interface of bone in contact with methyl-methacrylate in canines, illustrated that self-curing methyl methacrylate cement (as used in this experi-

ment) was well tolerated by osseous tissue and that the bone did grow in direct apposition to methacrylate without interposition of fibrocartilage. The plugs in these experiments were all rigidly pressfitted into drilled holes (except for those experiments in which cement was allowed to cure in situ).

No definite noxious effect from the heat of polymerization or from the monomer could be identified from the methyl methacrylate as used in these experiments. A typical histological morphology of the interface is shown in Fig.

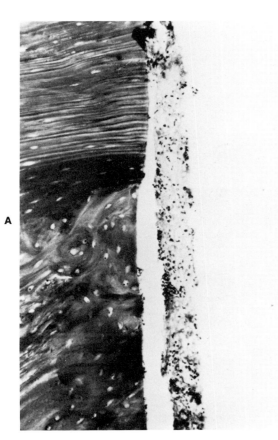

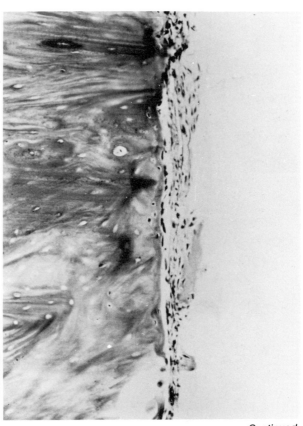

Continued.

Fig. 3-4. **A,** Four-day specimen showing layer of coagulum containing acute inflammatory cells interposed between wall of cortical defect and methyl methacrylate plug that occupied space to right. **B,** At 2 weeks, cement plug was separated from cortical bone within defect by very cellular fibrous tissue oriented perpendicular to long axis of cortex. **C,** At 4 weeks, fibrous layer was almost completely replaced by newly formed bone. Defect to right was filled with methyl methacrylate implant. NOTE: the empty lacunae within original cortical bone. Zone of dead bone is about 300 μ wide. NOTE: in this specimen methyl methacrylate was inserted similar to operating condition; that is, cement was polymerized in situ. NOTE: presence of giant cell reaction as well as impressions of cement on surface of fibrous layer now completely replaced by newly formed bone. **D,** Six-month specimen that shows small area of fibrous tissue between methyl methacrylate plug that occupied space to right and cortical bone. Also note semicircular impressions of cement in bone. **E,** Four-week specimen that contained Teflon plug zone of dead bone is noted within vicinity of implant presumably from trauma of surgery. **F,** At 4 weeks cortical defect that is allowed to heal without implantation of foreign material also demonstrates zone of cortical necrosis adjacent to defect. Line of demarcation between wall of defect and reactive new bone is clearly seen (**A** to **F** ×40). (Courtesy of Pawluk and Bassett.)

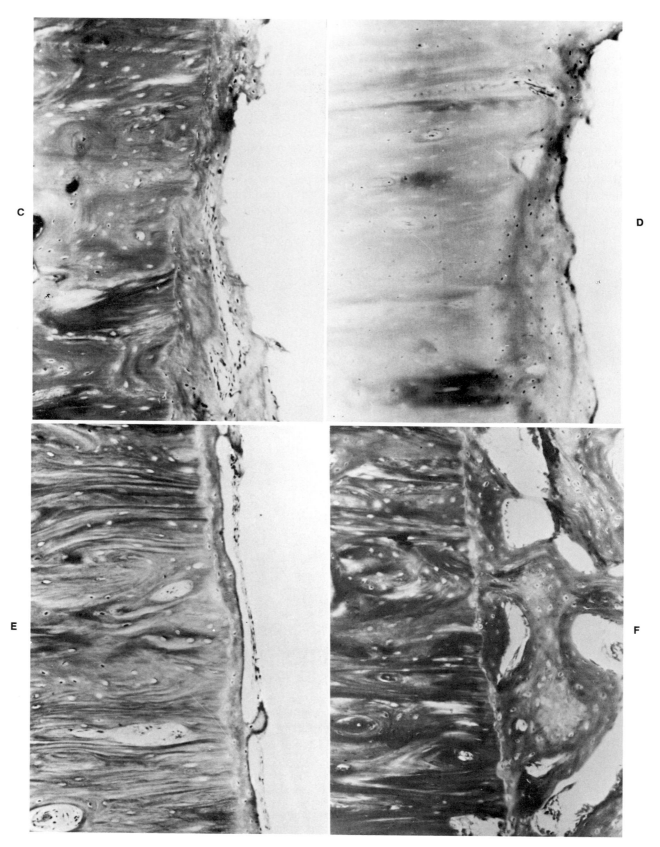

C

D

E

F

Fig. 3-4, cont'd. For legend see p. 71.

3-4 and compared with the histological changes in a drilled hole without any implant and one with a plug of Teflon.

Acetabulum. In the acetabulum the situation is somewhat different. Approximately 60% of postoperative radiographs show some evidence of demarcation—a phenomenon that is not found in the femur. This demarcation, which is nonprogressive (up to 10 to 12 years), represents a fibrous layer and metaplastic fibrocartilage caused by pressure.[44] It may be that the elastic behavior of cancellous bone of the acetabulum is responsible for the formation of this rather thick layer of fibrocartilage. In some areas of weight bearing the fibrocartilage is loose, thin, and perhaps not capable of weight bearing; but again, such a zone is in a transitional state and can be treated as obviously capable of weight bearing as if fibrous metaplasia into cartilage were taking place in these areas. This phenomenon explains why one may see a line of demarcation radiologically and yet clinically the result is successful.

Where fibrocartilage does not exist and a continuous sheet of giant cells is in direct contact with the cement, it may be that no weight bearing is taking place. Because of normal fat storage and the absence of collections of giant cells forming granulomatous material (similar to that of the femur), it is concluded that cement is well tolerated by bone, as long as it remains mechanically under load and stable within the osseous tissue.

Reactions to loose acrylic cement

The available literature is mainly unclear in describing the difference between the tissue responses of failed total hips and infected total hips (where those tissue responses had not previously been identified, and the failures were attributed to acrylic cement).[8,28,35,111] For example, loose fragments of cement, along with caseation cavitation and necrosis, are frequently observed in a loose cemented prosthesis where motion has been present for some time prior to surgical intervention. In the presence of infection, reactions are different in that usually signs of osteitis are present and microabscesses are frequently observed at the interface. In addition to infection, mechanical defects occurred in metal-to-metal total hip prostheses, which may suggest sensitivity to metal particles, especially chromium and cobalt particles.[72] It should be

emphasized that extensive tissue reaction with giant cell formation and caseation suggests the presence of loosening of cement fragments in the bone for a long time prior to surgical intervention (Fig. 3-5). Further, it is clear that cement particles are not birefringent, as birefringent material is related to the particles worn from polyethylene not from cement (Fig. 3-5). Unfortunately, since there is no specific stain technique available for acrylic cement (methyl methacrylate), the presence or absence of cement particles accompanying giant cells and macrophages cannot be verified.

Early loosening must be considered a complication of surgical technique. It is usually related to fragments of cement becoming mobile in a soft tissue bed; the bone shows increased osteoclastic activity and remodeling at the site with sequestrated acrylic "pearls" at the bed of the implant. If the loosening is of long standing (more than 2 years), a permanent organized tissue bed is produced with movable cement within it. This tissue usually exhibits tears accompanied by a fibrous exudate and an occasional zone of necrosis (Fig. 3-3 and 3-4). It has also been suggested that excessive load applied early during the "repair stage" is detrimental to fixation.[118] The greatest risk in securing a good fixation comes from insufficient immediate contact between cement and bone, leading to early motion and damage to both tissue and cement.

Cystic erosions encountered in the calcar region of the femur (after a successful arthroplasty of many years) may be attributed to microfractures in the cement and minor loosening at this heavily loaded zone. Occasional extensive bone absorption and cystic changes along the shaft may also be related to motion between the cement, and the bone. When motion is not severe (amplitude), the patient may be asymptomatic, but with the passage of time and further loosening, clinical failure will result.[26,65] Cracks and cleavage planes within the cement cone may allow pumping of minute cement or high-density polyethylene particles to occur, thus causing erosive changes in the bone; the macrophagic response is usually proportional to the amount and size of these particles. Usually, there are three types of foreign body giant cells: large giant cells, small giant cells, and the histiocytes. Perhaps these types of cells are all manifestations of the same phenomenon, but

73

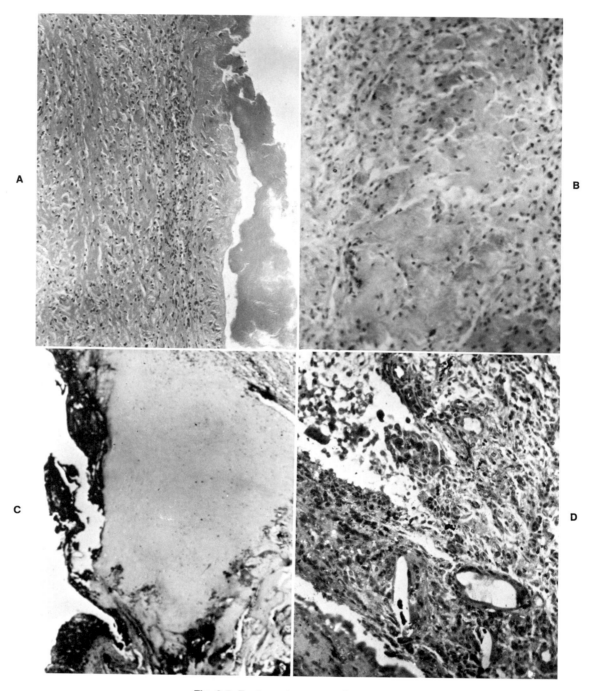

Fig. 3-5. For legend see opposite page.

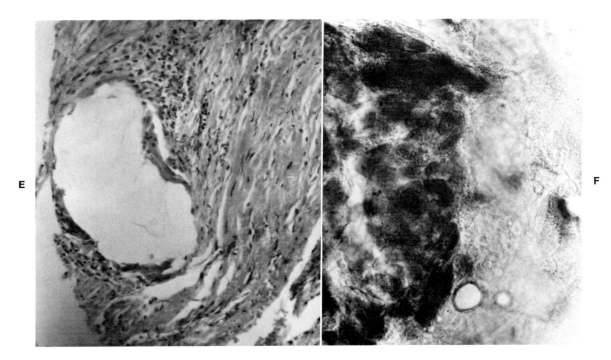

Fig. 3-5. A, Fibrinoid material found on surface of fibrous capsule is nonspecific to type of implant. It may be seen with loose prosthesis with or without cement. Severe fibrinoid material found in tissue may also suggest possibility of infection. This low-power photomicrograph is taken from loose Moore self-locking prosthesis. Specimen is from fibrous sleeve adjacent to stem of prosthesis. **B,** Intracellular amorphous material indicative of fibrinoid removed from tissue adjacent to loose cemented cup of total hip prosthesis. **C,** Caseation found in region of calcar. Severe caseous formation is evidence of motion between cement and bone, resulting in necrosis. No birefringent material was found. **D,** Considerable histiocytic reaction found in region of calcar. This histiocytic reaction is typical of loose cemented prosthesis. **E,** Foreign body granuloma reaction to loose cemented femoral prosthesis. Large void in field represents relatively large fragment of cement that has been removed from tissue during preparation. **F,** High-power magnification showing cluster of histiocytes. These cells usually contain acidophilic granular cytoplasm with tendency to cluster. If birefringent granules are seen within vicinity, most likely reaction relates to high-density polyethylene; without their presence, reaction must be considered secondary to loose fragments of cement. Occasionally these cells may appear as large sheet within field resembling pseudocarcinoma-type appearance.

the reactions to the different sizes and shapes of the particles result in different kinds of cells. It is possible that large, hollow foreign body giant cells are caused by large particles of acrylic cement and that most of the small giant cells contain particles of high-density polyethylene. More puzzling areas are the sheets of histiocytes, for the formation of which small particles of high-density polyethylene can only ocasionally be incriminated.[26]

In summary, the histology of tissue contact with cement that is rigidly fixed in the bone is entirely benign, and the occasional giant cells revealed in non-weight-bearing zones of the interface are the only suggestion of tissue response to cement. Any evidence of severe tissue response, such as severe giant cell reaction and caseous formation leading to bone cavitation, must elicit a suspicion of the mechanical loosening of the cement in the bone. Acrylic cement is not birefringent, and histologic evidence of birefringent material is indicative of wear debris from high-density polyethylene (Fig. 3-6). Where severe bone necrosis accompanies focal cell infiltration and fibrinoid necrosis, the possibility of infection (see Chapter 16) also must be considered.

FORCES ABOUT THE HIP

It is an established fact that the static force on the femoral head is greater than the weight of the body (Fig. 3-7)—during stance, perhaps

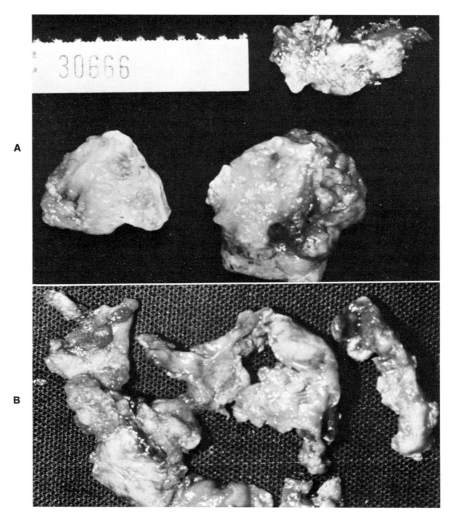

Fig. 3-6. A and **B,** Fibrous capsule formed around artificial hip joint usually contains plastic fragments, by-product of wear of high-density polyethylene. This tissue is usually firm and gritty. **C** to **E,** Large foreign body birefringent materials representing loose pieces of high-density polyethylene within fibrous capsule are seen. This specimen is taken from a hip following recurrent dislocation. NOTE: adjacent tissue is also refractile but not vascular.

two or three times greater (with the direction of the force being inclined 10 to 15 degrees from the midaxis of the body).[71,90]

Assuming that "maximum wear" occurs at the "maximum force location," Elson and Charnley, after their examination of worn-out Teflon acetabular cups, calculated the direction of the actual resultant force to be 10 to 15 degrees from the midaxis of the body. They determined that this was the most common direction of wear, although in a small percentage of their cases it was as much as ±20 degrees toward or away from the midline.[48]

Forces acting on the hip joint are influenced considerably by the pelvic angle and the position of the trunk and limbs.[82,108] With the pelvis in a normal walking attitude and the limbs symmetrically disposed, muscle forces range from 1 to 1.8 times the body weight, joint forces from 1.8 to 2.7 times the body weight; even small changes in the positions of the lever arms of the muscles involved will alter these forces considerably.[52] With simple calculations it has been shown that the load on the hip joint, when lying on the back and raising a leg 2 inches off the ground, is approximately twice that of the body

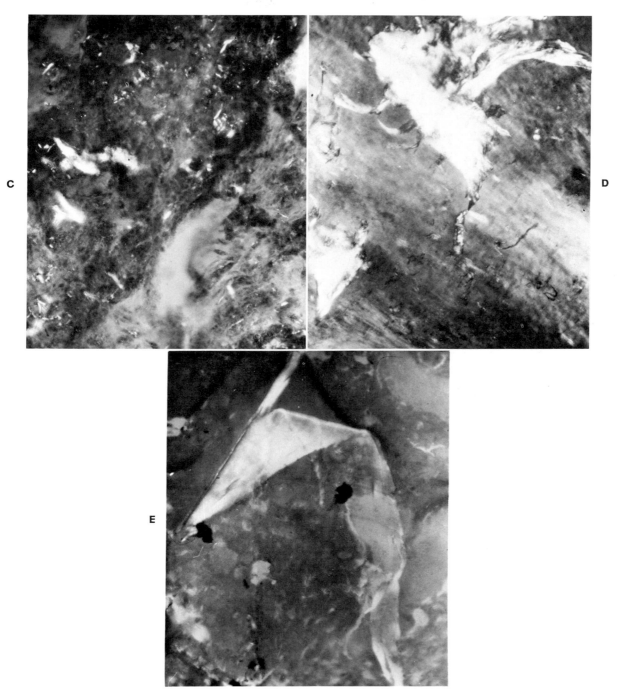

Fig. 3-6, cont'd. For legend see opposite page.

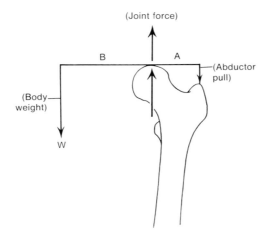

Fig. 3-7. Force on femoral head is equal to abductor pull (force) times *A* (distance) plus body weight times *B* (distance). Static force on femoral head is greater than weight of body, *W*, during stance, being two to three times greater in magnitude than body weight. NOTE: direction of abductor pull is shown in same direction as body weight for clarity.

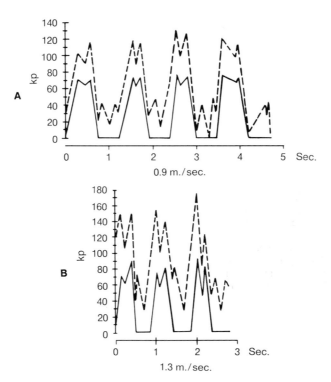

Fig. 3-8. While static force is considerably greater than body weight, even greater force is generated in dynamic situations such as acceleration and deceleration. Instrumented prosthesis indicates that with walking speed of 1.3 m./sec. maximum force of 3.8 times body weight is generated, **B**, and reduction of speed to 0.9 m./sec. diminished force on hip joint to 1.8 times body weight, **A.** (Modified from Rydell, M. W.: Acta Orthop. Scand. [Suppl.] **88**:Suppl., 1966.)

weight; obviously, then, the forces generated in the hip as the result of muscle action must be kept in mind when recommending exercises to the patient in the absence of weight bearing.[53] The clinical implication is a paradox: keeping a patient "non-weight bearing" while emphasizing active straight leg raise exercises.

While the static force is considerably greater than the body weight, an even greater force is generated in dynamic situations such as acceleration and deceleration.

The direct measurement of the forces acting across the hip joint was made in studies using an instrumented Moore self-locking prosthesis.[93,94] These studies showed that, at a walking speed of 1.3 m./sec., a maximum force of 3.8 times the body weight was generated; however, the reduction of the speed or distance to 0.9 m./sec. diminished the force on the hip to 1.8 times the body weight. This means that the weight forces on the hip joint were reduced by 50% by simply reducing the walking speed (Fig. 3-8). Dynamic data obtained with a force plate (to determine ground reaction) indicates that there may be an even larger amount of force being generated than can be revealed by an instrumented prosthesis. During the stance phase of the gait, the forces on the femoral head may be approximately five or six times the body weight, and the forces are at least equal to the body weight during the swing phase of the gait; this is because, in the "swing phase," the forces result from the mass of the limb and the muscular and ligamentous action producing the load on the joint, while in the "stance phase" the ground reaction is additionally responsible for the generation of the forces. It must be recognized that the pelvic angle and position of the trunk and limbs have a considerable effect on the forces. The forces acting on the abductor muscles and on the femoral head have been determined experimentally in a range of different "pelvic attitudes."[82] In these studies the position of the center of gravity of the body was determined by force measurement with simultaneous radiography to relate it to the skeleton. The forces were calculated using muscle positions, cadaveric dissections, and radiography of specimens. Calculations revealed that, with the pelvis in the normal walking attitude and limbs symmetrically disposed, muscle forces ranged from 1.0 to 1.8 times the body weight and joint forces from 1.8 to 2.7 times the body weight.

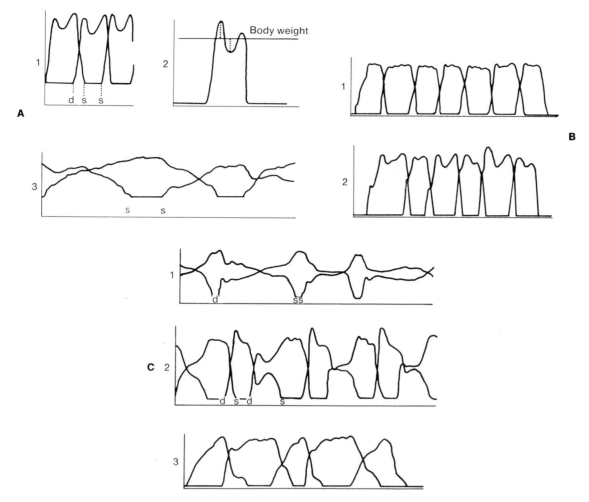

Fig. 3-9. A, Subject walking on recording platforms of gait recorder. *(1)* Characteristic trace in normal gait of young subject; *ds,* double support phase; *ss,* single support phase. *(2)* Level of body weight in relation to peaks caused by acceleration and deceleration of body mass. One millimeter vertical height equal to 5 pounds actual weight is recorded with both feet on one trace. *(3)* Short steps made very slowly. Part only of very long trace needing 20 steps to cover 11 feet. **B,** *(1)* Gait of elderly person (normal) or symmetrical arthritis of hips. *(2)* Notch on ascending limb of pulse probably indicating incoordination of knee extension. **C,** *(1)* Symmetrical slow progress of "alternate-standing" type. *(2)* Marked asymmetry of *ds* phase. Patient not stepping through with right foot, merely bringing one foot up to other and leading again with same foot. *(3)* Severe limp from unilateral hip disease. NOTE: for normal limb *ss* phase is too long to show "first and second peaks" of normal gait as seen in **A** *(1)*. (Modified from Charnley, J., and Pusso, R.: Clin. Orthop. **58:**153-164, 1968.)

The major pattern (quality) and amount (quantity) of forces in the hip joint may be recorded and analyzed in a clinical situation by a force plate[48,88] or a "gait recorder" that indicates the quantitative measure of force versus time in a tracing for an objective method of gait analysis.[32] This method is sensitive enough to produce, for example, an asymmetrical tracing in a case of bilateral hip disease, which clinically shows symmetrical involvement. In other words, such a recording can determine the type of gait pattern far more sensitively and objectively than can clinical observation or cinematography. These records can be made readily available for inspection in the patient's clinical record in order to evaluate and compare the pre- and postoperative status of the patient's gait pattern (Fig. 3-9).

Reduction of hip joint forces

Abnormal forces on the hip joint from disease (for example, congenital dysplasia of the hips,

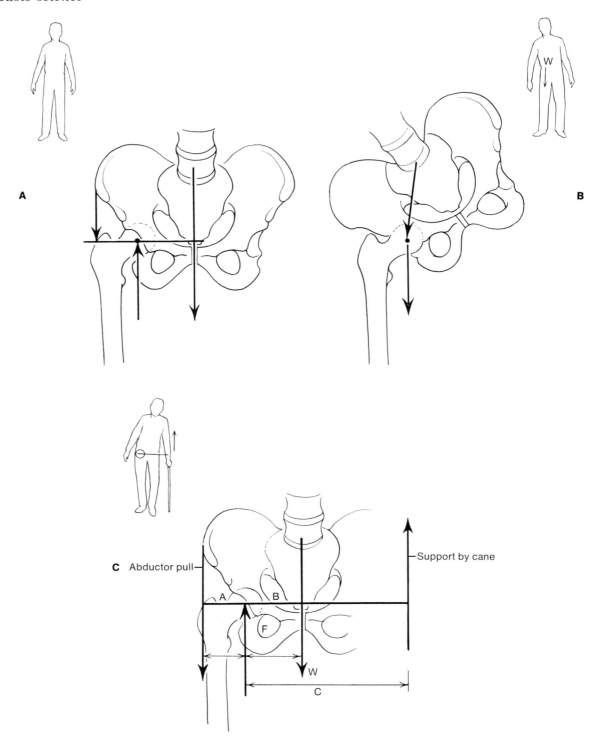

Fig. 3-10. A and **B,** Mechanics of painful hip may be changed by reduction of force generated by having pa-tient lean over affected hip. In this situation center of gravity moves laterally toward center of femoral head, thus shortening its lever arm. **B,** This action simply reduces magnitude of forces needed in abductor mus-cles to produce "balance," thus reducing net force across hip joint. **C,** Another means of reducing force, *F,* on hip joint is use of cane. Supporting force is provided by cane applied through favorable lever arm and greatly reduces force that abductors must exert to produce balance. In this diagram *A* represents abductor lever arm; *B,* body weight lever arm; and *C,* hip support (cane) lever arm.

osteoarthritis) or imbalanced muscles may lead to excess wear and tear, thus causing pain. It is logical therefore to reduce the load and the forces that generate pain in a malfunctioning hip joint in order to improve its function.

A simple example of changing the mechanics of a painful hip is the reduction of the force generated by having the patient lean over the affected hip. In this situation the center of gravity moves laterally toward the center of the femoral head, thus shortening its lever arm. This action simply reduces the magnitude of forces needed in the abductor muscles to produce "balance," thus reducing the net force across the hip joint (Fig. 3-10).

Another example of reduction of forces in the hip is increasing the weight-bearing surface in the joint itself by osteotomy—in which a major portion of the head is brought underneath the weight-bearing zone of the acetabulum (the logic for a varus osteotomy in congenital dysplasia of the hips). Even more logical is the reduction of stress in the hip by the obvious means of weight loss. Weight reduction is the simplest of all principles in reducing the force on the femoral head and thus the hip joint. Since for each pound of weight loss the force is reduced by approximately 2.5 to 3 pounds, a reduction of even a few pounds in weight is significant in reducing the force exerted across the hip joint (Fig. 3-11). Another means of reducing the weight placed on the hip joint is the use of a cane. Blount[7] and others have demonstrated the effectiveness of reducing the load on the hip by the use of a cane in the opposite hand (Fig. 3-10, *C*).

As noted previously, the reduction of force can also be achieved by reducing the speed of walking[87,89,93] and by the reconstruction of the joint at arthroplasty.

The restoration of hip function via lateralization of the abductor forces and medialization at the center of rotation of the hip has been advocated by Charnley.[22] (See Chapter 2: Surgical Approaches to the Hip.) The theory advanced is that by redistributing the forces about the hip joint, the socket load may be reduced, thus sparing the artificial joint from excessive stress, which might be of considerable importance in terms of wear, loosening, or fracture failures of the stem (Fig. 3-12). This reduction of load is achieved by (1) reducing the body-weight moment arm through maximal deepening of the acetabulum, thus moving the center of rotation medially and (2) increasing the gluteal moment arm via lateral transfer of the greater trochanter.

From the foregoing it can be noted that the shorter the body-weight moment arm, the less the pull of the abductors required to balance the pelvis; conversely, by lengthening the abductor moment arm, the gluteal tension required to balance the pelvis is reduced, and in this way the total load on the hip joint is also reduced (Fig. 3-13).

This mechanical situation can be illustrated by an attempt to balance a beam on a fulcrum, for example, balancing an 18-inch ruler on a fingertip (Fig. 3-14). As shown in the diagram, no extra force is needed to balance the ruler on the finger if the fulcrum point is exactly at the midpoint of the ruler (marked 9″). The weight transferred to the tip of the finger is equal to the weight of the ruler acting at point A. By transferring the finger (fulcrum) to point A′, we readily see that added force is required to balance the ruler. An even greater weight (force) is needed for balance if the distance between the weight and the fulcrum on the acting moment arm is further reduced (point A″); consequently, the forces on the fulcrum are also increased. This simple analogy demonstrates the importance of recognizing the moments of the forces about the hip in attempting to reduce the socket load (fingertip, in the experiment). When these principles are applied to hip arthroplasty, the lateral transposition of the trochanter does not merely "stretch" the elastic muscle fibers to provide stability. The stability produced by these means results in increased abductor moment arm, thus less demand from the abductor and consequently less of a load on the joint. It is not

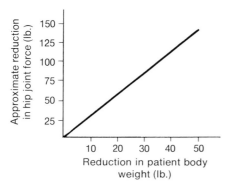

Fig. 3-11. Graph shows correlation between weight loss and hip joint force; reduction is by ratio of 1:3.

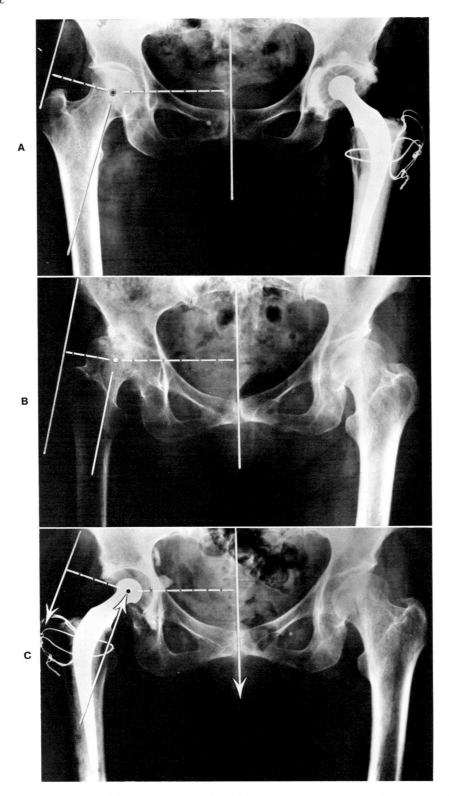

Fig. 3-12. Reduction of load following arthroplasty is achieved by reducing body weight moment arm through maximal deepening of acetabulum, thus moving center of rotation medially, and by increasing gluteal moment arm via lateral transfer of greater trochanter. **A,** Normal; **B,** osteoarthrosis; **C,** following arthroplasty.

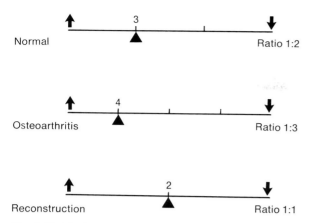

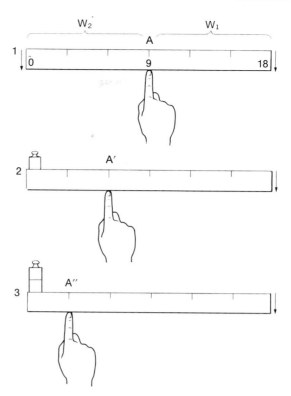

Fig. 3-13. Mechanical principles involved in arthroplasty are shown. Normal hip has ratio of about 1:2, but in osteoarthritis this ratio can change to 1:3 or more. By low-friction arthroplasty (deep socket, small head, and transposition of greater trochanter) it is possible to bring lever ratio to 1:1, thus reducing socket load. (Solid triangles represent socket load in each situation.)

commonly appreciated that the marked external rotation of the hip reduces the distance between the abductor tendons and the center of rotation of the hip; in other words, because of the effective shortening of the abductor moment arm, the muscle must act severely to compensate for this shortening. Therefore, by lateral transposition of the greater trochanter following removal of the external deforming force (short rotators), the effective neck length is increased, thus reducing the demand on the abductors.

As an added bonus in this concept of arthroplasty, with a small diameter head it is possible to place the hip's center of rotation further out medially. At surgery, additional elongation of the abductor moment arm and reduction in the "body-weight moment arm" can be conveniently achieved without excessive damage to the acetabular floor (by deepening).[41]

FRICTIONAL FORCE

The frictional forces acting on the acetabular component of total hip prostheses are dependent on several factors.

1. The magnitude of the resultant compressive force: 2½ to 3 times the body weight

2. The direction of the forces: 15 degrees inclined medially from the vertical

3. The frictional moment and the axes around which they act

4. The geometry of the prostheses (that is, ball

Fig. 3-14. Analogy of hip joint forces as related to changes in lever arm systems. *1,* Beam (18-inch ruler) is balanced on fingertip. Fulcrum point is exactly at midpoint of ruler. Weight transferred to tip of finger is equal to weight of ruler acting at that point *(W₁ + W₂). 2,* By transferring finger (fulcrum) to point *A'* added force is required to balance ruler. *3,* Even greater force is needed for balance if distance between weight and fulcrum on acting moment arm is further reduced (point *A''*). Consequently, forces on fulcrum are proportionately increased, that is, weight of ruler *(W₁ + W₂)* plus weight required to balance beam.

size: the frictional torque is the product of the frictional force acting tangentially to the surface times the radius of the ball; consequently, the smaller the radius, the smaller the frictional torque)

5. The coefficient of friction between the mating surfaces (metal on plastic has a lower frictional coefficient than metal-on-metal devices)

The frictional moments that act on the artificial hip joint have been measured by several investigators. Frictional moments must be considered both in dynamic and static modes, since both situations may apply to human hip joint function.

In the hip simulators using Ringer's solution, synovial fluid, or bovine serum, and under a variety of load conditions, the frictional moments have been measured, as listed in Table 3-5.[105]

83

Table 3-5. Frictional moments measured in Charnley and McKee-Farrar prostheses*

Type of prosthesis	Material of head	Material of cup	Diameter of head (millimeters)	Source of results	Lubricant	Frictional moment in newton-meters (pounds-force-inches) under	
						Constant load of 890 newtons (200 pounds force)	Load varying from 0-890 newtons (0-200 pounds force)
Charnley	Stainless steel	High-density polyethylene	23	Freeman and Swanson	Ringer's solution	0.4-1.2(4-11)	—
					Synovial fluid	0.47 (4.2)	—
				Wilson and Scales	Bovine serum	0.90 (8)	0 hr.: 1.1 (10) 500 hr.:0.67(6)
McKee-Farrar	Cobalt-chromium	Cobalt-chromium	41	Freeman and Swanson	Ringer's solution	17.4 (154)	8.5 (75)
					Bone fat	2.3 (20)	1.7 (15)
					Synovial fluid	8.9 (88)	7.9 (70)
				Wilson and Scales	Bovine serum	4.5 (40)	0 hr.:4.5 (40)
			35	Freeman and Swanson	Synovial fluid	2.7-4.4(24-39)	500 hr.:3.1 (27) —

*From Andersson, G. B. J., Freeman, M. A. R., and Swanson, S. A. V.: J. Bone Joint Surg. **54B**:590-599, 1972.

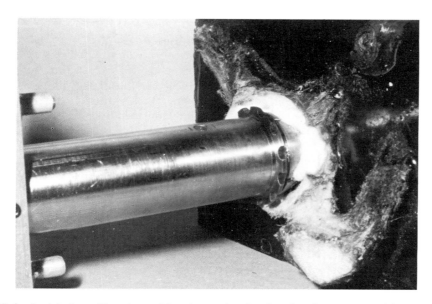

Fig. 3-15. In simulated conditions in our laboratory, pairs of cadaveric pelves were used for comparison of methods of fixation of acetabular component. In simulated conditions pelvis was fixed in epoxy glue (to right) base, while cup was subjected to torque and torn out of its bed. In simulated conditions coining of prepolymerized cement in cadaveric bone, prepared by multiple small holes, produced at least three times better fixation than procedure in which three anchor holes were only sources for fixation mechanism.[47] (See text.)

The strength of the fixation (bond) of the acetabular cup was measured in pairs of cadaveric hemipelves at our laboratory.[47] The figures obtained were in favorable agreement with studies by others (Fig. 3-15). In the experimental situation, cadaveric bone was used and surgical conditions were simulated. The lowest turning moment (in a static situation) required to twist a prosthetic socket loose out of its bone in the tests was 44.5 newton-meters (394 in./lb.), which is more than four times larger than the highest frictional moment (10.4 newton-meters or 92 in./lb. force); serum was used as the lubricant, and more than twice the highest frictional moment than was measured with Ringer's solution was needed. These observations suggest that the frictional moment exerted on the fixation of the cup is unlikely to approach the failure strength of the fixation (cup-cement or cement-bone interface). These conditions may not, however, represent either the surgical conditions, the development of necrosis following the polymerization of the cement (exothermic reaction), or the role played by cyclically applied frictional forces.

Differences in the coefficient of friction between the all metal and metal-plastic total hip designs of today are of such magnitude (Table 3-5) that it is safe to assume that metal-to-metal components will have a greater tendency to cause bone fatigue, thus leading to loosening, than metal-to-plastic designs. A low frictional moment in metal-to-metal prostheses is by far more dependent on the presence of a "designed" lubricating fluid film than in metal-to-plastic designs (mechanism of elastohydrodynamic lubrication); therefore the occasional marked increases in frictional torque resulting from "squeezed out" fluid film in metal-to-metal joints may be responsible for metallic seizures leading to the sudden onset of loosening.

Because the failures in clinical situations occur at the cement-bone interface, efforts are directed to (1) maximizing the bond strength at surgery and (2) preserving supporting bone at the site of fixation (providing the bone is healthy and in continuity). Special attention must be paid to preserving the bone close to the acetabular rim, since it is the periphery of the acetabulum that provides the greatest resistance against the frictional force.

Using a frictional torque comparator pendulum method, Charnley demonstrated the differences between the frictional torque in different prostheses. Tests were performed both in dry and wet conditions; the lowest level of frictional torque was obtained with a 22-mm. stainless steel head against high-density polyethylene and the highest by a metal-to-metal prosthesis of the McKee-Farrar type.[20]

The force required to initiate motion in most bearings is usually larger than that required to maintain it. At a low speed (that is, normal walking) it is expected that poor lubrication will give rise to stick-slip motion, or what is commonly known by engineers as "stiction." Static friction ("stiction friction") differs very little, under physiological conditions, from "dynamic friction" in metal-to-metal as well as metal-to-plastic prostheses, as long as there is a fluid film present between the two components. However, static friction increases significantly after a relatively long-standing period at high load. These frictional forces are usually at least 40 times higher than those generated in normal joints.[99]

FIXATION ELEMENTS AND METHODS

There are at least five conceivable ways by which total hip prosthetic components may be fixed to the bone. There are external plates and screws (fastening), intramedullary spike (stem), chemical adhesive bonding (glue), acrylic cement as a filler (grouting), and porous material (ingrowth of tissue).

Fixation by plate and screws

Fixation of artificial joints with a plate and screws has been discussed extensively in orthopaedic literature. This method has been criticized because of failures owing to varying stress concentrations of materials of different moduli of elasticity at the fixation site.[76] Loss of fixation as the result of motion at the plate-screw-bone site leads to a vicious cycle of bone absorption and necrosis, which, in turn, causes further absorption and necrosis, thus greater loosening.

At the site of fixation, a "shear force" is generated, which acts on the screws and ultimately causes failure at the screw-plate-bone junction. When the frictional resistance between a plate and the underlying bone disappears, the main part of the shearing force acting on the plate will be shifted onto one or more of the screws; the high concentration of stress with further bone necrosis at the site and increased motion leads to the failure of the screw. The entire system will eventually fail as the force is shifted onto the second screw and the pattern of stress concentration is repeated. When a screw is subjected to repeated loading and unloading following a successful operation (such as osteotomy for fracture fixation), the screw generally becomes loose and easily extractable at surgery. This, presumably, is because the bone absorbs under conditions of loading and unloading, allowing further motion of the screw within the bone (Fig. 3-16). However, when screws are inserted and rapid bone union takes place (so that the screw has never actually transmitted any major load), the screws may become tighter than when originally inserted. They may be so difficult to extract at reoperation that their heads may be sheared off in the attempt. This state of affairs may also suggest that bone growth onto the surface of some metals, that is, chromium-cobalt-molybdenum (Vitallium) alloy, has taken place without any intervening fibrous interposition, which is what makes the bond so much stronger. It must be recognized, however, that despite the difficulty of extraction of these screws, microscopically in most instances, some soft tissue has been interposed between the bone and the metal. This type of mechanical fixation is not predictable, since the state of the fixation is dependent on the magnitude and direction of the forces; therefore, in all cases, a fixation of the same magnitude cannot be reproduced for a permanent fixation of prosthetic devices.

Fixation by intramedullary spike (interference fit)

Spike impaction of a tapered stem produces an old engineering action known as "press fit" or interference fit. In a conventional prosthesis, for example, Moore self-locking prosthesis, weight bearing through the collar as well as through the tapered stem and the tip of the stem must be considered. The fenestration could conceivably carry some of the load also.

Load bearing via the collar. When a Thompson prosthesis is inserted by simple interference fit (without interpositioning material such as cement), the collar of the prosthesis rests against the cut end of the femur. It can be demonstrated that motion takes place between the collar of the prosthesis and the cut end of the femur during the loading and unloading of "walking cycles," the stem acting only as a stabilizing element to prevent the prosthesis from tilting. The motion between the prosthesis and the bone seems to be related to the difference of the modules of elasticity between the steel

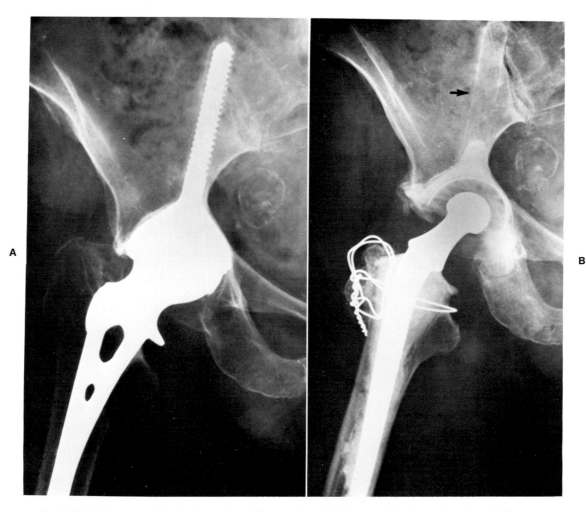

Fig. 3-16. A, Two years following insertion of Ring prosthesis in 64-year-old patient with osteoarthritis. NOTE: marks proximal and distal migration of prosthetic components. NOTE ALSO: lack of bony interdigitation with threads of screw. **B,** Immediately following low-friction arthroplasty. NOTE: smooth track following removal of Ring prosthesis (arrow). At surgery prosthesis was extracted with ease and without any need for turning cup counterclockwise in order to extract it. This is example of bone absorption under conditions of loading and unloading. High-stress concentration and fretting leads to bone necrosis.

and the bone:[100] the module of elasticity of steel is 2.8×10^7 lb./in.² (1.93×10^8 K.N./m.²), and for bone, approximately 2×10^6 lb./in.² (1.38×10^7 K.N./m.²). Since the load is transmitted via the collar and the stem length remains constant as the load is applied, the femur will be shortened by an amount that can be calculated from the load and the elastic modulus and the size of the section of the bone. Assuming that the entire load is transmitted via the collar, and assuming a 15-inch long femur with an external diameter of 1.25 in. and internal diameter of 0.5 in., it can be calculated that the contraction in length of the femur under a load of 150 lb. is 0.001 in.*

According to these calculations, every inch of femur will shorten under load by 0.000066 in.;

---

*Cross-section at area of bone $= \frac{\pi}{4}(1.25^2 - 0.5^2) = 1.026$ in.²

Axial load = 150 lb.; Compressive stress $\frac{150}{1.026} = 146$ lb./in.²

Modulus of elasticity $= 2.2 \times 10^6$ lb./in.² (ranging from 2.9×10^6 lb./in.² to 1.5×10^6 lb./in.²)

Strain $= \frac{146}{2.2 \times 10^6} = 66.3 \times 10^{-6} = 0.000066 \times 15 = 0.00099$ in. (or about $\frac{1}{1,000}$ in.)

87

keeping in mind that the 5-inch length of the stem of the prosthesis under load remains constant and that the corresponding segment of bone will shorten, there must therefore be a fretting movement of 0.00033 between the stem tip and the endosteal surface of the bone. Considering that the load of the hip joint for dynamic and static situations is three times that of the body weight, the actual displacement between the stem and the endosteal surface of the bone would be three times greater, that is, $^1/_{1,000}$ in. or 25 μ. The cyclic loading and unloading causing relative motion between metal and bone

has been inculpated as causing bone absorption. This phenomenon, well-known by engineers as "fretting," causes failure between dissimilar materials under loading conditions. Charnley proposed that this mode of failure under biological conditions could result even if there were no difference in the modulus of elasticity between the two materials (bone and steel); it can therefore be argued that this mode of failure would result even if the prosthesis was made of bone (with a similar modulus of elasticity) because of the persistence of motion (fretting) between the prosthesis and the bone.

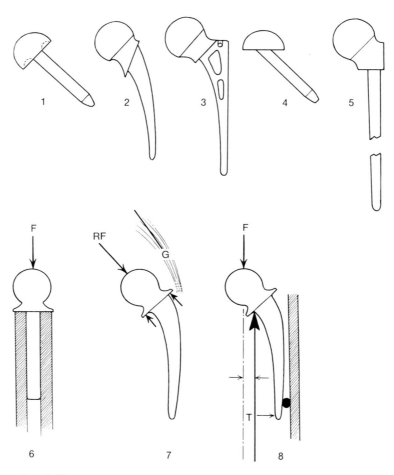

Fig. 3-17. Examples of different neck designs in several prostheses used in past by interference fit. *1,* Original Judet, *2,* Thompson, *3,* Moore self-locking, *4,* modified Judet, and *5,* Leinbach. Ideal inclination of neck depends entirely on efficiency of abductor mechanism. For example, *6* illustrates prosthesis with collar that is most efficient if abductor pull is not present; *7* illustrates that if abductor pull is normal, plane of collar should be at 90 degrees to resultant forces, *RF.* Compare direction of forces of *7* with *6. 8,* Illustrates resultant forces acting on intramedullary stem prosthesis. Vertical load, *F,* causes bending moment in absence of abductor muscle tending to turn prosthesis into varus direction. Force, *T,* neutralizes moment of force, *F,* tending to rotate prosthesis. Schematic drawing illustrates major compressive forces being present at calcar and lateral side of prosthesis.

When examining the loading of the upper femur via the collar of the prosthesis, the role played by the length of the neck must also be considered. If the resultant forces (pull of the abductors and the body weight load) are in equilibrium—with force directed to the neck of the femur—the length of the neck will have no effect on the forces applied to the cut end of the femur (Fig. 3-17). On the other hand, when the abductors are weak, the resultant forces would be more vertical and the long neck would increase the pressure on the calcar; conversely, a short neck would reduce the pressure caused by weight bearing.

It is also important to note that absorption of bone occurs under the vertical load as well as under the stress produced by any tangential movement; therefore the collar of the prosthesis must be ideally inclined so as to distribute the load throughout the cut surface of the femur and prohibit tangential movement. The ideal inclination, as already mentioned, will depend entirely on the efficiency of the abductor power. For example, if the abductor muscles and their epiphyses are normal, the plane of the collar should be at 90 degrees toward the resultant forces (Fig. 3-17),[19] but as the abductor system becomes more defective, the inclination of the collar must approach a more horizontal angle.

Load transmission via tapered stem. The previous discussion was relative to the assumption that the collar was the sole transmitter of the load. Now let us imagine a prosthesis without a collar, in which a tapered 5-inch stem is driven into the medullary cavity; as an example, one can calculate that if the tapering of the stem is $1:7$ (1 in. proximally to 0.14 in. at the tip) and a 120 lb. patient loads such a prosthesis, the total transverse force available to dilate the femoral canal will be $120 \times 3 \times 7 = 2,520$ lb. Assuming the surfaces to be plane, and assuming the wedge to be 5/16 in. (0.3126 in.) in thickness and the whole length (both medial and lateral surfaces) to be in firm contact with bone, the area of contact would be approximately $5 \times 2 \times 0.313$, equal to 3.13 in.^{2} given a stress on the bone of $3.13/2,520 = 800$ lb./in.^{2}. Quite obviously, the fretting movements (as the result of the "wedge action" of such a theoretical prosthesis) would be considerable, and failure would result from sinking, unless the cut end of the femur comes in contact with a collar that would prevent further subsidence of the pros-

thesis or further sinking stops in a new position owing to "lock wedge."

In addition to simple compressive forces acting on the femoral canal and the endosteal surface of the bone by the wedge action of a polished tapered stem, the shear loading may also be achieved by employing a prosthesis with a roughened exterior (serrations), with such a fixation that it would keep the stress below the bone's shear strength. Such a theoretical prosthesis may be impossible to extract (because of fibrous bone ingrowth) without damage to the bone should its removal become necessary.[13,31]

Weight bearing via the stem tip and fenestration. The best results in fixation by intramedullary interference fit are achieved in cases where weight transmission is shared by the collar and the tip of the stem as well as the bone of fenestration. This optimum situation is usually achieved when the prosthesis has fallen (tilted) into a varus or valgus orientation (Fig. 3-18). In these cases, a local strengthening of the cortex testifies to elements of weight-bearing phenomena (Wolff's law). This situation is often observed after a period of sinking and usually occurs in strong, active patients with good functional capacity.

It is conceivable, however, that the cancellous bone of the trochanteric region growing into the fenestration of Moore self-locking prosthesis might withstand some vertical stress and also resist the action of rotary forces (Fig. 3-18). Unfortunately, this has been observed in only a few cases because the fretting movement and high-stress concentration between the prosthesis and the bone cannot be entirely eliminated. When the bone in the fenestration is visible by x-ray films—and even when the fenestration is completely obliterated by bone—it is doubtful that a true state of locking exists. Despite difficulties encountered in the removal of such a prosthesis (that is, Moore self-locking prosthesis with bone growth or fenestration), definite motion between the prosthesis and the bone is frequently observed (Fig. 3-18).

Another fixation concept that is attractive to some surgeons is the use of a longer prosthetic stem to maximize fixation, but, as stated before, because the collar is the main weight-bearing region, the fact remains that the stem offers no advantage except to prevent a valgus-varus angulation. It can even be argued that an extremely long-stem prosthesis, such as the Match-

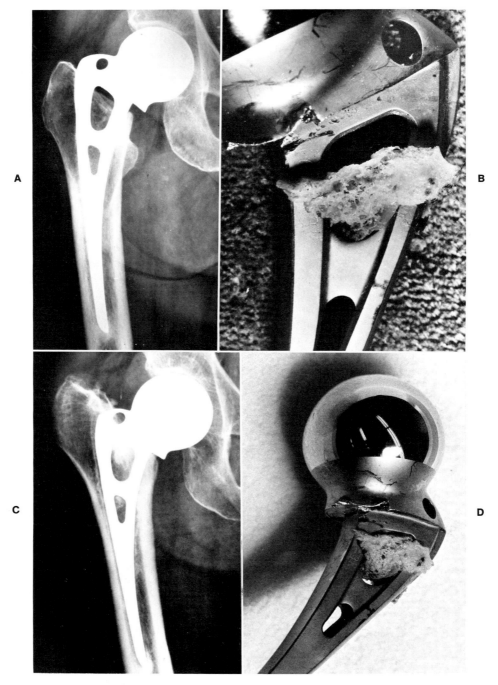

Fig. 3-18. A, Four years following successful Moore self-locking prosthesis inserted for fracture of neck of femur. Weight-bearing film shows space between top end of femur and collar of prosthesis. NOTE: weight-bearing zone at tip of prosthesis indicating fact that although weight bearing is eliminated from collar, it is shared by tip of stem and tapered segment of stem. **B,** Considerable violent trauma was necessary to extract this prosthesis despite gross motion (wobble) noted at surgery. **C,** Example of "sunk-in" prosthesis that has eventually stabilized itself by same mechanism shown in **A**. Observe extreme neck absorption prior to stabilization of prosthesis. It is presumed that stabilization was achieved by 3-point fixation of tapered segment and tip as well as bone of fenestration. **D,** Considerable difficulty experienced while extracting this prosthesis. No detectable motion was observed at surgery. (See text.)

et-Brown prosthesis, increases the amplitude of fretting movements. For example, the amplitude of fretting at the tip of a 15-inch stem is three times as much as at that of a 5-inch stem —thus a greater range of motion is transferred to a further distal zone with resultant increased fretting movement and bone necrosis without preventing loosening.[19]

Fixation by the use of glue

Arguments supporting the search for an ideal substance to act as an adhesive or glue may be conceived; however, a glue may not be practical[78] to apply because:

1. Chemical interaction would be needed between the substance and the bone—indicating that the "glue" must be partially water soluble.

2. The allergic and toxic effects of many available adhesives prohibit their use.

3. Adhesive mating parts must be tightly conjoined with a thin layer of adhesive in between them, but because of the variations in the sizes of human bones, a precise mating between the prosthetic and bone surfaces cannot be achieved (Fig. 3-19, *A*).

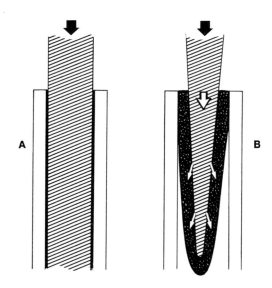

Fig. 3-19. Comparative mechanism of fixation by glue, **A,** and by grouting materials, **B. A,** Adhesive mating parts must be tightly conjoined with thin layer of adhesive between them. When grouting material such as acrylic cement is used, cavity is broached oversized and filled with doughlike material that makes accurate cast or mold of rough interior surface of bone. Thus inserted prosthesis acts as an integral part of cement, that is, "cement-prosthesis unit." Increased external surface area and greater resistance against compressive and shearing forces can be achieved, **B.**

4. With progressive chemical interaction, absorption of the material would ultimately occur —as living osseous tissue would replace or insulate it with fibrous tissue—leading to the failure of the chemical bond. Some experiments currently in progress suggest the possible usefulness of materials known as "bioglasses" to be successfully utilized as glue in a biological situation. These materials will form a direct bond to both soft and hard tissues.

Fixation by grouting "filler"

In contrast to a glue, an inert material such as quick-setting acrylic cement is interpositioned in bulk between the two parts and acts as a "grout" or a "filler." Therefore:

1. No chemical interaction is necessary between the cement and the bone. A thin layer of fibrous acellular-like base membrane or fibrocartilaginous membrane will act as an ultimate weight-bearing medium. This interposed layer's biological characteristics may become altered as a result of load bearing, but it remains noninvasive as long as the fixation is optimal between bone and cement (Fig. 3-19, *B*).

2. The bone cavity does not have to be perfectly shaped to accept the prosthesis; instead, it is broached "oversize" and then filled with the doughlike cement, which makes an accurate cast or mold of the rough interior of the bone.

3. The inserted prosthesis acts as an integral part of the cement, that is, cement-prosthesis unit.

4. As stated before, by increasing the total surface area of the cement (exterior), the cement-prosthesis unit presents a greater surface area with which to resist shearing forces under axial loads (Fig. 3-20).

5. The increased external surface area and greater resistance against the shearing forces presents an ideal situation for elderly patients with severe osteoporosis.

6. Undoubtedly, the interpositioning fibrous layer (regardless of how thin it is) must produce a relative movement between the cement and bone. However, the amplitude of the movement (coupled with the elastic behavior of the layer of bone) is of such a small degree that it has no deleterious effects (fretting) on the bond.

7. The rough exterior of the cement-prosthesis unit might be expected to produce a rasping action against the rough interior surface of the bone. This does not occur, however, because the

91

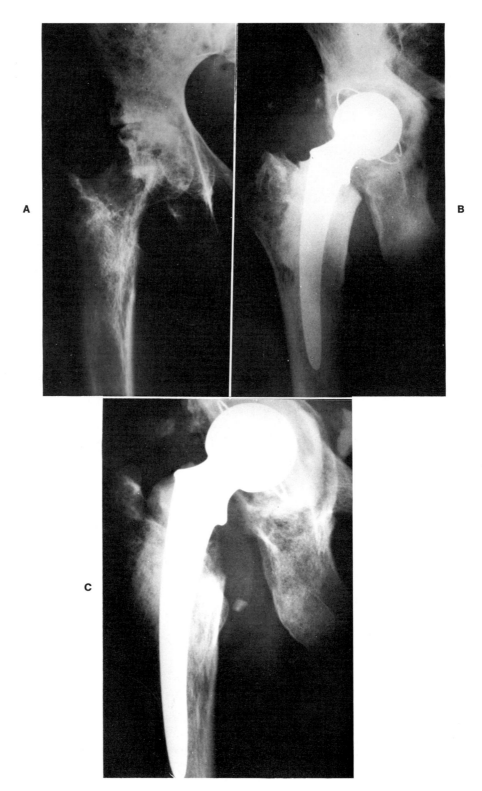

Fig. 3-20. For legend see opposite page.

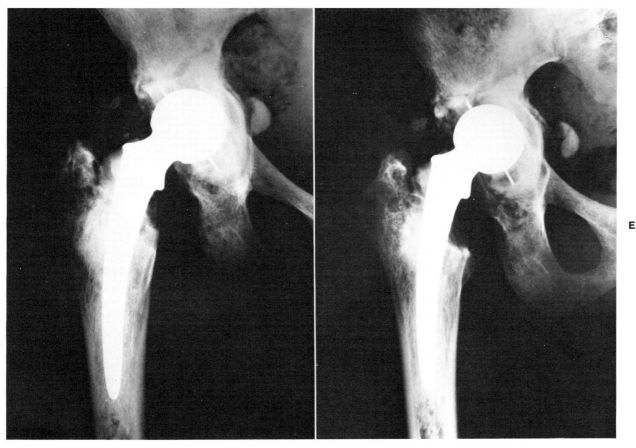

D

E

Fig. 3-20. By increasing total surface area of prosthesis by use of cement (cement-prosthesis unit), axial compressive and shearing forces are tolerated. **A,** Right hip of patient with sickle cell disease, avascular necrosis, and multiple infarcts. **B,** Six months after hip replacement. **C,** Fifteen months after hip replacement. **D,** Twenty-four months after surgery. **E,** Thirty months after surgery. NOTE: progressive bone absorption in region of calcar as well as progressive loosening around acetabulum. Despite precarious support by calcar, distal stem is still capable of weight bearing. This is good example of cement acting as "filler," transmitting load via tapered segment.

vertical and shearing stresses are neutralized by the very intimate "keying" of the fibrous layer filling the space between the two[13,31] (Fig. 3-21).

8. Regardless of the type of tissue presented at the interface (fibrous or metaplastic cartilage), thin or thick, the bone remains uninterrupted since no firm "gluing" exists between the two parts. Fig. 3-21 illustrates how the elastic behavior of the interface allows recoiling after the release of force in a nonconfined space.

The role of fixation via cement may be summarized as follows:

1. With acrylic cement, the total contact zone between the prosthesis and bone is increased, improving stress distribution from the prosthesis to the bone.

2. Compressive stresses, which approximate the failure limits of compressive bone strength, are considerably reduced.

3. Fretting—the cause of progressive implant loosening—is minimized when cement is used.

4. The elastic "fibrocartilaginous-bone layer" is an excellent medium for the transmission of a load—providing it acts as an "elastic system" at that level, allowing only "controlled motion" between cement and bone (Fig. 3-21).

Energy (peak) must be dissipated in viscoelastic or elastic elements or it will destroy the bone (damping effect). This analogy is similar to the analogous periodontal ligament in fixation of a tooth in the bone. The major argu-

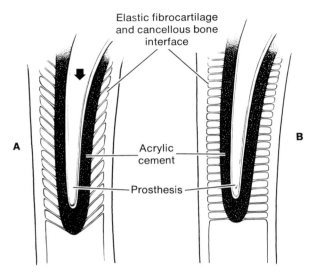

Elastic fibrocartilage
and cancellous bone
interface

A

B

Acrylic
cement

Prosthesis

Fig. 3-21. Elastic fibrocartilaginous bone layer works intimately at interface to produce excellent medium for transmission of load when cement is used. Successful fixation via such a medium will be permanent providing it acts as elastic system at that level allowing only controlled motion under, **A,** loading and, **B,** unloading. Energy must be dissipated in viscoelastic elements of interface or it will destroy bone. **A,** Schematic drawing of elastic behavior of loaded prosthetic cement interface. **B,** Illustrates the rocolle (system unloaded).

ment against cement is the requirement for a strict and perfect technique of application at the time of insertion—the bond must be perfect or failure will result. The bony support must also be adequate to withstand the compressive forces transmitted to it via the cement. Once the loosening is initiated, further bone damage and further loosening are the eventual outcomes, and the fixation will not usually be improved by nonoperative means. The other criticism of cement is its rather poor mechanical property in "tension" (see Modes of failure, pp. 109 and 127).

Fixation by porous material

Fixation has been a fundamental issue in total hip replacement during the past decade, and numerous investigations have explored the use of porous material into which bone could grow to provide a good fixation for total prosthetic devices. There are various materials and several processes for producing porous aggregates that serve this purpose; the processes are generally applicable to both metals and ceramics, but porous aggregates are usually derived from others, initially consolidated and shaped in molding dies under pressure. Along with several investigators, Galante has shown the feasibility of

using a sintered titanium fiber aggregate for the fixation of the prosthesis to the bone.[61] Mechanical fixation is provided by the bone growing into the void spaces of the metallic composite.

Laboratory experimentation has demonstrated the practicability of using the sintered titanium fiber aggregate with optimization of the pore size to allow adequate ingrowth of bone into the material; in clinical practice, however, one of the fundamental problems is the need for "immediate" fixation after the implantation of the artificial hip joint. Operations of this type are usually performed on older people and require early ambulation in order to avoid complications, therefore ingrowth fixation, which requires nonweight bearing for good results, is undesirable in this regard. Secondly, the "permanent fixation" is theoretically objectionable since mutilation would be required to remove such a prosthesis if it should become necessary.

This type of fixation for joint replacement is being evaluated in several centers. When a controlled mechanism for bone absorption or formation is established, this method may ultimately replace all other methods of fixation for a permanent bonding of the prosthesis to the bone.

DESIGN OF RECONSTRUCTION (OPERATION)

Whenever possible, arthroplasty procedures should include a change in the force distribution in the hip joint to reduce the total load on the artificial joint; this concept obviously differs from simply replacing the joint by a mechanical device. The principles of force redistribution have already been discussed and are of considerable importance—as pointed out by Pauwels, Paul, Charnley, Blount, and others.* It can be argued that the equalization of the ratio of levers (length of abductor lever divided by length of the body weight lever) is fundamental in reducing the demand on the abductors, despite many surgeons' "satisfaction" with total hip arthroplasty without an attempt to equalize the lever-arm system. The beneficial effect of reducing the forces acting on the hip joint has already been discussed, and an example of reduction of forces by surgery is illustrated (Figs. 3-13 and 3-14).

In a comparative study of the lever system after low-friction arthroplasty and McKee-Farrar arthroplasty, it was found that routine medializa-

---

*See references 3, 7, 23, 63, 87-90, 93, and 94.

tion of the socket and lateral transfer of the greater trochanter reduce the load on the artificial joint by about 12% of the body weight. While it is not absolutely essential to restore or improve the lever arms about the hip to obtain good results (limp-free walking and freedom from pain) following the replacement of the hip joint, it would seem safe to suppose that the reduction of the load on the socket by as much as 12% would have a beneficial effect on prolonged fixation and perhaps result in the reduction of metal fatigue and its rate of wear.[41]

The varus or valgus orientation of the stem in the shaft of the femur and the length of its neck undoubtedly affect the medialization of the center of rotation. It can be said that a short neck places the shaft further medially, thereby reducing the socket load, but a valgus position of the prosthesis in the shaft increases the socket load by decreasing the abductor moment (the distance between the center of the rotation of the head and the abductor pull). Obviously, the transfer of the greater trochanter's position can compensate (to some degree) for the valgus orientation of the stem in the shaft.

In the design of the low-friction arthroplasty procedure, several closely related ideas have been incorporated.

The principal features include:
1. Use of a small-diameter femoral head
2. Reconstruction of the hip joint through the lateral displacement of the abductor pull
3. Medialization of the center of rotation by deepening the socket

In addition to these procedures, allowance for subluxation, which the small head accomplishes, provides a "safety valve" for the fixation elements (see Chapter 17), thus reducing the forces transmitted to the fixed prosthesis.

Considering the influence of the unit load (pressure) and the relative velocity on the rate of wear of the bearing, the reduction of the load may be of considerable importance; therefore, in theory, any means of reducing the load will reduce the wear and prolong the life of the socket. While awaiting the results of studies on comparable wear rates and mechanical failure (for example, related to femoral head size), it is good practice to utilize measures that might prolong the life of the artificial joint in the body. With regard to wear and loosening, the results of the first 10 years of using Charnley's low-friction arthroplasty were encouraging enough to warrant the continued use of the existing design until data from other prosthetic types (with larger heads and without equalization of the lever-arm system) become available.

PROSTHESIS DESIGN FEATURES

Several interrelated aspects must be considered in the design of the total hip prosthesis.
1. Its anatomical adaptation and surgical feasibility
2. Reduction of forces acting on the artificial hip joint
3. Mechanical optimization of wear, friction, strength, and so on

Good clinical results obtained with a simple ball-and-socket design with surfaces exposed to the tissue fluid make it unnecessary to propose a more complicated design for an artificial hip joint—such as engineering bearings of a more complex nature, carrying lubricant sealed under a flexible diaphragm. The more complex joints proposed by engineers may have some attractive features, but present failure hazards—through exposing the tissue to foreign materials (that is, lubrication fluids)—are a risk and may engender unexpected reactions. As previously noted, a metal-to-metal bearing has its own limitations: friction is increased; surfaces may possibly seize; dissimilar metals may cause electrochemical reaction; and, since metals are hard and noncompliant, they do not lend themselves to the absorption of energy at the joint level.

Metal against plastic, on the other hand, produces a most satisfactory bearing for human artificial hip joints because of a very close coaptation occurring between the metal and the plastic, resulting in a "self-lubrication" bearing system. This mechanism, known as an "elasto-hydrodynamic system," eliminates the need for tissue fluid as a lubricant: such a system also reduces frictional torque, which is of primary concern in preventing loosening under extremely strenuous conditions.[12] The wear debris generated in this system (high-density polyethylene vs. metal) appears to be well tolerated by local tissue.[18,21]

In the present design of the prosthesis the following features must be considered: head size, socket design, neck design, and stem design.

Size of the head

The role of a small-diameter head in medialization has already been discussed. The variables relating to the head size include: load per unit area; frictional torque, distance required to be travelled during movement by a given point on the surface of the femoral head against the socket, thickness of the socket required to withstand wear, volume of wear debris (volumetric wear) generated influencing tissue reaction, and speed of penetration of the femoral head into the thickness of the socket (linear wear). These interrelated matters of design should be considered when choosing the size of the femoral head. Charnley has remained faithful to the 22-mm. femoral head because of his "Teflon wear" experience. He considers the small head an important feature of the design because it allows the surgeon to employ a thick plastic socket. The 22-mm. head has clinically proved satisfactory, without the risk of rapid penetration into the socket or fear of instability (see Chapter 17), allowing for a socket 10 mm. or more in thickness even where the anatomy is restricted by a small acetabulum. On the other hand, with a large femoral head—32 to 50 mm.—the socket must be thin; conceivably, elastic deformation under load may eventually disturb the fixation. Thick plastic may act as an energy absorber and enhance eventual fixation under the load.

It has been argued that a small head reduces the frictional torque, thus alleviating the strain at the bond; also, minor degrees of subluxation between the femoral head and the socket in extreme ranges of motion can occur, which reduce the force transmitted to the socket. As stated previously, a transient subluxation of the head against the posterior wall provides a "safety valve," allowing the head to escape from the socket more readily than a large femoral head.[23]

Socket design

The plastic socket must accommodate the femoral head with clearance enough to allow free movement but without excessive dimensions that will create a "sloppy fit." Sockets are generally manufactured by machinery, but recently plastic molding has been introduced as an acceptable method. When manufactured, the socket's concavity (articulating surface) is not mechanically polished and appears dull on inspection; polishing generally takes place after the socket has been implanted in the body by "bed-in" phenomena resulting from pressure and wear introduced via the femoral head. The thickness of the socket in any given situation is complementary to the diameter of the head; therefore in a design

with a small diameter head, a thicker plastic socket is possible, allowing for the anatomical restrictions caused by the smallness of the acetabulum.

Conceptually, an acentric concavity within the cup yielding an extra thickness of plastic in the weight-bearing area is an attractive idea, but its employment is usually complicated by the resultant undesirable features:

1. The inferior portion of the plastic remains thin, inviting possible plastic deformation.

2. With the extreme wear of the socket the femur neck will impinge on the socket rim, actually prying the socket loose before the full thickness of the socket is completely worn. Teflon sockets wore out; in most cases, loosening *preceded* complete socket wear.

The periphery of the socket may be serrated for additional fixation (as in the original Charnley design) or a smooth and broadened rim may be designed to facilitate the injection of cement into the acetabulum at insertion. Grooves on the outer aspect of the socket of commonly used prostheses are usually adequate for its fixation to the cement. As a rule, the greater the outer diameter of the socket, the better the fixation; this is because of the increased total contact surface and a greater radius to resist rotary forces. A radiographic wire marker clipped to the outer aspect of the cup assists in the measurement of wear and orientation.

Neck design

The prosthetic neck must be sufficiently strong (adequately thick) but should allow angular motion with no encroachment against the socket rim. Using a simple three-dimensional protractor, one can demonstrate the range of motion of an artificial hip joint when the socket is fixed at the basic 45 degrees orientation without forward or backward tilt. Using such a protractor, one can demonstrate that:

1. The smaller the diameter of the neck, the greater the range of motion without impingement against the socket

2. The greater the recession of the neck, the greater the range of motion without impingement against the socket

3. The greater the head-neck diameter ratio, the greater the range of motion without impingement

4. The smaller the socket depth-ball ratio, the greater the range of motion without impinge-

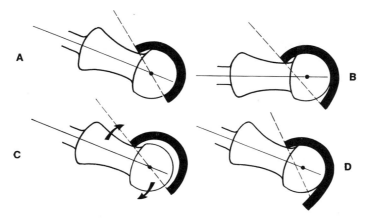

Fig. 3-22. Mechanism of dislocation by neck socket impingement. **A,** Neck socket contact (angle of dislocation) if center of ball is in same plane as mouth of cup. **B,** Greater stability of hip is achieved by placing head deep to edge of cup. **C,** Deepening of socket increases neck socket impingement but does not alter angle of dislocation (similar to angle of dislocation in **A**). **D,** Long posterior wall of prosthesis (Charnley prosthesis) allows subluxation without loss of contact between ball and socket.

ment (An elliptical neck, such as in the Aufranc-Turner or Chamfering prostheses [T-28], of the socket rim is also aimed at increased flexion without impingement.) (Fig. 3-22).

Simulating the range of motion of a total hip prosthesis with a three-dimensional protractor shows that any degree of abduction relieves the neck from impingement,[1,3] which is helpful, because in normal functional activities the hip joint assumes the position of abduction and some external rotation occurs as the flexion is maximized (Fig. 3-22). In Charnley's 22-mm. prosthetic head (in order to ensure strength at the junction of the sphere and the neck) the thinnest portion of the neck is placed inside the contour of the sphere. The range of angular motion is dependent on the diameter of the neck at its point of junction with the sphere. Because of this and because the bending moment on the neck is increased (the farther the narrow section of the neck is from the center of the ball), the best place for the narrowest part of the neck is inside the circumference of the ball (Figs. 3-22 and 3-23).

Increasing the depth of the socket by 2 mm. also increases its resistance to dislocation without changing the "angle of impingement," a fact that is often not considered when comparing the stability of a small head to that of a large one (Fig. 3-23). Additionally, an extended posterior wall is designed to augment stability in flexion, thus resistance (Fig. 3-24) against dislocation or subluxation (see Chapter 17). In a comparative study of the range of motion of various pros-

theses, Amstutz and his co-workers demonstrated that the neck-socket contact angle varies significantly in maximum flexion and abduction for different prostheses that were tested, and that the test results indicated that the performances of most of the prostheses were only marginally acceptable in flexion. Further, as expected, several millimeters of socket wear decreases the range of motion and thus may increase wear at the point of contact between the neck and the socket.[1,3] Although in practice "socket-rim wear" has not produced any problems (such as dislocation), these goniometric studies amplify the importance of orienting the components properly at surgery to avoid impingements in extreme ranges of motion such as neck-socket contact (Fig. 3-25).

Stem design

The intramedullary stem of a total hip prosthesis must have the following characteristics:

1. A configuration and size that fits the anatomical shape of the upper femur

2. Dimensions that do not exceed the narrowest segment of the shaft (isthmus)

3. A degree of tapering that facilitates cement injection

4. Resistance against rotational and compressive forces

5. A size (selected for a given case) that allows the use of acrylic cement as a thick layer—especially at the medial (concave) side of the prosthesis in the calcar region

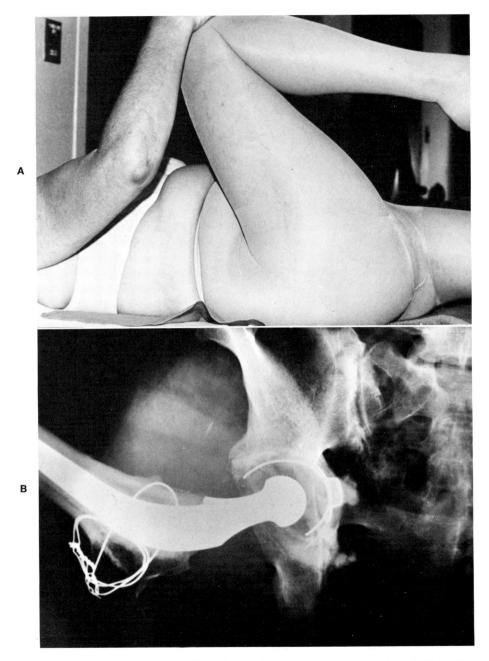

Fig. 3-23. A and **B,** Postoperative status of low-friction arthroplasty performed for osteoarthritis in 58-year-old woman who has achieved good range of motion following arthroplasty. **A,** With right hip in maximum flexion, anteroposterior radiograph of pelvis and hip is obtained. NOTE: head of prosthesis has remained within depth of socket, **B,** without subluxation despite flexion beyond 90 degrees. **C,** With left hip in maximum flexion (approximately 135 degrees) x-ray film, **D,** reveals head remaining completely within depth of socket. It is possible a few degrees of abduction and external rotation relieve neck socket impingement in addition to capsule, which tightens at extreme motions by twisting along its axis, thus retaining (stabilizing) head at depth of socket.

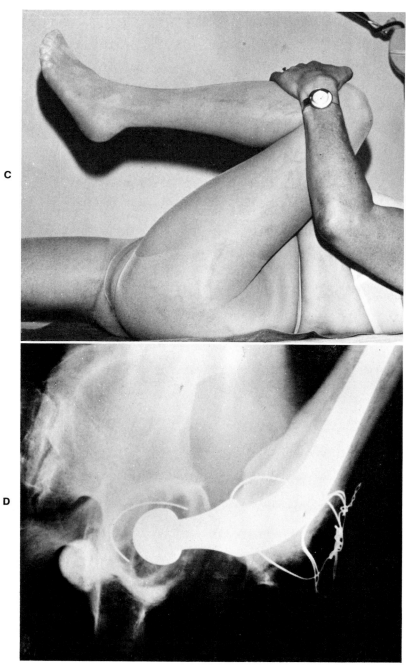

Fig. 3-23, cont'd. For legend see opposite page.

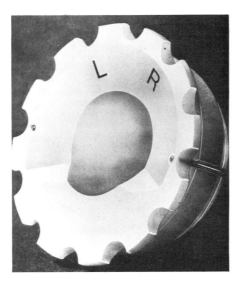

Fig. 3-24. Long posterior wall of socket provides platform for head, preventing momentary subluxation or dislocation in extreme ranges of flexion.

6. Sufficient strength to withstand cyclic long-term loading

7. A length that allows adequate fixation via its tapered segment, but not one that is so long that it jeopardizes optimal orientation in the canal (double curve of femur) (It should only be long enough to prevent varus and valgus tilt.)

Obviously, the design and shape of the stem influence the mechanical behavior of the prosthesis inside the shaft. The tensile stress (at the lateral surface) of the stem is directly proportional to the bending moment, but inversely related to the section modulus of the stem.

The metallurgical composition and processing of the stem may greatly influence its strength—an essential feature in total hip arthroplasty in heavy and younger patients. The continuous bending moments around the stem are influenced by the stem-shaft angle and the neck length of the prosthesis; so, in order to minimize

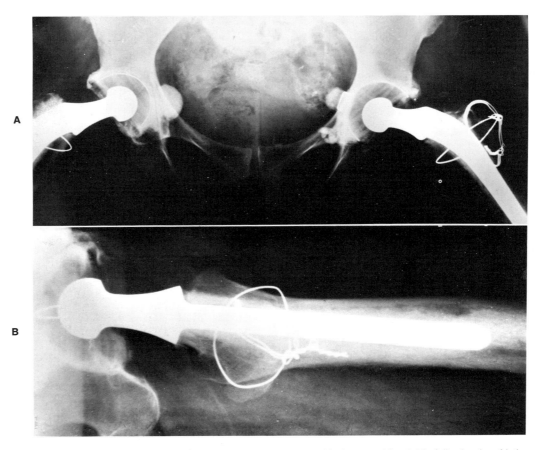

Fig. 3-25. A, Excellent range of motion is achieved in patient with rheumatoid arthritis following low-friction arthroplasty. This 36-year-old female was able to abduct to 45 degrees in each hip. **B,** Manfredi lateral radiograph of left hip illustrating position of "neutroversion" of both components.

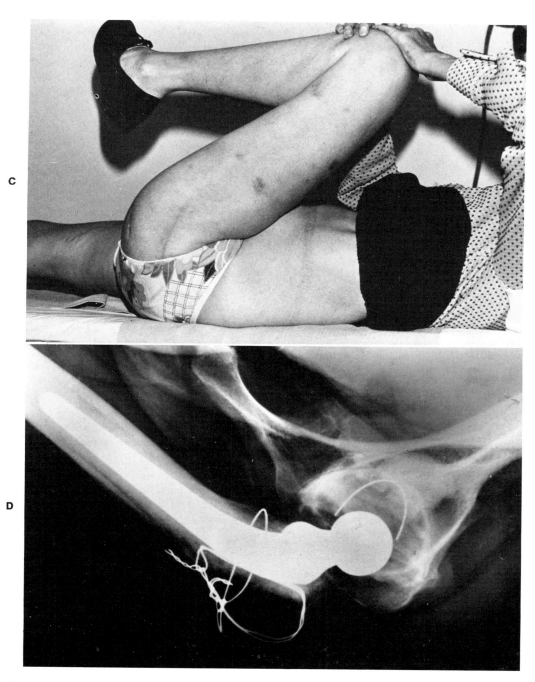

Fig. 3-25, cont'd. C, Extreme range of flexion of left hip 1 year following surgery. It should be noted that once hip reaches approximately 90 degrees of flexion, it assumes slight external rotation and abduction position, which should relieve impingement of neck against socket. **D,** Shoot-through (Manfredi lateral) radiograph is attempted while hip has remained in maximum flexion as in **C.** There is suggestion of possible migration of head out of depth of socket but supported by long posterior wall of socket. (See text.)

101

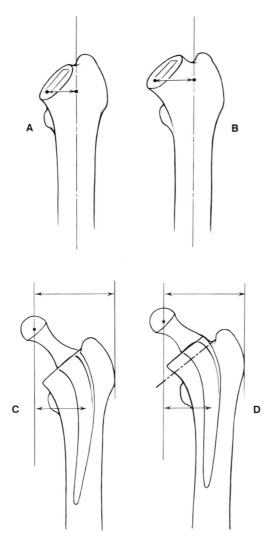

Fig. 3-26. A, Low- and, **B,** high-level amputation of neck for insertion of prosthesis. **C** and **D,** Short-neck prosthesis used with long femoral neck stump favorably compares with short-neck stump and long-neck prosthesis. Combination of short-neck prosthesis and long stump of neck is preferred. Bending moment created on both stems is same, **C** and **D;** however improved support by bone is achieved in **D.**

the bending stresses on the stem, there should be a minimum offset between the center of the head and the axis of the prosthetic stem (Fig. 3-26). The offset of the Charnley prosthesis in profile is considerably greater than either the Müller or McKee-Farrar designs[16,25] (Charnley, 4.3 cm.; Müller, 2.9 cm.; McKee, 2.6 cm.). (Charnley selected a 4.3 cm. offset in the original design, with a neck-shaft angle of 130 degrees.) Aiming for maximum deepening at sur-

gery, a shaft-neck angle of this size allows the head to reach the depth of the socket during adduction or abduction without impingement, particularly in a heavy, bony man with a considerably enlarged acetabulum and muscle bulk. Such a prosthesis still allows the surgeon to place a stem into the shaft in a favorable position, that is, a slight valgus orientation, without fear that the center of the head will be displaced too far out of the socket depth. At the present time, prostheses with a reduced shaft offset (that is, more neck-shaft valgus orientation) are preferred. The crux of the problem lies in the optimization of the neck-shaft angle, which would minimize the bending moments and also allow the head to reach the depth of the acetabulum with the stem in a slight valgus orientation. It is obviously useless to consider the strength of the prosthesis and its design outside the context of its fixation to the shaft of the femur with acrylic cement[22,59]; special attention must be paid not only to the prosthesis itself, but also to its support by the cement inside the medullary canal, especially in the calcar region. Failure results from the lack of fixation between cement and bone at the concave side of the prosthesis within the upper shaft of the femur; this must be borne in mind if the prosthesis' design is so thick that it fits flush, without space for cement insertion. A trapezoidal or cross-section, in addition to gradual tapering of the stem, seems to be an important aid in wedging the cement peripherally into the cortical and cancellous bone while it is being driven into the cemented canal. A prosthesis with a fin or phlange, for example, Charnley's cobra phlanged stem, provides the ability to forcibly inject cement into the upper and medial femoral canal, in addition to providing added strength on the tension side of the prosthesis. Because of the variation in the size of the femoral shaft in different individuals, it is advisable to choose a slightly smaller stem rather than the thickest possible stem that can be fitted to allow a slight valgus orientation or to avoid varus tendency, which often prevails in a tight canal; such a system provides an adequate thickness of cement on the concave side of the prosthesis where the most support is needed. It does not seem advantageous to increase the dimensions of the stem to a degree above the fatigue failure limits, since this reduces the thickness of the cement layer on the medial side (see "Modes of Failure of Total Hip Prostheses," p. 106).

WEAR, FRICTION, AND LUBRICATION IN ARTIFICIAL JOINTS

In the context of total hip replacement, the science concerned with lubrication, friction, and wear (tribology) is aimed at the design of a joint that performs satisfactorily with a minimum wear rate. Wear debris volume is a product of load and distance travel of rubbing surfaces. This influences the nature and extent of subsequent wear, which affects the overall performance of the artificial joint. In a biological environment such as the human hip joint, the potential hazards of short- or long-term body reaction to wear debris cannot be overemphasized.

Wear is defined as the deterioration of a surface owing to the usage of the mating surfaces; its nature may be adhesive, abrasive, or fatigue.

Adhesive wear is a result of the shearing of microwelds at the points of contact, so that a fragment is released from one or both surfaces as a by-product. Abrasive wear occurs at the high points between the mating surfaces with one scratching the other, releasing small fragments. Fatigue wear is due to a localized point of fatigue at the surface.

Wear is measured by:

1. The weight of the specimen before and after the test, or the measurement of the particulate matter released from the surfaces (When a continuous lubrication system is in use, the wear by-product can be filtered and the wear measured by the weight of the filter.)

2. The measurement of a replica of the surface of the worn segments

3. The direct measurement of the components' wear when removed from patients in clinical situations such as at surgery or in postmortem specimens (the most reliable measurement)

Wear and friction are entirely independent phenomena. Wear is the loss or removal of particles from the bearing surfaces following relative motion between them; friction, on the other hand, is the relative resistance to displacement of one surface to the other. Close studies indicate that friction shows no unique correlation with wear. In other words, low friction can coexist with a high wear rate and low wear with high friction. A good example is Teflon, which shows a low coefficient of friction but a high wear rate. Another example of an inverse relationship between wear and friction is the wear rate of a metal-against-metal prosthesis, which is low under biological conditions, but whose friction coefficient is high.[112]

The best material for total hip arthroplasty should have a low wear rate and a low friction coefficient, the latter being essential in reducing the torque of the artificial joint. Laboratory and clinical data suggest that high molecular weight polyethylene-against-metal appears to be an appropriate combination.

Laboratory wear of HDP (high-density polyethylene)

In the past decade there have been numerous laboratory investigational efforts using different methods of testing and lubrication to measure the wear rate of high-density polyethylene.* The accelerated wear machine is widely used to test this highly wear-resistant plastic and lubricants in industry, but the "accelerated wear" of artificial joints in the laboratory is not a true representation of the clinical situation, since neither the speed of wear nor the type of lubrication can be made to closely duplicate human conditions. This fact may be borne out by comparing recent in vivo calculations of wear with UMWHDP (ultra molecular weight high-density polyethylene) laboratory test results.

In addition to mechanical factors such as load and velocity, several other factors may affect the wear of an artificial hip joint, including:

1. The surface quality (finish) of the prosthetic component
2. The sphericity of the femoral head
3. The clearance between the ball and the socket
4. The diameter of the femoral head

Gold and Walker[62] reported various wear results by studying several types of prosthesis in the hip joint simulator. They found that the amount of frictional torque was proportional to the diameter (22 mm., 28 mm., and 32 mm.) of the prosthetic head. The wear of the plastic in all tests did not vary by a factor of more than 3.

The wear rates of the Charnley stainless steel and cobalt-chromium joints were about the same. The 28-mm. diameter head wore less than the 22-mm. head, whereas the 32-mm. head was no better than a 28-mm. head. There was no difference in wear between joints with a clearance of 0.004 in. and 0.020 in. A lack of sphericity of up to 450 microinches in the femoral com-

---

*See references 24, 29, 30, 34, 56-58, 97, and 111.

ponent did not cause any significant increase in wear. The ideal surface finish was considered to be 2 to 3 microinches.

Other studies, however, indicated that, of the conventionally available materials, Vitallium alloy against ultra-high molecular weight polyethylene offers the lowest wear rate; stainless steel produces a higher rate than Vitallium alloy, and titanium alloy produces the highest wear rate. Among the materials tested, "irradiated high-density polyethylene" showed an increased wear resistance; the wear of ceramics was very high in these tests, making it unsuitable for prosthetic replacement.[56-58]

Despite the poor prospects for ceramics (low tensile and poor yield strength), ceramic hardness is higher than metals and polymers. Therefore at present, considerable interest is being shown in developing these materials for bearing surfaces. Under investigation include high-purity alumina (aluminum oxide), which has shown a lower wear rate than chrome-cobalt alloys against high-density polyethylene.

Clinical wear of HDP (high-density polyethylene)

Radiographic studies of the wear rate of high molecular weight polyethylene sockets 9 to 10 years after surgery (in patients averaging 73 years of age) showed that the average rate of wear in 68% of them was 0.05 mm./yr., and more than 2.5 mm. of wear occurred in 15% in the 10 year follow-up. There appeared to be a diminution in the wear rate with the passage of time: in the second 5 years, wear was approximately 40% less than in the first 5 years. The patient's weight and physical activity did not show any direct relationship to the final amount of wear of the plastic[29,30]: in a study of 33 younger disabled patients (a group under 30 years of age in which 59 hips were followed for 38.4 months) the wear was rather high; a paradoxical finding was that the patients who were completely normal for their activities and age demonstrated less than the average wear of their group. The study of Charnley and Halley[29,30] is at the present time the longest term clinical material available on which to base our judgment on the wear rate of high-density polyethylene in humans (Figs. 3-27 and 3-28).

Based on these clinical studies, a wear at 5 mm. is considered crucial. Changing of the socket should be considered, despite the wall thickness

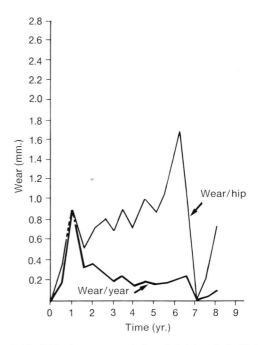

Fig. 3-27. Clinical wear at end of each total period of follow-up in 59 hip sockets in patients under 30 years of age. (Modified from Charnley, J., and Halley, D. K.: Clin. Orthop. **112:** 170-179, 1975.)

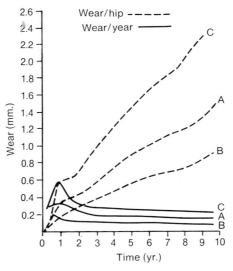

Fig. 3-28. Wear per hip and wear per year in 72 hip sockets in three groups of patients. *A,* Average amount of wear. *B,* Low-wear group. *C,* High-wear group. Average amounts of wear for 72 hip sockets, plotted annually in 9- to 10-year follow-up. Low-wear group sockets wearing up to 10 and including 1.5 mm. in 9 to 10 years. High-wear group socket wearing more than 1.5 mm. in 9 to 10 years. (Modified from Charnley, J., and Halley, D. K.: Clin. Orthop. **112:**170-179, 1975.)

of the Charnley cup (10 mm.). Following 5 mm. of wear, the neck-socket impingement is usually of such a degree that it may cause loosening of the bond (cement-bone junction); based on these clinical wear studies, the predicted times of need for surgical intervention (5 mm. wear) were estimated to be 54 years, 19.5 years, and 30 years in the three groups studied.[29,30]

The direction of wear in the majority of the cases of Teflon failure (where considerable wear took place within a short period of time) was a 10-degree inclination from the vertical toward the midline of the body and was considered the result of all the forces on the hip joint; however, in several instances, wear was inclined away from the vertical toward the lateral.[48] The direction of wear in high-density polyethylene in 9- and 10-year follow-ups cannot be fully documented because of the small amount of wear encountered, but it was rather interesting to find that the most common direction of wear, where it did occur, was upward and outward, followed in frequency by vertical wear.[29]

Laboratory and clinical experiences suggest that the McKee-Farrar total hip prosthesis produces less wear than other metal-to-plastic devices. An in-depth study of this prosthesis indicated three types of wear[111]: (1) initial surface scratching, (2) a new smooth surface forming, and (3) a pitting on the newly formed smooth surface (from No. 2).

The depth of wear was estimated by stylus profilometry to be about 1 micrometer; the volumetric wear was less than on any other metal-on-plastic prosthesis. These observations are significant because of the low volumetric wear, which may have an application in terms of the long-term dimensional stability of this prosthetic design.

Clinical and laboratory correlation

Laboratory wear measurements of high-density polyethylene are in accord with its excellent wear properties in artificial human hip joints.* Charnley observed that its wear rate in the laboratory is less than the 0.050 mm./yr. average rate of wear observed in clinical practice. The clinical and laboratory wear rates of Teflon (tetrafluoroethylene) were correlated at a walking activity of about 2.5 miles/day. The wear testing of high-density polyethylene produced in the laboratory

---

*See references 29, 30, 56-58, and 62.

is equivalent to the patient walking over 150 miles/day, yielding a relative wear of 0.15 mm./yr. in the hip. It is possible that the high-density polyethylene forms a protective layer on the rubbing surface, and it may be the presence or absence of this layer that explains the variable behavior of high-density polyethylene in different circumstances.

Over a period of 10 years of laboratory testing of high-density polyethylene, it was suggested that from a test standpoint, in certain circumstances, random motion with track repetition did reduce the rate of wear by nearly two orders of magnitude. High-density polyethylene was unaffected by the nature of the motion or the type of "water bond" lubricant used in the test. It was also concluded that high-density polyethylene demonstrates acquired resistance to wear as the result of changes in the polymer coating on the rubbing surfaces.[97,105]

The laboratory tests of high-density polyethylene in hip simulators may be criticized for not producing the type of wear seen in the prostheses removed from the patients, but in a scanning electron microscope study by Weightman and his associates[115] and in the hip simulator studies by Duff-Barklay and Spillman,[45] it was suggested that the estimated wear in the machine can be transposed on the performance of the human hip joint. An estimated 1 to 2.5 million cycles occur in the human hip joint per year; this suggests that 1,000 hours in the simulator at 30 cycles per minute (1.8 million cycles) is equivalent to approximately 1 year of wear in the human body. Based on this assumption, the overall depth wear rate in the simulated test of the Charnley prosthesis amounted to 0.006 in./yr.[45] Apparently the lack of abduction-adduction and rotation motion in the simulator did not affect surface wear, but there were obvious differences between the patterns of wear scratches in the simulator test and the prostheses removed from humans. Weightman and his associates[115] tested three prostheses (the Charnley, the Charnley-Müller, and the McKee), concluding that all are adequate in terms of wear resistance, and failure is not likely to occur from wear alone; however, the frictional torque among these prostheses was considerably different. The Charnley prosthesis produced the least frictional torque, hence loosening would presumably be less likely with it than with the other two (see "Frictional Force").

105

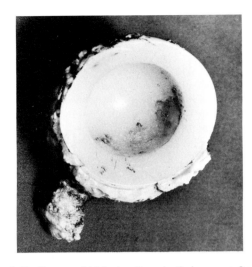

Fig. 3-29. Removed high-density polyethylene cup 2 years after surgery. NOTE: unusual loss of thickness of cup by wear. Large fragment of cement interposed between metal head and acetabulum cup with severe tissue reaction was present at surgery.

In clinical situations an interposed fragment of cement may dramatically accelerate the wear rate (Fig. 3-29).

MODES OF FAILURE OF TOTAL HIP PROSTHESES

Basically, failure of total hip prostheses may result from:

1. Biological failures such as infection and sensitivity
2. Technical failure such as poor cement technique and poor orientation of the components
3. Mechanical failure such as loosening, breakage, and defective materials

Biological causes have been discussed in Chapter 16 as well as in this chapter. Technical causes of failure have been discussed in Chapter 17. Mechanical failure may be the result of the acetabular or femoral loosening of the compo-

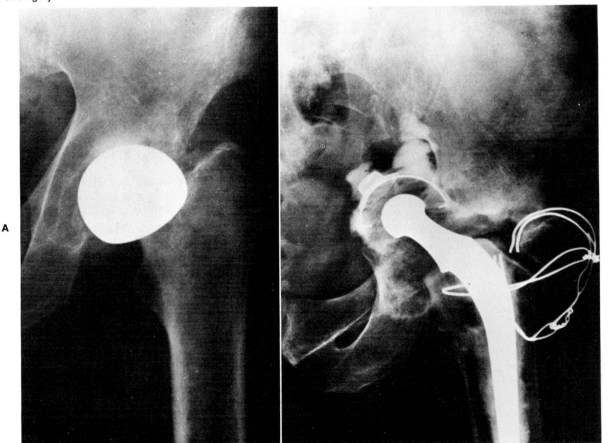

Fig. 3-30. A, Painful left cup arthroplasty originally performed for osteoarthritis in 64-year-old man. **B,** Three-month postoperative x-ray film. Excess deepening of acetabulum leads to fracture of floor, resulting in protrusion of components (see text).

nents with or without the mechanical failure of the prosthesis itself.

Acetabular loosening

A special reference was already made to the role of frictional torque causing acetabular loosening. It was suggested that, as a fundamental principle, prostheses must provide the least frictional torque possible at the bone to minimize bond failure and that a good cement technique must be used to ensure adequate and immediate fixation at surgery.[120]

If the radiological demarcation of cemented sockets can be taken as evidence of loosening of the acetabular component, a majority of hip replacement prostheses using high-density poly-ethylene sockets and methyl methacrylate cement for fixation show evidence of loosening. In a recent study of 141 hips covering up to 10.1 years of follow-up[44]:

1. Sixty-nine percent of 141 hips showed some type of demarcation, 9.2% of which were thought to be progressive.
2. Radiological demarcation did not always accompany failure, but progressive migration was considered serious in nature.
3. Thirty percent of the cases showed no demarcation even after 10 years, supporting the idea that a rigid and permanent fixation may be achieved by cement.

With more attention to technical details a better fixation may be achieved at surgery, with

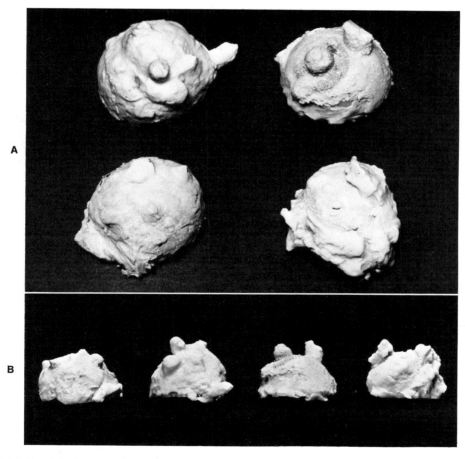

Fig. 3-31. Four failed cemented sockets removed at revision surgery probably share same common cause for loosening. Although considerable thickness of cement is present throughout sphere of acetabular component, smooth surface of exterior of cement indicates possibility of lack of pressure injection by cement or inadequate preparation of acetabulum at time of fixation. All these prostheses were metal-to-plastic type and had been inserted less than 2 years prior to revision surgery. NOTE: large projections of cement did not prevent loosening. (See text.) **A,** Top view, **B,** Side view.

107

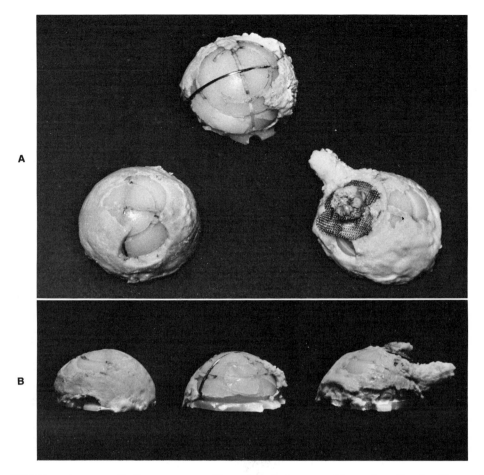

Fig. 3-32. Three loose prosthetic cups removed from patients because of loosening without evidence of infection. NOTE: absence of cement covering cups that were removed with ease at time of surgery: "poor cement technique." **A,** Top view; **B,** side view.

the hope of eliminating a number of radiological lucencies—but more importantly the progressive medial migration.

Generally, the mode of failure of fixation follows one of the following patterns:

1. Acute detachment of the prosthetic socket with complete dislodgment, owing to technical problems related to a poor mechanical fixation achieved at surgery
2. Acute interpelvic protrusion of the acetabular component (Fig. 3-30), also related to technical errors by excessive deepening or accident
3. Chronic slow medial or upward migration of the prosthesis, possibly the result of a technical error, but infection suspected
4. Progressive radiological demarcation and

alteration in the acetabular orientation with a history of technical difficulties must alert the surgeon to infection

Because of the lack of relationship between the thickness of cement used to fix the socket and the frequency of loss of fixation in clinical situations, the heat of polymerization of the cement cannot be incriminated as a cause of loosening, nor does there seem to be any relation between the patient's weight and activities and loosening; therefore the initial mechanical fixation by a good surgical technique and providing a good bony support at surgery are the only mechanisms by which one objectively may anticipate a permanent fixation without loosening. Three technical surgical details seem to be most important:

1. Providing adequate bony surface without

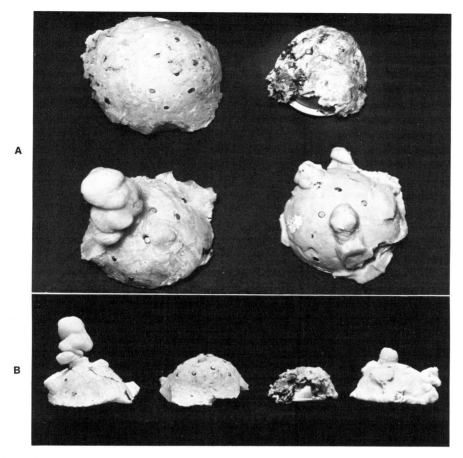

Fig. 3-33. Four acetabular cups removed because of loosening. NOTE: all four prostheses were McKee-Farrar type. Technical defect must have contributed to loosening in addition to high-frictional torque inherent in prosthesis. NOTE: studs of metal cup have protruded through cement mass, and exterior surface of cement is smooth in most areas. This indicates that metal reached bone at insertion obviating pressure injection exerted by operator onto cup. (See text.) **A,** Top view; **B,** side view.

the removal of firm subchondral bone from the acetabulum

2. Pressurizing the cement at the time of fixation (Fig. 3-31) and retaining cement uniformly between the cup and bony acetabulum (Figs. 3-32 and 3-33)

3. Providing many small irregular cavities, such as drill holes, in the subchondral bone for "keying" of the cement (As stated elsewhere, multiple small holes are better than few large ones.)

Femoral loosening

Any evidence of acrylic fractures must be considered accompanied by loosening of the femoral component,[114] which may be present in any of the following several modes (Fig. 3-34):

1. Subsidence of the entire prosthetic component, taking the core of cement with it distally

2. Pistoning of the stem in the acrylic core without distal migration[51] (Fig. 3-34, *D*) of the stem in relation to the cement core

3. Sinking of the prosthesis into the cement cone, leaving the cement cone behind, no fracture seen in the cement column

4. A gradual subsidence of the stem in the cement core resulting in a fracture at the tip of the cement column without further subsequent subsidence

5. A gradual radiological drift of the stem into a varus position, leaving a gap between the cement and the prosthesis at the convex side of the prosthesis (Fig. 3-34, *E*)

6. Proximal medial drift (migration) of the

109

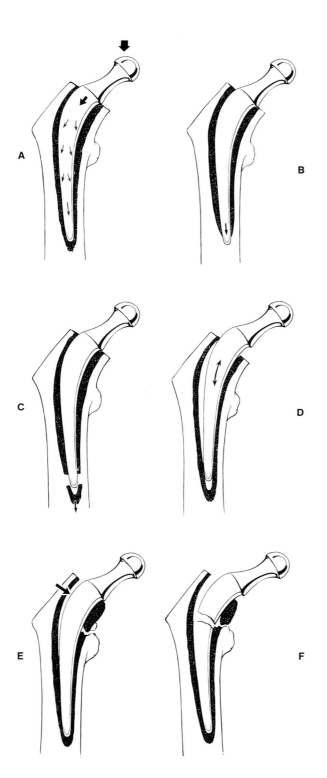

Fig. 3-34. Mode of failure of femoral fixation and stem. **A,** Compressive forces are transmitted via tapered segment of prosthesis onto cement and dissipated over large surface area of bone in this manner. Although distal end of stem conceiveably may transmit load, it is by far less important than tapered upper segment of stem. **B,** Possibility of minor subsidence of stem inside cement core without any consequence to fixation providing that subsidence is not severe. **C,** Gradual subsidence of stem in cement core resulting in fracture at tip of cement column, but prosthesis is stabilized in new position. This mode of failure of fixation also may remain satisfactory providing that new position of prosthesis inside core of cement is permanent. **D,** Pistoning of stem in acrylic core is possible without being manifested by x-ray films. This mode of failure of fixation is uncommon but may cause cystic errosions of bone without detection of loosening by x-ray films. **E,** Gradual radiological drift of stem into varus position may be documented by radiolucent zone appearing on convex side of upper femur (arrow). This usually coincides with bone absorption or cystic changes in region of calcar. **F,** Loss of proximal fixation following bone absorption at region of calcar leading to fracture of cement. Loss of support in this region leads to plastic deformation of stem (ultimately fatigue fracture). Stem fracture is product of increased bending moment such as in a cantilever beam. Fracture can only occur if distal stem is rigidly fixed in core of cement.

stem with rigid support distally, leading to plastic deformation of the stem or fatigue fracture of the stem produced by increased bending such as in a cantilever beam (Fig. 3-34, *F*)

Radiopaque cement has rendered the opportunity to observe significant fractures in the cement-bone junction, but unfortunately, standard x-ray films may not reveal microfractures when they occur; it is not possible to obtain a three-dimensional appearance of the prosthesis on a single x-ray plane.

Of the several modes of failure outlined in the preceding, the type of cement column fractured at the tip does not seem to be related to the inadequate bonding of the cement at the level distal to the stem tip, but since in most instances the fracture of the cement column takes place early and in vigorous, healthy individuals, it may be postulated that:

1. The stem has been loose in the cement track.
2. The stem becomes "end-loaded."
3. With end bearing at the stem tip, the acrylic cement is under tension.
4. Acrylic cement is poor in tension.
5. Acrylic fractures at the weakest point.
6. The entire stem subsides.
7. The cement track (the whole length) again comes under compression.
8. A new position of stability is achieved.

In the mode of failure that involves radiolucency in the convex side of the stem and a varus drift of the prosthesis, the mechanism may be attributed to the following causes:

1. Cement shrinkage, thus pulling away from the prosthesis
2. "Stem wobble" during insertion prior to full polymerization
3. Uneven distribution of the cement in the canal, thus leading to the fracture of a segment of cement at the lower level in the canal allowing further subsidence by shifting the entire prosthesis medially

The idea of shrinkage of the cement may be eliminated because of the fact that the cement is routinely used and in most cases loosening is not observed; the facts are also against the theory of shrinkage by the evidence of the small amount of volumetric changes occurring in the cement during polymerization (see Chapter 4). Stem wobble and uneven distribution of cement in an unsupported segment of bone is a real possibility in producing loosening.

Following the failure of the cement at the tip of the "cone," further subsidence will take place until the prosthesis is stabilized in the column of cement. This situation is usually accompanied by bone loss in the critical calcar zone. If the stem is not stabilized by this mechanism, further subsidence and thus failure of the prosthesis with additional loosening is inevitable.

The varus mode of loosening must be considered as the most serious mode of failure, especially where the upper portion of the prosthesis drifts into a varus position while the distal portion of the stem is rigidly fixed in the bone, generating a bending moment at the junction of the rigid column (distally) and a movable segment (proximally), leading to fatigue failure of the metal (Figs. 3-34, *E* and *F*, and 3-35). In this context a plastic deformation of metal to the point of yield (permanent) must be considered prior to fracture. For technical reasons it is advantageous to revise such a prosthesis prior to completion of the fracture, which makes the operation for removal of a distal fragment more difficult.

Fatigue failure of the acetabulum

Degeneration or degradation of the plastic as the result of fatigue similar to the fatigue of cement exposed to the internal environment under load is a theoretical possibility that cannot be entirely dismissed; however, there has been no definite report of fatigue or changes in the behavior of plastics in the past 10 years.

We consider containing the socket within the acetabulum an important feature in the prevention of plastic flow and deformation, which is a condition that contrasts with the unsupported high-density polyethylene used in most designs of total knee arthroplasty prostheses.

Fatigue failure of metal (stem breakage)

The problems of loosening and fatigue failure of the stem are closely interrelated. Fatigue failure of the stem is the product of repetitive cyclic load, normally initiated at a site of high tensile stress that usually resides at the lateral surface of the stem. Cracks are initiated and grow slowly across the stem until not enough metal is available to support the body weight, which is when the stem fractures at a fast pace. Cracks usually start at places where the stress is concentrated, that is, at any defect such as a scratch, notch, void, and so on. Fig. 3-36 illustrates the cross-section of a fractured pros-

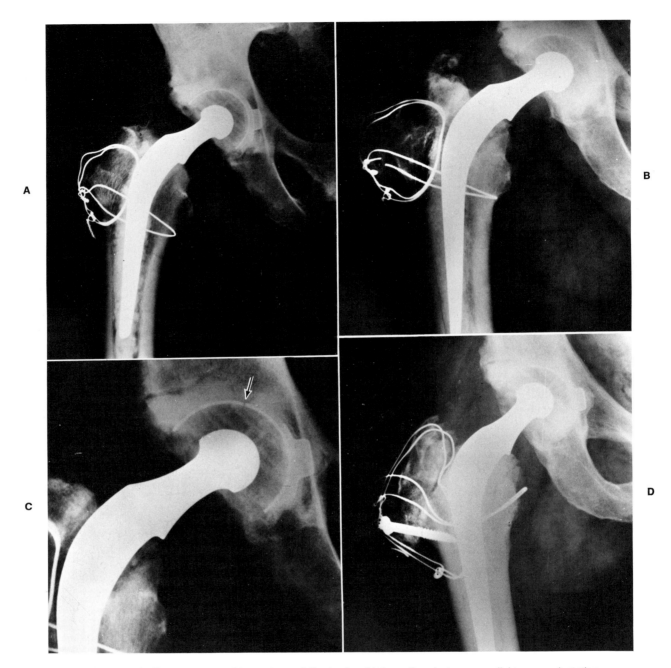

Fig. 3-35. A, Sixty-two–year–old man 1 year following low-friction arthroplasty. NOTE: slight varus orientation of stem in shaft. **B,** Loosening of upper end of prosthesis 3 years following surgery. Patient weighed 232 pounds, was extremely active, and played sports competitively. **C,** Close-up of same patient in **B.** NOTE: wire marker on cup is fractured (arrow), indicative of possible plastic deformation of wire under excess load. Femoral prosthesis is bent (plastic deformation) but not fractured. **D,** Six months following revision using heavy stem. Weight reduction succeeded (180 pounds at time of revision surgery).

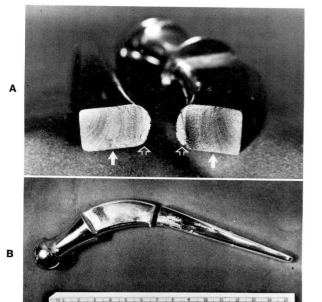

Fig. 3-36. Fatigue failure of stem is product of repetitive cyclic load usually initiated at site of high-tensile stress, which usually resides at lateral surface of stem. NOTE: cross-sectional area of fractured prosthesis that was removed in 215-pound male patient who enjoyed successful total arthroplasty for 5 years. Prosthesis had been inserted in varus orientation. Areas of slow and fast propagation of crack, **A,** (slow, solid arrow; fast, hollow arrow). **B,** Level of fractured stem (same prosthesis as shown in **A**).

Fig. 3-37. X-ray film of typical patient who sustained fractured stem. Prosthesis is drifted into varus direction, neck is markedly absorbed, radiolucent zone has appeared on lateral upper aspect of prosthesis between bone and stem, distal stem is rigidly fixed in bone. Patient's weight was 245 pounds at time of fracture, 3 years following surgery (arrow shows fracture site).

thesis and shows the areas of slow and fast propagation of the crack.

Since the fracture is the result of "excessive tensile stress" at the lateral surface of the prosthesis owing to the bending moment* and the load (patient's weight and activities), it is important to consider the possible factors that contribute to its appearance (Fig. 3-37). They are:

1. The neck shaft angle of the prosthesis; that is, the smaller the neck shaft angle the greater the stress
2. The neck length; that is, the longer the neck the greater the stress (Fig. 3-38)
3. The orientation of the stem in the canal; that is, the greater the angle of varus the greater the stress (Fig. 3-39)

---

*Bending moment: M, force; F, distance from; D, line of action. $M = F \times D$.

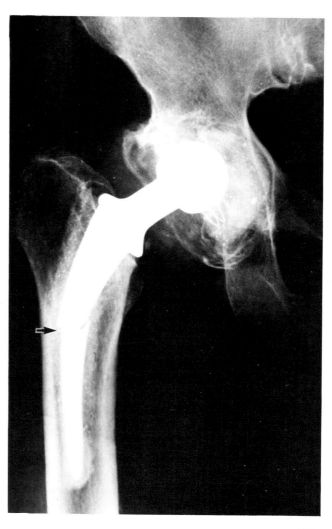

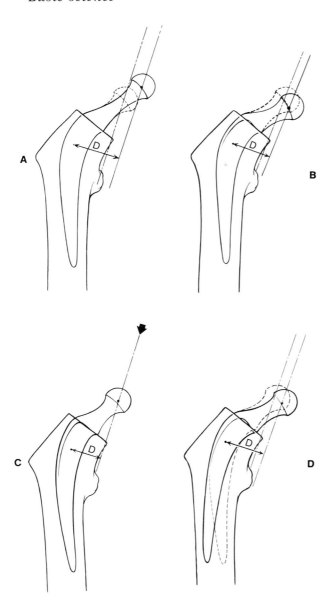

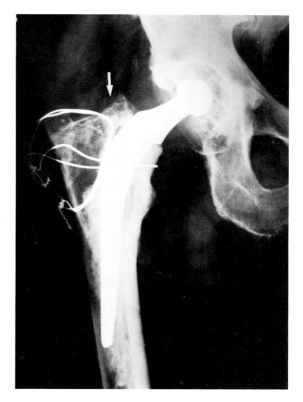

Fig. 3-39. Avoidable complication of varus orientation is demonstrated; greater trochanter is osteotomized, but prosthesis is inserted in marked varus orientation. By removal of bridge between bed of trochanter and neck, prosthesis could have been conveniently inserted without varus orientation. Arrow indicates bone bridge between trochanter and neck. (See Chapter 12.)

Fig. 3-38. A, Longer the neck of prosthesis, greater the distance, *D*, thus greater bending moment. **B,** Smaller the neck shaft angle, greater the distance, *D*, greater the bending moment on stem. **C,** Slight valgus orientation of stem in shaft; less distance, *D*, thus less bending moment on stem. **D,** More varus orientation of stem the more distance, *D*, thus increased bending moment on stem.

One must recognize that metallic devices with unlimited "fatigue life" (over 80,000 to 100,000 p.s.i.) may be introduced to circumvent the problem of "fatigue fractures." In that case loosening would become the most important problem that should be considered in tracing the initiation of a failure. Loosening is the result of motion tak-

ing place between different materials, such as cement and metal, which creates a stress fracture leading to further loosening. In a two-dimensional finite element analysis, McNiece and associates concluded that the basic question concerning bone is the level of interface shear stress and the degree of protection against slippage.[83] From their studies it became obvious that maximum interface shear occurs on the inferior surface of the stem-neck region and over the distal lateral surface at the tip of the stem, and that within these zones the largest concentration of values was predominantly in the calcar zone. These values of shear stress would be the minimum values that could prevent bond failure, but since impact forces could easily double these values, it appears that the bond strength between the stem and the acrylic cement should be at least 35 N-mm.^{2}. Although this is a good engineering bond (the same level as the ultimate shear stress of acrylic cement), in practice such a bonding between the metal and the cement would make the subsequent removal of the prosthesis impossible should it become necessary.

In a similar two-dimensional stress analysis the effect of some of the factors leading to early fatigue failure of the femoral stem in total hip replacement was studied.[5,60,79] This led to a similar conclusion that loss of proximal stem support at the level of the calcar femorale resulted in a level of stress on the stem that led to fatigue failure. The role of the load (body weight) and the range of cyclic stress played an important part in fatigue life under test conditions. Increasing (beefing up) the stem dimension at the middle-third level of the stem (the critical level, where maximum tensile forces are found) was suggested, although it should be emphasized that static testing in laboratories might be an oversimplification of the three-dimensional geometry of the stem and the forces that are applied to it as they occur in the body. So this model would only partially explain the early failure of the metal.

Many unresolved problems besides a failure-free stem must be considered for research. The unknown factors are basically related to the metallic alloy, design features, and lack of understanding of the complex mechanism of weight bearing in the upper femur, which is subjected to many stresses. It is also important to develop techniques for adequate anchoring of the prosthesis into the shaft of the femur. Basically none of the studies so far has been directed toward equalizing the moduli of elasticity between the prosthetic components and their fixation and bone, which may be equally important in the future design of the stem.

Based on the clinical analysis of stem failures today, one may search for the cause of failure in the following categories: excessive load, failure of support by the bone, loss of fixation at the cement-bone-metal interface, uneven stress distribution throughout the cement column, metallurgical causes, and failure of surgery.

Excessive load. Fatigue fracture of the femoral prosthesis is the product of a "successful arthroplasty" in a heavy, athletic, active patient in which the dimensions of a standard prosthesis have been used (Fig. 3-35). The valgus position of the prosthesis, while important by itself in reducing bending stresses, does not eliminate

the fracture. The support of the prosthesis by the cement on the medial aspect is most important; an extremely heavy stem in the upper portion would automatically reduce the amount of cement used, inviting further loosening problems that can initiate fatigue fractures. The anatomical advantages of a 130-degree shaft-neck angle are great enough to warrant its sole use in patients with a huge bony structure, in order to allow clearance between the neck and the rim of the acetabulum. Obviously, heavier prostheses should be designed for people who anticipate excess load by their weight or excess stress by the degree of their activities.

Based on the clinical examination of 17 fractures, the especially high-risk patients are males weighing over 170 pounds, especially those with a standard prosthesis whose early design (original standard stems) was not adequate. It was also concluded that the situation was compounded in most cases by inadequate cement support at the concavity of the upper femur. Charnley attributed the low incidence of fracture of the stem in long-term follow-up results to a good cementing technique.[25] The highest risk patients are those who are physically active, but because of their small bone size (narrow medullary canal) a large stem cannot be inserted. Patients with a severe disability in the opposite extremity are also at risk, owing to the likelihood of increased loads on the arthroplasty side. To overcome these problems, no patient should be accepted for arthroplasty whose weight is over 200 pounds.

Overactive patients should be warned to reduce their participation in certain kinds of activities such as contact sports. Technically, especially in large, bony men, the large-sized prosthesis, which can be accommodated in a neutral or slight valgus attitude, should be used. One should avoid using long-necked prostheses (whenever possible) or a varus orientation at surgery. The cement technique for the upper femur is demanding and a good fixation at the calcar level seems to be essential. Manufacturing control in the production of prostheses with a high-strength and high fatigue–resistant metal should also minimize the chance of stress fracture of the stem.

Failure of support by the bone. There is now substantial evidence that the loss of support by the bone is a fundamental cause of the failure of cement fixation in the calcar region, leading

115

to eventual failure of fixation at the concave side of the stem. Therefore, from the histological evaluation of the calcar region, it seems reasonable to suggest that the cystic erosion of bone in this region is due to slight movement between the cement and the bone. With the stress concentration at the calcar region and cement fragmentation causing tissue reaction such as bone resorption and necrosis, further varus subsidence of the prosthesis follows. The similarity between the periodontal disease and bone necrosis with the loosened cemented prosthesis is striking. In both instances, once loosening is initiated, a vicious cycle is created. The cement loses support and permits increased motion in the upper end of the prosthesis between the bone and the calcar at the concave side of the prosthesis, while the remainder of the prosthesis (the distal portion) may remain fixed in the bone (Fig. 3-34). As a solution to the problem, it seems reasonable to suggest a surgical technique that should include, in addition to a slight valgus orientation for the prosthesis, removal of the loose cancellous bone of the calcar region in order to provide strong support by the cement. Poor support by the bone, despite a valgus orientation of the stem, has been occasionally observed.[25]

Loss of fixation. As indicated earlier, the most important cause of the failure of the stem is the initiation of the loosening of the prosthesis in the shaft, especially in the upper region (with the medial side of the prosthesis at the calcar region). Although most loosenings may not terminate in failure by stem fracture, retrospective examination of most cases reveals early loosening prior to stem fracture (Fig. 3-35). Improper cementing, that is, varus orientation of the stem and lack of support by the cement at the concave side of the prosthesis (in the compression side), creates increased stresses on the metal and the cement as well as the bone, leading to failure of fixation in this region.[118]

Experimental studies[60] coupled with studies of clinically failed prostheses can aid in determining the area of high-stress concentration and the location of the fracture. In both clinical and laboratory situations the loss of fixation by the cement precedes the failure of metals; therefore it seems reasonable to assume that paying attention to the technical details of insertion and producing adequate support for the prosthesis at the calcar region to eliminate loosening are the first line of defense against fatigue fracture.

Uneven stress distribution (malposition). It is commonly agreed that most failed stems have been the product of loosening, improper cementing, and inadequate calcar support, but in most cases a varus positioning of the stem has also been noted, although it must be emphasized that the support conditions provided by the cement and the bone are more important than the simple orientation in the canal. In other words, a valgus orientation of the stem in the canal inadequately supported by cement and bone medially would still not prevent fracture when excess stress was imposed on it. In an experimental model prediction, a Charnley prosthesis was instrumented with foil strain gauges.[60] The instrumented prosthesis was implanted into a cadaveric femur in a valgus orientation; after the cement was set and static loads applied and the resulting strength was recorded, the computed stresses were quite comparable and consistent with a theoretical model. In the finite element analysis the stem in neutral position showed the lowest peak stresses. The stem in the valgus alignment with lateral cortical contact showed peak stresses approximately one-third higher than those of the stem in neutral position. If these experimental analyses are representative of conditions in the clinical situation, efforts must be made at surgery to avoid any degrees of varus orientation of the stem in the shaft, and it follows that a stem that is well centered in the shaft is mechanically superior to a valgus-oriented stem.

Metallurgical causes. Fatigue is an engineering term used to describe the failure of materials by a fluctuating stress, which if applied a sufficient number of times, will produce failure in the material. The stress required to produce failure is often much lower than that required to fracture the same material on a single application. While this principle is applicable to most machine elements and laboratory tests may produce the basic information regarding fatigue properties of the materials, the stress cycles that cause "fatigue failure" in biological situations are usually extremely complex. Gross appearance of a fatigue-fractured surface of metallic components such as a stem of total hip prosthesis shows two distinct regions: (1) a relatively smooth surface area with concentric markings described as clamshell, beach, or ripple markings, and (2) a surface area of rough granular appearance as if showing a cross-section of a multifilament cord. The smooth area is an indication of a slow propagation of the fatigue cracks, and the rough zone is indicative of the final fractured zone in a ruptured fashion (brittle) (Fig. 3-36). Most femoral components of total hip prostheses are made of annealed stainless steel, chromium-cobalt alloy, or titanium. Annealed stainless steel, cast chromium-cobalt alloys, and titanium have similar ultimate tensile strengths but the "yield stress" is much lower in annealed stainless steel than chromium-cobalt or titanium. Therefore in order to avoid plastic deformation (permanent) in annealed stainless steel, the stem must have a greater dimension than that of a similar design made of chromium-cobalt or titanium alloy (Tables 3-1 and 3-2).

A new alloy that is used in Europe and in the United States is a combination of cobalt, nickel, chromium, and molybdenum known as Protosul 10 or MP35N. This alloy is made in a "multiphase" state. The mechanical properties of this alloy are outstanding with a yield strength of 60,000 p.s.i. when fully annealed with elongation of 70%. With work, hardening, and heat treatment the yield strengths up to 300,000 p.s.i. and only 10% elongation is achieved. These characteristics make MP35N an ideal alloy (combining good properties of stainless steel and chromium-cobalt).

The problem of metal fatigue has been discussed by Grover,[64] who attributed the failure of fixation to fatigue wear of specific orthopaedic implants;[64] however, Calhoon and Paxton[9,10] concluded that failure was related to either metallurgical defects or improper design. A more recent study of 35 stainless steel and chromium-cobalt-molybdenum alloy devices showed that a very large number of these were defective or deficient; the defects were due to the presence of delta-ferrite in 316 L stainless steel, porosity in the cast chromium alloy or the presence of cracks and pits, and in some instances a low molybdenum content in the steel. A number of other mechanical explanations have been proffered for the failure of metal in orthopaedic surgery: a brittle fracture owing to stresses exceeding the ultimate strength of the material, the use of an alloy not resistant to corrosion was suggested by Colangelo and Green,[39] brittle fractures as the result of combined mechanical and electrochemical defects,[70] impact loading, fatigue tract propagation of 316 L stainless steel,[116] and the weakness of the bone at the region of the femoral calcar.[84] The effect of the grain size on the fatigue life of 316 L stainless

steel has been established, but it may be a significant factor in determining the strength of the stainless steel used for the stem of the femoral component. It is possible that a fine grain size is preferable and that maintenance of a fine and uniform grain size is possible by manufacturers. Galante and his associates[59] feel that strings of shrinkage porosity in cast chromium and cobalt alloy should be considered as flaws.[59] When a string length approaches an appreciable fraction of a millimeter, it must be considered as a progenitor of early failure, and large amounts of shrinkage porosity could be detrimental to the strength of the metal. Obviously, maintaining the highest standards of microstructural quality for the metal used in the stem of the prosthesis is imperative.

In regard to metallurgical studies, the main morphological characteristic of most of these fractures is obviously fatigue failure, but in most of the cases examined so far, a premature fatigue failure has occurred, probably owing to a combination of circumstances. These include inadequate quality controls in manufacture and flaws in the metallic structures; for example, 316 annealed stainless steel is unsuitable for a femoral stem, since loss of strength of this material can be expected under loading conditions; wrought cold-worked 316 stainless steel should be the material of choice, instead, when stainless steel is used.

One must be skeptical of the estimated fatigue limits for surgical metals[64]; exposure to the internal milieu of the body could significantly degrade fatigue strength and lead to corrosion fatigue much more readily than in air-tested specimens.

To summarize, the current concepts of femoral stem failure in total hip replacement are based on the studies of several investigators.[16,25,60] There appear to be three major avenues of exploration in detecting the causes of stem failure.

1. The study of the characteristics of fracture surfaces and their relation to metallurgical defects
2. The detailed observation of the metallic materials to detect flaws or defects
3. The understanding of the stresses to which these devices are subjected in actual use

Failure of surgical judgment, technique, and patient's cooperation. A patient weighing over 200 pounds should be refused for surgery until weight reduction is accomplished because the patients most susceptible to stem fractures are those who weigh over 170 pounds and are frequently active in vigorous athletic performance; they are usually careless in lifting heavy objects or in participating in sports that cause the prosthesis to be loaded beyond its fatigue endurance limit. The previous designs of prostheses (standard type up to 1973) were generally small and inadequate for large bony men; similarly, patients whose bone size is too small to allow a heavy prosthesis and those who will not limit their activities are also considered high-risk patients. Educating patients in this regard is essential. The cementing technique should include forceful packing of the canal following the removal of all loose bony trabeculae and fatty marrow. Special attention should be paid in preparing the canal in the region of calcar femorale to packing the cement well within the concave side of the prosthesis and femur. No "jarring" or "wobbling" is permitted when the prosthesis is being inserted, as this will produce a track in the cement that is larger than the size of the stem and initiate a piston action of the stem in the canal.

Any degrees of varus orientation of the stem will expose it to an excessive load (Fig. 3-39). Extreme valgus orientation is equally as disadvantageous extreme varus orientation, although a slightly valgus position will allow for a thick layer of cement in the calcar region at the concave side of the prosthesis. In selecting a prosthesis, ideally it should possess a shorter neck in valgus position (small center shaft offset) with an increased section modulus. An extremely large stem occupying the main space in the canal is not attractive since it obviates the thickness of cement in the calcar region, which is so essential for support of the prosthesis under compressive load. A high-level metallurgical study of fatigue-resistant metals is essential and a prerequisite in selecting a prosthesis.

SUMMARY OF ESSENTIALS

■ Concepts concerning biomaterials and biomechanics of the artificial joints are rapidly changing. New developments based on investigations in the laboratories and the correlations of these findings with clinical problems are both essential to the surgeon performing total hip arthroplasty. The problems concerning the surgeon include biomaterials and compatibility, forces about the hip joint, frictional forces, methods and elements of fixation, design of

reconstruction procedure, prosthetic design features, wear, friction and lubrication, and finally the mode of failure of devices is of particular concern in selecting the type of prosthesis and the method of surgery.

■ Unlike stationary devices that are used in fracture fixation, the total hip prostheses are expected to perform a mechanical function by transmission of weight, load, and translation of motion. Although it is possible as an engineering exercise to calculate the magnitude of forces and to conceptualize a design with expected behavior, such a model when applied to human function is not practical because of the body environment and undetermined nature of forces applied to such a system. On this premise therefore laboratory work has its limitations and can only be used as a guide for verification of some aspects of clinical application.

■ Because the development of implantable polymers (plastics) is relatively recent, the issue of their long-term, complete prosthetic acceptability has not been fully resolved. However, a large experience in thousands of humans following implantation as long as 20 years has shown that polymers are well tolerated. The metals, on the other hand, have a longer history of compatibility and are considered safe for repair and replacement surgery.

■ A simple ball-and-socket bearing is the most effective design for total hip joint arthroplasty, but in such a system in which particulate matters are released as the result of wear, it should not cause local or remote tissue reactions.

■ In vivo research should be directed toward the selection of biocompatible materials for the bearing joints but employing any new materials clinically must be done judiciously.

■ Materials selected for joint replacement should be adequately fatigue resistant in order to withstand weight-bearing stresses. Wear must be minimal, and the level of frictional resistance reduced to a minimum in order to protect the fixation from excess stress. It should also withstand corrosion and degradation in the hostile environment. Further, the weight-bearing element must be compliant and attenuate force and, above all, must have local and remote biological compatibility.

■ The metals commonly used for bearings in human artificial joints include stainless steel, chromium-cobalt-molybdenum, and titanium. The impurities in stainless steel prostheses may initiate corrosion, leading to failure of the implant; they can act as stress concentrators and along with corrosion may result in fatigue fracture.

■ Tissue reaction to long-term implantation of chromium alloys (chromium-cobalt-molybdenum) is minimal although it does occur. Analysis of tissue adjacent to this metal has revealed the ions of all three metals in this alloy.

- In an attempt to establish a quantitative method for tissue response to particles of foreign materials, a rating system has been developed based on the concentration of particles per field and inflammatory response by the adjacent tissue.
- Corrosion may be uniform, pitting, intragranular, and cracking type. In general, reactions to metals relate not only to the ionic behavior in a biological situation but also to the size, shape, movement, and other physical parameters of the implant itself. The type of tissue reaction may be classified as injury reaction, repair reaction, corrosion reaction, and reactions to the metal particles.
- Most plastics have provoked sarcomas when implanted in rats and mice. Experimental work has indicated that sarcomas are caused primarily by the size and the shape of the implant and not by their chemical nature. It is of special interest that, despite the extensive implantation of plastics in humans, no benign or malignant tumors have ever been reported as having been caused by these materials.
- Unlike Teflon and polyesters, gross and histological sections adjacent to implanted high-density polyethylene have revealed minimum to moderate inflammatory foreign body reaction. Up to 10 years follow-up the particles of high-density polyethylene have been well tolerated by the tissue.
- In connection with tissue reaction to polymethyl methacrylate (PMMA) one must differentiate between the state of rigidity and loosening of the cement. The early literature is mainly unclear in describing the difference between the tissue responses of failed total hips, such as loosening and infection, and rigidly fixed cement in the bone.
- An extensive tissue reaction with giant cell formation and caseation suggests the presence of loosening of cement fragments in the bone for some time prior to surgical intervention. Similarly, cystic erosions encountered in the calcar region should be attributed to loosening of cement at this heavily loaded zone. In contrast, the histology of cement that is rigidly fixed in the bone is entirely benign and the occasional giant cells revealed in non-weight-bearing zones of the interface are the only suggestion of tissue response to cement.
- It should be noted that acrylic cement is not birefringent, and histologically birefringent material is indicative of wear debris from high-density polyethylene.
- Forces acting on the hip joint are considerably influenced by the pelvic angle and the position of the trunk and limbs. With the pelvis in a normal walking attitude and the limbs symmetrically disposed, muscle forces range from 1 to 1.8 times the body weight and the joint forces from 1.8 to 2.7 times the body weight. The direction of the forces is inclined 10 to 15 degrees from the midaxis of the body.

- Hip joint stress may be reduced by changes in mechanics of the joint such as leaning over the affected hip, increasing the weight-bearing surface of the joint, and most importantly reducing the load by weight loss of the patient. Another example of reducing the force is the use of a cane held on the opposite side of diseased hip.
- Reduction of the hip joint forces by surgery may be achieved by lateralization of the abductor forces and medialization of the center of rotation of the hip. This phenomena may spare the artificial joint from excess stress, which might be considerably important in terms of wear, loosening, or fracture of the prosthesis. This reduction of force is achieved by (1) reducing the body-weight moment arm through deepening of the acetabulum and (2) increasing the gluteal moment arm via lateral transfer of the greater trochanter.
- The frictional forces acting on the acetabular component of total hip prostheses are dependent on several factors: the magnitude of the resultant compressive force, the direction of the force, the frictional moment and the axes around which they act, the geometry of the prosthesis, and the coefficient of friction between the mating surfaces.
- The difference in the coefficient of friction between the all metal and metal-plastic designs of hip prostheses are of such magnitude that it is safe to assume that metal-to-metal components will have a greater tendency to cause bone fatigue and loosening than metal-to-plastic designs.
- To prevent loosening (resistance against frictional forces) one should maximize the bond strength at surgery, preserve the supporting bone at the site of fixation, and use a system (prosthesis) with low frictional torque.
- Fixation of elements to the bone may be achieved by external plates and screws, intramedullary spike, chemical adhesive bonding, acrylic cement as a filler, and porous material or ingrowth.
- None of the methods described here are totally free of problems, but the most reliable method at the present time is the use of acrylic cement, which is used as a "grouting" or a filler to transmit the load.
- The design of reconstruction arthroplasty is an integral part of the prosthetic replacement, which should be directed toward the distribution of the load to prevent bone necrosis and loosening to reduce the total load on the artificial joint, thus protecting the artificial joint from excess wear and fatigue failure.
- In the design of the low-friction arthroplasty several closely related ideas have been incorporated: the use of a small diameter femoral head, the lateral displacement of the abductor pull, and the medialization of the center of the rotation of the hip.
- The design of the artificial joint should include the

119

anatomical adaptation and surgical feasibility, the reduction of forces acting on the artificial hip joint, and the mechanical optimization of wear, friction, strength, and so on.

■ In regard to the size of the femoral head, ranges between 22 to 28 seem optimal and allow the use of a thick plastic socket without the risk of rapid penetration into the socket or fear of instability. A transient subluxation of the head with a small (22 mm.) head prosthesis is possible and may provide a safety feature by allowing the head to escape from the socket, thus alleviating the fixation from excess stress. The plastic socket need not be highly polished but must allow clearance in articulating with the femoral head.

■ A radiographical wire marker clipped to the outer aspect of the cup assists in assessing the orientation as well as wear of the plastic.

■ In design of the neck one should consider adequate dimensions to be sufficiently strong but should allow angular motion with no encroachment against the socket rim. The smaller the diameter of the neck, the greater the range of motion without impingement; the greater the recession of the neck, the greater the range of motion without impingement; the greater the head-neck diameter ratio, the greater the range of motion without impingement; the smaller the socket depth-ball ratio, the greater the range of motion without impingement.

■ By increasing the depth of the socket it is possible to increase resistance against dislocation. A fact taken into consideration in Charnley's design of the prosthesis.

■ The design and shape of the stem of the prosthesis influence the mechanical behavior of the prosthesis inside the shaft. The tensile stress (at the lateral surface) of the stem is directly proportional to the bending moment but inversely related to the section modulus of the stem. The metallurgical composition and processing of the stem may greatly influence its strength, an essential feature in total hip arthroplasty in heavy and younger patients.

■ In anchoring the stem of a prosthesis one should recognize that the failure of the stem is largely dependent on the quality of fixation at surgery. With this in mind the prosthesis designed so thick that it fits flush, without space for cement insertion especially at the concave side of the prosthesis, may well fail because of the lack of support by cement. Thus it is advisable to chose a slightly smaller stem (rather than the thickest possible) to allow a slight valgus orientation or to avoid varus tendency and provide adequate thickness of cement on the concave side.

■ Although wear and friction are entirely independent phenomena, the best material for human joint arthroplasty should have a low wear rate and a low friction coefficient, the latter being essential in reducing torque. High molecular weight polyethylene against metal appears to be an appropriate combination.

■ In addition to mechanical factors such as load and velocity, other factors affecting the wear include the surface quality (finish), the sphericity of the femoral head, the clearance between the ball and the socket, and the diameter of the femoral head.

■ Most clinical and laboratory studies indicate that high-density polyethylene is suitable for weight bearing in artificial hip joints. The average wear in long-term (9 to 10 years) clinical studies is 0.15 mm. or less per year although some variation from the average is observed. A wear rate of 5 mm. is considered clinically crucial. Changing the socket should be considered if such a degree of wear occurs. The reason for surgical intervention is the neck socket impingement that will cause loosening of the bond. The need for surgical intervention is predicted to range from 19.5 years to 54 years in the groups studied.

■ Mechanical failure of a total hip prosthesis may result from biological, technical, and mechanical causes. Acetabular loosening as evidenced by radiological demarcation of the socket may accompany migration. This complication should be prevented by utilizing a "perfect technique" of cementing and a prosthesis with minimum frictional torque properties. At surgery one should provide adequate bony surface preparation without removal of firm subchondral bone.

■ Loosening of the femoral component may be manifested by subsidence of the entire prosthetic component, pistoning of the stem, sinking of the prosthesis into the cement cone, a gradual subsidence of the stem in the cement core resulting in fracture of the tip of the cement, a gradual drift into varus position, or a medial drift and rigid support distally.

■ The varus mode of loosening must be considered as the most serious mode of failure, especially where the upper portion of the prosthesis shifts into varus orientation but the distal portion is rigidly fixed in the bone, generating a bending moment at the junction of the rigid column (distally) and a movable segment (proximally) leading to fatigue failure of the stem.

■ The problems of loosening and fatigue failure of the stem are closely interrelated. Fatigue failure of the stem is the product of repetitive cyclic load usually initiated at the site of high tensile stress, which commonly resides at the lateral surface of the stem. Cracks are initiated and grow slowly across the stem until fracture occurs.

■ Since the fracture is the result of excessive tensile stress at the lateral surface of the prosthesis owing to the bending moment and the load, it is important to consider the contributing factors including

(1) the neck-shaft angle of the prosthesis, (2) the neck length, and (3) the orientation of the stem inside the medullary canal as well as metallurgical causes of failure including mechanical deficiencies of the stem dimension at the middle-third and especially at the tension side of the prosthesis (convex side).

■ Based on the clinical observations the causes of stem failure may include excessive load, failure of support by bone, loss of fixation at the cement-bone-metal interface, uneven stress distribution, metallurgical causes, and failure of surgery.

■ Of all causes of failure of total hip prosthesis, perhaps surgical technique and proper selection of patients are the most important aspects in preventing failure.

REFERENCES

1. Amstutz, H. C.: Practical considerations in the selection of materials and design for total hip replacement. In American Academy of Orthopaedic Surgeons: Instructional course lectures, vol. 23, St. Louis, 1974, The C. V. Mosby Co., pp. 169-178.
2. Amstutz, H. C., Lodwig, R. M., Schurman, D. J., and Hodgson, A. G.: Range of motion studies for total hip replacements. A comparative study with a new experimental apparatus, Clin. Orthop. **111:**124-130, 1975.
3. Amstutz, H. C., and Markolf, K. L.: Design features in total hip replacement. The Hip Society: The hip. Proceedings of the second open scientific meeting of The Hip Society, St. Louis, 1974, The C. V. Mosby Co., pp. 111-112.
4. Andersson, G. B. J., Freemen, M. A. R., and Swanson, S. A. V.: Loosening of the cemented acetabular cup in total hip replacements, J. Bone Joint Surg. **54B:**590-599, 1972.
5. Andriacchi, T. P., Galante, J. O., Belytschko, T. B., and Hampton, S.: A stress analysis of the femoral stem in total hip prostheses, J. Bone Joint Surg. **58A:**618-624, 1976.
6. Bloch, B., and Hastings, G. W.: Plastics in surgery, Springfield, Ill., 1967, Charles C Thomas, Publisher.
7. Blount, W. P.: Don't throw away the cane, J. Bone Joint Surg. **38A:**695, 1956.
8. Bullough, P. G.: Tissue reaction to wear debris generated from total hip replacements. In the Hip Society: The hip. Proceedings of the first open scientific meeting of The Hip Society, St. Louis, 1973, The C. V. Mosby Co., pp. 80-91.
9. Cahoon, J. R., and Paxton, H. W.: Metallurgical analysis of failed orthopedic implants, J. Biomed. Mater. Res. **2:**1-22, 1968.
10. Cahoon, J. R., and Paxton, H. W.: A Metallurgical survey of current orthopedic implants, J. Biomed. Mater. Res. **4:**223-244, 1970.
11. Calanan, J.: The use of inert plastic material in reconstructive surgery, Br. J. Plas. Surg. **16:**1-22, 1963.
12. Charnley, J.: The lubrication of animal joints in relation to surgical reconstruction by arthroplasty, Ann. Rheum. Dis. **19:**10-19, 1960.
13. Charnley, J.: The bonding of prostheses to bone by cement, J. Bone Joint Surg. **46B:**518-529, 1964.
14. Charnley, J.: A biomechanical analysis of the use of cement to anchor the femoral head prosthesis, J. Bone Joint Surg. **47B:**355-363, 1965.
15. Charnley, J.: An artificial bearing in the hip joint: implications in biological lubrication, Fed. Proc. **25:**1079, 1966.
16. Charnley, J.: Factors in design of hip arthroplasty. Symposium on lubrication and wear and living artificial human hip joints, vol. 6, London, 1968, Institution of Medical Engineers, pp. 104-112.
17. Charnley, J., Acrylic cement in orthopedic surgery, Baltimore, 1970, The Williams & Wilkins Co.
18. Charnley, J., editor: Total hip replacement, Clin. Orthop. **72:**1-344, 1970.
19. Charnley, J.: The fixation of prostheses in living bone. In Simpson, D. C., editor: The modern trends in biomechanics, vol. 1, New York, 1970, Appleton-Century-Crofts, pp. 52-80.
20. Charnley, J.: Comparison of dynamic frictional torque in different total hip implanting by a pendulum method, Internal Publication No. 35, Centre for Hip Surgery, Wrightington Hospital, England, December, 1971.
21. Charnley, J.: Low friction arthroplasty of the hip joint, J. Bone Joint Surg. **53B:**149, 1971.
22. Charnley, J.: The moments of force about the hip joint mechanism of the low friction arthroplasty, Internal Publication No. 40, Centre for Hip Surgery, Wrightington Hospital, England, August, 1972.
23. Charnley, J.: Biomechanical considerations in total hip prosthetic design. In The Hip Society: The hip. Proceedings of first open scientific meeting of The Hip Society, St. Louis, 1973, The C. V. Mosby Co., pp. 101-117.
24. Charnley, J.: The status of research into the wear of high molecular weight polyethylene in total hip replacement as of Jan. 1974. Internal Publication No. 49, Centre for Hip Surgery, Wrightington Hospital, England, March, 1974.
25. Charnley, J.: Fracture of femoral prosthesis in total hip replacement. A clinical study, Clin. Orthop. **111:**115-120, 1975.
26. Charnley, J. In Robert Jones lecture, combined meeting, London September, 1976.
27. Charnley, J., and Crawford, W. J.: Histology of

bone in contact with self-curing acrylic cement, J. Bone Joint Surg. **50B:**228, 1968.

28. Charnley, J., and Eftekhar, N.: Postoperative infection in total prosthetic replacement arthroplasty of the hip joint with special reference to the bacterial content of the air of the operating room, Br. J. Surg. **56:**641-649, 1969.

29. Charnley, J., and Halley, D. K.: Rate of wear in total hip replacement, Clin. Orthop. **112:**170-179, 1975.

30. Charnley, J., and Halley, D. K.: Rate of wear in the total hip replacement, Orthop. Dig. **2:**13-14, December 1976.

31. Charnley, J., and Kettlewell, J.: The elimination of slip between prosthesis and femur, J. Bone Joint Surg. **47B:**56-60, 1965.

32. Charnley, J., and Pusso, R., The recording and the analysis of gait in relation to surgery of the hip joint, Clin. Orthop. **58:**153-164, 1968.

33. Charnley, J., Follacci, F. M., and Hammond, B. T.: The long-term reaction of bone to self-curing acrylic cement, J. Bone Joint Surg. **50B:**822-829, 1968.

34. Charnley, J., Kramanger, A., and Longfield, M. D.: The optimum size of prosthetic heads in relation to the wear of plastic sockets in total replacement of the hip, Med. Biol. Eng. **7:**31-39, 1969.

35. Charosky, C. B., Bullough, T. G., and Wilson, P. D.: Total hip replacement failures, J. Bone and Joint Surg. **55A:**49-58, 1973.

36. Clarke, E. G. C., Hickman, J., Collins, D. H., and Scales, J. T.: Discussion of metals and synthetic materials in relation to tissues, R. Soc. Med. **46:**641-652, 1953.

37. Cohen, J., and Hammond, G.: Corrosion in a device for fracture fixation, J. Bone Joint Surg. **41A:**524-534, 1959.

38. Cohen, J., and Wulff, J.: Clinical failure caused by corrosion of a Vitallium plate, J. Bone Joint Surg. **54A:**617-628, 1972.

39. Colangelo, V. J., and Greene, N. D.: Corrosion and fracture of type 316 S.M.O. orthopedic implants, J. Biomed. Mater. Res. **3:**247-265, 1969.

40. Coleman, R. F., Herrington, J., and Scales, J. T.: Concentration of wear products in hair, blood and urine after total hip replacement, Br. Med. J. **1:**527-529, 1973.

41. Dall, D., and Charnley, J.: Comparison of the lever systems in low friction arthroplasty and the McKee-Farrar arthroplasty, Internal Publications No. 34, Centre for Hip Surgery, Wrightington Hospital, England, September, 1971.

42. Danckwardt-Lillieström, G.: Reaming of the medullary cavity and the effect on diaphyseal bone, a fluorochromic, microangiographic and histologic study on the rabbit tibia and dog femur, Acta Orthop. Scand. [Suppl.] **128:**Suppl. 1969.

43. Danckwardt-Lillieström, G., Lorenzi, G. L., and Olerud, S.: Intramedullary nailing after reaming: an investigation on the healing process in osteotomized rabbit tibias, Acta Orthop. Scand. [Suppl.] **134:**Suppl. 1970.

44. DeLee, J. G., and Charnley, J.: Radiological demarcation of cemented sockets in total hip replacement, Clin. Orthop. **121:**20-32, 1976.

45. Duff-Barclay, I., and Spillman, D. T.: Total human hip joint prostheses; a laboratory study of friction and wear. Inst. Mechn. Eng. Proc. **181** (3J):104, 1966-67.

46. Dumbleton, J. H., and Black, J.: An introduction to orthopedic materials, Springfield, Ill., 1975, Charles C Thomas, Publishers.

47. Eftekhar, N. S.: Mechanical failure in low-friction arthroplasty. In American Academy of Orthopaedic Surgeons: Instructional course lecture, vol. 23, St. Louis, 1974, The C. V. Mosby Co., pp. 230-242.

48. Elson, R., and Charnley, J.: The direction of the resultant force in total prosthetic replacement of the hip joint, Med. Biol. Eng. **6:**19-27, 1968.

49. Evans, E. M., Freeman, M. A. R., Miller, A. J., and Vernon-Roberts, B.: Metal sensitivity as a cause of bone necrosis and loosening of the prostheses in total joint replacement, J. Bone Joint Surg. **56B:**626-642, 1974.

50. Ferguson, A. B., Jr., Laing, P. G., and Hodge, E. S.: The ionization of metal implants in living tissues, J. Bone Joint Surg. **42A:**77-90, 1960.

51. Frankel, V. H.: Chairman, Committee on biomedical engineering, American Academy of Orthopaedic Surgeons (exhibit).

52. Frankel, V. H.: The femoral neck; function, fracture mechanisms, internal fixation, Springfield, Ill., Charles C Thomas, Publishers, 1960.

53. Frankel, V. H.: Biomechanics of the hip. In Tronzo, R. G., editor: Surgery of the hip joint, Philadelphia, 1973, Lea & Febiger, pp. 105-125.

54. Freeman, M. A. R., Swanson, S. A. V., and Heath, J. C.: Study of the wear particles produced from cobalt-chromium-molybdenum-manganese total joint replacement prostheses, Ann. Rheum. Dis. **28**[Suppl. 29], 1969.

55. Galante, J. O.: Personal communications.

56. Galante, J. O., and Rostoker, W.: Wear in total hip prostheses; an experimental evaluation of candidate materials, Acta Orthop. Scand. [Suppl.] **145:**Suppl. 1973.

57. Galante, J. O., and Rostoker, W.: Wear rates of candidate materials for total hip arthroplasty. In The Hip Society: The Hip. Proceedings of the first open scientific meeting of The Hip Society, St. Louis, 1973, The C. V. Mosby Co., pp. 67-78.

58. Galante, J., and Rostoker, W.: Materials, wear and potential late complications. In American Academy of Orthopaedic Surgeons: Instruction-

al course lectures, vol. 23, St. Louis, 1974, pp. 178-183.

59. Galante, J. O., Rostoker, W., and Doyle, J. M.: Failed femoral stems in total hip prostheses, J. Bone Joint Surg. **57A:**230-236, 1975.

60. Galante, J. O., Andriacchi, T., Rostoker, W., Schultz, A., and Belytschko, T.: Femoral stem failures in total hip replacements. In The Hip Society: The hip. Proceedings of the third open scientific meeting of The Hip Society, St. Louis, 1975, The C. V. Mosby Co., pp. 231-239.

61. Galante, J. O., Rostoker, W., Lueck, R., and Ray, R. D.: Sintered fiber metal composites as a basis for attachment of implants to bone, J. Bone Joint Surg. **53A:**101-114, 1971.

62. Gold, B. L., and Walker, P. S.: Variables affecting the friction and wear of metal-on-plastic total hip joints, Clin. Orthop. **100:**270-278, 1974.

63. Greenwald, A. S., and Nelson, C. L.: Biomechanics of the reconstructed hip, Orthop. Clin. North Am. **4:**435-447, 1973.

64. Grover, H. J.: Metal fatigues in some orthopedic implants, J. Materials, **1:**412, 1966.

65. Harris, W. H., Schiller, A. L., Scholler, J., Frieberg, R. A., and Scott, R.: Extensive localized bone resorption in femur following total hip replacement, J. Bone Joint Surg. **58A:**612-618, 1976.

66. Henrichsen, E., Jansen, K., and Krogh-Poulsen, W.: Experimental investigation of the tissue reaction to acrylic plastics, Acta Orthop. Scand. **22:**141-146, 1952.

67. Hoopes, J. E., Edgerton, M. T., and Shelley, W.: Organic synthetics for augmentation mammoplasty: their relation to breast cancer, Plast. Reconstr. Surg. **39:**263-270, 1967.

68. Hudack, S.: High chromium, low nickel steel in the operative fixation of fractures, Arch. Surg. **40:**867-884, 1940.

69. Hueper, W. C., and Conway, W. D.: Chemical carcinogenesis and cancers, Springfield, Ill., 1964, Charles C Thomas, Publisher, p. 353.

70. Hughes, A. N., and Jordan, B. A.: Metallurgical observations on some metallic surgical implants which failed in vivo, J. Biomed. Mater. Res. **6:**33-48, 1972.

71. Inman, V. T.: Functional aspects of the abductor muscles of the hip, J. Bone Joint Surg. **29:**607, 1947.

72. Jones, D. A., Lucas, H. K., O'Driscoll, M., Price, C. H. G., and Wibberly, B.: Cobalt toxicity after McKee hip arthroplasty, J. Bone Joint Surg. **57B:**289-296, 1975.

73. Kurokawa, K. M., Pawluk, R. J. and Eftekhar, N.: The response of canine bone to self-curing methyl methacrylate (unpublished data).

74. Laing, P. G.: Compatability of biomaterials, Orthop. Clin. North Am. **4:**249-273, 1973.

75. Laing, P. G., Ferguson, A. B., Jr., and Hodge, E. S.: Tissue reaction in rabbit muscle exposed to metallic implants, J. Biomed. Mater. Res. **1:**135-149, 1967.

76. Loomis, L. K.: Internal prosthesis for upper portion of the femur, J. Bone Joint Surg. **32A:**944-946, 1950.

77. Ludinghausen, M. V., Meister, P., and Probst, J.: Metallosis after osteosynthesis, Pathol. Eur. **5:**307-314, 1970.

78. Mandarino, M. P., Salvatore, J. E.: Ostamer: a polyurethane polymer: its use in fractures and diseased bone, J. Bone Joint Surg. **41A:**1542, 1959.

79. Markolf, K. L.: Discussion at The Hip Society. In the Hip Society: The hip. Proceedings of the third open scientific meeting of The hip society, St. Louis, 1975, The C. V. Mosby Co., p. 240-244.

80. McDougall, A.: Malignant tumor at site of bone plating, J. Bone Joint Surg. **38B:**709-713, 1956.

81. McKee, G. K.: McKee-Farrar total prosthetic replacement of the hip. In Jayson, M., editor: Total hip replacement, London, 1971, Sector Publishing, Ltd., pp. 47-67.

82. McLeish, R. D., and Charnley, J.: Abduction forces in the one legged stance, J. Biomech. **3:**191-209, 1970.

83. McNiece, G.:Personal communications.

84. Müller, M. E.: Total hip prosthesis, Clin. Orthop. **72:**46-68, 1970.

85. Oppenheimer, B. S., Oppenheimer, E. T., Danishefsky, I., Stout, A. P., and Eirich, F. R.: Further studies of polymers as carcinogenic agents in animals, Cancer Res. **15:**333-340, 1955.

86. Oppenheimer, B. S., Oppenheimer, E. T., Stout, A. P., Danishefsky, J., and Willhite, M.: Studies of the mechanism of carcinogenesis by plastic films, Acta. Un. Int. Canc., **15:**659-663, 1959.

87. Paul, J. P.: Biomechanics of the hip joint as clinical relevence, Proc. Roy. Soc. Med. **59:**943, 1966.

88. Paul, J. P.: Forces transmitted by joints in the human body, Proc. Inst. Mech. Eng. **181:**8, 1967.

89. Paul, J. P.: Forces at the human hip joint, Thesis, University of Chicago, 1967.

90. Pauwels, F.: Der Schenkelhalsbruch, ein Mechanisches Problem, Stuttgart, Ferdinand Enke Verlag, 1936.

91. Rook, A. J., Wilkinson, D. S., and Ebling, F. J. G.: Textbook of dermatology, vol. 1, ed. 2, Oxford, Blackwell Scientific Publications, 1972.

92. Rose, R. M., Schiller, A. L., and Radin, E. Z.: Corrosion accelerated mechanical failure of a Vitallium nail-plate, J. Bone Joint Surg. **54A:**854-862, 1972.

93. Rydell, M. W.: Forces in the hip joint. In Bio-

mechanics and related bioengineering topics, London, 1964, Pergamon Press Ltd.

94. Rydell, M. W.: Forces acting on the femoral head prosthesis: a study on strain gauge supplied prostheses living persons, Acta. Orthop. Scand. [Suppl.] **88:**Suppl., 1966.

95. Scales, J. T.: Aspects of medical physics. In Rotblatt, J., editor, London, 1966, Taylor and Francis Ltd., pp. 115-151.

96. Scales, J. T., Winter, G. D., and Shirley, H. T.: Corrosion of orthopedic implants, screws, plates, and femoral nail plates, J. Bone Joint Surg. **41B:** 810-820, 1959.

97. Seedhom, B. B., Dowson, D., and Wright, V.: Wear of solid phase formed high density polyethylene in relation to the life of artificial hips and knees, Wear **24:**35, 1973.

98. Siddons, A. H., and MacArthur, A. M.: Carcinomata developing at the site of foreign bodies in the lung, Br. J. Surg. **39:**542-545, 1951-52.

99. Simon, S. R., Paul, I. L., Rose, R. M., and Ridin, E. L.: "Stiction-friction" of total hip prostheses and its relationship to loosening, J. Bone Joint Surg. **57A:**226-230, 1975.

100. Smith, J. W., and Walmslay, R.: Factors affecting the elasticity of Bone, J. Anat. **93:**503, 1959.

101. Spealman, C. R., Main, R. J., Haag, H. B., and Larson, P. S.: Monomeric methyl methacrylate: studies on toxicity, Ind. Med. **14:**292-298, 1945.

102. Stinson, N. E.: The tissue reaction induced in rats and guinea pigs by polymethylmethacrylate (acrylic) and stainless steel, Br. J. Exper. Pathol. **45:**21-29, 1964.

103. Stinson, N. E.: Tissue reaction induced in guinea pigs by particulate polymethylmethacrylate, polyethylene and nylon of the same size range, Br. J. Exper. Pathol. **46:**135-146, 1965.

104. Swanson, S. A. V., and Freeman, M. A. R.: The scientific basis of joint replacement, New York, 1977, John Wiley & Sons.

105. Swanson, S. A. V., Freeman, M. R., and Heath, J. C.: Laboratory tests on total joint replacement prostheses, J. Bone Joint Surg. **55:**759-773, 1973.

106. Trueta, J.: Studies of the development and decay of the human frame, London, 1968, William Heineman, Ltd.

107. Trueta, J., and Cavadias, A. X.: Vascular changes caused by the Küntscher type of nailing. An experimental study in rabbits, J. Bone Joint Surg. **37B:**492-505, 1955.

108. University of California: Fundamental studies of human locomotion and other information relating to design of artificial limbs, Berkeley, California, 1947.

109. Venable, C. S., and Stuck, W. G.: Three years' experience with Vitallium in bone surgery, Ann. Surg. **114:**309-315, 1941.

110. Venable, C. S., Stuck, W. G., and Beach, A.: The effects on bone in presence of metals; based on electrolysis, Ann. Surg. **105:**917-938, 1937.

111. Walker, P. S., and Bullough, P. G.: The effects of friction and wear in artificial joints, Orthop. Clin. North Am. **4:**275-293, 1973.

112. Walker, P. S., and Erkman, M. J.: Metal-on-metal lubrication in artificial human joints, Wear **21:**377, 1972.

113. Walker, P. S., Salvati, E., and Hotzler, R. K.: The wear on McKee-Farrar total hip prostheses, J. Bone Joint Surg. **56A:**92-100, 1974.

114. Weber, F. A., and Charnley, J.: A radiological study of fractures of acrylic cement in relation to the stem of the femoral head prosthesis, J. Bone Joint Surg. **57B:**297-301, 1975.

115. Weightman, B. O., Rose, R. M., Paul, I. L., Simon, W. R., and Radin, E. L.: A comparative study of total hip replacement prostheses, J. Biomech. **6:**299-311, 1973.

116. Wheeler, K. R., and James, L. A.: Fatigue behavior of type 316 stainless steel under simulated body conditions, J. Biomed. Mater. Res. **5:** 267-281, 1971.

117. Willert, H. G., Frech, H. A. and Bechtel, A.: Measurements of the quantity of monomer leaching out of acrylic bone cement into the surrounding tissues during the process of polymerization, paper presented at the 166th National Meeting of the American Chemical Society, Chicago, Illinois, 1973.

118. Willert, H. G., Ludwig, J., and Semlitsch, M.: Reaction of bone to methacrylate after hip arthroplasty, J. Bone Joint Surg. **56A:**1368-1382, 1974.

119. Williams, D. F., and Roaf, R.: Implants in surgery, Philadelphia, 1973, W. B. Saunders Co.

120. Wilson, J. A., and Scales, J. T.: Loosening of the total hip replacements with cement fixation, Clin. Orthop. **72:**145-160, 1970.

121. Wiltse, L. L., Hall, R. H., and Stenehjem, J. C.: Experimental studies regarding the possible use of self-curing acrylic in orthopaedic surgery, J. Bone Joint Surg. **39A:**961-972, 1957.

122. Zierold, A. A.: Reaction of bone to various metals, Arch. Surg. **9:**365-412, 1924.

CHAPTER 4

Acrylic cement for fixation of total hip prostheses

There is no doubt that in orthopaedic surgery acrylic cement is going to be widely used in many different parts of the world; there is equally no doubt that its use by uninformed operators will produce complications which might seriously threaten its reputation and might hold back the progress of science.

SIR JOHN CHARNLEY

. . . Many surgeons thought that it was an adhesive, and many subconsciously still do, as indicated by the fact that it is still frequently called a "glue."

SIR JOHN CHARNLEY

A thorough understanding of the background and properties of self-curing acrylic cement is essential in order to appreciate the mechanism of fixation and the biological interaction between bone and cement and to understand problems that may arise from defective fixation of a total hip prosthesis related to the methods of fastening. Space limits a complete account of self-curing cement, but a comprehensive report of its use in orthopaedic surgery has been published by Charnley,[17] a source the reader is strongly urged to review.

HISTORICAL BACKGROUND

The chemical history of acrylic cement began with its first synthesis in 1843.[76] Ester-saturated ethyl methacrylate was prepared in 1865 and 1877, and its tendency to polymerize was observed at that time. Industrial techniques for polymerization of cement were developed by Rohm & Haas in Germany at the turn of the century, and by 1927 the first acrylic ester polymer produced commercially was made available. Methyl methacrylate (hereafter referred to as MMA) was developed in Britain principally by Hill and Crawford.[66] It can spontaneously polymerize, but the reaction is very slow. However, with heat, ultraviolet light, or chemical activating agents, polymerization is accelerated. Heat is used for commercial polymerization of MMA to form Plexiglas (Rohm & Haas), Perspex (ICI, Ltd.), and Lucite (DuPont).

Heat-cured MMA was first used in the human body as a denture base material in 1937.[96] Acrylic resin was first used in Germany during World War II and became available commercially as Rapid Paladon and subsequently as Simplex Pentocryl. Since then, acrylic cement has been used in medicine, dentistry, neurosurgery, thoracic surgery, plastic surgery, ophthalmology, otology, and other areas.[19,26] In 1946, the Judet brothers introduced the heat-cured material for replacement of the femoral head, the first clinical application of such a large-sized acrylic prosthesis in hip surgery.[59]

In 1940, Zander[106] first performed an acrylic cranioplasty in humans; since that time many reports have been published on its use in such surgery.*

In a recent publication by Cabanela and associates[11] a long-term follow-up of patients with MMA cranioplasties was reported. Dutton[33] also used MMA as intracranial investment, and in 1959 Knight[64] reported using self-curing MMA for over 10 years to stabilize the spine, especially the cervical spine, with considerable success.

*See references 8, 32, 36, 62, 86, 89, 93, 94, 104, and 105.

Among the first surgeons to use self-curing acrylic cement in hip surgery were Kiaer and Jansen of Copenhagen, prior to 1951. Kiaer[63] used MMA to fix the hip prosthesis into the upper femur. Subsequently, Haboush[46] at the Hospital for Joint Diseases in New York used self-curing MMA as a setting compound to distribute the load to the calcar of the prosthesis during extensive biomechanical analysis of the prosthetic femoral head replacement. However, he did not use the cement for transmitting the load through the intramedullary canal of the femur. Charnley's experience with acrylic cement started in 1958 after discussion with Dr. D. C. Smith, in charge of the Materials Laboratory of the Turner Dental School, Manchester University, England. He is responsible for the present popularity of the cement and for clarification of the principles and technique by which prosthetic replacement fixation can be successfully achieved.[14-17,24,25] McKee and Watson-Farrar[72] and Müller[77] have attributed their successes to Charnley's advocacy of self-curing acrylic cement during the early development of total hip surgery. The Food and Drug Administration in the United States considers acrylic cement as a "drug," and at the present time only one brand, Simplex cement, is approved for clinical use.*

CONSTITUENTS AND CHEMISTRY OF POLYMETHYL METHACRYLATE (PMMA)

The basic MMA polymer formula is $R \cdot CH_2 \cdot C(CH_3) \cdot COO(CH_3)$. The box at the right details the chemical formula. For orthopaedic surgery there are several acrylic products available, which usually consist of separately packaged liquid monomer and sterile polymer powder. The different brands vary in their chemical composition, powder:liquid ratio, and consistency of powder. CMW† is used in Europe, and Charnley's work is based solely on the use of CMW cement. The bone cement presently available in the United States is Simplex P radiopaque.* The powder of Simplex P consists of fine granules of prepolymerized polymethyl methacrylate (PMMA) (15% W/W), copolymerized MMA styrene (75% W/W), and barium sulfate (10%). PMMA is produced by an aqueous redox system and is free from initiator residues. MMA styrene

*Northill Plastics, Inc., London, England.
†CMW Laboratories, Ltd., Blackpool, England.

Basic formula of acrylic cement

$$(CH_2 : C[CH_3] \cdot COOH \cdot CH_3)$$

$$CH_2 = C \Big\langle {}^{R_1}_{COOR_2}$$

Acrylic acid results by replacing H for R_1 and R_2:

$$CH_2 = C \Big\langle {}^{H}_{COOH}$$

When one methyl is substituted at R_1, methacrylic acid results:

$$CH_2 = C \Big\langle {}^{CH_3}_{COOH}$$

The methyl acrylate and methyl methacrylate are thus produced with following formulas:

$$CH_2 = C \Big\langle {}^{H}_{COOCH_3}$$
Methyl acrylate (ester)

$$CH = C \Big\langle {}^{CH_3}_{COOCH_3}$$
Methyl methacrylate (ester)

The formula of polymethyl methacrylate follows:

$$-CH_2-C-CH_2-C-CH_2-C- \atop {}^{CH_3 \quad CH_3 \quad CH_3}_{COOCH_3 \quad COOCH_3 \quad COOCH_3}$$

copolymer is produced by dispersion using benzoyl peroxide as the polymerization initiator and tertiary dodecyl mercaptan as the chain regulator.[1] A cellulose derivative is used as a dispersing agent. This copolymer contains small quantities of initiator and modifier residues but is free from dispersing agent residues. The total weight of the radiopaque bone cement powder is 40 gm. per package; the powder without barium sulfate is also 40 gm. The latter, therefore, has relatively more prepolymerized PMMA (16.7% W/W) and MMA styrene copolymer (83.3% W/W).

The liquid monomer contains 97.4% V/V and has *N,N*-dimethyl-para-toluidine (DMPT) (2.6% V/V) and traces of hydroquinone (75 ± 15 ppm.). DMPT is the amine accelerator that permits the cold curing of acrylic cement; hydroquinone is added to prevent premature spontaneous polymerization of the monomer. The volume per vial is 20 ± 1 ml. The Simplex P is supplied already sterilized by gamma radiation. The liquid is sterilized by passing it through a Seitz bacterial filter.[1-3]

A suitable formulation for self-curing acrylic cement (according to Charnley and Smith[25]) consists of a liquid component of 97.9% MMA, 2% tertiary amine (dimethyl-p-toluidine) as initiator, and 0.1% hydroquinone as inhibitor.

The powder typically consists of 97% PMMA and 2% benzoyl peroxide as activator. Pigment and fillers constitute 1%.[25]

In collaboration with a dental manufacturing company (EMC), Charnley formulated the CMW cement used today in orthopaedic surgery. The powder is of low molecular weight in granular form (PMMA) with no other additives. The granules are formed in a dispersion medium by the "pearl polymerization" process. The liquid is first distilled to remove the hydroquinone inhibitor, which is then replaced by 0.02% ascorbic acid as an inhibitor; 1.2% dimethyl-p-toluidine is added as accelerator. Charnley felt that the use of ascorbic acid in place of hydroquinone was advantageous in its medical application.[17,25]

RADIOPACITY OF CEMENT

Radiopacity is an extremely important feature that should be preserved in all formulas for cement used in total hip surgery. Without this property the presence or amount of cement cannot be determined. The best radiographical density for the acetabulum was produced by the addition of 2.5 gm. barium sulfate to 40 gm. powder and double the amount of barium sulfate (5 gm.) for the shaft and femur. The barium sulfate is contained in two separate packets, each containing 2.5 gm. and each having been sterilized in its packet by gamma irradiation. Each is then added to the cement at the time of mixing. However, with Simplex P radiopaque cement barium sulfate is added to the powder at manufacture and constitutes a 10% W/W of the total polymer powder.

MECHANICAL AND PHYSICAL PROPERTIES

The mechanical properties have been determined by several investigators.[25,35,52,68] Charnley and Smith[25] evaluated self-curing acrylic cement as used in orthopaedic surgery and found a positive relationship between the mechanical properties of pure polymer and that used in actual surgery. Compared with heat-cured material containing a minimum of residual monomer, the tensile strength was reduced by 10% and the stiffness by 5% because of 2% residual monomer.[91] However, Charnley maintains that more important alterations in mechanical behavior result from porosity induced by mixing air in the mass of cement, or as happens at surgery, by inclusion of blood in the mass of cement during insertion. Barring inclusion of air or blood, the average following figures were presented[25]:

Compressive strength	15,000 p.s.i.
Flexural strength	15,000 p.s.i.
Tensile strength	10,000 p.s.i.
Modulus of elasticity	0.3 × 10⁶ p.s.i.

The mechanical properties of Simplex P acrylic cement mixed for orthopaedic use determined by Lee and co-workers[67] are listed in Table 4-1.

The average shearing strength of surgical Simplex P bone cement was found to be 5,762 ± 180 p.s.i.[102] whereas average shearing strength of compact bone is about 10,000 p.s.i. It was therefore concluded that surgical Simplex P does not resist shear forces as well as compact bone and should not be used as a substitute for bone when avoidable. The inclusion of 10% barium sulfate for radiographical purposes did not adversely affect the shear strength. This amount of barium was the same percentage by weight as that found in radiopaque Simplex

Table 4-1. Mechanical properties of acrylic cement as determined by Lee and Ling*

Parameters tested	Unit (newton/mm.²)	No. of specimens tested
Compression		
Ultimate stress	−77	
0.1% proof stress	−60	324
	2,270	
Tension		
Ultimate stress	25	24
Torsion		
Ultimate stress	37	
Modulus of rigidity	850	24
Shear		
Ultimate stress	41	42

*From Lee, A. J. C., Ling, R. S. M., and Wrighton, J. D.: Clin. Orthop. **95**:281-287, 1973.

127

Table 4-2. Strength imparted when Moore self-locking prosthesis was cemented *

Paired femurs tested	Condition tested	Load at failure†	Difference in lb.	Percent difference
Femur pair K (control)	Right with cement Left with cement	2,250 2,200	300	13
Femur pair C	Right with cement Left—no cement	1,150 500	+650	+130
Femur pair I	Right with cement Left—no cement	2,400 1,695	+750	+42

*From Buerkle, A. R., and Eftekhar, N. S.: Clin. Orthop. **111**:134-141, 1975.
†Inch pound.

Table 4-3. Recemented group*

Paired femurs tested	Condition tested	Load at failure†	Difference in lb.	Percent difference
Femur pair B (control)	Right—no conversion Left—with conversion	1,570 1,380	−190	−13
Femur pair F	Right—no conversion Left—with conversion	1,420 1,300	−120	−10
Femur pair E	Right—no conversion Left—with conversion‡	1,400 1,570	+170	+14

*Recementing of a prosthesis, that is, conversion of Eftekhar prosthesis to Charnley low-friction arthroplasty stem, did not alter load-bearing capacity of femur. From Buerkle, A. R., and Eftekhar, N. S.: Clin. Orthop. **111**:134-141, 1975.
†Inch pound.
‡Split into lesser trochanter during preparation of canal.

Table 4-4. Blood admixture group*

Paired femurs tested	Condition tested	Load at failure†	Difference in lb.	Percent difference
Femur pair L (control)	Right—with blood Left—with blood	950 1,450	500	42
Femur pair O	Right—no blood Left—with blood	1,740 1,725	−15	−1
Femur pair M	Right—no blood Left—with blood	1,420 1,190	−230	−18
Femur pair A	Right—no blood Left—with blood	1,570 1,810	+240	+14
Femur pair D	Right—no blood Left—with blood	930 920	−10	−1

*Blood admixture with cement had no substantial deleterious effect on fixation. From Buerkle, A. R., and Eftekhar, N. S.: Clin. Orthop. **111**:134-141, 1975.
†Inch pound.

Table 4-5. Catheter group*

Paired femurs tested	Condition tested	Load at failure†	Difference in lb.	Percent difference
Femur pair G (control)	Right—with catheter Left—with catheter	1,050 1,110	60	6
Femur pair H (control)	Right—no catheter Left—no catheter	1,830 1,560	270	17
Femur pair J	Right—no catheter Left—with catheter	1,220 1,550	+330	+24
Femur pair N	Right—no catheter Left—with catheter	960 800	−160	−18
Femur pair P	Right—no catheter Left—with catheter	420 480	+60	+13

*The use of a catheter at insertion of cement did not change load-bearing capacity of femur. From Buerkle, A. R., and Eftekhar, N. S.: Clin. Orthop. **111:**134-141, 1975.
†Inch pound.

P in clinical use. The shear force at failure increased slightly with increased time of curing. The curing periods in their experiments varied from 2 to 168 hours. All strengths were estimated to be approximately 25% lower than the upper limits of normal bone, and the stiffness five to ten times less.[25] Mechanical properties of cement were not significantly affected by a variation of mixing techniques studied by Lee and associates.[68] They suggested that in clinical practice the presence of blood in the cement may cause weakness, although the adverse effect was not significant. Lamination was minimized when the mixture of blood with cement was kept to a minimum and when the cement was under pressure.

In a recent study at our laboratories[9] the mechanical properties of a cemented stem were studied in the following situations: (1) venting the medullary canal with a catheter during the insertion of cement, (2) the inclusion of blood into cement during insertion, and (3) recementing a prosthesis. In addition, the strength imparted by cement to a prosthesis was evaluated. In this study, biological variables were minimized by the use of paired wet formalin-preserved femurs, one acting as control. A single static load was applied until failure. The results showed that the MMA-bone-metal system consistently produced good results with reasonable, but not careless, variations in technique. Venting the canal, recementing the prosthesis, or admixture with blood under these conditions did not alter the mechanical properties of the cement fixation (Tables 4-2 to 4-5 and Fig. 4-1).

Astleford and co-workers[4] evaluated the acetabular hole configuration of the prosthesis fixation in the pelvis as related to the strength of MMA. They concluded that the geometric configuration did not significantly affect the maximum shear load-carrying capabilities of the MMA.

Tests on stability of the mechanical properties of self-curing acrylic bone cement (both Simplex P and CMW) have revealed that storage of cement up to 2 years in bovine serum at 37° C. caused no significant deterioration or change in the mechanical properties (neither static properties nor compression fatigue behavior). Data on compression fatigue suggested that working stresses in the cement should be limited to less than 1.4×10^{-8} dynes/cm.^{2} to ensure long-term viability of any design or implantation technique.[57]

The effect of irradiation on acrylic cement, with special reference to fixation of pathological fractures, was studied by Eftekhar and Thurston.[35] Tests were undertaken to determine the mechanical properties of the two commonly used bone cements, Simplex P radiopaque and CMW, and the effect of irradiation on each. It was concluded that there was no significant difference in mechanical properties of irradiated and nonirradiated cement and that postoperative irradiation may be safely performed after fixation of pathological fractures or pathology of the pel-

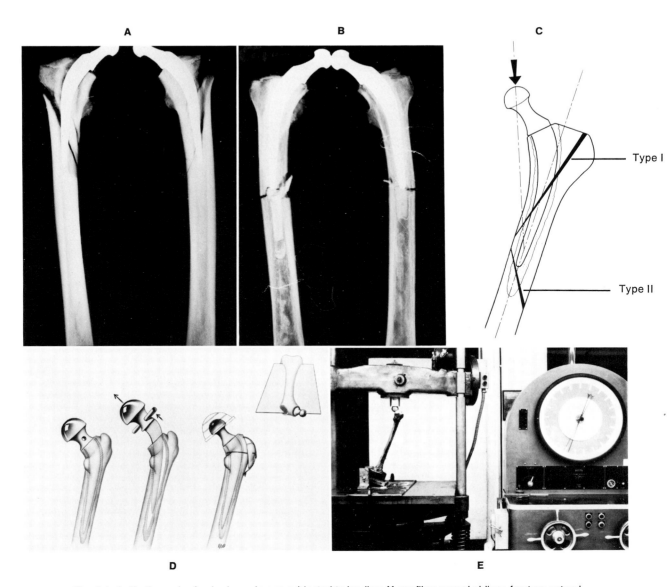

Fig. 4-1. A, Radiograph of paired specimens subjected to loading. X-ray films reveal oblique fracture extending from greater trochanter to medial cortex at level of tip of prosthesis. This mode of failure was by far more common in specimens tested. **B,** Post-test radiographs of femur with fracture of cement at level of tip of prosthesis. NOTE: reverse obliquity of fracture, which extends from medial side outward and distalward. **C,** Diagrammatic drawing of line of application of load. Direction of lines of fracture has occurred in two patterns: *Type I.* Prosthesis settled into varus. There was failure of trochanteric cancellous bone parallel to trochanteric line. *Type II.* Diaphyseal fracture of cortical bone was produced with reversed obliquity of fracture line beginning at tip of prosthesis. All specimens showed cement fractures at tip of prosthesis, at junction of stiff column with more elastic column of shaft. Twenty tests showed type I fractures, **A,** and eight showed type II fractures, **B.** All showed cement fractures at tip of stem of prosthesis. **D,** Charnley's low-friction arthroplasty stem (standard) compared with author's stem. Latter design is similar to Charnley's standard stem but 10% proportionately larger in all dimensions. In recementing tests Eftekhar prosthesis was knocked out of channel, and Charnley stem cemented in place using only small amount of cement. *Inset,* Transcondylar plane (neutroversion) of preparation of femur. **E,** Testing setup using a Baldwin, 10-ton press. NOTE: for testing, femoral condyles were placed in epoxy molds. Long axis of bone was placed at 20 degrees to vertical in press to produce resultant joint force of one-legged stance plus normal varus inclination of femur. Rate of loading was slow, 400 lb./min. At fatigue, or shatter, failure the force noted on scale would drop despite continued compression. End point was taken as peak force applied.

130

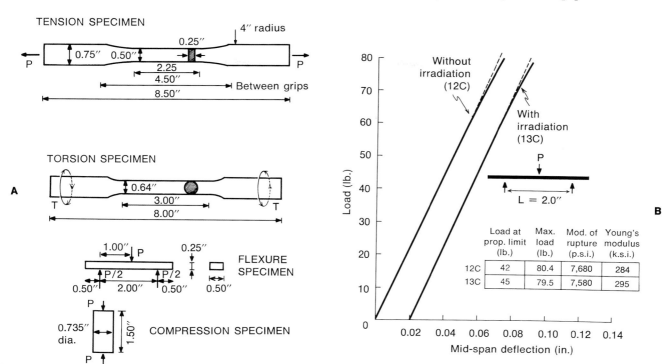

Fig. 4-2. A, Tests were conducted for both CMW and Simplex cements with and without barium sulfates and with and without irradiation. Specimens were molded by hand in molds machined from Teflon stock. Dimension and arrangement for tension, torsion, and compression specimens are shown. **B,** Typical load-deflection curve using irradiated and nonirradiated specimens.[35]

vis without adverse effects on the mechanical properties of the cement (Fig. 4-2).

LOSS OF MONOMER BY EVAPORATION AND LEACHING

Loss of monomer during mixing was studied by Charnley and Smith[25] and Lee and associates.[67,68] The major monomer loss from evaporation of acrylic cement dough appears to take place during periods of mixing of the dough rather than at the final stage of mixing (from surface of the bolus prior to insertion) (Tables 4-6 to 4-8). It is of special interest that, irrespective of the amount of beating in preparation, cement became stronger with the passage of time up to 1 week following polymerization. A very satisfactory mechanical strength of MMA was observed in a specimen examined 7½ years after implantation.[68]

PMMA monomer is a very volatile substance. Its solubility in water is about 1.5% at 30° C., and it is rapidly eliminated from the body. The total concentration of leached-out monomer

Table 4-6. Mean monomer loss in gm./½ min. during mixing at different mixing frequencies

No. of cements	Beat frequency/min.	Mean monomer loss in gm./½ min. during mixing
22	60	0.133
12	120	0.213
7	184	0.355
29	260	0.436

Table 4-7. Monomer loss at polymerization testing three different commercially available acrylics*

Type of cement	Total loss over 1½ min.	Loss/min.
Simplex	0.165 gm.	0.055 gm.
Simplex opaque	0.192 gm.	0.064 gm.
CMW opaque	0.273 gm.	0.091 gm.

*From Lee, A. J. C., Ling, R. S. M., and Wrighton, J. D.: Clin. Orthop. **95:**281-287, 1973.

must therefore be low.[17] The residual monomer in self-curing acrylic cement is measured by a calorimetric test using potassium permanganate. With this test, Smith and Bains[90] showed that two specimens of acrylic cement showed no further loss of monomer after 36 hours' immersion in distilled water at 37° C. With heat-cured cement, the leaching of the monomer was completed experimentally at 17 hours in large volumes of water at 37° C. and also after a similar period in a large group of volunteer patients. Smith examined four types of self-curing acrylic cement from different manufacturers for residual monomer from 1 hour to 58 weeks after curing. The four products demonstrated that fall in residual monomer was related to the "after-cure" process of further polymerization of the cement. The four specimens started the test with retained monomer ranging from 3.5% to 1.9%. The residual monomer contents fell slightly over the period of the test, and for all specimens the drop

Table 4-8. Total monomer loss in gm./15 min. at different mixing frequencies*

Beat frequency/min.	Monomer loss in gm.
60	0.85-1.28
120	1.01-1.96
184	1.67-2.24
260	2.4-3.4

*From Lee, A. J. C., Ling, R. S. M., and Wrighton, J. D.: Clin. Orthop. **95:**281-287, 1973.

averaged 0.3% over 58 weeks.[17] Monomer loss by evaporation from acrylic cement dough takes place to a significant degree only during periods in which the dough is being mixed and cannot be significantly altered following the mixing period. If the cement mass was left undisturbed until implantation, the concentration of monomer at the surface became low, but manipulation of the mass (during insertion into the medullary cavity of the femur, for example) would expose the deeper layer of the dough, and thus the monomer, to the bone surface.[67] It is logical to suggest a vigorous mixing during doughing time to rid the cement of monomer. It should continue until cement is pasty and thick and starts giving "fine hairs" from the surface.

Residual activator (benzoyl peroxide) in the powder was also determined. Two of four specimens started with peroxide contents of approximately 0.35%, which fell in the first 58 weeks to a final value of about 0.05%, which fell over 58 weeks to a final level of 0.02%.[91]

WORKING TIME AND SETTING TIME CHARACTERISTICS

At surgery, the full amount of liquid monomer is added to the preweighed polymer and thoroughly mixed with a spoon. For about 30 seconds there appears to be insufficient liquid for the powder, but the mass soon becomes further liquefied and then rubbery. With mixing and aeration tenacious "hairs" form, indicating readiness for removal from the bowl. When hairs

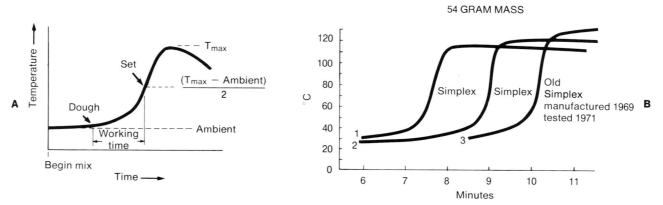

Fig. 4-3. A, Setting and working time characteristics of cement and its relationship to exothermic reaction. **B,** Illustrates effect of storage on setting characteristics of acrylic cement. Examples presented here: *1,* Simplex fresh, 1969; *2,* Simplex fresh, 1971; *3,* old Simplex manufactured in 1969 tested in 1971 using a 54-gm. mass. (Adapted from Amstutz, H. C., and Gruen, T. In Ahstrom, J. P., editor: Current practice in orthopaedic surgery, 1973, St. Louis, 1973, The C. V. Mosby Co.)

no longer form, the glistening liquidlike appearance disappears, and a soft doughlike consistency allows removal from the bowl by scraping. The working time of the cement is approximately 2 to 4 minutes. During this period the surgeon inserts it into the bone (Chapter 12). The setting characteristics (Fig. 4-3, *A*) of commer-

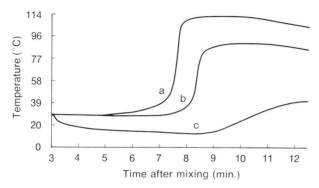

Fig. 4-4. Effect of ambient temperature on setting characteristics of polymethyl methacrylate (PMMA). *a,* Thermal profile of mass center polymerizing at room temperature. *b,* Thermal profile of center. *c,* Periphery of mass setting with plastic bag immersed in ice water. (Adapted from Amstutz, H. C., and Gruen, T. In Ahstrom, J. P., editor: Current practice in orthopaedic surgery, 1973, St. Louis, 1973, The C. V. Mosby Co.)

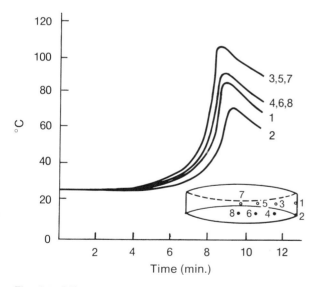

Fig. 4-5. Differences observed in temperature rise with respect to location in setting cement. Cement is insulating material and capable of withstanding large temperature gradient. At surface considerable heat can be conducted away by prosthesis or bone; at interior mass of cement temperature rise is considerably greater. (Adapted from Meyer, P. R., Lautenschlager, E. P., and Moore, B. K.: J. Bone Joint Surg. **55A:**149-156, 1973.)

cially available cements vary from brand to brand, batch to batch, and with the age of the liquid monomer (Fig. 4-3, *B*). An increase in ambient temperature will decrease the working time of the dough; setting time (usually 12 to 13 minutes) depends on humidity, molecular weight of the polymer, texture of the powder, proportion of activator and initiator, proportion of liquid to powder. Meyer and associates[75] concluded that in one batch of MMA tested, the surface temperature of the setting cement never exceeded 70° C.; the setting time was prolonged by lowering the ambient temperature, decreasing the powder : liquid ratio, and increasing the mass of cement. Although working time is not altered materially by changing powder : liquid ratio, rise in maximum temperature is noted when excess monomer is employed (Fig. 4-3, *A*). As a rule, CMW cement sets in about two-thirds the time of Simplex P. The most significant and practically important factor is a decreased working time with rises in ambient temperature. Most investigators have concluded that batch-to-batch variations in cement composition should be expected.[21,68,71,75] Setting characteristics of cement as related to exothermic temperature and working time are shown in Figs. 4-3 to 4-6 and Tables 4-9 and 4-10.

INSTRUCTIONS FOR MIXING AT SURGERY

A dose is prepared by mixing the entire contents of one packet of powder (a mixture of PMMA, styrene copolymer, and barium sulfate), 40 gm., and one ampule of the liquid monomer (MMA), 20 ml. Depending on the surgical procedure and technique, one or two doses are required. Each dose is mixed separately when used sequentially.

Preparation

Since the outer surface of the ampule of the liquid component is not sterile, it is recommended that the ampule be sterilized before use by submersion in a cold sterilizing solution.

While the outer surface of the packet containing the powder component is sterilized at time of packaging, it is recommended that the entire package be submerged in a cold sterilizing solution for 18 hours to check for possible leaks in the overwrap and resultant contamination of the packet of powder. The cold sterilizing solutions recommended are 2% glutaraldehyde

133

Fig. 4-6. A, At low magnification of cut surface of acrylic cement (prepared at surgery) elongated void in the internal mass of bolus can be seen (scanning electron microscopy). **B,** Higher magnification of **A** shows features of surface of void, revealing small spheres of polymer on internal surface (scanning electron microscopy). **C,** Moderate magnification of cement-bone interface, showing blob of cement at upper right corner of field. NOTE: characteristic feature of cement surface—spheres of polymer (scanning electron microscopy). **D,** High-power magnification of cement in contact with polymethyl methacrylate cement. NOTE: intimacy of cement with trabeculae. Note also healed fractured trabeculae (center of the field) presumably from trauma at surgery. **E,** Scanning electron microscopy of PMMA cement-bone interface. Close coaptation of cement with bone in specimen is observed. Polymeric spheres again are seen here. (Courtesy James Pugh, Ph.D.)

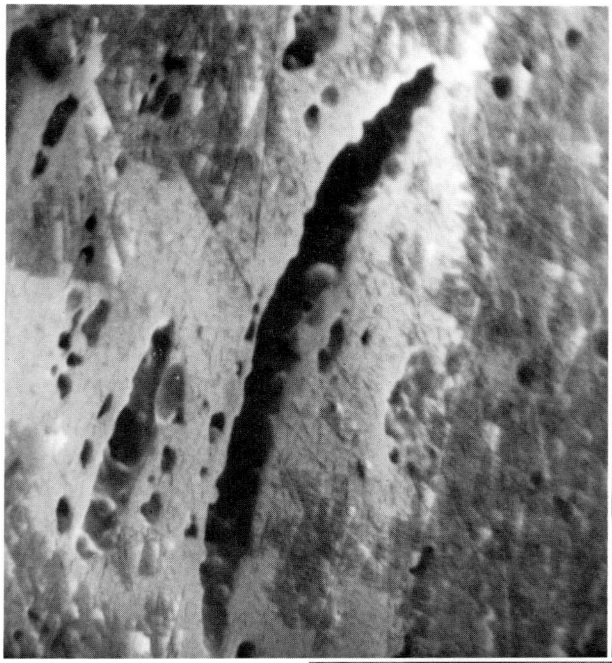

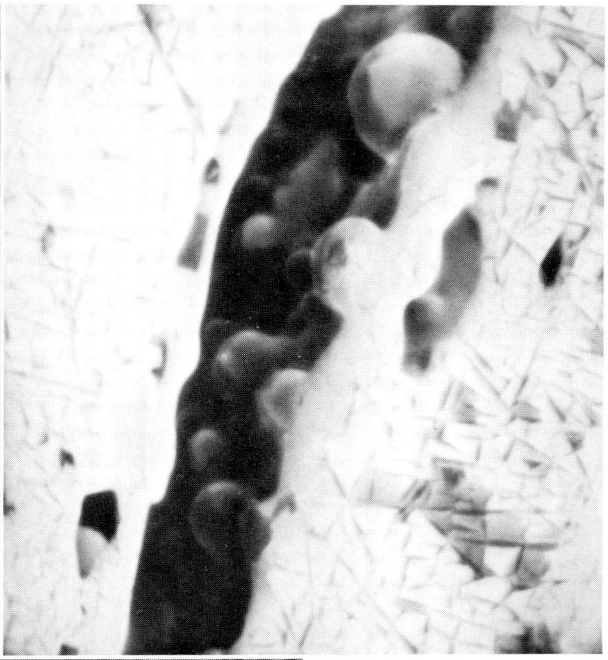

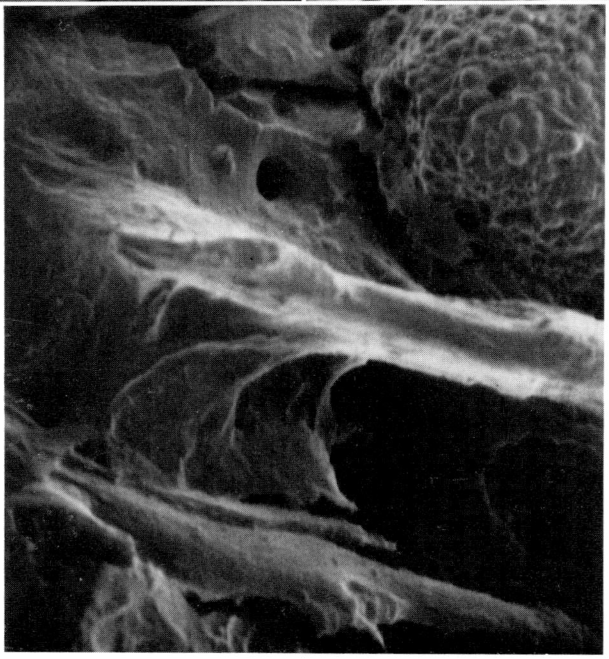

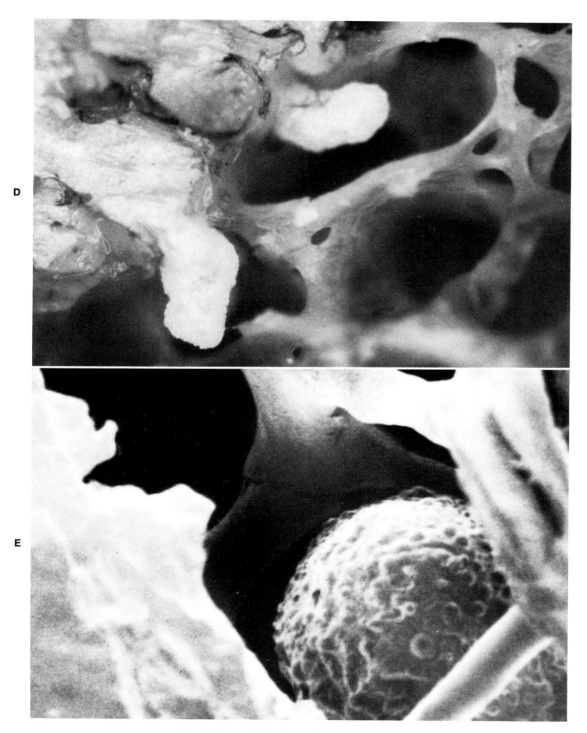

Fig. 4-6, cont'd. For legend see opposite page.

Table 4-9. Effect of ambient temperature of setting properties of acrylic cement*

Ambient temperature (°C.)	Dough time (min.)	Set time (min.)	Working time (min.)	T_{max}† (°C.)
4	34.0	60.0	26.0	53
15	10.5	21.5	11.0	89
20	4.5	13.0	8.5	101
25	3.0	8.0	5.0	107
30	2.0	5.0	3.0	111
37	1.0	3.0	2.0	125

*From Meyer, P. R., Jr., Lautenschlager, E. P., and Moore, B. K.: J. Bone Joint Surg. **55A:**149-156, 1973.
†Measured in center of 36-gm. specimen, 10 mm. thick, mixed at P/L = 2.0, and placed in a 60-mm. diameter Teflon mold.

Table 4-10. Effect of thickness and weight on setting properties*

Thickness (mm.)	Weight (gm.)	Set time (min.)	T_{max} (°C.)
10	36	8.0	107
6	22	7.0	86
3	11	6.2	60

*Ambient temperature = 25° C. All specimens set in 60-mm. Teflon mold. T_{max} measured in center of disk at a depth of 5, 3, and 1.5 mm., respectively. From Meyer, P. R., Jr., Lautenschlager, E. P., and Moore, B. K.: J. Bone Joint Surg. **55A:**149-156, 1973.

aqueous solution and, 0.13% benzalkonium chloride aqueous solution. For convenience we use a 2% tincture of iodine in 70% alcohol.

To mix, empty the entire contents of the packet containing the powder component into a stainless steel mixing bowl. Add the entire contents of the ampule containing the liquid component. *Add the liquid component to the powder, not the powder to the liquid.* Stir with a stainless steel spoon in a stainless steel or porcelain bowl, until the powder is completely saturated with the liquid. *Continue stirring until a doughlike mass is formed that does not stick or adhere to the rubber gloves of the operator.* The doughlike mass (at completion of doughing time) is then ready for manipulation. The mixing and manipulation process should be at least 4 minutes in duration for Simplex P radiopaque cement. The mixing and kneading time required to obtain a proper consistency for application to bone is best determined by the experience of the surgeon under working conditions. Mixing should resume if cement adheres to the rubber glove. All the cement must be removed from the bowl. If more than one unit of cement (40 gm. powder and 20 ml. liquid) is needed, the contents of two packets of powder are emptied into the mixing bowl, then two ampules (20 ml. each) are emptied simultaneously into the powder, thus 40 ml. of monomer are used. As stated before, the setting time may be divided into doughing time and working time; working time is calculated from the time that dough is "not sticky" to "hard set." To reduce setting time by reducing the monomer amount will reduce working time at the expense of increasing doughing time. An informed surgeon is not likely to be caught by surprise if a sloppy mixing technique results in loss of 3 or 4 ml. of monomer.

RISE OF TEMPERATURE AND DENATURING OF PROTEIN

The degree of temperature elevation in the polymerizing cement mass is directly proportional to the size of the mass and to the ambient temperature. For example, a mass 1 inch in diameter may become too hot to hold in the hand. The temperature in the center of such a mass may rise to the boiling point, whereas the exterior temperature may be somewhat lower. When cement is used in conjunction with the prosthesis, considerable heat may be absorbed by metal and plastic, thus diminishing the surface temperature. Occasionally, however, one may see darkening of the blood adjacent to a thick layer of cement, suggesting heat denaturation of hemoglobin. When rise in temperature can be palpated, the working time is cut; thus cement becomes too hard to allow insertion of cement or prosthesis, and the surgeon is well advised to discard it (Figs. 4-4 and 4-5).

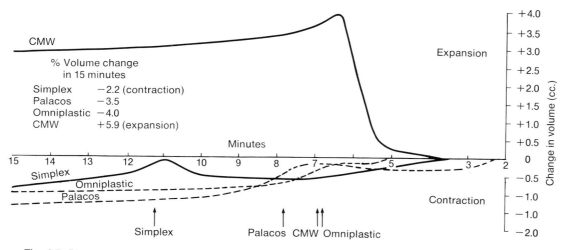

Fig. 4-7. Dimensional changes of four commonly used orthopaedic cements: Simplex, Palacos, CMW, and Omniplastic. (Adapted from Amstutz, H. C., and Gruen, T. In Ahstrom, J. P., editor: Current practice in orthopaedic surgery, 1973, St. Louis, 1973, The C. V. Mosby Co.)

DIMENSIONAL CHANGES DURING POLYMERIZATION OF ACRYLIC CEMENT

Shrinkage of the acrylic cement mass following polymerization is expected. This shrinkage of pure monomer is approximately 20% with an increase in density from 0.94 gm./cm.[3] to 1.19 gm./cm.[3] after polymerization.[1,6] When the bulk of cement is polymerized, shrinkage of the final mass is attributed to volumetric shrinkage of the liquid component. Since in orthopaedics acrylic (combined liquid and powder) liquid comprises only one third of the total mass, the shrinkage of the mass should be approximately 7%. Smith[91] observed that polymerization shrinkage with dental cement was concentrated in a localized area not uniform throughout the mass. Volumetric changes of CMW cement were determined by Charnley.[17] Several other investigators conducted similar studies and concluded that Simplex P, Omniplastic, and Palacos initially contracted, then expanded minimally, and finally contracted 2.2%, 4%, and 3.5%, respectively[17,52,101] (Fig. 4-7). The expansion of CMW was considerably greater; the net dimensional change after 15 minutes was 5.9%. Ideally, it would be beneficial if the cement would expand and penetrate into the bony interstices for a better fixation. In 1957, Wiltse[103] reported a shrinkage of about 6% by volume. Charnley[25] concluded that the air bubbles trapped in the mix during preparation were responsible for expansion of the volume of cement and compensated for shrinkage of the total mass. This is the basis for his recommendation of vigorous beating for aeration.[17]

MICROSTRUCTURE OF PMMA CEMENT

The powder of PMMA is composed of two forms of PMMA, one consisting of tiny spherical beads formed by the suspension polymerization method and the other of finely ground amorphous PMMA. In surgical Simplex P, as stated before, 83.8% of the polymer is MMA styrene copolymer, whereas in CMW the polymer is pure PMMA.

Charnley basically described polymerized cement as having a biphasic structure consisting of aggregates of small spheres or granules of the previously described polymer (powder) cemented together by recently polymerized monomer (liquid) (Fig. 4-6). The balls of polymer are from 10 to 80 μ in diameter and are said to be responsible for the semicircular impression on the surface of endosteal bone. Cameron and associates[13] also examined the structure of polymethyl methacrylate (CMW). Their observations corroborated Charnley's conclusion that the cement mass is an aggregate of previously polymerized polymer granules stuck together with recently polymerized monomer. Charosky and Walker,[27] on the other hand, using scanning electron microscopy, concluded that the cast surfaces and polished sections of two different types of cement (Simplex P and

137

CMW) demonstrate spherical domes 5 to 30 μ in diameter. The domes are bubbles in the material seen in polished sections. They concluded that the cement probably is a monophasic material.

The presence of bubbles and voids in the texture of the cement is clearly seen under the microscope. In studying the porosity of self-curing acrylic cement, Smith and co-workers[91] observed two types of porosities: (1) large irregular voids, which were attributed to polymerization contraction, and (2) fine spherical bubbles similar to those of gaseous porosity in heat-cured materials. They cited work showing that acrylic monomer can contain up to 10% dissolved air by volume, and there is a suggestion that these bubbles are caused by the separation of dissolved air as the monomer solidifies.

STERILIZATION OF SELF-CURING ACRYLIC CEMENT

Sterilization of the cement poses certain technical problems. The liquid monomer possesses some self-sterilization power as verified by Charnley.[17] With exposure to monomer, cultures of *Staphylococcus aureus* were sterilized in 1 minute, but spore bearers required 4 days. Towers[98] found that *Staphylococcus aerogenes* survived up to 20 minutes' exposure, while the spore-forming *Bacillus cereus* was viable up to 14 days' exposure. Because of self-polymerization, sterilization of monomer by autoclaving or gamma radiation is not possible. Seitz filtration is used for purification.

Based on laboratory tests, it was concluded that over a period of weeks, common organisms tend to die out spontaneously in acrylic cement powder.[17] This is consistent with observations made in 1962 by Hullinger, who did not encounter any growth of organisms in tissue cultures to which unsterilized Palacos powder had been added.[54,55,91] Charnley felt that formaldehyde vapor was quite safe for sterilization of powder. He recommended double-wrapped polyethylene packaging and placing a porous packet containing formaldehyde vapor within each pack, to be thrown away when the pack is opened. The powder may also be sterilized by gamma rays, which also prolong the setting time by approximately 2 minutes. Irradiation of the mixed barium sulfate and cement powder must be avoided, however, since this prolongs the setting time by 20 minutes or more.[17,25] Simplex

P powder as supplied for surgical use is sterilized with 2.5 megarads from a cobalt 60 source. It is suggested that the packet containing the cement powder be soaked in a 2% iodine solution prior to opening its exterior polyethylene wrap for delivery to the surgical field.

MECHANICAL FIXATION BY ACRYLIC CEMENT

Some of the principles involved in mechanical fixation have been detailed in Chapter 3.

The term "glue" has often been used by uninitiated surgeons using the cement in the field of replacement surgery. Distinction between a "glue" and a "filler" is not merely semantic but based on real differences in mechanisms by which the two operate. Understanding how acrylic cement can transfer the load from the stem of a prosthesis to the shaft of the femur and diffuse the load onto the endosteal surface of the bone is the sine qua non of correct application of the cement. When used as a stiff paste or dough, it has space-filling properties not possessed by the thin liquid characteristic of glue. If a prosthesis were glued to the bone, it would be advantageous to have a tight mechanical fit using the thinnest possible layer of glue. The stem would be wet with the glue and then driven firmly into a tight bed. In this situation, obviously the surfaces must be shaped to make an accurate fit, which is not possible in this surgery. Also, glue depends on a chemical reaction for adhesion, and a thin adhesive could not withstand the incumbent stresses. On the other hand, a filler, or cement, does not require any chemical interaction between the two, with cement serving as an interface. Thus an accurate fit between bone surface and prosthesis is not required, since the cement fills in bulk inaccuracies and gaps between the two structures. In this context, therefore, the cement is used thickly, with the mechanical advantage of withstanding a considerable amount of stress. Indeed, a thin layer may weaken and become brittle, inevitably fragmenting.

Because most forces in the hip are compressive, this material is most suitable for bonding, since its best mechanical property is compressive strength. By interdigitation of the cement into the bone during cyclic loading and unloading of the transmission of body weight, the whole surface of the interior of the bone is subjected to the load, thus preventing stress concentration at any given area of contact. Therefore shearing forces between prosthesis and bone are reduced by the absence of friction between the two surfaces. Lack of motion prevents fretting movements that cause bone necrosis. The most common cause of failure of fixation is principally related to the stress concentration often produced by "mechanical-interference-fit" (also known as Press-fit) of implants in bone.

It must be recognized that inability to understand the mechanism by which cement functions led to the failure of early surgeons to achieve successful results.[46,63] Apparently they used a small amount of cement only to improve the seating of the collar of the prosthesis against the cut surface of the femoral neck. This also explains the failure of fixation when cement was delicately applied to the upper femur. Failure will occur if the surgeon does not appreciate that interosseous injection of cement provides adequate thickness and bonding over a relatively large surface area. My personal criticism of using a cement gun is based on the fear of inadequate peripheral injection of the cement because pressure is not built up behind the column. Fixation of a prosthesis into the medullary canal is analogous to a flagpole being pushed into a hole filled with wet concrete. The larger the volume of concrete and the greater interdigitation of its surface with the ground, the more stability against compressive and shearing stresses is provided for the flagpole.

Charnley is credited with the discovery of the concept of using cement as a filler rather than an adhesive. He contended that it forms an accurate filling for cavities of the interior surface of the bone. Thus it transmits the load evenly over a fairly large area between the outer surface of the metal and the inner surface of the bone.[14,15,18]

SYSTEMIC AND LOCAL SIDE EFFECTS

Reports have appeared in the literature concerning four interrelated aspects of monomeric effects: (1) toxicity studies, (2) lowering of blood pressure and cardiac arrest, (3) fat embolization, and (4) allergic reaction.

Toxicity studies

Wiltse and co-workers[103] observed no harmful effects when an amount of MMA cement equivalent to a dose in humans of 2 pounds was implanted in animals. Thus they concluded that

the toxicity of MMA was not very high. When dogs were given large doses in an intravenous drop over a period of 19 seconds, the fatal dose calculated from the blood volume was 125 mg./L.[53,54] Injection of pure monomer into the veins of experimental animals such as guinea pigs, rabbits, and rats produced vascular irregularities and eventual cardiac arrest and death, showing that monomer is cytotoxic.[31,52,73] When injected intravenously in rabbits, a monomeric dose of 0.03 ml./kg. body weight produced a sudden and transient fall in arterial blood pressure.[59] Although Homsey was able to produce localized pulmonary hemorrhage in dogs after intravenous administration of 5 mg./100 ml., morbidity did not occur in the animals even when a dose of 50 mg./100 ml. was given for as long as a year. However, when the dose was increased to 125 mg./100 ml., the blood pressure dropped severely, and the animal died of respiratory failure.[52] Homsey further investigated the MMA in clinical use and found that its level in the central venous system reached a maximum of 1.26 mg./100 ml., preceding by 1 to 3 minutes the heat generation of hand-held acrylic. The monomer was also detected in expired anesthetic air.[51,52] The effect of pulmonary changes reported by Homsey have not been found in routine radiological examination of the human chest.[29,30]

Charnley explicitly discussed the papers presented by Henrichsen and co-workers,[48] Wiltse and co-workers,[103] Scales,[87] Reitz,[85] and Homsey and co-workers[52,53] in his monograph on acrylic cement.[17] He suggested that the widespread bone and animal death related to intramedullary filling in experimental animals should be carefully considered and compared when small doses are introduced in human bone at the time of total hip arthroplasty. Fortunately, because cement is fully polymerized in 15 minutes and there is only minimal residual monomer at the time of full polymerization, tissue is exposed to a negligible amount of monomer.

Histological and hemodynamically toxic effects of MMA monomer were also studied by Holland and associates.[50] From their animal experimentation, they concluded that the toxic effects were dose related. When MMA was injected into dogs in the range of 59 mg./100 ml. by three different routes (portal vein, carotid artery, thoracic aorta), histological changes of congestion, edema, hemorrhage, degeneration, and/or necrosis were observed in the lungs, liver, and kidneys, depending on the route of injection. These authors were unable, however, to demonstrate histological changes in the brain, heart, gastrointestinal tract, or spleen.

Blood clearance of MMA and acute pulmonary toxicity in dogs after simulated arthroplasty and intravenous injections have been studied. Clearance of ^{14}C-labeled monomer from the blood was determined in beagles during simulated hip arthroplasties and after intravenous injection of the monomer. Blood clearance was found to be rapid, with the lungs apparently functioning as a major clearing organ for MMA. Decreased pulmonary function (documented by decreased P_{O_2}, elevated P_{CO_2}, and metabolic acidosis) occurred only when the dose of monomer was more than 35 times the amount liberated in humans during total hip replacement procedures.[73]

Lowering of blood pressure and cardiac arrest

Charnley showed the effect of monomer on blood pressure in the human after implantation of acrylic cement. He considered this lowering effect to be transient and recovery uneventful when it appears during anesthesia; he suggested no special precautions during surgery at the time of cement insertion based on his extensive experiences. However, he recommended aeration of the mix during cement preparation to rid it of excess monomer and leaving the bolus of cement undisturbed at the time of insertion to prevent bringing interior monomer to the surface of the bolus just prior to its insertion.[12]

In recent literature, several isolated cardiac arrests and sudden deaths have been attributed to the monomer lowering the blood pressure and causing circulatory collapse. However, controversy still exists as to the cause of death in these cases.*

Fearn and co-workers[38] and Phillips and co-workers[83] reported their experiences with changes in systolic blood pressure during total hip replacement operations. Fearn cited systolic blood pressure changes in 45 patients during total hip replacement with cement. At the acetabular stage of the operation, blood pressure rose in 16 patients (35%), fell in 24 (53%), and

---

*See references 10, 28, 43-45, 47, 61, 74, 78, 80, 81, and 84.

remained unchanged in 5 (12%). He found that when the femur was packed with cement, the systolic blood pressure rose in 24 (54%), fell in 20 (44%), and remained steady in one patient (2%). Phillips and associates[83] also measured arterial blood pressure, central venous pressure, ECGs, blood gases, and intrafemoral pressure in patients undergoing total hip replacement. They measured monomer level in blood samples taken during the operation and demonstrated that there was usually a substantial fall in arterial blood pressure following the introduction of cement into the upper end of the femur, but rarely after introducing the cement into the acetabulum. Packing cement into the femoral canal resulted in a rise of intramedullary pressure as much as 1,900 mm. Hg. They concluded that the rise in medullary canal pressure did not appear to be responsible for the fall in blood pressure. They felt that the time relationship between the two phenomena was inconsistent with a reflex effect via baroreceptors in the bone. The measurement of monomer level in the blood was small only after acetabular implantation, but relatively large after introducing the cement into the femoral canal. They concluded that the fall in blood pressure had always been transient and should not be considered a cause for alarm during total hip replacement.

The cardiovascular effect of MMA was studied by Ellis and associates,[37] who compared the effects of the liquid components of commercial acrylic cement and pure MMA monomer on mean arterial blood pressure, central venous pressure, heart rate, and cardiac output. They concluded that the cardiovascular disturbance is caused by monomeric MMA alone, rather than by any other constituents in the liquid monomer. Berman and associates[5] evaluated the blood pressure lowering effect of monomer in 12 normovolemic and hypovolemic dogs and concluded that the monomer influenced arterial blood pressure and cardiac output as well as peripheral resistance. Furthermore, it was concluded that the monomer produced vasodilation of the small blood vessels and that peripheral resistance and blood pressure were decreased in both normovolemic and hypovolemic dogs. There was, however, a significant increase in cardiac output of normovolemic dogs, but a decrease in hypovolemic dogs (Fig. 4-8).

McMaster and associates,[74] in their study of

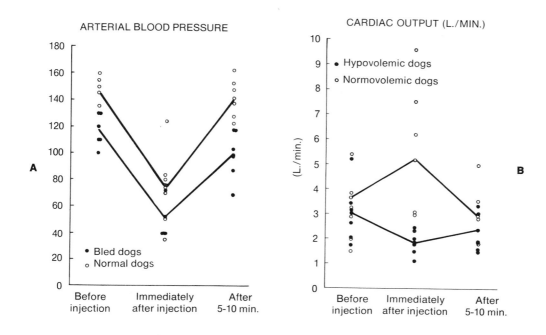

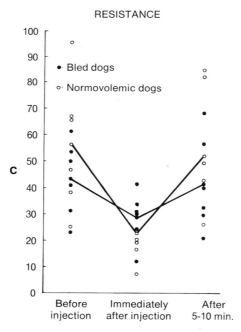

Fig. 4-8. A, Graph of arterial blood pressure in normovolemic and hypovolemic dogs showing lower initial blood pressure in hypovolemic dogs but equal decrease in blood pressure after administration of monomer. **B,** Graph of cardiac output in normovolemic and hypovolemic dogs showing rise in cardiac output in normovolemic dogs, and decrease in hypovolemic dogs. **C,** Peripheral resistance in normovolemic and hypovolemic dogs showing greater decrease in resistance in normovolemic dogs. (Adapted from Berman, A. T., Price, H. L., and Hahn, J. F.: Clin. Orthop. **100:**265-269, 1974.)

the blood pressure lowering effect of MMA monomer, concluded that with intravenously injected MMA the depletion of blood volume potentiates the lowering of blood pressure. Therefore these authors felt that peripheral vasodilation with myocardial depression is the main mechanism by which peripheral arterial blood pressure is lowered, thus confirming the findings of Charnley and Smith[25] and Homsey.[52,54]

It is clear from presently available literature that the pathophysiology of blood pressure lowering by monomer is not fully understood, and the cause of cardiac arrest attributed to implantation of MMA is not being fully investigated.[97] It is agreed, however, that hemorrhagic shock and inadequate blood replacement might have been a predisposing factor in the severe blood pressure lowering effect of circulating monomer in many cases of operative death.

Because embolization of monomer as a cause of death in humans has not been documented, it is logical to presume a mechanical migration of air or fat or both as the etiological factor for a drop in blood pressure. This view is augmented by the fact that fall in pressure is not often seen when the cement is inserted into the acetabulum but usually is present when it is inserted into the femur. Furthermore, this does not occur in all patients. In addition, during bilateral operations on the same patient, only one hip surgery may cause blood pressure lowering. It must also be recognized that blood pressure lowering occurs in humans even with a smaller dose of monomer as compared with animal experimentation such as Homsey's. This theory of the erratic occurrence of fall in blood pressure owing to air and fat embolization would also explain the rapid onset of drop in blood pressure after insertion of cement into the bone causes extrusion of the fat and air into the circulation.[69]

Fat embolization

McLaughlin and co-workers[73] established that lung parenchyma functions as the major clearing tissue for MMA monomer following intramedullary cement insertion. A decreased pulmonary function (as measured by decreased P_{O_2}) occurred only when the monomer was more than 35 times the equivalent of the amount liberated in humans during total hip replacement. However, fat particles in the lung have been histologically demonstrated in several autopsies.[28] In some cases, air and fat were noted in pelvic veins and coronary vessels.[56] Fat embolization has been experimentally produced in animals following reaming of the medullary canal, and marrow tissue has been observed in blood samples from the femoral vein during reaming in animals. The elevation of pressure within the medullary canal has been blamed for massive mobilization of fat and marrow, especially the pressure created by the impact of the acrylic cement into the canal of the femur. Based on these observations, venting has been suggested by some investigators in order to reduce the pressure in the femur. Ohnsorge[79] experimentally recorded a pressure rise of 4.2 atm. (61.7 p.s.i.) during insertion of the prosthesis into acrylic cement. The pressure could be reduced to 1.4 atm. (20.6 p.s.i.) if a drill hole was made in the femoral cortex. Tronzo and co-workers[99] measured the intramedullary pressure of the femoral canal during total hip replacement in 12 patients and found transitory pressure changes. It was high when the femoral prosthesis was inserted without cement, higher when the MMA was forced into the cavity, and highest when the femoral prosthesis was finally positioned into the cement. He concluded that although venting of the femur proximally was ineffective, a distal vent prevented the rise in pressure, and suggested that distal venting is a good prophylactic procedure against embolization or cardiac arrest. After a comprehensive review of the literature and a clinical prospective study on physiological emboli changes observed during total hip replacement, Jones[58] concluded that fat embolization occurs with introduction of the femoral component and can be prevented by distal venting of the femur at the time of insertion of the cement. Alternatively, a plastic suction tube may be inserted as a method of venting the femoral canal during packing of the cement in order to eliminate the problem of fat embolization. Because of animal experimental work and personal preferences of those teaching in educational centers, venting has become a popular procedure. Based on Charnley's larger experiences, as well as our own, we have found it unnecessary. We prefer to have the anesthetic agents discontinued 2 to 3 minutes prior to the insertion of cement into the acetabulum and femur, with the patient maintained on pure oxygen at the time of cement insertion. Every effort is exercised to keep the patient normotensive and normovolemic prior to insertion of cement. At this time, approximately 3,000 low-friction arthroplasties have been performed at the New York Orthopaedic Hospital without venting the femur; no substantial hypotensive episodes have been observed, and there have not been any cardiac arrests as the result of cement insertion into the femur.

Many articles continue to appear that speculate on the causes of cardiac arrest associated with use of the cement. Suggested causes include fat embolism and toxic effect of monomer, as well as air embolism with subsequent neurogenic reflex starting in the lungs. Herndon and associates[49] reviewed the literature in 1974 and did an in-depth study. They noted 28 deaths, 20 of which had a postoperative autopsy; in 16 of these, fat emboli were found, some of which were massive. Three of the 16 also had documented bone marrow emboli, some of which were associated with both pulmonary and systemic fat emboli, while others were associated with acute myocardial infarction, pulmonary emboli, and suggestion of air emboli.

The true incidence of fat embolization in patients who died of sudden circulatory collapse is not known. Similarly, the incidence of pulmonary fat embolism in patients who survived cardiac arrest by resuscitation during the operation cannot be defined. Herndon and associates[49] studied 34 unselected patients in an attempt to quantify the incidence of fat embolism. They demonstrated the phenomena associated with fat embolization in most patients during the procedure, although none of these patients exhibited clinical or laboratory evidence of the fat embolism syndrome. They used an ultrasound probe over the femoral vein and performed serial analysis of venous blood fat. Computer energy–density spectrum analysis of the sounds was recorded by the ultrasound probe. "Chirps" were heard during insertion of the femoral component in all patients. Individual chirps lasting 2 to 5 milliseconds occurred every 10 to 15 milliseconds. Mean duration of activity was 4.2 minutes. Chirps were rarely heard during seating of the acetabular component, reaming, or insertion of cement into the femur. Blood samples* taken during peak ultrasound activity

*The fat emboli were counted in the blood samples by two histological techniques, and the plasma was analyzed for triglycerides before and after filtration.

showed 79 globules per high-power field by cryostat test (contrasted with a control of 1.7), or 360 globules per high-power field by the Millipore filter test (control, 6.8), and a mean drop in triglycerides of 27.8 mg./100 ml. (control, +1.2) after filtration. They concluded that although no clinical evidence of fat embolism was observed, venting of the femoral medullary canal at insertion of the femoral stem reduced the amount of fat emboli.

Kallos and associates[60] demonstrated that femoral medullary pressures and pulmonary embolization of medullary contents during insertion of cement and medullary rods in greyhounds were considerable. In three animals they found that insertion of cement into the femoral shaft resulted in medullary pressures between 290 and 900 torr, with the appearance of medullary contents in the lungs within 10 to 120 seconds. They also could prevent this phenomenon by drilling the shaft to release the pressure at the time of insertion.

Allergic reactions

Obscure complications at times have been attributed to allergic reactions to MMA, including radiological changes of bone simulating those of osteitis, wounds from which no organisms can be grown, mechanical loosening of the prosthesis, and unexplained pain after total hip replacement. Following a detailed study of the literature and based on his extensive experience with MMA, Charnley[17] concluded that allergic reactions are exceedingly rare. An occasional isolated allergic reaction, however, cannot be denied.

Numerous sensitivity studies are available in dental literature,* mostly relating to heat-cured acrylic. Sensitivity to acrylic resins has been studied by skin testing to demonstrate a true sensitivity in patients who had symptomatic reactions to their acrylic dentures. A single exposure for a sensitized individual working with the dental material may produce dermatitis that may last for several weeks or months. Fries and associates[42] collected 13 cases of contact dermatitis attributed to handling MMA; Fries himself was a victim. They tested a variety of commercially available gloves for penetration of monomeric MMA and suggested that most of these gloves were inadequate in protecting a

*See references 7, 39, 41, 42, and 65.

sensitive individual's skin and that improved surgical gloves were needed to prevent penetration of MMA monomer. They recommended that sensitive individuals add an extra pair of gloves, to be removed at once after handling cement. It has been suggested that the monomer may permeate rubber surgical gloves to produce contact dermatitis,[82] and the possibility of reactions to additives of PMMA has also been argued. It is suggested that benzoyl peroxide can occasionally cause sensitivity.[41] Charnley[17] proposed avoiding hydroquinone stabilizer (used in Simplex P) and replacing it with ascorbic acid (as in CMW). In addition to hydroquinone and benzoyl peroxide, dimethyl-p-toluidine may also be allergenic.[12]

SAFETY AND COMPATIBILITY

Acrylic cement has been used in its present form for over 20 years (other than hip replacement), and thousands of patients have had two or more doses of implanted material, some for up to 15 years. Certainly no animal experimentation is available, or will ever be available, conclusively superior to extensive human experiences already existing. Charnley has the longest available follow-ups of patients after total hip arthroplasty and has reported his experiences in early cases of low-friction arthroplasty with details related to the compatibility and clinical results achieved.[21,23,26] He also studied the histological details of bone in contact with cement, both in early and long-range follow-ups, presenting evidence that clinically, radiologically, and histologically, cement appears to be safe and physiologically well tolerated by the osseous tissue.[17,19,20,22] (See Chapter 3.)

Numerous reports on clinical results of total hip replacement from different centers in the world have become available.[95,100] (See Chapter 15.)

Convery and associates[29] studied in detail the relative safety of PMMA, comparing two groups of patients undergoing Charnley low-friction arthroplasty and other methods of total hip replacement, the former with the use of MMA and the latter without. It was concluded that the postoperative alterations, erythrocyte sedimentation rate, serum glutamic-oxyloacetic transaminase (SGOT), and lactic acid dehydrogenase (LDH) were related to the surgical intervention and not to the use of cement. Postoperative serum alkaline phosphatase was increased over

the preoperative level and remained elevated for up to 12 months in all patients. This was attributed to the formation of ectopic bone rather than hepatic toxicity of the cement. Intraoperative alterations in cardiovascular function were attributed to the use of cement. In one patient in the cemented group there was evidence of myocardial depression.

For further comments on application, see Chapters 3, 15, and 16.

CLINICAL OBSERVATIONS

I[34] reported a long-term study on the first series of Charnley low-friction total arthroplasties performed at Wrightington. This study related to 256 low-friction arthroplasties, with 7 to 8 years' follow-up. Operations were performed between November 1962 (the first acetabular component with high-density polyethylene) and December 1963. It was an unselected series of only 138 hips in 120 patients who qualified for the strict long-term study. A clinical and radiological study at 6 months, 5 years, and 7 to 8 years based on clinical and radiological evaluation was particularly scanned for late appearance of mechanical or biological incompatibility. The results of this study were most encouraging. Freedom from pain and mobility after surgery were remarkable, and there was no evidence of complications that could be attributed to the cement. These patients were subsequently studied at 9 and 10 years after surgery. Patients in this series who survived and were included in the long-term study showed no further changes.[21,23] The same group (mostly now in their 70s and 80s) was recently evaluated after 12 to 15 years following surgery by Sir John Charnley at Wrightington Hospital. They revealed no evidence of failure that could be attributed to the use of acrylic cement or any evidence of a pathological state of the bone related to the use of MMA.*

For more information on cement and tissue compatibility see Chapter 3.

---

*Personal communications.

SUMMARY OF ESSENTIALS

■ Acrylic cement was first synthesized in 1843. In 1937 its heat-cured form was first used in humans as denture base material. Judet introduced the heat-cured femoral head replacement in 1946, and Zander first performed an acrylic cranioplasty in

1940. Its early use in hip surgery by Kiaer in 1952 and Haboush is of special interest.

- Charnley is credited with formulation and elucidation of the principles involved in the use of acrylic cement in orthopaedic surgery today. His analysis of the mechanism by which fixation is achieved is one of the greatest single milestones in the history of orthopaedic surgery of this century.

- The chemistry and constituents of the cement must be suitable for effective use. Its liquid component is methyl methacrylate (MMA), a tertiary amine that acts as an initiator and an inhibitor. The powder typically consists of polymethyl methacrylate (PMMA) and an activator.

- Radiopacity is an essential feature of the acrylic cement used in orthopaedic surgery, without which the presence and amount of cement cannot be determined in hip surgery. Barium sulfate is an acceptable ingredient producing radiopacity.

- Considering the mechanical properties of the cement, acrylic cement is an excellent material under compression but weak in tension or shear strength. Of many variables that can alter the mechanical properties of cement, the technical aspects of its application seem to be the greatest influence.

- Working time and setting time characteristics of acrylic cement vary in different cement brands and among the circumstances of its use. These variables include ambient temperature, ratio of monomer to polymer, humidity, molecular weight of the polymer, texture of the polymer, proportions of activator and initiator, and degree of aeration. Mixing and insertion instructions must be accurately followed to achieve optimum results.

- Temperature elevation in the polymerizing cement mass is directly proportional to the size of the mass. Under normal circumstances, the heat of polymerization and dimensional changes during polymerization do not appear to interfere with clinical fixation.

- Acrylic cement should not be considered an adhesive glue because it possesses no adhesive properties by chemical interaction between bone and cement. It acts as a filler when it is used in conjunction with the prosthetic component. When used as a stiff dough (paste), it has space-filling properties, thus eliminating the need for an accurate fit between the prosthesis and bone required when adhesives are used. Because most forces in the hip are compressive and acrylic is most suitable for bonding, it makes an ideal grouting media for fixation of the prosthesis. Cement fills the cavities of the interior bone surfaces and allows transmission of the load evenly over a fairly large area between the prosthesis and the inner surface of the bone.

- Four aspects of systemic and local toxicity of cement may be considered: (1) toxicity studies and animal experimentations, (2) blood pressure lowering effect and cardiac arrest, (3) fat embolization, and (4) allergic reactions.

- Based on available clinical evaluation of a large number of patients with total hip replacement and other procedures involving the use of acrylic cement over 20 years in thousands of patients, cement may be considered an acceptable and biologically compatible material in total hip arthroplasty.

REFERENCES

1. Amstutz, H. C., and Gruen, T.: Prosthetic fixation with polymethyl methacrylate. In: Proceedings of National Academy of Science Symposium on Internal Structural Prosthetics, 1973, pp. 52-57.
2. Amstutz, H. C., and Gruen, T.: Clinical application of polymethyl methacrylate for total joint replacement, Curr. Pract. Orthop. Surg. **5:**158-182, 1973.
3. Amstutz, H. C., Lurie, L., and Bullough, P.: Skeletal fixation with self-curing polymethyl methacrylate, Clin. Orthop. **84:**163-178, 1972.
4. Astleford, W. J., Asher, M. A., Lindholm, U.S., and Rockwood, C. A., Jr.: Some physical and mechanical factors affecting the simple shear strength of methyl methacrylate, Clin. Orthop. **108:**145-148, 1975.
5. Berman, A. T., Price, H. L., and Hahn, J. F.: The cardiovascular effects of methyl methacrylate in dogs, Clin. Orthop. **100:**265-269, 1974.
6. Blumenthal, L. M.: Recent German developments in the field of dental resins, F.I.A.T. Report No. 1185, May, 1947.
7. Borzelleca, J. F., Larson, P. S., Henninger, G. R., Jr., et al.: Studies on the chronic oral toxicity of monomeric ethyl acrylate and methyl methacrylate, Toxicol. Appl. Pharmacol. **6:**29-36, 1964.
8. Bricolo, A., Benati, A., and Bazzan, A.: Cranioplastiche con ressiva acrilica, con rete di acciaio inossidokile pesante e con framenti di teca, Renerva Neurochir. **11:**208-211, 1967.
9. Buerkle, A. R., and Eftekhar, N. S.: Fixation of the femoral head prosthesis with methyl methacrylate, Clin. Orthop. **111:**134-141, 1975.
10. Burgess, D. M.: Cardiac arrest and bone cement, Br. Med. J. **3:**588, 1970.
11. Cabanela, M. E., et al.: The fate of patients with methyl methacrylate cranioplasty, J. Bone Joint Surg. **54A:**278-281, 1972.
12. Calnan, C. D. and Stevenson, C. J.: Studies in contact dermatitis, XV Dental materials, Trans. St. John's Hosp. Derm. Soc. **49:**9-26, 1963.
13. Cameron, H. U., Mills, R. H., Jackson, R. W., and Macnab, I.: The structure of polymethyl methacrylate cement, Clin. Orthop. **100:**287-291, 1974.

14. Charnley, J.: Anchorage of femoral head prosthesis to the shaft of the femur, J. Bone Joint Surg. **42B:**28-30, 1960.
15. Charnley, J.: The bonding of prostheses to bone by cement, J. Bone Joint Surg. **46B:**518-529, 1964.
16. Charnley, J.: A biomechanical analysis of the use of cement to anchor the femoral head prosthesis, J. Bone Joint Surg. **47B:**354-363, 1965.
17. Charnley, J.: Acrylic cement in orthopaedic surgery, Baltimore, 1970, The Williams & Wilkins Co.
18. Charnley, J.: The fixation of prostheses in living bone. Simpson, D. C., editor: In modern trends in biomechanics, New York, 1970, Appleton-Century-Crofts.
19. Charnley, J.: The reaction of bone to self-curing acrylic cement. A long-term histological study in man, J. Bone Joint Surg. **52B:**340-353, 1970.
20. Charnley, J., guest editor: Total hip replacement (Symposium), Clin. Orthop. **72:**1-204, 1970.
21. Charnley, J.: Long-term results of low-friction arthroplasty of the hip as a primary intervention, J. Bone Joint Surg. **54B:**61-76, 1972.
22. Charnley, J., and Crawford, W. J.: Histology of bone in contact with self-curing acrylic cement, J. Bone Joint Surg. **50B:**228, 1968.
23. Charnley, J., and Cupic, Z.: The nine- and ten-year results of the low-friction arthroplasty of the hip, Clin. Orthop. **95:**9-25, 1973.
24. Charnley, J., and Kettlewell, J.: The elimination of slip between prosthesis and femur, J. Bone Joint Surg. **47B:**56-60, 1965.
25. Charnley, J., and Smith, D. C.: The physical and chemical properties of self-curing acrylic cement, Internal Publication No. 16, 1968, Center for Hip Surgery, Wrightington Hospital, England.
26. Charnley, J., Follacci, F. M., and Hammond, B. T.: The long-term reaction of bone to self-curing acrylic cement, J. Bone Joint Surg. **50B:**822-829, 1968.
27. Charosky, C. B., and Walker, P. S.: The microstructure of polymethyl methacrylate cement, Clin. Orthop. **91:**221-224, 1973.
28. Cohen, C. A., and Smith, T. C.: The intraoperative hazard of acrylic bone cement: report of a case, Anesthesiology **35:**547-549, 1971.
29. Convery, F. R., Gunn, D. R., Hughes, J. D., and Martin, W. E.: The relative safety of polymethyl methacrylate, J. Bone Joint Surg. **57A:**57-64, 1975.
30. Daniel, W. W., Coventry, M. B., and Miller, W. E.: Pulmonary complications after total hip arthroplasty with Charnley prosthesis as revealed by chest roentgenograms, J. Bone Joint Surg. **54A:**282-283, 1972.
31. Deichmann, W.: Toxicity of methyl, ethyl, and N-butyl methacrylate, J. Ind. Hyg. Toxicol. **23:**343-351, 1941.
32. Dodge, H. W., Jr., and Craig, W. M.: Acrylic cranioplasty: a newer rapid method for repair of cranial defects; preliminary report, Proc. Staff Meet. Mayo Clin. **28:**256-257, 1953.
33. Dutton, J.: Acrylic investment of intracranial aneurysms, J. Neurosurg. **31:**652-657, December, 1969.
34. Eftekhar, N.: Charnley "low-friction torque" arthroplasty. A study of long-term results, Clin. Orthop. **81:**93-104, 1971.
35. Eftekhar, N. S., and Thurston, C. W.: Effect of irradiation on acrylic cement with special reference to fixation of pathological fractures, J. Biomech. **8:**53-56, 1975.
36. Elkins, C. W., and Cameron, J. E.: Cranioplasty with acrylic plates, J. Neurosurg. **3:**199-205, 1946.
37. Ellis, R. H., and Mulvein, J.: The cardiovascular effects of methyl methacrylate, J. Bone Joint Surg. **56B:**59-61, 1974.
38. Fearn, C. B. D'A., Burgidge, H. C., and Bentley, G.: Effect of methyl methacrylate cement on systolic blood pressure in operations for total hip replacement, J. Bone Joint Surg. **55B:**210, 1973.
39. Fisher, A. A.: Allergic sensitization of the skin and oral mucosa to acrylic denture materials, J.A.M.A. **156:**238-242, 1954.
40. Fisher, A. A.: Allergic sensitization of the skin and oral mucosa to acrylic resin denture materials, J. Prosthet. Dent. **6:**593, 1956.
41. Fisher, A. A.: Contact dermatitis, Philadelphia, 1967, Lea & Febiger.
42. Fries, I. B., Fisher, A. A., and Salvati, E. A.: Contact dermatitis in surgeons from methyl methacrylate bone cement, J. Bone Joint Surg. **57A:**547-549, 1975.
43. Frost, P. M. I.: Cardiac arrest and bone cement, Br. J. Med. **3:**524, 1970.
44. Gresham, G. A., and Kuczynski, A.: Cardiac arrest and bone cement, Br. Med. J. **3:**465, 1970.
45. Gresham, G. A., Kuczynski, A., and Rosborough, D.: Fatal fat embolism following replacement arthroplasty for transcervical fractures of femur, Br. Med. J. **2:**617-619, 1971.
46. Haboush, E. J.: A new operation for arthroplasty of the hip based on biomechanics, photoelasticity, fast-setting dental acrylic, and other considerations, Bull. Hosp. Joint Dis. **14:**242-277, 1953.
47. Harris, N. H.: Cardiac arrest and bone cement, Br. Med. J. **3:**523, 1970.
48. Henrichsen, E., Jansen, K., and Krough-Poulson, W.: Experimental investigation of the tissue reaction to acrylic plastics, Acta Orthop. Scand. **22:**141-146, 1953.

49. Herndon, J. H., Bechtol, C. O., and Crickenberger, D. P.: Fat embolism during total hip replacement. A prospective study, J. Bone Joint Surg. **56A:**1350-1362, 1974.

50. Holland, C. J., Kim, K. C., Malik, M. I., and Ritter, M. A.: A histologic and hemodynamic study of the toxic effects of monomeric methyl methacrylate, Clin. Orthop. **90:**262-270, 1973.

51. Homsey, C. A.: Prosthesis seating compounds of rapid cure acrylic polymer. Paper presented at the National Academy of Science–American Academy of Orthopaedic Surgeons Joint Workshop on Total Hip Replacement and Skeletal Attachment, Washington, D.C., November, 1969.

52. Homsey, C. A., Tullos, H. S., Anderson, M. S., Diferrante, N. M., and King, J. W.: Some physiological aspects of prosthesis stabilization with acrylic polymer, Clin. Orthop. **83:**317-328, 1972.

53. Homsey, C. A., Tullos, H. S., and King, J. W.: Evaluation of rapid-cure acrylic compound for prosthesis stabilization, Clin. Orthop. **67:**169-171, 1969.

54. Homsey, C. A., Tullos, H. S., and King, J. W.: Physiological sequel from implantation of rapid-cure acrylic compounds, J. Bone Joint Surg. **51A:**805, 1969.

55. Hullinger, L.: Untersuchungen uber die Wirkung von Kunstharzen (Palacos und Ostamer) in Gewbekulturen, Arch. Orthop. Unfallchair. **54:**581, 1962.

56. Hyland, J., and Robbins, R. H. C.: Cardiac arrest and bone cement, Br. Med. J. **4:**176-177, 1970.

57. Jaffe, W. L., Rose, R. M., and Radin, E. L.: On the stability of the mechanical properties of self-curing acrylic bone cement, J. Bone Joint Surg. **56A:**1711-1714, 1974.

58. Jones, R. H.: Physiologic emboli changes observed during total hip replacement arthroplasty, Clin. Orthop. **112:**192-200, 1975.

59. Judet, J., and Judet, R.: The use of an artificial femoral head for arthroplasty of the hip joint, J. Bone Joint Surg. **32B:**166-173, 1950.

60. Kallos, T., Enis, J. E., Gollan, F., and Davis, J. H.: Intramedullary pressure and pulmonary embolism of femoral medullary contents in dogs during insertion of bone cement and a prosthesis, J. Bone Joint Surg. **56A:**1363-1367, 1974.

61. Kepes, E. R., Underwood, P. S., and Becsey, L.: Intraoperative death associated with acrylic bone cement, J.A.M.A. **222:**576-577, 1972.

62. Kerr, A. S.: The use of acrylic resin plates for the repair of skull defects, J. Neurol. Neurosurg. Psychiatry **6:**158, 1943.

63. Kiaer, S.: Hip arthroplasty with acrylic prosthesis, Acta Orthop. Scand. **22:**126-140, 1952.

64. Knight, G.: Paraspinal acrylic inlays in the treatment of cervical and lumbar spondylosis and other conditions, Lancet **2:**147, 1959.

65. Lawrence, W. H., Bass, G. E., Purcell, W. P., and Autian, J.: Use of mathematical models in the study of structure toxicity relationships of dental compounds. I. Esters of acrylic and methacrylic acids, J. Dent. Res. **51:**526-535, 1972.

66. Lazansky, M. G.: Materials for total hip replacement, Part I: Methyl methacrylate: chemical properties and clinical uses. In American Academy of Orthopaedic Surgeons: Instructional course lectures, vol. 23, St. Louis, 1974, The C. V. Mosby Co., pp. 164-169.

67. Lee, A. J. C., and Ling, R. S. M.: Further studies of monomer loss by evaporation during the preparation of acrylic cement for use in orthopaedic surgery, Clin. Orthop. **106:**122-125, 1975.

68. Lee, A. J. C., Ling, R. S. M., and Wrighton, J. D.: Some properties of polymethylmethacrylate with reference to its use in orthopaedic surgery, Clin. Orthop. **95:**281-287, 1973.

69. Ling, R. S. M., and James, M. L.: Blood pressure and bone cement, Br. Med. J. **2:**404, 1971.

70. Loshaek, S., and Fox, T. G.: Cross-linked polymers. I. Factors influencing the efficiency of cross-linking in copolymers of methyl methacrylate and glycol dimethacrylates, J. Am. Chem. Soc. **75:**3544-3550, 1953.

71. Luskin, L. S., and Myers, R. J.: Acrylic ester polymers. In Encyclopedia of polymer science and technology, vol. 1, New York, 1964, John Wiley & Sons, Inc.

72. McKee, G. K., and Watson-Farrar, J.: Replacement of arthritic hips by the McKee-Farrar prosthesis, J. Bone Joint Surg. **48B:**245-259, 1966.

73. McLaughlin, R., et al.: Blood clearance and acute pulmonary toxicity of methyl methacrylate in dogs after simulated arthroplasty and intravenous injection, J. Bone Joint Surg. **55A:**1621-1628, 1973.

74. McMaster, W. C., Bradley, G., and Waugh, T. R.: Blood pressure lowering effect of methyl methacrylate monomer. Potentiation by blood volume deficit, Clin. Orthop. **98:**254-257, 1974.

75. Meyer, P. R., Jr., Lautenschlager, E. P., and Moore, B. K.: On the setting properties of acrylic bone cement, J. Bone Joint Surg. **55A:**149-156, 1973.

76. Miles, D. C., and Buston, J. H.: Polymer technology, New York, 1965, Chemical Publishing Co., Inc.

77. Müller, M. E.: Total hip prostheses, Clin. Orthop. **72:**46-68, 1970.

78. Newens, A. F., and Volz, R. G.: Severe hypotension during prosthetic hip surgery with

acrylic bone cement, Anesthesiology **36**:298-300, 1972.

79. Ohnsorge, J.: Some aspects of polymerizing bone cement, J. Bone Joint Surg. **53B**:758-759, 1971.

80. Parsons, D. W.: Cardiac arrest and bone cement, Br. Med. J. **3**:710, 1970.

81. Peebles, D. J., Ellis, R. H., Stride, S. D. K., and Simpson, B. R. J.: Cardiovascular effects of methyl methacrylate cement, Br. Med. J. **1**:349-351, 1972.

82. Pegum, J. S., and Medhurst, F. A.: Contact dermatitis from penetration of rubber gloves by acrylic monomer, Br. Med. J. **2**:141-143, 1971.

83. Phillips, H., Lettin, A. W. F., and Cole, P. V.: Cardiovascular effects of implanted acrylic cement, J. Bone Joint Surg. **55B**:210, 1973.

84. Powell, J. N., McGrath, P. J., Lahiri, S. K., and Hill, P.: Cardiac arrest associated with bone cement, Br. Med. J. **3**:326, 1970.

85. Reitz, K. A.: Polymer osteosynthesis, Acta Chir. Scand. Supp. **3**:388, 1968.

86. Roberts, A. C.: The surgical application of autopolymerizing acrylic resin, Biomed. Eng. **2**:392, 1967.

87. Scales, J. T.: Biomechanics and related bioengineering topics. Oxford, 1965, Pergamon Press, p. 219.

88. Sevitt, S.: Fat embolism in patients with fractured hips, Br. Med. J. **2**:257-262, 1972.

89. Small, J. M., and Graham, M. P.: Acrylic resin for the closure of skull defects. Preliminary report, Br. J. Surg. **33**:106-113, 1945.

90. Smith, D. C., and Bains, M. E. D.: The detection and estimation of residual monomer in polymethyl methacrylate, J. Dent. Res. **35**:16-24, 1956.

91. Smith, D. L., and Schoonover, I. C.: Direct filling resins: dimensional changes resulting from polymerization shrinkage and water sorption, J. Am. Dent. Assoc. **46**:540-544, 1953.

92. Spealman, C. R., Main, R. J., Haag, H. B., and Larson, P. S.: Monomeric methylmethacrylate; studies on toxicity, Indust. Med. **14**:292-298, 1945.

93. Spence, W. T.: Form-fitting plastic cranioplasty, J. Neurosurg. **11**:219-225, 1954.

94. Spence, W. T.: Ten years' experience using form-fitting plastic for cranioplasty, Bull. Georgetown Univ. Med. Cent. **10**:154-160, 1957.

95. Stinchfield, F. E., guest editor: Statistics on total hip replacement, Clin. Orthop. **95**:1-262, 1973.

96. Sweeney, W. T.: Acrylic resins in prosthetic dentistry, Dent. Clin. North Am. **2**:593, 1958.

97. Thomas, T. A., Sutherland, I. C., and Waterhouse, T. D.: Cold curing acrylic bone cement: a clinical study of the cardiovascular side effects during hip joint replacement, Anesthesiology **26**:298-303, 1971.

98. Towers, A. G.: Viability of common pathogens in cold-curing acrylic resin used in orthopaedic surgery, Br. Med. J. **2**:1046-1047, 1966.

99. Tronzo, R. G., Kallos, T., and Wyche, M. Q.: Elevation of instramedullary pressure when methyl methacrylate is inserted in total hip arthroplasty, J. Bone Joint Surg. **56A**:714-718, 1974.

100. Urist, M. R.: Acrylic cement stabilized joint replacements, Curr. Probl. Surg. November, 1975, pp. 1-54.

101. Walker, P. S., and Bienenstock, M.: Fixation properties of acrylic cement, Rev. Hosp. Spec. Surg. **1**:27, 1971.

102. Wilde, A. H., and Greenwald, A. S.: Shear strength of self-curing acrylic cement, Clin. Orthop. **106**:126-130, 1975.

103. Wiltse, L. L., Hall, R. H., and Stenehjem, J. C.: Experimental studies regarding the possible use of self-curing acrylic in orthopaedic surgery, J. Bone Joint Surg. **39A**:961-972, 1957.

104. Woolf, J. I., and Walker, A. E.: Cranioplasty. Collective review, Int. Abstr. Surg. **81**:1-23, 1945.

105. Woringer, E., Schweig, B., Brogly, G., and Schneider, J.: Nouvelle techniques ultra-rapide pour la réfection de brèches ossenses craniennes à la résine acrylique: avantages de la résine acryliques sur le tantale, Rev. Neurol. **85**:527-535, 1951.

106. Zander, Cited by Kleinschmidt, O.: Plexiglas zur Deckung von Schädellücken, Chirurg. **13**:273-277, 1941.

PART TWO

GENERAL SURGICAL PRINCIPLES

CHAPTER 5

General surgical considerations

Our prime concerns in doing constructive hip surgery
or any surgery for that matter are:
- to handle the tissue gently,
- to approach the short dissection with sure anatomic
  knowledge that we are leaving an adequate
  neurovascular supply to the remaining tissue,
- to support the life of the repair,
- to surgically close such exposure with non-traumatizing
  sutures that will keep the tissue opposed through the
  functional ranges of motion that will eventually be
  required.

OTTO E. AUFRANC

not how *quickly,* but how *well* done

motto of DR. SUMNER L. KOCH

The orthopaedic surgeon performing hip replacement is bound, as all surgeons are, by principles that include a careful evaluation of the whole patient, well-founded indications for the specific surgical intervention, aseptic technique, and absolute precision if a successful result is to be expected. Complications after total hip replacement are at times disastrous to the patient, and a total failure may mean a resection pseudarthrosis. This is exemplified by an infected total hip replacement or conditions of iatrogenic pathology of the pelvis or femur following total hip replacement. Because of the magnitude of the problem when serious complications arise, prevention, not salvage after complications, should be emphasized and special attention should be given to all detailed specifics of technique to include pre- and postoperative care of the patient. (For specifics, see Chapters 6 to 11.)

SURGICAL AND NURSING CARE OF ELDERLY PATIENTS

Although the need exists, there are few pieces of orthopaedic literature emphasizing the importance of preoperative nursing care of elderly patients who will undergo "elective surgery"; there are many psychological and physical problems related to this particular group of patients that need special attention.[1,2,4,7] Most patients undergoing total hip replacement are in their 60s and 70s, with an occasional patient in his 80s. Unlike traumatic cases, patients being considered for major elective surgery are not particularly high surgical risks, but they do constitute a group with special needs. Wilder and Fishbein[8] report a study of 207 patients (over 80 years of age) followed for 30 days after surgery in which the overall mortality rate was 33.3%; they also found that mortality by speciality, such as orthopaedic surgery, was as high as 31.7%. Scott[6] and associates (in a study of 1,300 major operations on patients over 70 years of age) found the overall mortality rate to be 13.8%; however, this was reduced to 6.5% if patients with calculated operative complications were preoperatively excluded. This high degree of mortality is unacceptable when performing elective surgery such as total hip replacement and is obviously related to the "emergency nature" of the operation in older people, that is, preexisting complications accompanying surgery and/or serious complications that may occur after surgery in abdominal or neurological operations. Preoperative preparation and diagnostic errors have at times been blamed for the high rate of mortality in elderly patients, and these figures on mortality are totally unacceptable when considering elective surgery such as total hip re-

151

placement. However, as in our own series, approximately 25% of all patients develop a minor or major complication following total hip replacement; the mortality rate is estimated to be about 1%. (See Chapters 15 to 17.)

It is evident that the mortality rate in older patients can be reduced if detailed attention is given to all medical aspects, specifically to the systemic review and proper consultations, which should include anesthesia management and appropriate rehabilitation programs. When a severely debilitated patient is considered for surgery, this patient must be identified and special care rendered. A very old patient should begin ambulation earlier than the routine would normally require. In general, older patients tolerate the stress better than young patients, but this initial tolerance soon gives way to the dangers of shock and death. For example, following fracture of the hip the older patient may not complain as much as a younger person, but if the fracture is not immobilized, he soon may lapse into shock.

Social aspects are of great concern to the patient and his confidence in the surgeon and staff is augmented if the following issues are discussed prior to surgery:

1. Desire to return to his home as soon as possible after surgery

2. Experiencing loneliness in the hospital

3. Apprehension concerning spouse (or other relatives) remaining alone in the home environment

4. Resentment of lack of self-sufficiency, that is, being unable to reach for the telephone, picking up eyeglasses, and so on owing to confinement in bed

5. Sense of loss pertaining to useful or familiar objects—either because the hospital does not furnish them per se or because their hospital stay was not properly planned by themselves and/or relatives and friends

Many details of patient-centered surgical nursing care must be considered. Among these are transference of cheerful confidence to the patient when explaining the details of what to expect from surgery (if the patient is seeking information). It is also essential to listen carefully and to be sensitive to minor details that are obviously "important" to an elderly patient; respect and awareness of his great sense of vulnerability will engender understanding of his demands and antagonism. Personal feelings concerning

the patient's requests must be avoided; if the patient requests a specific type of cereal for breakfast or a particular type of vitamin or drinking water, these must be cheerfully provided rather than antagonistically withheld. If the older patient's demands are ignored, an undesirable situation may arise in which he loses confidence in the staff and hospital, thus making the problem of nursing care an even more complicated procedure. It can be terrifying to a confined older patient if his demands are not immediately met when he is asking for help. As a rule, older patients are short-tempered, and often their mental confusion, agitation, and inability to cooperate causes argumentative struggles between the patient and the nursing staff. Medications that the patient customarily takes should not be altered if at all possible; often he is accustomed to a specific brand name, which should be provided.

On admission, the patient should be educated concerning the rehabilitation process, including the details of transfer from bed, use of a bedpan, and other assisting devices. Postoperative necessities should be foreseen; back care is most essential. A pneumatic alternating pressure mattress or a sheepskin may be needed to protect sensitive skin during the first postoperative days; wrinkles in bed sheets at contact areas, particularly at the heels and elbows, potentiate skin breakage. Patients with back pain require a regular change in position. A trapeze and overhead frame are essential for older patients so that they can help lift themselves to use the bedpan and for back care. As stated, usual habits (though seemingly minor) are extremely important to older people, such as coffee or other beverage with meals or in the evening; on occasion, a pipe or cigar may be extremely important.

Excessive emphasis on the patient's "side effects" is unnecessary, since their overall well-being must come first. Breathing exercises, basic arm and leg exercises, and tightening of the abdominal and gluteal muscles (fanny clapping) are useful and psychologically important to patients who expect to actively assist in quick recovery from their surgery. On the other hand, as we shall see later, there is no need for a carefully planned or regimented physiotherapy program. The general strengthening exercise program should include the methods of turning and lifting up for positioning as well as demonstration of sitting out of bed during the postoperative course. In addition to physiotherapy, the use of a walker or crutches elevates the patient's self-confidence as well as restores a working relationship with other patients who are often forgetful (physiotherapy is unable to continuously attend them above and beyond the regular twice-a-day visit). Generally, it is better for older patients to begin ambulation with a walker (because they feel more confident with it) than with crutches; there is no reason to fear that they will not master a cane after a walker.

Long-range home transfer plans must be made; prior to the operation a realistic assessment should be made of (1) the patient's views, (2) the feasibility of second institutional care, or (3) home care with housekeeping assistance. Every older patient is individual in his needs, and an experienced senior nurse in charge of the ward carries the greatest responsibility in identifying these needs. If the patient's hearing or vision is impaired, this must be clearly marked on the chart and all nurses informed of proper care of the patient. Daily hospital visits are essential by house staff and the attending physician, particularly for the older person; an early perfunctory visit by an inexperienced staff member is an insufficient response to the patient's needs. Ideally, the surgeon should do his rounds on older patients later in the day (when questions and problems about routine activities have arisen). If the surgeon will not be visiting the patient for 1 or 2 days or another surgeon will be covering his service, this should be discussed with the patient. The surgeon's rounds on aged patients should include a daily neurological evaluation of the lower extremities to search for footdrop—as well as thromboembolism—since these patients may not be aware of relevant symptoms.

Most older patients need more reassurance than younger patients; they should be told what to expect after surgery; that is, the difference between incision pain and actual hip pain should be explained—for many patients expect total freedom from pain immediately after surgery and worry about postoperative pain. Many older patients develop some degree of psychosis or unusual responses to their relatives and friends, which often disturbs them when it is brought to their attention by visitors. Loss of memory may occur and the patient may not be aware of the time or date; other patients may be extremely confused for a few days, and these

patients and their families must be specifically reassured and supportive treatment instituted.

During daily visits the position of the hip must be examined, since the patient may not complain of the pain in the hip associated with dislocation; only examination of the knee position and extremity length would reveal this complication. For example, occasionally a patient will discard the abduction brace and even ignore the details of postoperative management: In this case, empathy and proper psychology are more effective than dogmatism and threats. Patients thrive on praise for their good performance rather than criticism of what they have done incorrectly. Similarly, as in handling children, criticism can be dangerous and nonconstructive.

Incontinence, urinary or fecal, is an extreme embarrassment to older patients following surgery; when this occurs, it should be handled without amplification by an experienced nurse who will be supportive rather than critical. An indwelling catheter will control urinary incontinence and add to the convenience of the patient. The dressing must be observed daily, and if adhesive tape causes itching, it must be adjusted. Following the first ambulation attempt, light-headedness and dizziness is quite natural and should be discussed with the patient so that he is not discouraged from further ambulation.

In the original interview, basic information about the surgery, potential risks, and complications is provided. It is a good idea to have the family present while discussing the proposed operation and, generally, the patient should be told as much as he wishes to know—but only relevant matters should be discussed. Older persons often have deep-seated fears and may not be inquisitive about the details; it is therefore unnecessary to "overstate" the risks and agitate the patient by drawing a "dark picture" of the worst possible outcome and then advise him to go ahead with surgery! If a cardiopulmonary or other systemic condition makes the patient a high risk, he should, of course, be fully informed and given guidance in making the decision with his relatives. To expose all possible hazards and leave an older person to make his "own decision" regarding surgery is not enough. It is often helpful for the surgeon to say that if the patient were his own relative he would—or would not—recommend surgery. Before entering the hospital, a fearful person is often helped by visiting one or two older patients who have already undergone

153

the same type of surgery and discussing the details with them.

OPERATIVE TIME VS. SURGICAL SKILL

The speed of surgery and minimization of wasted time improves with a surgeon's experience. There is a tendency in the beginner to attempt to break the time record for a given surgical procedure or to use shortcuts, but nowhere in orthopaedic surgery is the meticulous attention to technical details more important than in total hip surgery. Adequate preparation of the bones of the femur and acetabulum is essential in order to achieve proper orientation of the components for good functional performance and a long-lasting fixation. "Shortcutting" to gain time during any vital part of the operation will produce poor or even catastrophic results, which might require further surgical intervention and add to the misery of the patient. Indeed, with modern anesthesia and adequate operative care of the wound, there is no justification for shortening the operative period by 15 to 30 minutes at the risk of compromising technique. In older patients whose functional life expectancy is relatively short, performing a less-than-perfect operation is totally unjustifiable, especially since these older patients may not be able to withstand a second corrective procedure. In younger patients, on the other hand, projected years of physiological demand leave no room for compromise.

In general, operative time for total hip replacement should be between 60 and 90 minutes in a well-equipped and organized center, assuming a standard uncomplicated anatomy exists, that is, a straightforward osteoarthrosis. Depending on the severity of the case and difficulties of technical problems, operative time may extend to 180 minutes. Roentgenograms do not necessarily indicate the ease or difficulty of a case; however, they may point out the pace, and operative time should be planned accordingly. A standard rule and lesson for the beginner is to emphasize skill and proper execution of technique rather than shortening operative time.

PROPER PREPARATION OF THE BONE AND INSERTION OF THE COMPONENTS

In the forthcoming chapters, the details of technique will be discussed. At this point it is essential to emphasize that the artificial hip joint will work only if properly implanted and rigidly fixed to the bone in order to provide lifetime service to the patient. Being too scrupulous or gentle in preparing the bone may be ineffective and time-consuming; on the other hand, being too bold and inadvertently traumatizing the tissue may lead to serious complications, such as fractures of the femur or perforation of the pelvis, with catastrophic results. A commonsense approach is the key to surgical technique; it is important to evaluate difficulties at each step and to redirect the approach if necessary. It is useless to insert a prosthesis that could later become loose or fractured as a result of defective technique; only meticulous attention to all details will ensure permanent fixation. A surgeon must be certain that any modification of a time-tested procedure at any stage is for technical improvement and not a violation of the previously stated principles.

IRRIGATION, SUCTION, AND DEBRIDEMENT

Generally, irrigation might be of value during the operation (1) to keep the tissue moistened and to remove debris from the wound, (2) following cementing of each of the components, and (3) at the time of wound closure. Débridement of the muscle fibers (usually the gluteus maximus if detached and devitalized) may be indicated. While irrigation is useful to remove the particles and cement fragments mechanically, swabbing the wound throughout is the most effective way of keeping it clean. A strong suction tip inserted into the femoral canal and acetabulum might be useful; however, tight packing of the interior of the bone with dry swabs (both in the femur and the acetabulum) at the final stage provides a dry bed for fixation of the cement. Antibiotic deposit into the "bed" of the bone prior to cement insertion is not recommended, although irrigation with an antibiotic solution is a "rational exercise"; however, scientific proof has not been established concerning its effectiveness (see Chapter 6). Copious irrigation with large amounts of solution must be considered with caution—soaking the draping from "oversaturation" may add more contamination risks than is derived from its benefits.

DRAINAGE OF THE WOUND AND HEMATOMAS

A Hemovac draining tube inserted at surgery is removed 48 to 72 hours after surgery. While drains are routinely used deep to the fascia, it is also suggested that they be used superficial to the fascia. The dressing is not changed post-operatively for at least 4 or 5 days unless there are specific reasons. Clinically diagnosed hematomas (indicated by fullness of the thigh) that are not draining should not be disturbed, but the patient's activities should be curtailed until the hematoma subsides. Ice packs to the hip region will make the patient comfortable; needling is not indicated.

Spontaneous draining of a hematoma into the wound is best handled by reoperation and evacuation in the operating room under general anesthesia in absolutely sterile conditions. If anticoagulants are the causative agent, treatment must be reversed at once and the patient's activities stopped until the hematoma is completely dissolved. A draining (leaking) hematoma is a potentially dangerous problem from the standpoint of infection; it is not enough to place the patient on antibiotics and "observe" the wound. After diagnosis is made, the wound should be covered with a sterile dressing and the patient prepared for evacuation and closure of the wound under anesthesia. If fascia is sealed off and not disturbed, a careful, formal draping technique, similar to that used in total hip replacement technique, is essential. The wound must be copiously irrigated, clots removed, and the wound closed carefully (using retention sutures).

STUDY OF ANATOMY AND REHEARSAL

Detailed, prior knowledge of surgical anatomy of the hip is essential in order to comprehend the approaches to the hip joint and to minimize damage to the vital structures; avoidance of damage to the muscles, which basically provide the hip function, is essential. Since the abductor mechanism is the key source of power in the hip, its fibers must be protected, and the relationship of these muscles to the anterior and posterior groups of muscles must be fully understood. Each surgeon will learn the anatomy not only by study of the normal but by evaluating the pathological conditions at surgery, by the sense of touch and utilizing instrument, and most importantly, by appraisal of difficult situations. For example, when a maximum exposure cannot be obtained, sometimes an alteration of only 10 or 15 degrees of flexion of the hip may provide it; in another case delivery of the

upper femur out of the wound by a lever might be the solution. At any given point during surgery the surgeon must reexamine the possibility of improving the exposure; this can also be achieved by removing the assistant's fingers from the wound; adjusting the self-retaining retractors; swabbing the blood from the surface; stabilizing the limb in a certain degree of abduction, adduction, or rotation; or having the table leveled to a more convenient position.

By continuous study of the surgical wound and surgical anatomy, obstacles and unpredicted nuisances (such as fractures of the femur and pelvis) are eliminated. Indeed, this learning leads to surgical "common sense," which will inspire confidence to advance or retreat when necessary—actions based on knowledge, not fear. As a general rule, no tissue should be removed unnecessarily during exposure of the wound. However, as much capsule of the joint may be excised as is necessary in order to obtain maximum exposure; with the exception of the abductor mechanism, any muscle may be released to achieve a fully mobile hip without residual deformity. Use of a bony skeleton and dissection of a cadaveric hip are emphasized as commencement exercises for the beginner, but perhaps having assisted in several operations (prior to performing a first operation) is even more valuable. All of the following contribute to the surgeon's awareness of correct placement of the incision along the lines of approach to the joint: study of the surface anatomy of the hip joint and observation of the bony prominences of the anterosuperior spine, the crest of the ilium, the location of the greater trochanter; palpation of the abductor muscles (gluteus medius and minimus); and orientation of the gluteus maximus from the sacrum investing the buttock into the lateral aspect of the shaft. These anatomical relations may be appraised and compared with the opposite side prior to surgical draping; once again, it would be advantageous for the surgeon to practice the entire procedure (including handling of the cement fixation) on a cadaveric hip prior to surgery.

SKIN INCISION AND WOUND EXPOSURE

Numerous methods for skin preparation have been recommended; one that is practical and applicable to the immediate surgical environment must be selected. Since the patient is usually in the hospital for more than 48 hours prior

155

to surgery, it is advisable to wash the surgical area (with hexachlorophene or a similar antiseptic soap) as he showers at least twice a day to combat the general bacterial population of the skin; repeated bathing of the skin of staphylococcal carriers with hexachlorophene emulsion reduces the number of staphylococci, and the rate of their dispersion in the environment (see Chapter 6). On the night before surgery the groin should be washed and pubic hair clipped (shaving often scratches the skin, which enhances colonization of organisms); it is best to remove hair from the entire extremity—from groin to foot. The toenails are clipped and all nail polish is removed. Toweling of the hip area and lower extremity prior to moving the patient to the operating room is a sensible, although not essential, procedure. Defatting of the skin with ether (or a similar defatting agent such as Freon) and application of 2% tincture of iodine are both of paramount importance prior to draping; an iodine patch test performed the night before surgery will determine a possible allergic reaction to iodine. This phenomenon must be extremely uncommon, since we have rarely observed it. The painted iodine must be left on the skin and not removed; in our experience this has not caused skin burn, although it may occur in areas of pooling (such as the buttocks) if the patient lies in it. Often, "frictional burns," created by careless removal of the "transfer sheet," have been mistaken for iodine burns.

At surgery, skin edges must be handled with care, and a perfect skin closure is essential. Insulation by towels is helpful in eliminating trauma to the skin edges and prevention of surface contamination by skin contaminants. The towel clip method using turkish towels is effective, but the end of the incision should not be cut short by application of the distal and proximal towel clips; the clips should not crush the skin edges.

The skin incision length must be adequate, and it is psychologically important to the patient that the surgeon produce symmetrical incisions in bilateral replacements. Correct placement of the incision is of great value in producing maximum exposure with a minimum length incision; however, if the incision is misplaced, a generous length must be provided to prevent undue trauma during surgery. Prolonged overretraction of the skin over the corners by additional instrumentation may cause skin ischemia and lead to delayed healing; it is always advisable to make

a longer incision rather than struggle for a better exposure. It is worth remembering that postoperatively a patient does not discuss the length, location, or type of approach to his joint; patients do complain, however, regarding the reasons for the failure of an operation owing to complications, that is, fractures of the shaft of the femur occurring during surgery, infections, and hematomas that occurred as a result of excessive struggle in performing surgery through a limited exposure. It is advisable for the novice to use a longer incision (with experience, they will shorten), and it is better to have a longer incision from the beginning than to add to its length during the procedure. A longer incision is used when surgical difficulty is anticipated; the entire length of the skin incision must be utilized as the deeper layers are incised. When an adhesive plastic drape has been used, after its removal and prior to closure of the fat retention sutures, reapplication of 2% tincture of iodine to the skin is advisable since, during surgery, bacteria of the deep layers may be brought to the surface with removal of the adhesive plastic drape. Previous operative scars in close proximity to the hip joint create a nuisance, yet must be handled intelligently; this is a common pitfall for surgeons performing a correction of a previously failed surgery. Often a surgeon may place the incision too anteriorly or posteriorly (which are almost, but not precisely, the perfect location for the second surgery) in order to avoid previous incisions. Although it is a good principle to ignore old scars about the hip, a new incision must be made where it is best suited for the exposure of the hip. We have found that when a new incision has been made within the vicinity of an old incision at almost any angle or location, it has been safe and there has been no ischemic necrosis about the hip, as sometimes is expected when incisions cross each other. The good supply of skin flaps, and abundant anastomotic circulation about the hip allows the surgeon to make almost any type of incision (from the anterior ilioinguinal ligament to the region of the ischium) without fear of necrosis. Cauterization of bleeders close to the epidermis must be avoided lest skin edge necrosis develop; usually the bleeders close to the epidermis are controlled by towel clips applied to the skin edges. A continuous running mattress stitch with 3-0 nylon has been found to be adequate for closure; however, subcuticular closure, as well as interrupted mattress sutures, may be utilized at the discretion of the surgeon. Skin closure must be done by the surgeon and not left to the more junior members of the team.

SUBCUTANEOUS FAT

When entering the subcutaneous fat along the incision, skin towels must be applied prior to entering deeper layers of fat. Deepening of the incision in the fat must constantly be checked against the greater trochanter and the midlateral shaft. Undercutting of the fat and separating the fat from fascia are common exercises that should be resisted; much of the error in misplacement of the skin can be improved by appropriate cutting of the fat layer. Occasional irrigation of the fat decreases drying out of the tissue and may minimize cell death. A thin person may be in just as much danger of infection as a very obese person with heavy deposits of adipose tissue in the hip region. In both extreme cases, a meticulous approximation of fat and retention of the tension within this tissue is essential to prevent accumulation of seroma or production of fat necrosis, which may evacuate into the dressing —a common source of contamination of the wound. While interrupted 2-0 catgut may be adequate to close the fat layer, retention sutures fastened over thick foam pads (popularized by Charnley) have proved to be a superior method of closure after total hip arthroplasty (see Chapter 12). The fat sutures are applied—but tightened—over the sponges following the closure of the skin edges. While it is possible that lateral femoral cutaneous nerves may be damaged during the exposure of the hip joint (in the anterior approach), there is no cutaneous nerve of any importance in the area of the hip when it is approached laterally or posterolaterally. In an obese patient with fat thickness of more than 1 inch, it is advisable to have a separate drain tube applied superficial to the fascia in the fat layer. The fat layer must be considered as a separate compartment from the hip joint; therefore a tight fascial closure and elimination of dead space is a constant feature of wound closure technique. There is no excuse for relegation of this important part of the operation to the most junior member of the operative team.

FASCIA AND TENDONS

Because of the importance of the abductor muscle, its tendinous attachment to the greater trochanter must never be removed without a bony fragment. Reattachment of tendon by itself

is not satisfactory and leads to a defective result. Meticulous technique and careful detailed consideration must be given to reattachment of the greater trochanter to restore a good and powerful abductor mechanism for the hip.

The deep fascia of the thigh, basically a deep envelope separating the skin from the hip joint proper, must be respected as a very important structure. Opening of this fascia at midline with reference to the iliotibial tract and careful repair of this structure following surgery (1) produces stability for the hip and (2) separates the superficial inflammatory process and drainage from the deep structures. Special emphasis is placed on proximal closure of the fascia. The gluteal fascia is often thin and its exposure generally requires considerable retraction of the fat by an assistant. This is a common site of hematoma formation; the use of nonabsorbable suture material gives the fascia a chance for complete healing. If the fascia has been incised in a T-shape manner, this must be repaired carefully prior to the closure of the remainder of the fascia. The tendinous insertion of iliopsoas, adductor, and external rotator muscles may be released in order to correct fixed deformities during total hip arthroplasty; these tendons should be disinserted next to the bone to minimize bleeding. Like adductors and rotators, the iliopsoas tendon may be released from the lesser trochanter. The blood supply or accompanying vessels should be coagulated following removal of these tendons from their insertions. Commonly, the artery accompanying the piriformis may retract and cause a hematoma. The iliopsoas tendon can be readily visualized by external rotation and thus removed from the lesser trochanter and its vicinity. The adductors longus and brevis may be disinserted from the pubis by subcutaneous tenotomy. As stated, none of the tendons about the hip (unless the gluteus medius inadvertently has been disinserted without bone) require resuturing, since the purpose of tenotomies about the hip during the construction is to release the contracture and to correct deformity. A compression dressing applied to the groin area will assist in tamponade of the bleeders following adductor tenotomy.

HANDLING OF OTHER SOFT TISSUES

At times considerable force is required to retract the planes of the muscles and fascia for insertion of instruments and location of the prosthetic components; this is especially true in large and muscular males and if the greater trochanter has not been removed as a part of the routine surgical technique. During excessive retraction of the anterior structures, femoral nerve palsy can be produced, especially with a defective anterior wall of the acetabulum as in a dysplastic hip. The sciatic nerve may also be in danger if marked anatomical distortion and an excessive posterior scar is present. For example, in severe protrusion of the head and neck into the pelvis, the greater trochanter is displaced medially and within the vicinity of the sciatic nerve, thus a careless osteotomy of the greater trochanter renders danger to the sciatic nerve. In these cases it is good to palpate the nerve or to be guided by the existing fat surrounding the nerve. The anterior or posterior fibers of the very important "gluteus medius" may be damaged during the exposure of the hip joint without the removal of the greater trochanter, leading to scar formation and a weak abductor mechanism. Likewise, excessive retraction or trauma at the interval between the tensor fascia femoris muscle anteriorly and the anterior border of the gluteus medius may damage the nerve to the tensor fascia femoris, thus eliminating an important, yet less appreciated, structure of the hip joint. The muscle bundles of the gluteus maximus, which are occasionally detached from their parent bundles, must be excised if they appear devitalized. Since particles of cement are potentially irritants if deposited loosely in the soft tissue about the hip, irrigation with isotonic solution must be done. Irrigation of the muscles and other soft tissue deep to the fascia seems advisable during at least two stages of the operation—prior to closure and after cementing of the acetabular cup and the femoral component.

HANDLING OF THE GREATER TROCHANTER

The greater trochanter must be osteotomized at the appropriate level to obtain optimal size. An excessively large trochanter carries the vastus lateralis ridge with it producing a large "bump" on the outer aspect of the femur and occasionally is difficult to reattach onto the lateral aspect of the shaft. On the other hand, an excessively small trochanter may be difficult to handle—producing less than optimal coaptation of the surfaces for union, thereby escaping through the wires utilized for its fixation. The

trochanter must be handled gently from the time of its removal to the final stage of its reattachment. Only when it is removed at an optimal size and shape will the greatest degree fixation occur. A fragmented trochanter is not only difficult to reattach but also may be disengaged from its fixation wires, promoting a weak abductor mechanism and inviting dislocation of the prosthesis. Often, patients require an undesirably lengthy rehabilitation period to achieve healing of the trochanter. If excessively osteoporotic (as in rheumatoid arthritis), a larger size trochanter should be removed and greater care and attention used during its retraction and reattachment. Reattachment of the greater trochanter requires attention to details; appropriate orientation of the fibers of the gluteus medius should be oriented to preserve its fiber length and direction in a normal (physical) manner. Furthermore, a maximum coaptation between the inner surface and the outer aspect of the shaft of the femur must be obtained; handling will be discussed in detail later. A firm reattachment is of major importance with respect to a successful hip replacement through a lateral approach. Wires used for reattachment must not be scarred or nicked, and rewiring on a model or bone is advisable prior to clinical experience. If inadequate fixation of the trochanter is recognized at surgery, the patient must be protected postoperatively by 2 to 3 weeks bedrest (see Chapters 11 and 12).

SHAFT OF THE FEMUR AND THE ACETABULUM

The details of handling the shaft and the acetabulum will be discussed in subsequent chapters; however, it is basic and essential to regard the bony structures as supportive devices and to avoid damaging them (which may lead to failure of the prosthetic components). Replacement of the bony structure may be compared to the embedding of a flagpole in concrete. If the surrounding ground is weak, the flagpole will fail in spite of the strength of its materials; so, too, if the bony structures are weakened, failure of the prosthesis may occur. Removal of a previously inserted nail and plate or prosthesis may weaken the shaft of the femur, which would then require special attention; if excessive trauma is induced at the time of removal of the previously inserted device, a retreat may be necessary. Excessive damage to the floor of the acetabulum may lead to an unfortunate medial migration of the entire component, for which no solution is available at this time. Careless and/or eccentric use of the reamers or inappropriate use of drills may fracture or remove a part of the bony acetabulum and lead to subsequent loosening of the components. Special attention to preparation details of the upper femur and acetabulum is the sine qua non of good replacement surgery. While it is essential to preserve as much bony stalk as possible, removal of osteophytes must be done appropriately to prevent their functioning as a fulcrum on the periphery of the acetabulum and upper femur, facilitating dislocation. Bleeding, both in the upper femur and in the acetabulum, is best controlled by tightly packing the canal or the acetabular cavity with a large swab guaze tightly inserted into these cavities. This procedure is similar to that of a dentist packing cavities prior to application of the filling material. It is always impressive that maintaining pressure on these swabs for a period of 1 to 2 minutes leads to an almost dry surface, which is so desirable for cement application. A swab soaked in 2% tincture of iodine may be used in the bone cavities where previous prostheses had been inserted; this surgical disinfection may be useful if there is any suspicion of low-grade subclinical infection.

A maximum exposure is absolutely essential. Nowhere in the practice of orthopaedic surgery is so-called "keyhole surgery" more dangerous than in total hip arthroplasty. When the surgeon must struggle throughout the procedure to obtain exposure, more time is lost than would have been necessary to obtain good exposure at the outset of surgery; more blood loss is encountered, and the job is never done with greatest efficiency. It is far better to lose time in exposing the hip joint adequately and then to regain this time during the actual implantation. As a working rule, in performing this operation routinely we allocate two thirds of the working time for exposure and closure of the wound and only one-third to preparation of the bone and actual implantation of the prosthesis.

ORGANIZATIONAL FACILITIES TO PERFORM TOTAL HIP REPLACEMENT

To my knowledge, Sir John Charnley has been the only proponent of "specialized centers" for total hip surgery.[2] His enthusiasm stems from his experiences with the evolution and growth of the Centre for Hip Surgery at Wrightington Hospital.

Despite his great contributions and success—not only in Great Britain, but throughout the world—no other such center for dealing exclusively with surgery of the hip joint has yet been organized. Obviously, in order to duplicate such a center, comprehensive geographical planning and total devotion of time and leadership would be required. The economical impact on the private practice of most surgeons is perhaps at the root of unwillingness for the organization of such a center in the United States.

There are probably between 700,000 and 1,000,000 people with osteoarthritis—in addition to those with degenerative disease of the hip joint resulting from trauma, rheumatoid arthritis, and a variety of other afflictions—half of whom may require reconstructive surgery at some point. Some estimate that one third of the major reconstructive surgery in orthopaedic practice is related to the hip.

With life expectancy increased to 72 years of age for males and 78 years of age for females and approximately 20,000,000 Americans now over 65 years of age, we can readily see the increasing numbers of potential candidates for total hip surgery. According to Kelgren and Lawrence's field sampling in Great Britain, the incidence of arthrosis of the hip requiring arthroplasty was probably 100,000 to 200,000. Therefore we have come to recognize that the heavy load created by total hip replacement surgery (not counting total joint replacement in shoulders, knees, and elbows) calls for definite institutional reform. Furthermore, future "repair" or "maintenance" work imposed by failure of total hips might add to the cumulative number of patients requiring hip surgery.

Many older people living out the last decade of their lives could benefit from treatment of their hip disabilities. From a humanitarian point of view alone, they should be made more mobile and less confined in their advanced years; it is therefore inhumane to refuse them surgery because we lack organizational facilities and hospitals to accommodate them. In some areas of Great Britain and in nonprivate institutions in the United States, elderly people must wait for many months until they are admitted for this type of elective surgery.

Among the many advantages one expects

from a highly centralized and specialized facility for surgery are lower costs, reduction of surgical complications, and, above all, improved quality of care coupled with technical surgical perfection and minimum morbidity. This would be enhanced by optimum productivity provided by maximum use of facilities, and it would provide for an economy of effort on the part of the surgeon when he performs these operations daily. In a unit such as Wrightington Centre for Hip Surgery, six hip arthroplasties are performed in one operating room each workday—18 arthroplasties in three operating rooms. Minimum staff members are required because the routine is not interrupted by unexpected work such as trauma. Still, the staff can provide excellent patient care and render adequate clinical and basic research in the field.[3] A correlative, vivid example of maximum efficiency is displayed in bilateral operations performed during the same anesthesia and made practical because the superior organization provides a quick turnover; thus two operations may be performed during the same anesthesia without undue strain on the patient or the surgical staff.[5]

Because this type of surgery is elective and patients are not forced to accept a "compromise solution" to their problems, they are willing to travel to obtain the best possible care. Practitioners and other sources of referral would be encouraged to refer patients to a center (such as Wrightington) in view of the consistently good results and excellence of care. Therefore the reputation of such a center would attract patients from a wide geographical area.

It is now estimated that total hip replacement is one of the most commonly performed elective orthopaedic procedures in most parts of the world as well as in the United States. Yet, despite the frequency of these operations, there has been no trend toward specialization, which would provide continuous care and service. Charnley stated that "to consider the insertion of a total hip replacement into a patient 25 years of age in 1971, without having a 'service station' provided and organized for 1986, is like selling motorcars without providing mechanics and workshops." We have already seen the experiences of some surgeons who, having performed such operations in community hospitals, now find themselves under considerable pressure in dealing with complications such as infections and technical problems. It is obvious that at

this point patients who are referred to the centers for further corrective surgery have become resentful—since the new challenge is of much greater magnitude than the original procedure—and centers can offer limited or no help in further treatment because of the technical complexity of the involved problems.

Evidently, major universities and medical centers have been unwilling to devote a portion of their postgraduate training to this area—because of polarization of patients, patient load, and the need for reorganization of their staffing —despite the increased need for patient care imposed by the number of total hip operations being performed.

While it is not possible to have all total hip replacements performed in centers, if located in major cities, centers could conceivably serve not only to reduce the hospital workload but also be used as "training grounds" for orthopaedic surgeons at the postgraduate level—for these centers would attract those who are willing to devote their future work (or at least a major portion of it) to this type of surgery in order to acquire superior skills. Such centers would also free community hospital facilities for other types of work, as well as providing better overall patient care and, naturally, guarantee future "repair work."

It is my impression that if a center cannot be devoted exclusively to this type of practice, then "pooling" of patients among a group of orthopaedic surgeons practicing in one hospital would be a reasonable compromise. This group would learn from each other how best to cope with potential complications and failures, as well as being able to offer better total patient care. The popular trend of the so-called group practice in the United States may be a model for "pooling" among practicing orthopaedic surgeons rather than by a hospital-oriented group.

It would be regrettable if a procedure such as total hip replacement was used by a university and/or hospital only to attract residents to their training program (with the promise that they would be doing a "certain number" of total hip replacements by the time they were through with training). Since total hip surgery constitutes a bulk of surgical procedures, this may be a "selling point" to the young physician eager to enter into a training program in orthopaedic surgery. Operations of this magnitude should not be performed by a junior resident who has devoted insufficient time to the procedure and does not yet understand the scope of the problems lying beyond mere technical ability to perform an operation.

At the New York Orthopaedic Hospital at the Columbia–Presbyterian Medical Center, a junior resident in our training program is in charge of pre- and postoperative patient care (under the supervision of the senior resident on the hip service), in addition to being present at all operations and acting as second assistant. The overall supervision and responsibility belong to the attending physician. Routine orders are established in the pre- and postoperative periods, and a medical consultant evaluates the patient daily. This general pattern provides the junior resident with a familiarity of pre- and postoperative management of the patient; thus the daily resident's rounds are bound to be extremely helpful in identifying complications, early recording, and management.

A senior resident spends a period of 6 weeks exclusively and 6 weeks partially on the hip service; on completion of his residency during the third year he will have performed from 20 to 30 technically uncomplicated total hip procedures—assisted in all of them by an experienced attending surgeon. (He is discouraged from performing more complex procedures, even in the final year of his training.) Additionally, he has acquired experience through rotation and by having assisted in all cases during this period; it is believed that by this time he is qualified to select appropriate patients for total hip procedures and aware of his limitations in taking up more technically complicated cases.

Basic training is offered to one or two postgraduate trainees, with a fellowship for the entire year; such a person, who is usually the mainstay of the organization of postgraduate training, not only participates in most operations but conducts daily rounds with the senior and junior residents. Supervised and assisted, he performs between 200 and 300 arthroplasties during this year and also supervises and assists in operations performed by staff or residents; he generally becomes qualified to perform complicated procedures toward the end of his fellowship.

It would be a great advantage to have all hip patients located in one special area of the hospital since this promotes efficiency, better staff training, and is psychologically better for the ambulatory patients who may derive benefits by sharing with others their similar experiences. There should be one or more operating rooms devoted to performing only this type of surgery, thereby providing maximum speed and efficiency.

In summary, I support the concept of superspecialization whenever possible, as advocated by Charnley.[3] If we take into account the frequency of such operations, the basic need for technical excellence, and humanitarian consideration of older people, the necessity of a team approach to such a problem can be readily recognized and should be acknowledged by authorities in the field of orthopaedic education. Furthermore, costs and complications would be minimized and the staff could devote adequate time to documentation, recording, and cooperating with the mechanical engineering staff to develop practical solutions to technical and mechanical problems. It is further believed that this system would offer superior training in orthopaedic surgery both at pre- and postgraduate levels, and, above all, provide better patient care and the assurance of further available treatment in the future if it becomes necessary.

SUMMARY OF ESSENTIALS

- Because complications after total hip replacements at times are disastrous and failure of the operation results in severe disability, greater attention must be directed toward prevention than treatment of complications. Keeping the complications constantly in mind, a proper planning of preoperative, operative, and postoperative management of elderly patients undergoing total hip replacement is essential.

- As surgeons, orthopaedists are bound by principles that include a careful evaluation of the "whole patient" and well-founded indications for the specific surgical intervention with aseptic technique and absolute precision if a successful result is to be expected.

- The importance of preoperative and postoperative nursing care of elderly patients undergoing elective surgery such as total hip replacement, both in regard to psychological and physical problems, must be dealt with and appraised with special attention to the needs of this specific group of patients by an experienced staff. Obviously, older people are potentially more prone to complications and postoperative complications that are in inverse proportion to the excellence of postoperative care.

- Preoperative preparation and diagnostic errors

have at times been blamed for the high rate of mortality in surgery in elderly patients. This mortality rate can be reduced if detailed attention is given to all medical aspects, especially to the systemic review and proper consultations that should include anesthetic management and appropriate rehabilitation programs.

■ In general, older patients tolerate the stress better than young patients, but this initial tolerance soon gives way to the dangers of shock and demise. Therefore prompt attention toward rectifying complications of surgery in this age group must be emphasized.

■ Social and psychological aspects concerning patients undergoing major elective surgery and the details of arrangements regarding postoperative accommodations must be worked out prior to the contemplated surgery. Many details of surgical nursing care must be considered. Among these are transference of cheerful confidence to the patient when explaining the details of what to expect from surgery.

■ On admission the details of rehabilitation including transfer from bed and the use of assistive devices are helpful in a smooth and uncomplicated postoperative management. Excessive emphasis on side effects of drugs or potential complications of the operation are unnecessary, and especially during the postoperative course medications must be judiciously used for the relief of the pain and the patient's comfort.

■ Daily visits by a surgical team should include not only attention to the physical disabilities but also to the patient's mental attitude toward the progress made in the postoperative course; criticism can be dangerous and nonconstructive. Urinary or fecal incontinence is an extreme embarrassment to older patients. When this occurs, it should be handled without amplification and with support rather than criticism. An indwelling catheter will control urinary incontinence and is a convenience for the patient.

■ In the original interview it is a good idea to have the family present while discussing the proposed operation. The patient should be told as much as he or she wishes to know, but only relevant matters should be discussed. Older persons often have deep-seated fears and may not be inquisitive about the details. It is therefore unnecessary to overstate the risks of the operation and agitate the patient. Transference of cheerful confidence is essential.

■ As a principle of surgery, the speed of surgery to minimize the waste of time will improve with the surgeon's experience. There is a tendency in the beginner to attempt to break the time record for a given surgical procedure. This temptation must be resisted in doing a total hip replacement. A "perfect technique," and not a "fast technique," is the goal. Taking shortcuts to gain time during the vital part of the operation will produce poor, or even catastrophic, results requiring further surgical intervention with added misery to the patient.

■ The speed at surgery must be geared to the circumstances, which include the surgical facilities, the experience of the surgeon performing the operation, and the anatomical abnormalities requiring specific attentions.

■ Being too scrupulous or gentle in preparing the bone may be ineffective and time-consuming. On the other hand, being too bold and inadvertently traumatizing the tissue may lead to serious complications. Modifications of time-tested procedures must be done only with "good logic" behind them. Violation of "established principles" is a grave responsibility the surgeon must bear in mind.

■ The tissue must be handled gently and support of life of repair must be kept in mind. Irrigation with isotonic solutions and removal of debris and necrotized tissue are good principles of successful surgery.

■ The routine use of drainage of the wound with a suction drain is to be encouraged both deep to the fascia and superficial to the fascia. A hematoma must never be drained or aspirated at the bedside. Spontaneous drainage of a hematoma into the wound is best handled by reoperation and evacuation in the operating room under general anesthesia in absolutely sterile conditions.

■ A draining (leaking) hematoma is potentially dangerous from the standpoint of infection and must be treated vigorously and handled as an emergency situation.

■ The study of anatomy and rehearsal prior to surgery is essential for the beginner. Participation in several surgical procedures as an assistant would not only familiarize the surgeon with the procedure but also give him a better understanding of unpredicted difficulties that may arise during this operation.

■ Preparation of the skin prior to surgery with surgical soap and meticulous clipping of the hair must be exercised with supervision. The use of 2% tincture of iodine and proper draping techniques is of paramount importance in performing the operation. The skin incision must be adequate and placed with care. The correct placement of the incision is of great value, similar to a good closure of the skin to prevent infection.

■ The use of retention sutures have dramatically improved the quality of wound healing after total hip arthroplasty. When handling the wound closure, the surgeon must consider a thin person to be as potentially susceptible to infection as an obese person. In both extreme cases a meticulous approximation of fat and retention sutures is essential to prevent the accumulation of seroma or hematoma. It is a bad principle to relegate the wound closure to the most junior member of the operating team.

- The greater trochanter must be handled with care and meticulous detailed technique for reattachment must be employed. The tendon of the abductor must never be removed partially or totally without a bony fragment since the repair in this instance is impossible.

- At times, considerable force is required to retract the planes of the muscles and fascia for insertion of instruments or prostheses in heavy muscled men. The best way to expose the hip joint is by using a technique that minimizes trauma to the muscle or the neurovascular structure of the hip joint. In this regard, removal of the trochanter facilitates exposure without undue damage to the soft tissue or bone.

- A meticulous preparation of the bony acetabulum and femur produces the opportunity to implant the prosthesis with optimal fixation at surgery—a poorly fixed prosthesis at surgery will remain poorly fixed to the bone. A maximum exposure is absolutely essential. Nowhere in the practice of surgery in "keyhole" surgery more dangerous than in performing total hip replacement where optimal fixation of the components is a guarantee to success of the operation.

- Despite the great emphasis on centralization of the operation of total hip arthroplasty, the prevalence of osteoarthrosis and rheumatoid arthritis requiring these operations, and emphasis on perfection and improved technique and "repair work" that may be required following this operation, there are only a few centers in the world dealing exclusively with the surgery of the hip joint. Among the many advantages one expects from a highly centralized and specialized facility for surgery of this type are lower costs, reduction of surgical complications, and, above all, improved quality of care coupled with technical surgical perfection with minimum morbidity.

- While it is not possible at the present time to have all total hip replacements performed in specialized centers, the centers could conceivably serve to reduce the hospital workload and become a training ground for the orthopaedic surgeons at the postgraduate level to attract those who are willing to devote their future work to this type of surgery. This goal could also be reached by pooling the patients among a group of surgeons practicing in one hospital and devoting their time and effort to the organization of facilities for this type of work within their own hospital.

- It would be a great advantage to have all hip patients located in one special area of the hospital since this promotes efficiency, better staff training, and is psychologically better for the ambulatory patients who may derive benefit by sharing with others their similar experiences.

- If we take into account the frequency of the operations such as total hip replacement and the need for basic technical excellence and humanitarian considerations of older people, the necessity of a team approach to such a problem can be readily recognized and should be acknowledged by authorities in the field of orthopaedic education. Costs and complications would be minimized and the staff could devote adequate time to documentation, recording, and cooperating with the mechanical engineering staff to develop practical solutions to technical and mechanical problems. Such a system would obviously provide a superior training in orthopaedic surgery both at pre- and postgraduate levels, and, above all, better patient care and assurance of further available treatment in the future if it becomes necessary.

REFERENCES

1. Aufranc, O. E.: Preoperative and postoperative treatment of the patient with reconstructive surgery of the hip, Clin. Orthop. **38:**40-44, 1965.
2. Aufranc, O. E.: Constructive surgery of the hip, St. Louis, 1962, The C. V. Mosby Co.
3. Charnley, J.: Personal communications.
4. Dolkart, R. E.: Medical considerations of orthopaedic surgery in the elderly patient, J. Bone Joint Surg. **47A:**1041-1042, 1965.
5. Jaffe, W. L., and Charnley, J.: Bilateral Charnley low-friction arthroplasty as a single operative procedure, Bull. Hosp. Joint Dis. **32:**198-214, 1971.
6. Scott, D. L.: Anaesthetic experiences in 1300 major geriatric operations, Br. J. Anaesth. **33:**354-370, 1961.
7. Viikari, S. J., and Vaalasti, T.: Surgery in aged persons, Ann. Chir. Gynecol. Fenn. **48:**19-30, 1959.
8. Wilder, R. J., and Fishbein, R. H.: Operative experience with patients over 80 years of age, Surg. Gynecol. Obstet. **113:**205-212, 1961.

CHAPTER 6

Prevention of infection

The greater the ignorance, the greater dogmatism.

SIR WILLIAM OSLER

The septic property of the atmosphere depended on
minute organisms suspended in it.

LORD LISTER

. . . This argument suggests that infections following bone
operations are exogenous, and that they are therefore preventable.

SIR JOHN CHARNLEY

GENERAL COMMENTS

The first report on aseptic technique was
made by Joseph Lister over 100 years ago in
1867. Clinical benefits were immediately forthcoming as a result of his discovery of aseptic
methods, isolation methods, and antimicrobial
agents. Lister's work strengthened the defenses
against bacterial infection, and subsequently
extensive work has been done in an attempt to
trace the causes of infections that occur in clean
surgical operations performed in ultramodern
operating rooms. Although listerism abolished
fulminating and epidemic hospital sepsis such
as clostridial infections ("hospital gangrene"),
infections caused by mildly pathogenic organisms such as staphylococci have remained common. At the present time, the literature on
wound infection and operating room prevention
methods is voluminous and many examples are
available both in general surgical literature*
and orthopaedic literature.† Progress made in
the sciences of bacteriology and the use of anti-
biosis over the past three decades (since the use
of antibiotics in surgery) has considerably reduced the mortality rates from postoperative
infections. However, the role played by antibiotics to prevent infection remains controversial mostly in general surgical experience. Additionally, continuous changes in bacterial ecology
and the increasing incidence of gram-negative

organisms not previously considered pathogenic
have emerged; in this context, fulminating infections caused by fungi have appeared at times,
resulting in the patient's death.[20,56]

The cost of infection and resultant disability,
both to the patient and society, is so great that
every effort should be made toward a sound prevention rather than treatment after the fact. In
Altemier's[10] 1967 study of 1,391,200 patients
with infection, there was an estimated cost of
$7,000.00 per patient for each infection or
$9.8 million in that year. While these costs are
examples of minor infections reflecting general
surgical experiences, the cost of each infected
total hip must be well above $50,000.00, and
perhaps 10 times greater in certain difficult and
complex infections (see Chapter 16). Beyond
the cost to the patient and the social impact,
the misery and resultant lifelong disability is of
the greatest concern.

In this section we will consider the highlights
of documented studies and their role in prevention of sepsis in major reconstructive surgery
such as total hip replacement. The clinical diagnosis and management of infection following
total hip replacement will be found in Chapter
16.

BACTERIAL INVASION VS. HOST
RESISTANCE

Two groups of factors play a part in the critical "disease-producing dose" of organisms: (1)
the number of infecting organisms at the site of

---

*See references 1, 90, 117, 136, and 137.
†See references 35, 39, 87, 106, 152, and 153.

the wound and (2) the virulence of organisms in relation to the host or to a given tissue. This time-honored explanation may be considered from yet another angle, which is the measure of the ability of a given host to deal effectively with a certain number of bacteria within a given space. Burke[30,32] has emphasized that it is not the actual number of organisms within a unit space of tissue that matters, but the number that can be dealt with effectively by the host's defense mechanisms during a given period of time; disease develops when the local concentration of bacteria exceeds the level that can be dealt with by the body. Therefore development of postoperative wound infection depends not only on the number of bacteria that enter the wound during surgery and on the exact physiological state of the patient and the wound itself but also on the "chance association" of bacteria landing on an area with sufficiently reduced resistance to cause infection. A localized reduction in host resistance is at least as important as bacterial contamination (Fig. 6-1) and it might therefore be interpreted that the number of wound infections after surgery would not fall to zero in clinical medicine until bacterial contamination is completely eliminated. Consequently, any efforts aimed at further reduction of postoperative infection must concentrate on host responses, while still holding down bacterial contamination and recognizing that almost any bacteria may become pathogenic under a certain set of circumstances.[65] It follows that no longer can one identify a harmless saprophyte merely by its morphological characteristics.[102]

In 1956, Elek and Conen[65] reported that over a million viable pathogenic staphylococci were necessary to produce infection by intradermal injection in human volunteers. However, the infection-causing number could be reduced to 100 viable organisms (a 10,000-fold decrease) if a silk stitch was inserted as well.

Charnley's[39,40] experiences suggest that in total hip replacement the wound can be infected with a dosage of organisms that is far less than previously imagined; for example, one infected dust particle may produce infection. The massive foreign body that is an integral feature of total hip replacement procedure is believed to be a contributing factor in the development of postsurgical wound infections.

In addition to "dose-related" virulence of bacterial infection, failure of defense mechanisms of the body that upset the bacteria-host equilibrium must be seriously considered as fundamental factors in producing infection. As a rule, the first line of defense against invading organisms is the "operative condition" of the "portal of entry." Once the organism reaches beyond this point, the body fluid and cells dynamically produce defense mechanisms against the invasion.[77] Among these defenses are the condition of surfaces and cavities, the cell type, nature of local secretion, drainage, pH, dryness, and so on. It is shown quantitatively that local defense systems destroy bacteria in a great proportion and that levels of viable bacteria reaching the bloodstream are approximately 10,000 times less than those controlled locally at the portal of entry.[100] It may be that the number of organisms destroyed at the site must be even greater, since Alexander and co-workers[4,5] have shown that bacteria may survive and even multiply after phagocytosis within the leukocyte.[5,7] In addition to leukocytes, wandering macrophages, as well as fixed macrophages of the reticuloendothelial system, enter the defense mechanism and act where leukocytes have failed. With failure to eliminate the bacteria at this point, their entry into the lymph nodes and bloodstream becomes imminent. However, macrophages in the spleen (or Kupffer's cells) still may eliminate them from blood circulation. While the battle between the invading organisms and cellular response is in progress, the host's humoral defense system is activated, the final and most decisive element in controlling the invading organisms.[4]

SURGICAL TREATMENT BY MASSIVE IMPLANTATIONS

With reference to foreign materials in the surgical wound adding to the risk and extent of

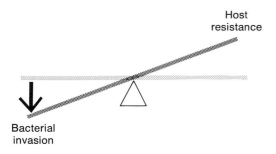

Fig. 6-1. Clinical infection is imminent when host resistance is weakened in favor of bacterial invasion. Loss of balance in favor of invading organism shown.

165

infection, experiments such as those by Elek and Cohen[65] (see p. 173) classically demonstrate causal relationships. Edlich and his co-workers[59] have unequivocally documented the role of percutaneous sutures in causing infection. For example, it is shown that taping skin (as compared with suturing) has reduced the wound infection rate in experimental animals.[36] It is of special interest that not only the presence of foreign material but also its physical characteristics[6,67,107] in experimental wound infection studies have reduced the level of host response.

Early experiences with the implantation of artificial joints proved that these surgical conditions are particularly favorable to infection, as evidenced by a high incidence of infection in the developmental era of total joint replacement. In previous publications, Charnley and Eftekhar,[40] Wilson and co-workers,[170] Amstutz,[11] and others reported a high incidence of wound infection when no extra precautions were exercised in the ordinary operating room environment. These surgeons had not experienced a comparable increase when dealing with ordinary operations. The following suggestions were offered as an explanation for such an increased susceptibility: (1) The condition of a ball-and-socket with a dead space left at surgery might favor survival of organisms. (2) Bacteria may be destroyed by tissue when it is immobilized (as in arthrodesis) but survive in conditions of mobility such as total hip replacement. (3) The plastics used may favor or, indeed, enhance the resistance of mildly pathogenic organisms. (4) Uniqueness of late-appearing infection with sinus formation may be the result of plastic used in the artificial joint. (5) Devitalized tissue adjacent to the cement may be a particularly suitable environment for proliferation of organisms. (6) The size of the implant is much greater than those previously used in orthopaedic surgery.

TERMINOLOGY OF SEPSIS

The true incidence of infection in surgery may not be possible to determine because of lack of a specific definition of infection. For example, positive cultures may be obtained from wounds that heal primarily without drainage— likewise, heat, redness, and swelling may be present in a postoperative wound even with some purulent exudate from which no organism may be cultured. Therefore a workable definition of wound infection applicable to the clinical

situation is one that partly disregards the bacteriology but greatly emphasizes the clinical situation[1,44]: (1) *uninfected wound*—heals primarily without drainage, (2) *definitely infected wound*—discharges pus even if culture is negative, and (3) *possibly infected wound*—inflamed but without drainage or a positive culture but may show nonpurulent drainage.

Confusion has arisen in the past because it has been stated that an organism must be a pathogen to cause disease, and nonpathogens or saprophytic organisms are merely contaminants. One commonly finds the term "contaminants" in bacteriological reports. Confusion has also arisen in defining infection according to the organism found in the wound itself. This problem is compounded by using the term "virulent," as measured by the number of organisms required to kill members of a particular animal species under standardized conditions in a definite period of time. Since the so-called nonpathogenic organisms have not been incriminated and yet are frequently seen in the wounds, the question of rejection of the plastics without infection has often been discussed among surgeons. Like Charnley, we have concluded that rejection or sensitivity to the acrylic cement must be exceedingly rare and an infected wound without a positive culture from the wound is not related to the cement reaction but rather is a failure of "bacteriological methods" to identify the organism. Many of the so-called nonpathogenic organisms are seen in an infected total hip replacement, and vast knowledge may be required of surgeons in dealing with these organisms in the future. These organisms are usually of low virulence and often are difficult to culture by routine methods of bacteriology.

Bacteriology of the sepsis in combined early and late infection in one study of 85 infected total hip replacements reported: 33 were caused by *Staphylococcus aureus,* 4 by *Staphylococcus albus,* 1 by *Pseudomonas* organisms, 6 by *Proteus* bacilli, and 5 by coliform bacilli.[39] As indicated, *Staphylococcus aureus,* coagulase positive, remains the most common offending organism in producing infection in total hip replacements. It has also been found that *Staphylococcus aureus* is responsible for both early and late infection. In 18% of early cases the wound has been "sterile" despite the presence of clinical infection.[39,40] Infections produced by coliform bacilli (12%) usually occurred in the early

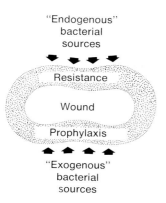

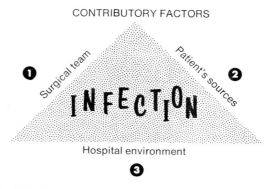

Fig. 6-2. In multifactorial sources of infection, both endogenous and exogenous sources of bacteria must be considered. By increasing local resistance of tissue and prophylaxic measures, wounds may be protected from those bacterial sources.

Fig. 6-3. All contributory factors to surgical infection must be considered: *(1)* surgical team, *(2)* patient's own sources, and *(3)* hospital environment in order to find means of prophylaxis.

group; in late infections, however, 41% of the cases had a sinus or organisms of low pathogenic nature responsible for infection. These factors are of considerable importance in planning the antibiotic prophylaxis in total hip replacement.

SOURCES OF SURGICAL INFECTION AND PROPHYLAXIS

In view of the many contributing factors in surgical infections, methods of prophylaxis and treatment must be considered separately, emphasizing different means of prophylaxis and treatment according to different etiological factors. Only understanding of all the factors contributing to surgical infections will lead to an intelligent means of prophylaxis[63] (Figs. 6-2 and 6-3).

The patient's sources

Experimentally, it has been shown that wounds become infected from infections elsewhere in the body[101] (Fig. 6-4). While this mode of wound infection is not common following surgery, it is a possibility that should be kept in mind.

As much consideration must be given to the factors related to the patient as to those related to the environment. One cannot deny that total hip replacement with massive implantation of a foreign body in a 65-year-old woman with rheumatoid disease, severe debility, and previous steroid therapy carries a much higher risk for surgical sepsis when compared with an otherwise healthy 12-year-old girl undergoing an

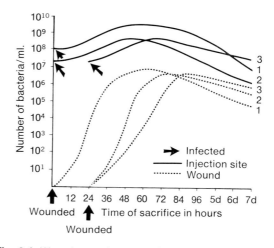

Fig. 6-4. Wounds may become infected from infection elsewhere. Quantitative distribution of staphylococci after subcutaneous injection with wounding of animal: *(1)* simultaneous wounding with injection, *(2)* 24 hours after injection animal was wounded, and *(3)* 24 hours after wounding animal was injected. (Modified from Krizek, T. J., and Davis, J. H.: J. Trauma **6:**239-248, 1966.)

appendectomy. Without adequate statistical proof, old age, obesity, and diabetes have all been suggested as favoring infection in general surgical experiences.[1,117]

In addition to a poor state of nutrition and steroid therapy, alternate sources of infection such as skin, urinary tract, and pulmonary lesions must be considered. Efforts should be made to isolate the organisms from the joints if there has been previous evidence of infection or repeated aspiration and injection with corticosteroids.

167

A genitourinary consultation is at times essential, and a symptomatic prostate gland should be evaluated preoperatively. Since many patients require catheterization postoperatively, prophylactic urinary antibiotics in patients with a previous history of urinary tract infection may be indicated. Urinary tract infection may be one of the most significant sources of infection following total hip replacement.[13,92] Postoperative urinary retention must be treated by indwelling catheterization performed by trained personnel adequately instructed in aseptic techniques. Suppressive therapy, such as sulfisoxazole (Gantrisin), nitrofurantoin (Furadantin), or similar drugs has been recommended. The patient's fluid intake has to be maintained at a high level, and when the catheter is removed, cultures and sensitivities should be obtained; if any evidence of active urinary tract infection is found, the operation must be postponed and appropriate antibiotics should be administered.

Chronic obstructive pulmonary disease theoretically may be the source of infection. In practice, it is not easy to identify the active stage of a chronic lung disease; however, if there is any evidence of exacerbation of chronic pulmonary disease, surgery must be postponed until the pulmonary state is fully evaluated. General surgical experiences have suggested that hospitalized patients become colonized with antibiotic-resistant staphylococci.[150]

Also, it has been shown that an increase in infection rate could be related to the preoperative hospital stay.[1] Increase in staphylococcal infections has been attributed to an extended preoperative stay of the patient prior to surgery[150] and that "staph-carrier state" increased directly with increased length of hospitalization,

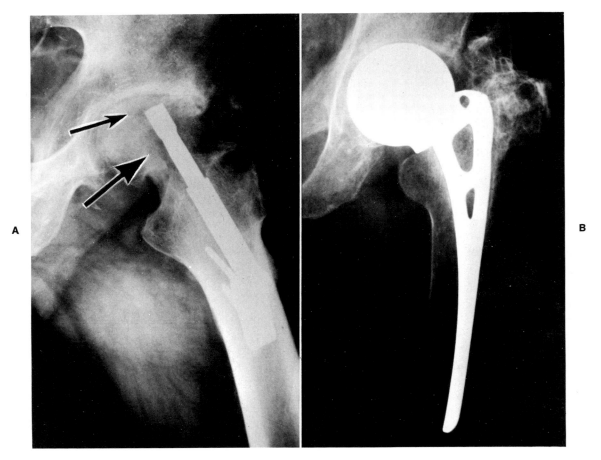

Fig. 6-5. A, Irregular patchy radiolucencies (arrows) (punched-out lesions) are indicative of osteitis. Patchy radiolucencies also must be regarded as highly suspicious for infection. **B,** Neither severe osteoporosis nor heterotopic bone formation as the result of previous surgery is indicative of infection.

which was accordingly proportional to the infection rate in these patients.[168] It should be noted that, while a lengthy preoperative stay is not a common factor in total hip replacement surgery, transferring a rheumatoid arthritic patient from a medical ward for surgery undoubtedly carries the added risk outlined previously. Furthermore, those patients who require a longer preoperative hospital stay may indeed have a complex range susceptibility such as debilitating soft tissue atrophy, rheumatoid arthritis, diabetes, and old age (necessitating lengthy hospital stay prior to surgery), thus predisposing these patients to infection.

Previous hip surgery

The presence or history of previous infection in the hip must be evaluated prior to total hip replacement. Infection is usually determined by several diagnostic measures including white blood count, erythrocyte sedimentation rate, appearance of infection on radiographs, gross appearance of infection at surgery, a smear (made at surgery), and finally, cellular morphology at operation[64] (see Chapter 16). Some surgeons recommend routine aspiration of all hips having had previous operations. At our institution, we have not found this to be a reliable method—so unless infection is highly suspected and an arthrogram is indicated, we do not recommend routine multiple aspiration of

the hip prior to operation. A sedimentation rate of about 40 mm./hr. or more is considered significant and suggestive of infection. These patients deserve scrutiny and aspiration of their joints prior to surgery.

A careful examination of the radiographs is helpful in screening infected cases. Localized patchy radiolucency or irregular punched-out lesions adjacent to the implant are highly suggestive of infection. However, the presence of heterotopic bone formation or generalized osteoporosis is not representative of infection. Furthermore, so-called onion skin appearance surrounding the stem of the prosthesis is considered nonspecific and, in many cases, is caused by motion rather than infection (Fig. 6-5).

At surgery, the presence of hypertrophic, grayish synovial tissue, necrotic debris, or purulent fluid in the hip joint is considered important in arriving at a diagnosis of infection. A differential diagnosis based purely on cellular morphology might not be possible; it is only helpful if polymorphonuclear cells are present. A Gram's stain for bacteria and cellular morphology is useful in establishing the presence or absence of infection. Since the final decision regarding the presence of infection is often made at the time of surgery, it is of greatest importance that the patient be fully informed of such a possibility beforehand (see Chapter 16) (Fig. 6-6).

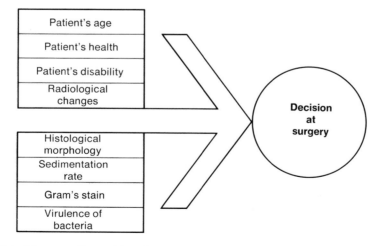

Fig. 6-6. Final decision regarding revision of suspected infected hip must be based on patient's age, health, disability, radiological changes, and elevated sedimentation rate. However, most important feature is histological morphology, positive Gram's stain, and nature of virulence of bacteria suspected at surgery that may lead to final decision (see text).

The operating room and surgical environment

The surgical environment includes factors such as gowns, masks, and gloves, as well as the surgical facilities such as construction of the operating room and ventilation methods. A substantial reduction in air contamination in the operating room can be achieved by prohibiting entry of ward clothes and bedding into the operating room and by preventing unnecessary movements of the staff.[1,58,60,137] A small proportion of *Staphylococcus aureus* carriers has been recognized as dispersers. In a surgical team, "dispersers" or "spreaders" may be particularly dangerous if the organisms they shed are highly virulent. The chance that the team includes a dangerous disperser increases the risk of additional contamination; thus the surgical team must be kept as small as possible and no one whose presence is not essential should be admitted to the operating room. Unfortunately, the method of detecting dispersers is too complicated for routine use. Moreover, as "carrier" and "disperser" functions are not consistent and since frequent tests would be necessary to find all dispersers in the team, it is not always possible to eliminate the sporadic dispersers from the operating room environment.[117]

There is some doubt that bacteria are ever freely suspended in the air; it is more generally accepted that they are airborne on particles of dust or on desquamating epithelium shed from the skin. Airborne particles most likely to contaminate a wound are those that are heavy enough to settle in less than 1 hour; these particles are usually over 10 μ in size and frequently carry clusters of organisms. Particles as small as 1 μ (the size of bacterial spores) remain suspended in the air for a long time and are less likely to seed a wound in large numbers and cause infection.

The cost of installation and maintenance of an air filtration unit for an operating room, therefore, can be minimized without sacrificing efficiency by filtering air for particles no smaller than 1 μ.[37,39,60,62] Some particles that carry bacteria are generated in the operating room during the operation. Infected dust particles are principally epithelial scales shed from the skin of personnel and come from body areas such as the perineum as well as from exposed parts such as the face or, a very obvious source, the nasopharynx (Fig. 6-7). Obviously, the generation of

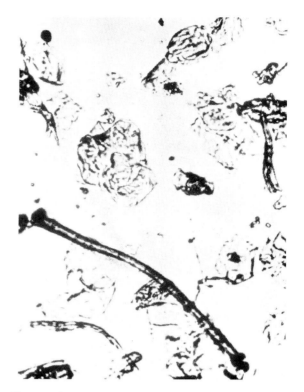

Fig. 6-7. Shape and size of most particles found in conventional operating rooms. Most frequent and dangerous particles are ones shed from personnel within operating room, which at times may contain viable organisms.

infected dust particles inside the operating room is not controlled by conventional ventilation systems. The greater the number of persons in the operating room, the greater the emission rate of infected particles. To dilute the concentration of infected dust particles, the volume of filtered air entering the room should be commensurate with the number of persons and the rate of particle emission. Some operations demand a large team of surgeons and it is frequently necessary that individuals other than team members be present for teaching or other purposes. Bacteriologically, clean air in a conventional operating room involves a more subtle planning than mere installation of a high-quality ventilation system based upon conventional methods, and it does not suffice simply to increase air changes two or three times or to install air filters that remove all particles of any size. This only raises the cost and the result will not prevent airborne contamination of an open wound. In an operating "enclosure" it is possible to bacteriologically isolate persons who are in direct contact with the open wound without in-

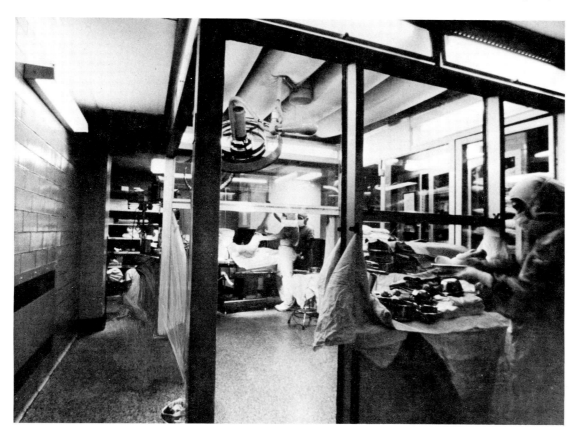

Fig. 6-8. Vertical flow enclosure within standard operating room. NOTE: post filter cloth tubes suspended from ceiling and special light to produce minimal obstruction for airflow. In background induction room is shown where patient is anesthetized and prepared for surgery prior to entry to enclosure. (Operating room K at Presbyterian Hospital at Columbia Presbyterian Medical Center, New York, N.Y.)

hibiting communication with others in the room (Fig. 6-8).

In an enclosure, clean air can be admitted at a rate that produces a positive movement of air in a predetermined direction, but the "ideal" in laminar-flow ventilation is difficult to achieve in practice. The major obstacle is turbulence resulting when air strikes stationary objects—the higher the flow, the greater the turbulence. There are also special problems of inordinate cooling of wounds from evaporation when the air flow is very fast. Therefore it has been suggested that the rate of admission of clean air to the enclosure should be such as to produce a positive movement of air that would prevent air from rising toward the ceiling by thermal convection. Following the development of a prototype clean air enclosure, Charnley[37] proposed a permanent installation made of glass, approximately 7 × 7 feet, with a ceiling height of 10 feet. Clean air enters the enclosure through HEPA* filters from an opening in the ceiling. The bottom edges of the enclosure rest upon metal feet, leaving a space for air to escape to the surrounding room at the floor level. Vertical edges of the glass plate forming the enclosure are separated by gaps of ⅛ inch to encourage escape of air and abolish dead air space in corners. The area of 7 × 7 feet was chosen as the smallest enclosure in which hip joint surgery can be performed conveniently. However, large rooms could be designed (and might be preferred) for accommodation of a larger surgical team. The entrance of the enclosure is covered by sterile curtains and the vertical air speed is increased to a maximum, thereby creating a positive pressure inside the enclosure that forces

---

*High-efficiency particulate air; referred to as absolute filters that are 99.97% effective on the DOP test.

air out through the open (service hatch) area at the foot of the enclosure. Surgical instruments needed for an operation are planned carefully prior to surgery and divided into separate trays that are prewrapped and autoclaved inside cloth bags. When required, the contents are inserted through the service hatch of the enclosure (Fig. 6-8).

Based on the foregoing, it should be clear that the effectiveness of a unidirectional air conditioning system—and the amount of air conditioning needed for a given situation—is dependent not only on the amount of air that enters the enclosure, but also on the amount of bacteria-laden particles generated by personnel within the room. It has been shown that a person may shed from 100,000 to 30,000,000 particles per minute and from 3,000 to 5,000 microorganisms per minute, depending on the activity and the effectiveness of clothing acting as a barrier to these particles.* It is also documented that because of direct attack on airborne bacteria (listerian concept) and equipment sterilization, wound infection has been reduced in an uncomplicated operation (such as herniorrhaphy) to only 1.9%.[137] While this rate of infection might be satisfactory to some surgeons dealing with herniorrhaphy, it is totally unacceptable to other surgeons dealing with total hip replacement. It is therefore our opinion that this rate should not be considered the "irreducible minimum"; elimination of *all* bacteria from the wound is essential. Airborne bacteria are still a large part of the inoculum of open wounds in conventional operating rooms. In a conventional operating room 30,000 to 60,000 organisms per hour may sediment into the 3 to 4 mm.[2] sterile field of a major operation.[151]

EXTREME AIR FILTRATION AND WOUND INFECTION

It is of historical interest that in the United States in 1930 the Chemical Warfare Service required further improvement in previously approved air filters for use in masks against newer chemical and biological warfare. During the early 1950s, the Atomic Energy Commission further refined the filters, which led to the development of HEPA filters. The primary purpose was to rid air of radioactive submicron particles.[14,163] The principle of laminar airflow was proposed by Whitefield and, subsequently, widely used by NASA contractors for protection of microelectronics and spacecraft components.[68,162,163] In a recent publication, Turner[155] summarized the background of clean-air–laminar-airflow rooms and evaluated the clinical results obtained by their installation and application for surgery. A laminar-airflow room has been in use at Batta Memorial Hospital, Albuquerque, New Mexico, since January of 1966.[155]

Following extensive bacteriological study of air-sampling techniques and colony counts on settle plates, several investigators have demonstrated the effect of clean-air systems on bacterial content of the air and degrees of wound contamination.*

Charnley[37,39,40] pioneered concepts of surgical environmental control after a continuous surveillance of case studies at Wrightington Hip Centre and attempts to correlate air cleanliness with rates of infection. He attempted control of the environment by use of an insulator "enclosure," irrespective of the state of the air within the main part of the operating room. With this technique only the surgical team was in the vicinity of the wound; the anesthetist and other personnel were excluded. The instruments were presented in a preprogrammed fashion and were not exposed to the air in the operating room. Air expired by members of the surgical team was drawn away by a suction system fitted inside ordinary masks.[38] Early results of this improved operating room were encouraging. In a subsequent study in 1969, further confirmation of favorable results by improved air cleanliness in the enclosure was reported.[40] With this new operating room, it became apparent that a unique set of data was available for study: (1) The degree of air contamination was controlled and recorded. (2) One operation was repeatedly performed by a team of surgeons following the same protocol throughout. (3) Most of the patients were in good health and in their 60s and 70s. (4) No prophylactic antibiotics were used throughout the study. (5) Last, and perhaps most important, the entire environment could be controlled with regard to traffic and other variables, which undoubtedly were not controlled in other studies.

In a recent communication, Charnley[39] sum-

---

*See references 14, 48, 50, 55, 75, 126, 128, and 138.

*See references 3, 11, 12, 26-28, 45, 46, 70, 71, 76, 81-83, 89, 93, 112, 114, 120, 133, 139-141, 146-148, and 164-167.

marized a 10-year experience with clean-air operating room systems, including a background experience of 10,000 total hip replacements. It was concluded that although air cleanliness in the operating room is important, it is not the only factor determining infection rate. Despite the fact that air cleanliness was 25 times better than in a modern operating room, the infection rate was reduced only by 50%. Therefore it may be concluded that the dosage of an organism necessary to produce infection must be less than previously imagined, refuting the experimental work of Elek and Conen.[65] Although more acceptable air cleanliness improved the statistics when infection rate was high (over 1%), it could not further reduce it below the level of 1%, which can be statistically documented.[39,105,106]

THE USE OF A CLEAN-AIR ENCLOSURE IS A "RATIONAL" DISCIPLINE

Even without unduly emphasizing air cleanliness, the use of a surgical enclosure itself will improve discipline in operating room traffic. It is our impression that the infection rate has been reduced in many centers by instituting a "critical discipline" (even without the use of a special clean-air enclosure per se), eliminating unnecessary personnel and controlling movement in the operating room. Our own rate of infection at The New York Orthopaedic Hospital in the first 1,100 cases, without any special enclosure but with very strict control of traffic and the use of prophylactic antibiotics, was very gratifying and the rate of infection was below 0.5%.[60] Obviously, with the infection rate at this level, it is not possible to attribute causes solely to one factor, and it requires a very large number of operations in order to make figures statistically significant.

A logical solution is to design an enclosure that isolates the surgical team from circulating personnel and spectators. The air entering the enclosure would be free of particles greater than 2 to 3 μ in diameter. Air pressure would be slightly positive and relatively unidirectional. Even if turbulence does occur within the enclosure, it would be acceptable since it is relatively clean. The surgical team does not contribute much to air contamination since they utilize impermeable all-investing gowns and hoods and a body exhaust system. This, then, would be a "nonlaminar-flow," slightly "turbulent" enclo-

sure, without the expensive equipment necessary for ultrafiltration and laminar-flow maintenance. Filtration of air particles less than 1 to 2 μ is not necessary because smaller particles do not appear to carry organisms, and bacteria are not suspended in air by themselves. Similarly, a horizontal-flow room may be designed to be installed in a conventional operating room without the necessity of altering existing structural changes within the room. The walls may be removable (for those surgeons who prefer to work without them), and existing operating lights may be used.[121-127] While the cost and "scientific proof" of air cleanliness have been challenged, the concept of exposing the surgical wound only to sterile air is a fundamental principle in surgery if we surgeons accept aseptic techniques as essential in surgery. Despite early opposition, especially from hospital administrators and general surgeons who usually are not dealing with ultraclean cases involving massive implantation of foreign bodies, clean air technology continues to grow in the areas of surgery where infection could bring about the most catastrophic results. There is now abundant literature available to demonstrate a marked reduction of wound contamination by the use of clean-air systems.* This in itself is sufficiently encouraging and adequate to recommend the use of these systems in total hip replacement surgery.

THE USE OF ULTRAVIOLET LIGHT IN OPERATING ROOMS

In order to provide clean air in the operating room at Duke University, Hart installed ultraviolet lights over 40 years ago (early 1936). This method has been effective at Duke University in reducing the number of airborne bacteria during the surgical procedure.[84,85] Eliminating 75% to 90% of viable bacteria by the settle plate method[1,9,23,48,85] was found to be effective in reduction of the wound infection rate in the ultra clean cases. A National Research Council (NRC)[1] study evaluating ultraviolet light concluded that a statistically significant reduction of postoperative wound infections was observed following clean, refined operations. The main body of this report, however, did not encourage the use of ultraviolet light, although average postoperative infection rate was reduced from

---

*See references 69, 91, 126, 147, and 148.

3.8% to 2.9%. Such an average drop might not have been impressive but represented a 24% improvement for the five hospitals under study with the range of improvement as high as 44% in one of the participating hospitals. Goldner, referring to Dr. Hart's work, concluded that the use of ultraviolet light in operating rooms is the simplest, most economical, and least involved method of obtaining a relatively clean air environment. Goldner and associates[79,80] have produced suggestive evidence of favorable results in the use of ultraviolet light in performing total hip replacements. Lowell[109] has also demonstrated a marked reduction in bacterial contamination with the use of ultraviolet lights. His statistical data, like others, suffer from lack of adequate numbers of cases and the multifactorial nature of total hip replacement operations.

SURGICAL SCRUB, SKIN DISINFECTION, AND GLOVING

The surgical scrub is a routine practice, accepted by most surgeons as a principle in prophylaxis against infection. It is regarded as an additionally protective step toward preparation in gloving for surgery. Because gloves may be torn or punctured during an operation, the added protection of a high-quality surgical glove, or a double pair of gloves, is essential in handling surgical wounds involving instrumentation and soft tissue and bone. It is now an accepted fact that the 10-minute hand scrub is an unneces-

sary ritual, although in a comparison of several agents, Dineen[52] showed differences between 5- and 10-minute scrubs (Fig. 6-9). It has been suggested that a 1-minute scrub may be adequate because of the slight differential in bacterial count on the fingertips of those examined after 1 minute of scrubbing and those examined up to 2 hours after scrubbing. Studies of Bernard[21] have also shown that reduction in bacterial counts of 85% (with 3-, 5-, or 10-minute scrubs) showed no difference among the various lengths of scrubs.

Because most gloves are found to be punctured by the end of an operation, it is essential to have the gloves frequently checked throughout the operation for obvious tears and perforations. The frequent change of gloves during surgery is a good and rational discipline. In a study of 100 operative procedures[34] it has been noted that one or more glove punctures occurred in 70% of the operations.

Others[42] have also documented the frequent puncture of gloves by evidence of blood seeping through the puncture site and have even demonstrated the bacterial counts of *Staphylococcus aureus* as reaching as high as 18,000.

Although no scientific report can be found in which the source of infection following surgery was traced to the punctured glove, it is a rational discipline to avoid puncturing the gloves during the operation and to replace them as soon as any puncture is detected. With regard to this

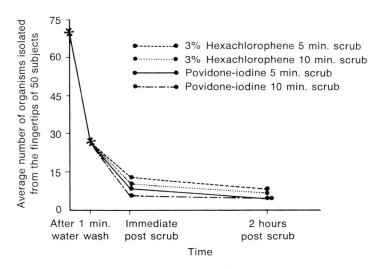

Fig. 6-9. Comparison of 5- to 10-minute surgical scrub on skin counts obtained from 50 subjects using different agents. *Indicates drop in bacterial population after 1 min. wash. (Adapted from Dineen, P.: Surg. Gynecol. Obstet. **199:**1181-1184, 1969.)

mode of transmission of bacteria, regardless of sterility of the surgeon's hands (at the end of the scrub period), the chances that they will remain sterile by the end of the operation (as the result of sweating and self-contamination within the surgical gloves) remain remarkably high. By the same basis, some surgical antiseptic soap left on the hands at the end of the scrub period may produce some disinfecting effect.

Surgeons must insist that all surgical members wear two pairs of high-quality gloves.

A most important source of exogenous infection is wound contamination via the surgeon's hands or soiling of the wound by contamination during postoperative recovery. The first 24 hours are perhaps the most critical following surgery in terms of direct contamination; after this period natural epithelial formation provides a barrier and the skin is self-protected. In a primary wound closure without drainage, purely from the bacteriological point of view a dressing is perhaps unnecessary after a few hours of skin closure.[86] Nevertheless, total hip replacement wounds are subject to considerable movement; elderly patients are commonly restless after surgery, and the chances of self-inoculation are high. A logical approach is to seal the wound after operation in order to prevent self-induced traumatic lesions or contaminations, as well as contamination of superficial minor hematomas in the early postoperative course.

Hair at the site of operation has been incriminated as an important source of contamination during surgery; the time and method of removal of hairs affects bacterial colonization at the site. Razor preparation of the operative site must be regarded as a potential danger for contamination.[149] It was found that the infection rate was 3.1% when routine preparation was within 24 hours before operation—20% if razor preparation exceeded 24 hours prior to operation. When use of a chemical depilatory (Surgex) was employed, it was found that the infection rates were 0.6% compared to 5.6% in which a razor was used to remove hair from the operative site.

Cruse,[49] in a series of 20,105 operations, found that clipping the hair at the surgical site was a useful method that could reduce wound infection from 2.3% (in those operations in which the site had been shaved) to 1.9% (where the hair had been clipped) and 0.9% if *no* attempt had been made to remove the hairs. It

was concluded that the percentile differences were due to trauma caused by the razor, which generated a port of entry for the exogenous bacteria with the injured tissues serving as a culture medium for bacterial growth.

SURGICAL MASKS

Surgical masks, like gowns and draping, have come under scrutiny in other patients to control exogenous bacterial contamination. It has been conclusively demonstrated that the nasopharynx can occasionally serve as a source of wound infections in patients (though not commonly).[151] Masks may decrease the amount of contamination by 90%. Dineen,[54] like others,[74] has shown that cloth masks are not efficient and that bacteria may escape easily through a thin cloth mask. Even though direct transference of organisms from the nasopharynx may be a rare cause of exogenous infection in the operating room, since personnel in the operating room may act as carriers, and since detection of all carriers is impossible, the use of conventional double masks or a vacuum system installed within the mask is a rational discipline for the operating room. The use of an all-investing gown and mask in addition to suction respirators has become increasingly popular after its original advocacy by Charnley.[38] There are a number of these units now available, some carrying their own communication system for teaching purposes. Although these units are initially somewhat cumbersome and complicated to those without adequate training, they have the advantage of being cool despite impermeable material used in their design.[116]

GOWN AND TEXTILE

The conventional permeable textile used for the operating room gown constitutes a serious weakness in the clean–air room theory, since the wound can be contaminated by direct contact and not through the air route.[8,39-41,103]

In a previous study we found that the cloth used for the surgical gown was inadequate.[41] Light microscopy revealed perforations of 1 to 50 μ, large enough to allow particles and bacteria to pass through (Fig. 6-10). This was thought to be particularly significant in operations such as total hip replacement when an instrument so frequently comes in contact with the surgeon's gown, especially at the time of manipulation of the limb and reduction of the

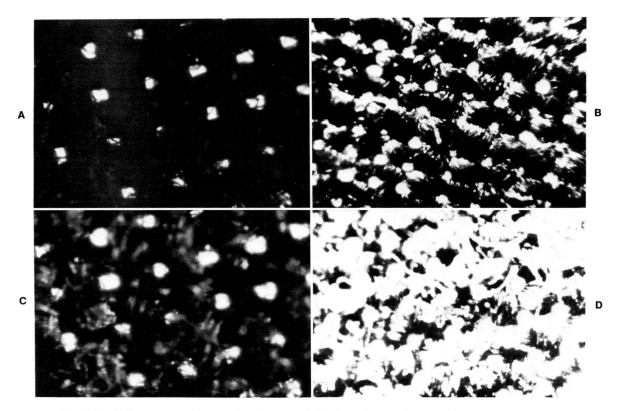

Fig. 6-10. **A,** Gown material (conventional balloon cloth) of excellent quality with tightly woven texture under light microscope. **B,** Same material as **A** but different brand showing less tightness of texture, thus allowing greater penetration. **C,** Prior to laundering conventional balloon cloth gown material. Perforation size ranging from 1 to 50 μ. **D,** Same material as shown in **C** but following heavy laundering procedure. Size of apertures now ranging from 100 to 1,000 μ. (From Eftekhar, N. S.: Clin. Orthop. **96:**188-194, 1973.)

Table 6-1. Colony counts in gown tests

No. of colonies/test	No. of tests	Total colony count
0	110	0
1–3	67	120
4–5	8	34
6–10	13	97
>10	2	47
Totals 0–26	200	298

Table 6-2. Type of organism and frequency

Type	Frequency (%)*
Coagulase-negative staphylococci	75
Coagulase-negative staphylococci + other organisms	12
Staphylococcus aureus	3
Bacillus sp. (aerobic spore-bearer)	5
Gram-positive bacilli (diphtheroid-like organisms)	4
Yeast	1

*Percent of 90 positive gown tests. (From Charnley, J., and Eftekhar, N.: Lancet **1:**72-174, 1969.)

prosthesis. A study was then initiated in which the front of the gown was examined bacteriologically at the end of each operation. The results of these studies are recorded in Tables 6-1 and 6-2, which illustrate the type and frequency of organisms recovered by this method.[41] Based on these findings, special attention was then given to the design of the gown using im-

permeable material. Since heat generated by the body was almost intolerable when impermeable gowns were worn, a ventilation system was installed within the gown that produced a considerably cooler environment. As a precautionary measure, a sterile jacket of finely woven cloth

176

worn over the gown or a plastic apron worn under the gown is a reasonable alternative to an all-investing gown and hood made of impermeable material. In early studies we considered the use of an improved surgical gown and mask in combination with the use of pullout sutures for wound closures as the most important factors in reducing the infection rate to below 1.5%.[40]

CHEMOPROPHYLAXIS IN TOTAL HIP REPLACEMENT
Background of recent interest

A review of surgical experiences and attempts to assess the role of antibiotics in the prevention of bone infections reveals their possible effectiveness in lowering the incidence of postoperative wound infections; this is in sharp contrast with some experiences reporting unsatisfactory results. In some contemporary reviews it has even been suggested that the widespread use of prophylactic antibiotics is often more harmful than beneficial; there are those who have suggested that their use increases the chance of infection. Most of these reports, unfortunately, relate to retrospective studies and involve the use of several antibiotics and various types of surgery. In most cases, the times that antibiotics were administered was not well defined; in some, they had been given only postoperatively.*

Early use of antibiotics (whether used prophylactically or therapeutically) is important for successful infection control and has been well established both clinically and in the laboratory (Burke).[31] The first few hours following contamination seem to be critical;[118] in fact, according to Burke's observations, to be most effective the antimicrobial agent must be present *before* lodgment takes place.[31] The effectiveness of antimicrobial agents is not only largely dependent on the bacterial sensitivity to them, but also on adequate serum and tissue levels of these agents. In many retrospective studies[1,51,130,153] where the prophylactic benefits of antibiotics were debated, the time the antibiotic was given was not known, 'or it was not administered during the critical period as outlined by Burke; in most instances it actually was given as an aftermath to bacterial lodgment.

Studies in favor of the use of systemic anti-

biotics in orthopaedic surgery by Fogelberg and associates,[72] Boyd and associates,[25] Pavel and associates,[132] Ericson and associates,[66] and Welch and associates[161] are worth noting. Unfortunately, these studies may not be regarded as conclusive owing to inadequate numbers of observations, length of follow-up, dissimilarity of clinical situations, or uncontrolled studies in most instances.

Based on experiments and available encouraging results obtained with antibiotics, most surgeons in the United States (better than 87%)[131] are using antibiotic prophylaxis in performing total hip replacement. Whether this trend continues—or the emergence of persistent species and delayed sepsis will abolish the present popularity—awaits future clinical research.

There have been surprisingly few perspective studies with random selection of patients following administration of antibiotics. In the study by Bernard and Cole,[23] the value of short-term prophylaxis in patients with a high risk of infection was demonstrated; their work included potentially contaminated wounds (including abdominal surgery), but the infection rate was lowered from 27% to 8% when chloramphenicol and penicillin were used as prophylactic agents.

Experimental studies by Alexander and associates,[7] Burke[31] and Bowers and associates,[24] as well as Polk and Lopez-Mayor[134] have shown that antibiotics may reduce infection during bacterial contamination of the wound. Wilson and associates[169] concluded that a hematoma can be penetrated by antibiotics if administered up to 4 days after its formation. Others have also shown that antibiotics are capable of penetrating the interstitial fluid (and even clots) if given within bactericidal levels.[15,18,129,157,160]

From the studies of Nelson and his co-workers,[122] it was found that both lincomycin hydrochloride and sodium oxacillin are able to penetrate the area of aspirating tubes within the depth of the wound, and they are found in measurable quantities regardless of the size and depth of the wound. This correlates with previous studies that have shown that antibiotics are capable of penetrating interstitial fluid, wound fluid, and fibrin clots in bactericidal levels.[17,19,95,115] The Nelson studies also substantiate the importance of antibiotics in intravenous intermittent administration over a 48-hour postoperative period.

Nelson and co-workers[122] have shown the

---

*See references 16, 22, 33, 51, 96, 108, 110, 130, 135, 142-144, and 152-154.

ability of antibiotics to penetrate a hematoma and thereby play an important role in preventing infection during the first few days following surgery. The extent of penetration and the efficacy of antibiotics in hematomas, wound fluids, and bones depends on the type of antibiotic and the mode of its administration.

The selection of an antibiotic must be based on three factors:

1. Organism susceptibility in the environment (the hospital)
2. Ability to affect the broadest spectrum of bacteria
3. Its bactericidal and bacteriostatic properties

Burke[31] has demonstrated that the most propitious time to administer intravenous antibacterial agents is 3 to 4 hours before bacterial lodgment has occurred.

One of the criticisms against the widespread use of antibiotics has been the possibility of change in the structure of the bacterial population responsible for nosocomial infections and the emergence of virulent bacterial species that had previously been considered nonpathogenic.[2,94] Furthermore, the possibility of toxicity and sensitivity produced by these agents increases potential danger to the patient.[113]

Altemeier[10] has studied and criticized the widespread use of antibiotics as causing changes in the patterns of infecting organisms. These changes include:

1. Increased incidence of gram-negative infections
2. Superimposed infections developing during use of antibiotics
3. Increased incidence of gram-negative infections by bacteria of low virulence
4. Mixed bacterial infections
5. Infections by *Candida albicans*
6. Increasing numbers of infections from L-forms and other atypical bacterial forms (The significance of L-forms in pathogenesis of infection is not fully understood.[113])

Systemic use of antibiotics

Prophylactic use of antibiotics in efforts to prevent infection has found a definite indication in clinical situations: (1) where potential and actual incidence of infection is of such a magnitude that their use is warranted and (2) the agent used is neither toxic nor allergenic and can be used in usual dosage and routes.

Systemic use of antibiotic prophylaxis is still controversial in general surgical practice, as well as in all orthopaedic procedures. As yet, there is no objective scientific evidence for the absolute usefulness of their routine prophylactic use. With increasing popularity the use of antibiotic prophylactic agents is now well accepted in "high-risk" operations such as total hip replacement. A properly designed prospective double-blind study with maximum controlled variables and follow-up is needed to identify the merits of this approach.

We feel it is beneficial and must be used; it is a rational approach if administered in the perioperative period—the so-called danger period—and is especially necessary when absolute control of the environment is not feasible. Transient bacteremia is not uncommon, and further endogenous sources of infection are not always obvious in the patient. Therefore the patient should be given extra protection by "umbrella" antibiotics for 12 hours before surgery, during surgery, and for 5 days after surgery. This view is especially supported by the fact that hematogenous seeding of organisms is a real possibility, especially in patients with rheumatoid arthritis.

The use of antibiotics is prophylactically indicated where there is danger of infection, provided that the agent is appropriate for the particular type of potential infection and when the operation is of severe magnitude. Particularly where a completely sterile environment or a sterile wound cannot be maintained, these drugs must be given in adequate doses prior to the time of potential contamination. The choice of a specific antibiotic for prophylaxis must be determined by prevalence of the organism in a given institution based on periodic surveillance of sensitivity patterns. For example, prior to 1972, at our institution most staphylococci (over 85%) were sensitive to penicillin. Penicillin was obviously the prophylactic drug of choice. However, subsequent emergence of more than 65% penicillin-resistant staphylococci necessitated the logical change of the prophylactic drug to sodium oxacillin and ampicillin. The boxed material represents a suggested preoperative, operative, and postoperative regimen for routine prophylaxis by common antibiotics.

Local application by irrigation

There is much evidence to support the efficacy of systemic antibiotic administration. How-

Suggested preoperative antibiotic regimen

Penicillin
    600 units IM, 6 PM, h.s., 6 AM
Ampicillin/oxacillin
    500 mg. ampicillin IM, 6 PM, h.s., 6 AM
    500 mg. oxacillin IM, 6 PM, h.s., 6 AM
Tetracycline
    100 mg. IM, 6 PM, h.s., 6 AM
Cephalosporins
    500 mg. cefazolin, IM, 6 PM, h.s., 6 AM
Lincomycin
    600 mg. IM, 6 PM, h.s., 6 AM

Suggested intraoperative antibiotic regimen

Penicillin
    1 million units IV during surgery
Oxacillin
    1 gm. IV push, 1 gm. IV during surgery
Tetracycline
    100 mg. IV during surgery
Cephalosporins
    1 gm. IV push, 1 gm. IV during surgery
Lincomycin
    1,200 mg. IV during surgery

Suggested postoperative antibiotic regimen

Penicillin
    1 million units/1,000 ml. IV fluids q.6h., or penicillin G 600,000 units IM q.6h. for 5 days
Ampicillin/oxacilin
    Oxacillin 500 mg. IV or by mouth q.6h. for 5 days and ampicillin 500 mg. IV or by mouth q.6h. for 5 days
Tetracycline
    100 mg. IV or 250 mg. by mouth q.6h. for 5 days
Cephalosporins
    Cephalothin 1 gm. IV q.4h. or cephalexin 500 mg. by mouth q.6h. for 5 days
Lincomycin
    600 mg. IM b.i.d. or 500 mg. by mouth q.6h. for 5 days

ever, none of the clinical studies has statistical data supporting the local usefulness of these agents, despite experimental work supporting their effectiveness.* It is perhaps unlikely that such agents permeate the tissue or are more effective than washing the wound with physiological solutions, as they are in contact with the wound for only a very short period. An appropriate level of antibiotics administered intraoperatively and thoroughly penetrating the tissue seems a more effective approach.[134] For local use of antibiotics in the past, penicillin G was widely used. In recent years, however, antibiotics that give a broader spectrum bacteria coverage have become more popular. Spraying the wound during surgery with a mixture of neomycin, bacitracin, and polymixin has been suggested to reduce the incidence of staphylococcal infection; the use of this method in neurosurgery was followed by a reduction of major infections.[73] Lazansky[104] and Müller[119] were early advocates for using local antibiotics in total hip replacement. However, further experience is required to evaluate the place for local prophylactic antibiotic solutions and to compare their effectiveness with electrolyte solutions in total hip replacement.

Any useful prophylactic antibiotic must combat *Staphylococcus aureus,* the most common cause of orthopaedic wound infections. In operations of long duration, with considerably deep incisions and a high frequency of deeply seated hematomas from the bone, a considerable concentration of antibiotics in the wound might provide an additional margin of safety to the patient.

The use of antibiotic-impregnated cement

A recent and very important development in the field of infection prevention is the use of antibiotics mixed with cement at the time of insertion. In early studies of wound infection we failed to produce data to show the efficacy of antibiotics used as a depot of 1 gm. penicillin and 1 gm. streptomycin pulverized into the acetabulum and femur just prior to cement insertion.[40] The concept of antibiotic-impregnated cement originated in Germany, where Buchholz[29] advocated the use of a gentamicin-Palacos combination when revising infected previous total hip operations. A success rate of 50% to 70% was reported by this method. At the present

---

*See references 47, 78, 110, 145, and 158.

179

time, however, there is no clinical evidence to substantiate the prophylactic role of antibiotic-impregnated cement in total hip arthroplasty. A number of studies so far have attempted to identify its individual role in inhibition of bacterial growth and possible alterations in the mechanical properties of such mixtures.[88,98,99,111,159]

It has been shown that acrylic cement without antibiotics had no bacteriostatic effect on *Staphylococcus aureus, Escherichia coli,* and *Pseudomonas.* Hessert and Ruchdeschel[88] showed that ampicillin and gentamicin added to methyl methacrylate were released in effective quantities, but tetracycline lost its antibacterial properties when added to methyl methacrylate cement. Also, these investigators showed that acrylic cement had no bacteriocidal or bacteriostatic action against *Staphylococcus aureus, Bacillus cereus, Escherichia coli,* and *Pseudomonas.* Marks and co-workers[111] studies clearly demonstrated that oxacillin, gentamicin, and cefazolin are stable in both types of cement (Simplex or Palacos) and diffuse from the cement in an active form over a prolonged period of time. Oxacillin, cefazolin, and gentamicin were stable in acrylic cement and were released in a microbiologically active form. The three antibiotics diffused from the Palacos in larger amounts daily and for a significantly longer time than from the Simplex. This indicates that the type of cement used in combination with antibiotics is very important. Palacos may be preferred because of its larger pore size in comparison with Simplex as demonstrated by scanning electron microscopy.

Bacteriostatic concentrations of oxacillin in wound hematomas were measured for 14 days after implantation of an oxacillin-Simplex combination in dogs. A high bacteriocidal concentration of antibiotics was measured in the surrounding bone for 21 days after implantation, the highest level ($127 \ \mu$g./g.) observed 24 hours after implantation. It decreased over the 3-week experimental period but continued to be bacteriocidal up to $52 \ \mu$g./gm. of bone. In a separate study by Kolczun and co-workers[98,99] following infusion of 2 gm. oxacillin, concentration was $7.66 \ \mu$g./gm.; therefore this study indicates that concentrations of antibiotics observed in surrounding bone are many times greater than the level that can be achieved by intravenous infusions.

Possible alterations of the mechanical proper-

ties of cement when mixed with antibiotics have been studied. These tests have shown that the addition to cement of powdered oxacillin, cefazolin, or gentamicin had no significant influence on the compressive or tensile strength —either at the time of mixture or after 40 days of waterbath treatment. However, adding aqueous solutions of antibiotics to acrylic cement not only interfered with the early prepolymerizing process during mixing but also resulted in a mechanically weakened cement. It was demonstrated that the alteration is due to the water and not the antibiotic itself.

One of the objections to using an antibiotic-cement combination is the possibility of serious complications from an allergic reaction to these materials, which may eventually necessitate removal of the entire combination of the cement and antibiotics with obvious consequences. These aspects have not been studied or reported at the present time.

It may be summarized that at the present time there is no objective evidence to support reduction of the rate of infection in total hip replacements by combining antibiotics with cement. Extensive clinical studies are needed to evaluate the merits and disadvantages of this procedure.

ANTIBIOTIC PROPHYLAXIS VS. HEMATOGENOUS INFECTIONS

An increasing number of observations are being made that indicate that hematogenous seeding of implants does exist. This can only occasionally be fully proved by identifying the same organism in the "source," the blood, and in the hip. Nevertheless, a sudden onset of pain in a previously pain-free hip concurrent with infection elsewhere in the body is highly suggestive of hematogenous infection. Prophylaxis on a long-term basis therefore is justifiable in a "danger situation" when a severe bacteremia may occur. "Danger situations" are those where substantial manipulation or trauma of areas with bacterial flora may cause bacteremia or where an obvious infected area of the body may release a large number of bacteria into the bloodstream. The choice of antibiotics is dependent on the particular lesion or flora. Most common offending bacteria of the anatomical region under treatment must be combatted. Because of the prevalence of *Staphylococcus aureus* in hematogenous infections, an antistaphylococcal antibiotic such as oxacillin or preferably cephalothin administered intravenously is justifiable in an emergency situation until the organism from the "remote source" is identified. Oral antibiotics maintain a good blood level and may be administered once the type of organism and sensitivity pattern are established.

THE CONTROVERSY OF CLEAN AIR AND ANTIBIOTICS IN TOTAL HIP REPLACEMENT

The effectiveness of clean air or antibiotics in preventing infection in total hip surgery has been the most controversial issue in recent years.[43,61,102] There are no data of significance to support either as a preferable means of prophylaxis, and the controversy is compounded by the emotionalism of surgeons advocating either method based on the following:

1. Multifactorial nature of infection
2. Definition of clinical infection and clean air in the operating room
3. Inadequate statistical interpretation of results
4. Development of late wound infections
5. Use of antibiotics for prophylaxis in combination with clean-air rooms
6. Introduction of protective measures in the operating room such as the body exhaust system, special masks, and gowns

The debate is exacerbated by the fact that the true incidence of infection following total hip replacement in general practice in a conventional operating room remains unknown.

The rationale for using a clean-air room and antibiotics has been discussed previously. The roles of a massive foreign body and the heat of polymerizing cement have been emphasized. How the use of plastic, mobility of the artificial joint, and the large dead space may contribute to the survival of organisms were also discussed. It was emphasized that unless germ-free clean air can be maintained in the vicinity of the wound, contamination during surgery is inevitable. Even then, the patient's own contamination sources, for which less extrinsic control is available, have not been taken into account, for example, skin, blood, and previous surgery. In this context, patients with rheumatoid disease are particularly prone to endogenous contamination because of the nature of their arthritis.[97]

The dilemma of statistics and their interpretation

Perhaps the greatest difficulty in judging the efficacy of antibiotics or clean air lies in the evaluation of statistics: the size of the sample and the complexity of the definition of wound infection—especially in view of late-appearing infections in this type of surgery. Lidwell and associates[105] and others[106] state that in order to demonstrate a significant fall of the infection rate (from 3% to 1.5%), studies of 800 operations in a control group and 800 operations in an experimental group would be required; to prove the significance of one factor for a rate below 1.5%, a sample of 5,000 operations of precisely the same type is essential. As a practical demonstration, a series of 1,750 operations grouped in blocks of 100 were studied. The rate of infection in these blocks varied from 0.0% (ninth block)

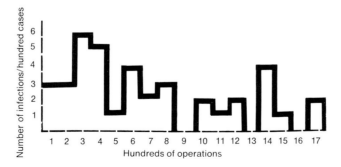

Fig. 6-11. Number of infections in 1,700 cases demonstrated in contiguous block of 100 cases. It is clearly demonstrated that while a greater number of infections have occurred in blocks on second and third 100 cases, as well as 14, no infection occurred during the ninth, thirteenth, or sixteenth block. It is essential to recognize this statistical fact in reporting incidence of infection in small series of cases. (Modified from Charnley, J., and Eftekhar, N.: Br. J. Surg. **56:**641-649, 1969.)

181

to 6% (third block) (Fig. 6-11). There were no obvious reasons to explain these differences. These findings make it imperative for us not to accept statistics from fewer than 500 samples to determine an infection rate of less than 3%.

Late appearance of infection

Interpretation of the rate of infection in total hip replacement is made especially difficult by the high incidence of infection occurring months after surgery. Of the five infections that appeared in the first 1,500 operations at the New York Orthopaedic Hospital, one manifested itself in less than 3 months, the other in 14 months, and the third at 18 months after surgery. The remaining two infections appeared 4 years following implantation of the prosthesis. Because of late-appearing infection, therefore, figures from an institutional sample were not validated until several years later.[39,40]

Results of a questionnaire

To identify the scope of the problem and document it statistically, the author distributed a questionnaire to members of The Hip Society (American) requesting the following:
1. Number of total hip procedures performed
2. Number of operations with a minimum of 1 year follow-up
3. Respective rate of infection
4. Use of systemic or local antibiotics
5. Opinions on the necessity of a clean-air room in total hip replacement procedures

The selection of only The Hip Society members was thought theoretically objectionable, but practical, since most surgeons were intimately involved with their cases and their special interest in hip surgery documentation made follow-up possible. It was further thought that a cooperative study would render the risk of introducing error: (1) because of the dissimilarity of samples; (2) unrecorded factors in retrospective studies might have occurred; and (3) the experiences of the community orthopaedic surgeon could not have been included.

Of the 25 members who responded to the questionnaire, only 18 institutions' statistics qualified for inclusion. The results were arbitrarily divided into three categories: A, B, and C. (See Tables 6-3 to 6-5.)

Category A. This category included seven institutions where the number of operations performed ranged between 100 and 500. The rate of infection ranged from 0.5% to 5%, with a minimum of 1-year follow-up and had no statistical significance. The following trends were observed in this group: (1) a much greater rate of infection was encountered in the first 100 operations than in the subsequent 300 or 400; (2) a higher rate of infection was noted in patients whose surgeons had performed fewer than 200 operations; and (3) the highest rate of infection—5.1%—was noted in 147 operations at an institution that used neither clean air nor antibiotics and felt that a clean-air room was not necessary. Two of the seven institutions in this category used clean-air rooms. Six of the seven used systemic antibiotics, and five of the seven used local antibiotics. It is interesting to note that the institutions with the highest rate of infection represented the least experience by number of operations and rarely used clean air and/or antibiotics. This group also expressed the most vehement views both for and against the

Table 6-3. Category A: 100 to 500 hip operations

Institution	I. Total hip procedures	II. Minimal 1-yr. follow-up	Number of infections		Clean air	Antibiotics		Clean air essential?
			In I	In II		Systemic	Local	
A	456	266	5	2	No	Yes	Yes	No
B	325	342	3	3	Yes	Yes	Yes	Yes
C	350	250	1	1	No	Yes	Yes	No
D	205	150	3	3	No	Yes	Yes	No
E	147	116	7	6	No	No	No	No
F	100	55	2	1	Yes	Yes	Yes	Yes
G	100	60	1	1	No	Yes	No	Yes
Totals 7	1,783	1,239	22	17	Yes (2) No (5)	Yes (6) No (1)	Yes (5) No (2)	Yes (3) No (4)

use of a clean-air room as essential in total hip replacement procedures. Three institutions were in favor of the clean-air room and four were against it.

Category B. Four institutions with from 600 to 900 operations were grouped in this category. The infection rate was 0.6% to 1.6%. Without any emphasis on statistical significance, this group represented some interesting features.

1. The rate of infection was acceptable, under 2%.
2. Two of the institutions used a clean-air room, one wished to obtain a clean-air room, and the fourth used ultraviolet light.
3. All but one used systemic antibiotics, and all four used local antibiotics.

Category C. This category included six institutions and was the most important from a statistical standpoint.

All institutions were located in the United States, with the exception of one, data from which were obtained from a recent publication.[39] The number of infections in this category ranged from 0.3% for institution P to 2.3% for institution Q. The rates of infection for institutions L and Q are now adjusted to 0.5% and 1.4%, respectively. The former claims that lack of a clean-air room in the first 188 operations was responsible for the 7% rate of infection, and the latter relates that the absence of systemic antibiotics in their first 147 operations led to the incidence of 4.7%.

To evaluate the influence of clean air on sepsis, category C could conveniently be divided into two groups: users and nonusers of clean-air rooms. It is clearly demonstrated that there is no difference in infection rates between the users and nonusers of clean-air rooms. It must be noted that all three institutions without a clean-air room used local and systemic antibiotics.

All three improved their operating room con-

Table 6-4. Category B: 500 to 1,000 hip operations

Institution	I. Total hip procedures	II. Minimal 1-yr. follow-up	Number of infections		Clean air	Antibiotics		Clean air essential?
			In I	In II		Systemic	Local	
H	900	700	6	4	Yes	Yes	Yes	Yes
I	700	450	2	2	Yes	No	Yes	Questionable
J	639	483	5	5	No	Yes	Yes	No
K*	600	500	8	8	No	Yes	Yes	No
Totals 4	2,839	2,133	21	19	Yes (2) No (2)	Yes (3) No (1)	Yes (4) No (0)	Yes (1) No (2) Questionable (1)

*Institution K uses ultraviolet light.

Table 6-5. Category C: over 1,000 hip operations

Institution	I. Total hip procedures	II. Minimal 1-yr. follow-up	Number of infections		Clean air	Antibiotics		Clean air essential?
			In I	In II		Systemic	Local	
L*	6,800	5,800		85	Yes	No	No	Yes
M	5,000	2,012		14	No	Yes	Yes	No
N	1,974	1,200	8	6	Yes	Yes	Yes	Yes
O	1,400	1,100	14	11	Yes	Yes	No	No
P	1,100	800	4	3	No	Yes	Yes	Yes
Q	1,007	652	15	14	No	Yes	Yes	No
Totals 6	17,281	11,564	41	133	Yes (3) No (3)	Yes (5) No (1)	Yes (4) No (2)	Yes (3) No (3)

*Institution not in the United States. Figures represented taken from a recent publication.[39]

ditions by eliminating unnecessary traffic, developing higher standards of technique, and upgrading their ventilating system when a total hip replacement program was instituted at their hospitals. It must be noted that two of the three users of a clean-air room also used prophylactic antibiotics, one locally, the other systematically.

Only institution L, with the most numerous operating experience in the world, continues to operate without antibiotics. Paradoxically, two of three nonusers of a clean-air room (that is, five of the six institutions performing the greatest number of hip replacement operations) now use a clean-air room for total hip replacement operations, despite their low infection rate.

To summarize, these cooperative statistical data, based on the experiences of seventeen major training institutions and 21,903 total hip arthroplasties, was nonconclusive in proving the advantages of clean air over antibiotics or vice versa. Eight of the seventeen institutions used a special clean-air room, and nine did not; fourteen used systemic antibiotics, and three did not; eleven used local antibiotic irrigations, and six did not; nine felt a special clean-air room was essential, and eight felt it was not.

It is apparent that with the advent of total hip arthroplasty, orthopaedic surgeons have become more aware of the relationship between environmental control and wound infection. Credit belongs to Charnley for his contributions in this area.

It is evident from available data that acrylic cement has not contributed to increasing the infection rate in orthopaedic surgery; this is apparent from the comments of surgeons participating in this study. It is also comforting to know that special precautions were being taken in the operating room where total hip replacement surgery was performed.

If the figures of the six institutions that performed more than 1,000 total hip replacements can be taken as evidence, the infection rate was lower than 1% 1 year following surgery; perhaps it would not have been more than 4% if a longer follow-up study were done. There was no difference in the infection rate between users and nonusers of clean-air rooms; all nonusers, however, routinely used systemic and local antibiotics. The significance of this in relation to late-appearing infections could not be determined from available data. The size of the sample is the most significant factor in interpreting the incidence of wound infection—keeping in mind that only 40% to 50% of the total number of infections appeared within 1 year.[39,40,61]

The views expressed in the questionnaire by members of The Hip Society led to the conclusion that the clean-air room was considered a "rational discipline"—and perhaps "essential" where it is difficult to control traffic in the operating room, especially in teaching institutions. It was felt, however, that further clinical investigation would be necessary to prove the absolute necessity of a clean air room; similar views were expressed with regard to the use of local and systemic prophylactic antibiotics.

ACKNOWLEDGMENTS

The author wishes to thank the members of The Hip Society for their cooperation in this survey, which provided the data* for this section: Drs. Harlan Amstutz, Otto E. Aufranc, William H. Bickel, Walter P. Blount, Mark B. Coventry, Charles M. Everts, Albert B. Ferguson, Jr., William H. Harris, John J. Hinchey, William W. Howe, Jr., Floyd H. Jergesen, Richard C. Johnston, Joe W. King, Mark G. Lazansky, Irwin S. Leinbach, J. Vernon Luck, E. M. Lunceford, Jr., Donald E. McCollum, Henry J. Mankin, William R. Murray, Augusto Sarmiento, Frank E. Stinchfield, Fredrick R. Thompson, Marshall R. Urist, and Phillip D. Wilson, Jr.

SUMMARY OF ESSENTIALS

- Although listerism abolished fulminating and epidemic hospital sepsis, such as clostridial infections, infections caused by mildly pathogenic organisms (such as staphylococci) have remained common.
- Concerning the problem of infection control, three factors are to be considered: (1) the number of infecting organisms at the site of the wound; (2) the virulence of the organisms; and (3) the chance association of bacteria with an area of sufficiently reduced resistance.
- A localized or systemic reduction in host resistance is at least as important as bacterial contamination. Consequently, any effort aimed at the reduction of postoperative infection must concentrate on host responses as well as reducing bacterial contamination, recognizing that almost any bacteria may become pathogenic under certain sets of circumstances. Thus no longer can one identify a harmless saprophyte merely by its morphological characteristics.
- Undoubtedly, early experiences have suggested

---

*Data were recently updated to include 38,000 operations without any significant alteration in the results or conclusions presented in this chapter.

that a high incidence of wound infection may be expected when performing total hip replacements if extra precautionary measures are not exercised in ordinary operating rooms.

■ In view of the lack of a clear definition and multifactorial elements of wound infection, methods of prevention are not well defined. However, a sound prophylaxis must be directed toward the patient's sources of contamination, environmental sources of contamination, and, as well, contamination of the wound by the surgical team.

■ Among other things, old age, obesity, diabetes, poor state of nutrition, and steroid therapy increase the chances of infection. Above all, the urinary tract, pulmonary lesions, silent sources of infection (especially skin), must be examined and treated prior to total hip replacement. In this regard, a history of previous infection in the hip joint must be verified and evaluated prior to contemplated surgery.

■ Patients with an elevated sedimentation rate of over 40 mm./hr., a history of previous drainage, or radiological changes suggestive of infection must be considered with caution for selection for total hip replacement in order to minimize infection problems.

■ At surgery, the presence of hypertrophic granuloma, necrotic debris, or purulent fluid, especially at the site of previous operations, coupled with a positive Gram's stain and evidence of acute inflammatory cells must be regarded as important in terminating an operation without replacement, with the hope of eradicating infection prior to replacement surgery at a later date.

■ Special emphasis should be placed on prevention of infection in the surgical environment, which includes factors such as gowns, masks, and gloves, as well as the surgical facilities.

■ A substantial reduction of air contamination is achieved by the use of clean-air enclosure, and by prohibiting entry of unnecessary personnel within the vicinity of the surgical wound. The chance that the team includes a "dangerous disperser" increases the risk of additional contamination. Since "carriers" and "dispersers" are not consistent and elimination of all carriers from the environment is not possible, elimination of unnecessary personnel from the surgical environment is a good discipline.

■ Because bacteria are generated by, and are proportional to, the number of personnel within the room, bacteria-containing particles may be kept to a minimum by the use of a clean-air enclosure. The volume of filtered air entering the enclosure should be commensurate with the number of persons present and the rate of their particle emission.

■ The surgical environment should provide a positive unidirectional movement of air in a predetermined direction, disregarding the laminar nature of the flow because of turbulence resulting from the air striking stationary objects.

■ Even without unduly emphasizing air cleanliness, the use of a surgical enclosure will improve discipline in the operating room traffic pattern. This, of course, is critical in eliminating unnecessary uncontrollable traffic within teaching institutions.

■ In the design of operating rooms, a logical plan would be to install enclosures with positive unidirectional (vertical or horizontal) airflow that is nonlaminar but slightly turbulent, with collapsible (removable) walls that could accommodate equipment within the room.

■ Filtration of air particles (of less than 1 to 2 μ) is not necessary because smaller particles do not appear to carry organisms, and bacteria are not suspended in the air by themselves.

■ A substantial reduction of air contamination in the operating room may also be achieved by the use of ultraviolet lights. However, the use of an enclosure itself seems to be a superior method because of the insulating character of the enclosure.

■ As a fundamental protective measure in performing total hip replacement, special attention to the textile and design of the gown is necessary to eliminate personnel-generated bacteria permeating the gown and contacting the instruments used in total hip arthroplasty.

■ A significant reduction of bacterial contamination via this route may be achieved by an all-investing hood and gown with a ventilation system incorporated within the gown. A sterile jacket of finely woven cloth worn over the gown or plastic apron worn under the gown are reasonable alternatives to an all-investing gown and hood made of impermeable material.

■ The use of chemoprophylaxis in total hip replacement has become a controversial issue, but increasing numbers of surgeons performing these operations are using systemic and/or local antibiotics. Experimental and clinical data are now available and endorse the usefulness of these agents, especially during the "danger period" perioperatively. The rationale for use of systemic antibiotics and prophylactic agents is that most wounds, despite precautions, may become contaminated by the end of a long operative procedure involving many manipulative procedures.

■ Transient bacteremia is not uncommon and hematogenous seeding of organisms in a low-resistant patient is a real possibility. The choice of the specific antibiotics must be based on prevalence of organisms in a given institution, and the type of organism commonly found in infected total hip replacements.

■ A combination of antibiotics effective against both gram-negative and gram-positive organisms should

185

be selected. It should affect the broadest spectrum of bacteria, bactericidally and bacteriostatically. It has been suggested that the most propitious time to administer antibacterial agents is 3 to 4 hours before bacterial lodgment occurs.

■ Widespread use of antibiotics has been criticized for causing changes in the pattern of infecting organisms, including increased incidence of gram-negative infections; superimposed infections developing during antibiotic use; increased incidence of gram-negative infections by bacteria of low virulence; mixed bacterial infections; infections by *Candida albicans;* and increasing numbers of infections from L-forms and other atypical bacterial forms.

■ Similar to the systemic use of antibiotics, their local use has also remained controversial. It is suggested that they may be no more effective than balanced electrolyte solutions used for mechanical irrigation and removal of debris from the wound; proof of their usefulness must await the conclusion of further clinical studies.

■ A recent and important development is the use of antibiotic-impregnated cement. Again, however, no hard data are available to substantiate their role. A number of studies thus far conducted have indicated that the effective bactericidal and bacteriostatic properties of antibiotics do not change the mechanical properties of cement (antibiotics used in powder form). Possible allergic reactions to such a mixture may be their greatest and most serious drawback, thereby generating criticism of this method of prophylaxis.

■ At the present time, controversy over the use of clean air and antibiotics is based on the multifactorial nature of infections; definition of clinical infection; clean air in an operating room; inadequate statistical interpretation of the results, development of late wound infections; the use of antibiotics for prophylaxis in combination with clean-air rooms; and the introduction of protective measures in the operating room (in addition to clean air and antibiotics) such as the body exhaust system, special masks, and gowns.

■ While the debate continues, conclusions were derived from cooperative statistical studies to identify the scope of the problem and document the present state of the art. The experiences of 17 major training institutions and 21,903 total hip arthroplasties indicated no conclusive evidence as to the advantages of clean air over antibiotics or vice versa.

■ It was apparent that with the advent of total hip arthroplasty, orthopaedic surgeons would be using some form of environmental control in their operating room in addition to systemic and/or local antibiotics. *Surgeons using neither antibiotics nor clean-air rooms are encountering a much higher rate of infection.* While at the present time further well-controlled clinical investigations are necessary to prove the absolute necessity of clean-air rooms and antibiotics, their use is obviously essential in performing total hip arthroplasty.

■ Prevention of infection is a multifaceted and complex problem. A germ-free human is not healthy; a germ-free patient is not possible. No single technique, prophylaxis measure, or germicide alone can produce an "infection-free" situation. Attention to a countless number of details is necessary for a sure path toward the best!

REFERENCES

1. Ad Hoc Committee of the Committee on Trauma, Division of Medical Sciences, National Academy of Sciences–National Research Council: Postoperative wound infection; the influences of ultraviolet irradiation on the operating time and influence of various other factors, Ann. Surg. **160**(2)(Suppl.): 1-192, 1964.
2. Adler, J. L., Burke, J. P., and Finland, M.: Infection and antibiotic usage at Boston City Hospital, January, 1970, Arch. Intern. Med. **127:**460-465, 1971.
3. Aglietti, P., Salvati, E. A., Wilson, P. D., Jr., and Kutner, L. J.: Effect of a surgical horizontal unidirectional filtered air flow unit on wound bacterial contamination and wound healing, Clin. Orthop. **101:**99-104, 1974.
4. Alexander, J. W., and Good, R. A.: Immunobiology for surgeons, Philadelphia, 1970, W. B. Saunders Co.
5. Alexander, J. W., and Meakins, J. L.: Natural defense mechanism in clinical sepsis, J. Surg. Res. **11:**148-61, 1971.
6. Alexander, J. W., Kaplan, J. Z., and Altemeier, W. A.: Role of suture materials in the development of wound infections, Ann. Surg. **165:**192-199, 1967.
7. Alexander, J. W., Sykes, N. S., Mitchell, M. M., and Fisher, M. W.: Concentration of selected intravenously administered antibiotics in experimental surgical wounds, J. Trauma **13:**423-34, 1973.
8. Alford, D. J., Ritter, M. A., French, M. L. V., and Hart, J. B.: The operating room gown as a barrier to bacterial shedding, Am. J. Surg. **125:**589-591, 1973.
9. Allen, B. L., Jr., Higgins, M. V., and Goldner, J. L.: Current status of ultraviolet radiation in operating room. In The Hip Society: Proceedings of the second open scientific meeting of The Hip Society, St. Louis, 1974, The C. V. Mosby Co., pp. 289-300.
10. Altemeier, W. A.: The significance of infection in trauma, Bull. Am. Coll. Surg. pp. 7-16, February, 1972.

11. Amstutz, H. C.: Treatment of sepsis in total hip replacement. In American Academy of Orthopaedic Surgeons: Instructional course lectures, vol. 23, St. Louis, 1974, The C. V. Mosby Co., p. 248.

12. Amstutz, H. C.: High velocity directional air flow systems (HVDAFS). Status of "clean air rooms," West. J. Med. **122**(2):154-155, 1975.

13. Amstutz, H. C., Irvine, R. D., and Johnson, B. L., Jr.: The relationship of genitourinary urinary tract procedures and deep sepsis after total hip replacements, Surg. Gynecol. Obstet. **139**(5):701-706, 1974.

14. Austin, P. R.: Design and operation of clean rooms, ed. 1, Detroit, Detroit Business News Publishing Co.

15. Baker, G., and Hung, T. K.: Penicillin concentration in experimental wounds, Am. J. Surg. **115**:531-534, 1968.

16. Barnes, J., Pace, W. G., Trump, D. S., and Ellison, E. H.: Prophylactic postoperative antibiotics, Arch. Surg. **79**:190-196, 1959.

17. Barza, M., and Weinstein, L. Penetration of antibiotics into fibrin loci in vivo, I. J. Infect. Dis. **129**:59-65, 1974.

18. Barza, M., Brusch, J., Bergeron, M. G., and Weinstein, L.: Penetration of antibiotics into fibrin loci in vivo. II, J. Infect. Dis. **129**:66-72, 1974.

19. Barza, M., Brusch, J., Bergeron, M. G. and Weinstein, L.: Penetration of antibiotics into fibrin loci in vivo. III, J. Infect. Dis. **129**:73-78, 1974.

20. Benner, E. J.: The use and abuse of antibiotics—1967, J. Bone Joint Surg. **49A**:977-988, 1967.

21. Bernard, H. R.: The effect of scrub time on hand antisepsis using providone-iodine surgical scrub for 3-, 5-, 10-minute scrubs. In Polk, H. C., and Ehrenkranz, N. J., editors: Therapeutic advances and new clinical implications: medical and surgical antisepsis with betadine microbicides, Norwalk, Conn., 1972, Purdue Frederick Co., pp. 95-97.

22. Bernard, H. R., and Cole, W. R.: The prophylaxis of surgical infection: the effect of prophylactic drugs on the incidence of infection following potentially contaminated operations, Surgery **58**:151-7, 1964.

23. Bernard, H. R., Cole, W. R., and Gravens, D. L.: Reduction of iatrogenic bacterial contamination in operating rooms, Ann. Surg. **165**:609-613, 1967.

24. Bowers, W. H., Wilson, F. C., and Greene, W. B.: Antibiotic prophylaxis in experimental bone infections, J. Bone Joint Surg. **55A**:795-807, 1973.

25. Boyd, R. J., Burk, J. F., and Colton, T.: A double-blind clinical trial of prophylactic antibiotics in hip fractures, J. Bone Joint Surg. **55A**:1251-1258, 1973.

26. Brady, L. P., Enneking, W. F., and Franco, J. A.: The effect of operating room environment on the infection rate after Charnley low-friction total hip replacement, J. Bone Joint Surg. **57A**:80-83, 1975.

27. Buchberg, H.: Management of the air environment of operating rooms. In American Academy of Orthopaedic Surgeons: Instructional Course Lectures, vol. 23, St. Louis, 1974, The C. V. Mosby Co., pp. 244-245.

28. Buchberg, H., Amstutz, H. C., Wright, J. D., and Lodgwig, R. M.: Evaluation and optimum use of directed horizontal filtered air flow for surgeries, Clin. Orthop. **111**:151-155, 1975.

29. Buchholz, H. W., and Siegel, A.: Erfahrungen mit refobacin Palacos in der Prosthesenchirurgie Actuel, Traumatol. **3**:233-239, 1973.

30. Burke, J. E.: Identification of the sources of staphylococci contaminating the surgical wound during operation, Ann. Surg. **158**:898-904, 1963.

31. Burke, J. F.: The effective period of preventive antibiotic action in experimental incisions and dermal lesions, Surgery **50**:161-168, 1961.

32. Burke, J. F.: Factors predisposing to infection in surgical patients. In Maibach, G., editor: Skin bacteria and their role in infection, New York, 1965, McGraw-Hill Book Co. pp. 143-156.

33. Busch, H., and Lane, M.: Chemotherapy, ed. 1, Chicago, 1967, Year Book Medical Publishers, Inc.

34. Butterfield, W. C.: Puncture wounds in surgical gloves, Conn. Med. J. **34**:180-181, 1970.

35. Cardenal, F. A., and Aufranc, O. E.: Incidence of wound infection in hip surgery, J. Bone Joint Surg. **44A**:1266, 1962.

36. Carpendale, M. T., and Sereda, W.: The role of the percutaneous suture in surgical wound infection, Surgery **58**:672-677, 1965.

37. Charnley, J.: A sterile air operating theater enclosure, Br. J. Surg. **51**:195-202, 1964.

38. Charnley, J.: Instructions for using the Charnley ventilated operating gown and mask. Internal Publication No. 22 Center for Hip Surgery, Wrightington, England, 1969.

39. Charnley, J.: Postoperative infection after total hip replacement with special reference to air contamination in the operating room, Clin. Orthop. **87**:167-87, September, 1972.

40. Charnley, J., and Eftekhar, N.: Postoperative infection in total prosthetic replacement arthroplasty of the hip-joint, with special reference to the bacterial content of the air of the operating room, Br. J. Surg. **56**:641-649, September, 1969.

41. Charnley, J., and Eftekhar, N.: Penetration of

gown material by organisms from the surgeon's body, Lancet **1:**172-174, 1969.

42. Cole, W. R., and Bernard, H. R.: Inadequacies of present methods of surgical skin preparation, Arch. Surg. **89:**215-222, 1964.

43. Committee on operating room environment: Special air systems for operating rooms, Bull. Am. Coll. Surg. **57:**18, May, 1972.

44. Committee on operating room environment of American College of Surgeons: Definition of surgical microbiologic clean air, Bull. Am. Coll. Surg. **61:**19-21, January, 1976.

45. Cook, R., and Boyd, N. A.: Reduction of the microbial contamination of surgical wound areas by sterile laminar air flow, Br. J. Surg. **58:**48-52, 1971.

46. Coriell, L. L., Blakemore, W. S., and McGarrity, G. J.: Medical applications of dust free rooms. II. Elimination of airborne bacteria from an operating theater, J.A.M.A. **203:**1038-1046, 1968.

47. Costen, D. F., Nach, R. J., and Spinzia, J.: An experimental and clinical study of the effectiveness of antibiotic wound irrigation in preventing infection, Surg. Gynecol. Obstet. **18:**783-787, 1964.

48. Cown, W. B., and Kethley, T. W.: In Proceedings, Fifth Annual Technical Meeting, Boston, Mass., 1966.

49. Cruse, P. J. E.: Postoperative study of 20,105 surgical wounds with emphasis on use of topical antibiotics and prophylactic antibiotics. Paper presented at the Fourth Symposium on Control of Surgical infection, Washington, D.C., November 10, 1972.

50. Davies, R. R., and Noble, W. C.: Dispersal of bacteria and desquamated skin, Lancet **2:**1295-1297, 1962.

51. Derian, P. S., and Green, B. M.: Postoperative wound infection—five year review of 1,163 consecutive operative orthopedic patients, Am. Surg. **32:**388-390, 1966.

52. Dineen, P.: An evaluation of the duration of the surgical scrub, Surg. Gynecol. Obstet. **199:**1181-1184, 1969.

53. Dineen, P.: Penetration of surgical draping material by bacteria, J.A.M.A. **43:**82-85, 1969.

54. Dineen, P.: Microbial filtration by surgical masks, Surg. Gynecol. Obstet. **133:**812-814, 1971.

55. Dineen, P.: The role of impervious gowns and drapes in preventing surgical infection, Clin. Orthop. **96:**210-212, 1973.

56. Drill, V. A.: Pharmacology in medicine, ed. 2, New York, 1958, McGraw-Hill Book Co.

57. Dubuc, F., Guimont, A., Roy, L., and Ferland, J. J.: A study of some factors which contribute to surgical wound contamination, Clin. Orthop. **96:**176-178, 1973.

58. Duguid, J. P., and Wallace, A. T.: Air infection with dust liberated from clothing, Lancet **2:**845-49, 1948.

59. Edlich, R. F., Tsung, M. S., Rogers, W., Rogers, P., and Wangensteen, O. H.: Studies in management of contaminated wound. I. Technique of closure of such wounds together with a note on a reproducible experimental model, J. Surg. Res. **8:**585-592, 1968.

60. Eftekhar, N. S., The surgeon and clean air in the operating room, Clin. Orthop. **96:**188-194, 1973.

61. Eftekhar, N. S.: Controversy of clean air and total hip replacement in the hip. In The Hip Society: Proceedings of the second open scientific meeting of The Hip Society, 1974, St. Louis, 1974, The C. V. Mosby Co., pp. 266-270.

62. Eftekhar, N. S.: Operating room design, ventilation clothing as factors in infection control, Hosp. Top., February, 1972.

63. Eftekhar, N. S.: Sepsis in total hip replacement: prevention and management. In American Academy of Orthopaedic Surgeons: Instructional course lectures, vol. 23, St. Louis, 1974, The C. V. Mosby Co., pp. 253-265.

64. Eftekhar, N. S., Smith, D. M., Henry, J. H., and Stinchfield, F. E.: Revision arthroplasty using Charnley low friction arthroplasty technic, with reference to specifics of technic and comparison of results with primary low friction arthroplasty, Clin. Orthop. **95:**48-59, 1973.

65. Elek, S. D., and Conen, P. E.: The virulence of *Staphylococcus pyogenes* for man: a study of the problems of wound infection, Br. J. Exp. Pathol. **38:**573-586, 1957.

66. Erickson, C., Lidgren, L., and Lindberg, L.: Cloxacillin in the prophylaxis of postoperative infections of the hip, J. Bone Joint Surg. **55A:**808-813, 1973.

67. Everett, W. G.: Suture materials in general surgery, Prog. Surg. **8:**14-37, 1970.

68. Favero, M. S., Puleo, J. R., Marshall, J. H., and Oxborrow, G. S.: Comparison of contamination levels among hospital operating rooms and industrial clean rooms, Appl. Microbiol. **16:**480-486, 1968.

69. Feigan, A.: The case for clean air. Presented at American Academy of Orthopaedic Surgeons meeting, audiovisual section, 1975.

70. Fitzgerald, R. H., and Washington, J. A., Jr.: Contamination of the operative wound, Orthop. Clin. North Am. **6:**1105-1114, 1975.

71. Fitzgerald, R. H., Peterson, L. F. A., Washington, J. A., II, Van Scoy, R. E., and Coventry, M. B.: Bacterial colonization of wounds and sepsis in total hip arthroplasty, J. Bone Joint Surg. **55A:**1242-1250, 1973.

72. Fogelberg, E. V., Zitzmann, E. K., and Stinchfield, F. E.: Prophylactic penicillin in ortho-

paedic surgery, J. Bone Joint Surg. **52A:**95-98, 1970.

73. Forbes, G. B.: Staphylococcal infection of operation wounds with special reference to topical antibiotic prophylaxis, Lancet **2:**505-509, 1961.

74. Ford, C. R., Peterson, D. E., and Mitchell, C. R.: An appraisal of the role of surgical face masks, Am. J. Surg. **113:**787-790, 1967.

75. Ford, C. R., Peterson, D. E., Mitchell, C. R.: Microbial studies in the air in the operating room, J. Surg. Res. **7:**376-382, 1967.

76. Fox, D. G., and Baldwin, M.: Contamination levels in a laminar flow operating room, Hospitals **42:**108-112, 1968.

77. Francis, T.: Response of the host to the parasite, In Dubos, R. J., editor: Bacterial and mycotic infections in man, ed. 2, Philadelphia, 1962, J. B. Lippincott Co.

78. Gingrass, R. P., Close, A. S., and Ellison, E. H.: The effect of various topical and parenteral agents on the prevention of infection in experimental contaminated wounds, J. Trauma **4:**763-783, 1964.

79. Goldner, J. L., and Allen, B. L.: Ultraviolet in orthopaedic operating room at Duke University, thirty-five years experience, 1937 to 1973, Clin. Orthop. **96:**195-205, 1973.

80. Goldner, J. L., and Lowell, J. D.: Ultraviolet light in orthopaedic operating suites, Presented at American Academy of Orthopaedic Surgeon's Meeting, scientific exhibit, 1975.

81. Goodrich, E. O., and Whitfield, W. W.: Air environment in the operating room, Bull. Am. Coll. Surg. **55:**7-10, June, 1970.

82. Goodrich, E. O., Whitfield, W. W., Blakemore, W. S., and Beck, W. C.: Laminar clean air flow in operating rooms, Bull. Am. Coll. Surg. **58:**9-14, July, 1973.

83. Gould, J. C., Bone, F. J., and Scott, J. H. S.: The bacteriology of surgical theaters with and without unidirectional air flow, Bull. Int. Soc. Surg. **33:**53-60, 1974.

84. Hart, D.: Sterilization of the air in the operating room by special bactericidal radiant energy, J. Thorac. Cardiovasc. Surg. **6:**45, 1963.

85. Hart, D., and Nicks, J.: Ultraviolet radiation in the operating room; intensities used and bactericidal effects, Arch. Surg. **82:**449-65, 1961.

86. Heifetz, C. J., Richards, F. O., and Lawrence, M. S.: Comparison of wound healing with and without dressings, Arch. Surg. **65:**746-51, 1952.

87. Henderson, E. D., and Kornblum, S. S.: Studies on the epidemiology of staphylococcal wound infections in previously clean surgical cases on an orthopaedic service. In American Academy of Orthopaedic Surgeons: Instructional course lectures, vol. 18, St. Louis, 1961, The C. V. Mosby Co., pp. 282-287.

88. Hessert, G. R., and Ruchdeschel, G.: Antibio-tiche Wirksamkeit von Mischungen des Polymethylmethacrylates mit antibiotica, Arch. Orthop. Unfallchir. **68:**249-254, 1970.

89. Hopton, D. S.: Investigation of wound protection by a sterile laminar air curtain, J. R. Coll. Surg. Edinb. **19:**98-103, 1974.

90. Illingworth, C., editor: Wound healing: a symposium based on the Lister Centenary Scientific Meeting (Gasgow, 1965), Boston, 1966, Little, Brown, & Co.

91. Irvine, R. D., and Amstutz, H.: Studies of airborne bacteria in the operating room, Surg. Forum **23:**457-459, 1972.

92. Irvine, R., Johnson, B. L., and Amstutz, H. C.: The relationship of genitourinary tract and deep sepsis after total hip arthroplasty and the role of DHFAS in reduction of wound site organisms, Surg. Gynecol. Obstet. **139:**701-706, 1974.

93. Johnson, B. L.: Prevention and treatment of sepsis: bacteriologic analysis of "laminar flow" operating room and the use of antibiotics. In American Academy of Orthopaedic Surgeons: Instructional course lectures, vol. 23, St. Louis, 1974, The C. V. Mosby Co., pp. 246-248.

94. Johnson, J. E.: Wound infections, Postgrad. Med. **50:**126-132, 1971.

95. Joos, R. W., Kading, W. H., and Hall, W. H.: Effect of antibiotics on growth of staphylocci in plasma clots, Am. J. Med. Sci. **253:**305-311, 1967.

96. Karl, R. C., Mertz, J. J., Veith, F. J., and Dineen, T.: Prophylactic antimicrobial drugs in surgery, N. Engl. J. Med. **275:**305-308, 1966.

97. Kellgren, J. H., Ball, J., Fairbrother, R. W., and Barnes, K. L.: Suppurative arthritis complicating rheumatoid arthritis, Br. Med. J. **1:**1193-1200, 1958.

98. Kolczun, M. C., and Nelson, C. L.: Antibiotics in bone. In The Hip Society: Proceedings of the second open scientific meeting of The Hip Society, 1974, St. Louis, 1974, The C. V. Mosby Co., pp. 206-230.

99. Kolczun, M. C., Nelson, C. L., McHenry, M. C., Gavan, T. L., and Pinovich, T.: Antibiotic concentration in human bone, a preliminary report, J. Bone Joint Surg. **56A:**305-310, 1974.

100. Krizek, T. J., and Davis, J. H.: The role of the red cell in subcutaneous infection, J. Trauma **5:**85-95, 1965.

101. Krizek, T. J., and Davis, J. H.: Endogenous wound infection, J. Trauma **6:**239-248, 1966.

102. Laufman, H.: The surgeon views environmental controls in the operating room, Hosp. Top. **47:**73-78, 1969.

103. Laufman, H., Eudy, W. W., Vendernoot, B. A., Liu, D., and Harris, C. A.: Strikethrough of moist contamination by woven and nonwoven surgical materials, Ann. Surg. **181:**857-862, 1975.

104. Lazansky, M.: Complications revisited. The debit side of total hip replacement, Clin. Orthop. **95**:96-103, 1973.
105. Lidwell, O. M., William, R. E. O., and Schuter, R. A., editors: Methods of investigation and analysis of results—infection in hospitals. Symposium of UNESCO and the WHO, Oxford, 1963, Blackwell Scientific Publications, Ltd.
106. Lindbom, G., and Laurell, G.: Studies on the epidemiology of staphylococcal infections, Acta Pathol. Microbiol. Scand. **69**:237-245, 1967.
107. Localio, S. A., Casale, W., and Hinton, J. W.: Wound healing; experimental and statistical study; bacteriology and pathology in relation to suture material, Surg. Gynecol. Obstet. **77**:481-492, 1943.
108. Louria, D. B., and Brayton, R. G.: The efficacy of penicillin regimens, J.A.M.A. **186**:987-990, 1963.
109. Lowell, D.: Personal communications.
110. Maguire, W. B.: The use of antibiotics, locally and systemically in orthopaedic surgery, Med. J. Aust. **2**:412-414, 1964.
111. Marks, K. E., Nelson, C. L., and Lautenschlager, E. P.: Antibiotic-impregnated acrylic bone cement, J. Bone Joint Surg. **58A**:358-364, 1976.
112. Marsh, R. C., and Nelson, J. P.: Comparing surgical clean room filters, Contemp. Surg. **7**:33-34, December, 1975.
113. Martin, W. J.: Complication of antibiotic therapy in the management of bacterial infections, Lancet **86**:159-168, 1966.
114. McDade, J. J., Whitcomb, J. G., Rypka, E. W., Whitfield, W. J., and Franklin, C. M.: Microbiological studies conducted in a vertical laminar air flow surgery, J.A.M.A. **203**:125-30, 1968.
115. McFadden, H. W., Jr.: Assay of antibiotic levels in body fluids. Antimicrobial susceptibility testing. Commission on Continuing Education, Council on Microbial Microbiology, American Society of Clinical Pathology, 1971.
116. McLauchlan, J., Pilcher, M. F., Trexler, P. C., and Whalley, R. C.: The surgical isolator, Br. Med. J. **1**(1):322-324, 1974.
117. Medical Research Council Report: Aseptic methods in the operating suite, Lancet, **1**:705-709; 763-768; 831-839, 1968.
118. Miles, A. A., Miles E. M., and Burke, J.: The value and duration of defense reactions of the skin to the primary lodgement of bacteria, Br. J. Exp. Pathol. **38**:79-96, 1957.
119. Müller, M. E.: Total hip prosthesis, Clin. Orthop. **72**:46-68, 1970.
120. Murray, W. R.: Total hip replacement in nonspecialized environment in the hip. In The Hip Society Proceedings of the second open scientific meeting of The Hip Society, 1974, St. Louis, 1974, The C. V. Mosby Co., pp. 271-288.
121. Nelson, C. L.: Clean air and the total hip arthroplasty, Orthop. Clin. North Am. **4**:533-538, 1973.
122. Nelson, C. L., Bergfeld, J. A., Schwartz, J., Kolczun, M.: Antibiotics in human hematoma and wound fluid, Clin. Orthop. **108**:138-144, 1975.
123. Nelson, J. P.: Bacterial studies in a horizontal flow operating room clean room, J. Bone Joint Surg. **57A**:137, 1975.
124. Nelson, J. P.: The prevention of orthopaedic surgical sepsis, Orthop. Dig. **4**:14-24, 1976.
125. Nelson, J. P., Glassburn, A. R., Jr., Talbott, R. D., and McElhinney, J. P.: Horizontal flow operating room, Cleve. Clin. Q. **40**:191-202, 1973.
126. Nelson, J. P., Glassburn, A. R., Talbott, R., and McElhinney, J. P.: Clean room operating rooms, Clin. Orthop. **96**:179-187, Oct. 1973.
127. Nelson, J. P., Glassburn, A. R., Jr., Talbott, R. D., and McElhinney, J. P.: Horizontal flow clean room—bacteriologic studies, Rocky Mt. Med. J. **72**:243-246, 1975.
128. Noble, W. C., Lidwell, O. M., and Kingston, D.: The size distribution of airborne particle carrying micro-organisms, J. Hyg. (Camb.)**61**:358-391, 1963.
129. O'Connell, C. J., and Plaut, M. E.: Fibrin penetration by penicillin in vitro simulation of intravenous therapy, J. Lab. Clin. Med. **73**:258-265, 1969.
130. Olix, M. L., Klug, T. J., Coleman, C. R., and Smith, W. S.: Prophylactic penicillin and streptomycin in elective operations on bones, joints and tendons, Surg. Forum **10**:818-819, 1960.
131. O. R. survey signs most orthopaedic surgeons use regularly, Orthop. Rev. **3**:56-57, 1974.
132. Pavel, A., Smith, R. L. Ballard, A., and Laren, I. J.: Prophylactic antibiotics in clean orthopaedic surgery, J. Bone Joint Surg. **56A**:777-782, 1974.
133. Peers, J. G.: Cleanup techniques in the operating room, Arch. Surg. **107**:596-599, 1973.
134. Polk, H. C., Jr., and Lopez-Mayor, J. F.: Postoperative wound infection—a prospective study of determinant factors and prevention, Surgery **66**:97-103, 1969.
135. Prothero, H. R., Parkes, J. C., and Stinchfield, F. E.: Complications after low-back fusion in 1,000 patients—a comparison of two series one decade apart, J. Bone Joint Surg. **48A**:57-65, 1966.
136. Public Health Laboratory Service Report: Incidence of surgical wound infection in England and Wales, Lancet **2**:659-663, 1960.
137. Ravitch, M. M., editor: Current problems in surgery—biology of surgical infection, Chicago, 1973, Yearbook Medical Publishers, Inc.

138. Riemensnider, D. K.: Spacecraft sterilization technology, NASA SP-**108**:97, 1966.

139. Ritter, M. A., French, M. L. V., and Hart, J. B.: Microbiological studies in a horizontal wall-less laminar air flow operating room during actual surgery, Clin. Orthop. **97**:16-18, 1973.

140. Ritter, M. A., French, M. L. V., and Eitzen, H. E.: Bacterial contamination of the surgical knife, Clin. Orthop. **108**:158-160, 1975.

141. Ritter, M. A., Eitzen, H., French, M. L. V., and Hart, J. B.: The operating room environment as affected by people and the surgical face mask, Clin. Orthop. **111**:147-150, 1975.

142. Rocha, H.: Postoperative wound infection—a control study of antibiotic prophylaxis, Arch. Surg. **85**:456-459, 1962.

143. Ruedy, J.: An overview—antibiotics, Clin. Orthop. **96**:31-35, 1973.

144. Sanchez-Ubida, R., Fernand, E., and Rousselot, L. M.: Complication rate in general surgical cases—the value of penicillin and streptomycin as postoperative prophylaxis—a study of 511 cases, N. Engl. J. Med. **259**:1045-1050, 1958.

145. Scherr, D. D., Dodd, T. A., and Buckingham, W. W., Jr.: Prophylactic use of topical antibiotic irrigation in uninfected surgical wounds; a microbiological evaluation, J. Bone Joint Surg. **54A**:634-640, 1972.

146. Schonholtz, G. J.: Maintenance of aseptic barriers in the conventional operating room, J. Bone Joint Surg. **58A**:439-445, 1976.

147. Scott, C. C.: Laminar-linear flow system of ventilation, Lancet **1**:989-995, 1970.

148. Scott, C. C., and Guthrie, T. D.: Environmental tests of linear flow ventilation for an operating theater, Br. J. Surg. **62**:462-467, 1975.

149. Seropian, R., and Reynolds, B. M.: Wound infections after preoperative depilatory vs. razor preparation, Am. J. Surg. **121**:251-254, 1971.

150. Snider, S. R.: Clean wound infections: epidemiology and bacteriology, Surgery **64**:728-35, 1968.

151. Sompolinsky, D., Hermann, Z., Oeding, P., and Rippon, J. E.: A series of postoperative infections, J. Infect. Dis. **100**:1-11, 1957.

152. Stevens, D. B.: Postoperative orthopaedic infections—a study of etiological mechanisms, J. Bone Joint Surg. **46A**:96-102, 1964.

153. Tachdjian, M. O., and Compere, E. L.: Postoperative wound infections in orthopaedic surgery, evaluation of prophylactic antibiotics, J. Int. Coll. Surg. **28**:797-805, 1957.

154. Taylor, G. W.: Preventive use of antibiotics in surgery, Br. Med. Bull. **16**:51-54, 1960.

155. Turner, R. S.: Laminar air flow. Its original surgical application and long-term results, J. Bone Joint Surg. **56A**:430-435, 1974.

156. Wardle, M. D., Nelson, J. P., LaLime, P., and Davidson, C. S.: A surgeon body—exhaust clean air operating room system, Orthop. Rev. **3**:43-51, 1974.

157. Waterman, N. G., and Kastan, L. B.: Interstitial fluid and serum antibiotic concentrations, Arch. Surg. **105**:192-196, 1972.

158. Waterman, N. G., Howell, R. S., and Babich, M.: The effect of a prophylactic topical antibiotic (cephalothin) on the incidence of wound infection, Arch. Surg. **97**:365-370, 1968.

159. Weinstein, A. M., Bingham, D. N., Sauer, B. W., and Lunceford, E. M.: The effect of high pressure insertion and antibiotic inclusions upon the mechanical properties of polymethylmethacrylate, Clin. Orthop. **121**:67-73, 1976.

160. Weinstein, L., Daikos, G. K., and Perrin, T. S.: Studies on the relationship of tissue fluids and blood levels of penicillin, J. Lab. Clin. Med. **38**:712-718, 1951.

161. Welch, R. B., Taylor, L. W., and Garnet, W.: The prophylactic effect of clean air systems and antibiotics in total hip replacement surgery, Orthop. Rev. **5**(11):27-34, 1976.

162. Whitcomb, J. G., and Clapper, W. E.: Ultra-clean operating room, Am. J. Surg. **112**:681-685, 1966.

163. Whitfield, W. J.: A new approach to clean room design, SC-4673 (RR) Scandia Corp., 1962.

164. Whyte, W., and Shaw, B. H.: Comparison of ventilation systems in operating rooms, Bull. Soc. Int. Surg. **33**:42-52, 1974.

165. Whyte, W., Shaw, B. H., and Barnes, R.: A bacteriologic evaluation of laminar flow systems for orthopaedic surgery, J. Hyg. (Camb.) **559**:64, 1973.

166. Whyte, W., Shaw, B. H., and Freeman, M. A. R.: An evaluation of a partial-walled laminar-flow operating room, J. Hyg. (Camb.) **73**:61-74, 1974.

167. Wiley, A. M., and Barnett, M.: The prevention of surgical sepsis: clean surgeons and clean air, Clin. Orthop. **96**:168-178, 1973.

168. Williams, R. E. O., Jevons, M. D., Shooter, R. A., Hunter, C. J. W., Girling, J. A., Griffiths, J. D., and Taylor, G. W.: Nasal staphylococcal and sepsis in hospital patients, Br. Med. J. **2**:658-662, 1959.

169. Wilson, F. C., Worcester, J. N., Coleman, P. D., and Byrd, W. E.: Antibiotic penetration of experimental bone hematomas, J. Bone Joint Surg. **53A**:1622-1628, 1971.

170. Wilson, P. D., Jr., Amstutz, H. C., Czerniecki, A., Salvati, F. A., and Mendes, D. G.: Total hip replacement with fixation by acrylic cement: a preliminary study of 100 consecutive McKee-Farrar prosthetic replacements, J. Bone Joint Surg. **54A**:207-236, 1972.

CHAPTER 7

Thromboembolic disease and its prevention

The unknown and known risks from any therapeutic or diagnostic procedure must always be balanced against the seriousness of the offending condition requiring it.

P. D. WILSON, Jr.

Thromboembolic disease is a leading cause of morbidity and death following total hip replacement. Owing to better recognition of the problem, its reported incidence is rapidly increasing. Additionally, the increase in elective surgery performed on older patients and the increase in the extent of surgery performed in the face of underlying cardiovascular abnormalities followed by immobilization will contribute to an even higher incidence of thromboembolic disease with an associated risk of fatal outcome. Consequently, to the orthopaedic surgeon performing total hip replacement, this is a critical issue.

It is currently estimated that each year there are between 50,000 and 200,000 fatal pulmonary emboli cases and 300,000 cases of deep vein thrombosis requiring hospitalization in the United States alone. These also contribute as an ancillary factor to an untold number of deaths. When applied to total hip replacement, thromboembolic involvement is no longer a disease, but rather a complication of many pathological states that may accompany total hip replacement. Virchow postulated a triad of features leading to the development of thrombosis: (1) stasis, (2) hypercoagulability, and (3) local damage to the vessel walls.[14] One or more of these predisposing factors always occur in total hip replacement. The horizontal position of the lower extremities allows considerable venous stasis in the calf and thigh.[16] Stasis is usually enhanced during the operation[40,45]; 50% blood flow reduction in the external iliac and popliteal veins during induction of anesthesia by thiopental has been shown.[8]

Wessler and his associates[61-63] have clearly shown hypercoagulability to be associated with thrombosis. Their experimental work demonstrated massive thrombosis in vascular segments containing stagnant blood quite far from the site of infusion of thrombin-free serum. Likewise, the prophylactic efficacy of low-dose heparin suggested hypercoagulability as a major contributing factor to thromboembolism during the postoperative period.[20,28] Undoubtedly, platelets play an important role in the production of thrombi; damage of the vessel walls and endothelium may predispose to the adhesion and aggregation of platelets, with subsequent thrombus formation.[4,6,7,43]

In recent years, new techniques for objective evaluation, diagnosis, and proper prophylactic/therapeutic management have been emphasized. In deep vein thrombosis the four most important advances in diagnosis have been (1) roentgenographic phlebography, (2) the labeled fibrinogen uptake test, (3) impedance or occlusion plethysmography, and (4) augmented ultrasound techniques based on the Doppler effect. These advanced diagnostic techniques have been developed concurrent with the appearance of excellent clinical studies evaluating the prophylactic efficacy of a variety of older and newer agents. Total hip replacement has offered an opportunity to study thromboembolic disease, not only because it is a commonly performed operation on older patients, but also because the operation involves the proximal limb and pelvis and requires postoperative bedrest.

In 1959 Sevitt and his co-workers[56,57] published the first study showing the efficacy of prophylaxis in thromboembolic disease in hip fracture patients using oral anticoagulants. Considerable advances have been made since then to define the proper use of these agents as a preventive measure in thromboembolic disease following hip surgery. The prophylactic use of low-dose heparin was first studied by Sharnoff and reported in 1966.[58] Heparin works by augmenting the effect of antithrombin 3 (heparin factor), a potent naturally occurring inhibitor of activated factor X and thrombin, and by decreasing platelet adhesiveness.

Coumadin is a proven antithrombotic, interfering with the hepatic synthesis of clotting factors by depressing vitamin K activity. Dextran, a branched polysaccharide of bacterial origin, alters platelet function and also disturbs the structure of a fibrin clot formed in its presence. Dextran preparations with an *average* molecular weight of 40,000 to 70,000 are used to prevent deep vein thrombosis and pulmonary embolism; dextran's effectiveness has been reported in patients with hip fractures and elective hip operations as well as in general surgical, urological, and gynecological procedures.[1,18] Despite its efficacy, however, routine prophylactic administration has not gained wide acceptance because of the frequent side effects, high cost, and need for intravenous administration. In contrast to dextran, newer agents that interfere with platelet adhesiveness, such as aspirin, are attractive because of ease of administration, fewer side effects, and low cost. Similarly, hydroxychloroquine and sulfinpyrazone have shown promise, but clinical trials at the present time are inadequate.[1,39,49,50,52]

Besides chemical agents, physical modalities such as external pneumatic compression and electrical stimulation of the calves during operation have been used, but further clinical studies are required to confirm claims of efficacy and feasibility of application to large numbers of cases in the prevention of thromboembolic disease.

The single most critical complication associated with anticoagulation is hemorrhage at the surgical site or in a remote area. This complication must be considered a serious one, and its incidence may be minimized by scrupulous patient selection: the exclusion of any patient with hemorrhagic diathesis or thrombocytopenia, coincidental gastrointestinal bleeding, history of recently active peptic ulcers or ulcerative colitis, diabetic retinopathy, or uncontrolled and severe hypertension. It is essential that anticoagulation be well controlled throughout the prophylactic period. Ideally, for safety's sake, one person must be responsible for the anticoagulation of each patient; this should not be a rotating task for the resident or attending physician covering a particular date. The medical consultant is invaluable in this regard. All noninvasive physical measures are important, such as elevating the foot of the bed, muscle exercises, and antiembolic stockings. Early ambulation appreciably reduces the threat of thromboembolic disease, and if the patient is able, standing and walking should begin as soon as possible after operation.

INCIDENCE OF THROMBOEMBOLIC DISEASE

In the past, the true incidence of thromboembolic disease was underestimated because investigations were usually based on grossly inaccurate diagnoses. The proclivity of the surgeon to deny a high incidence of thromboembolism is directly related to awareness and search for this condition. To determine the precise incidence of thromboembolic disease following total hip replacement, the method of diagnosis, the age group (comprising a higher risk factor at advanced age), and methods of prophylaxis must be considered. Death after sudden onset of chest pain has often been attributed to myocardial disease, but in many instances autopsy proved conclusively that death was due to pulmonary embolism (while the surgeon or internist was concentrating on a cardiac etiology). Autopsy studies of patients who died after a hip fracture, for example, demonstrated that pulmonary embolism was the cause of death in 38% of 247 cases.[60] As stated before, any patient over 40 years of age is at risk; younger patients incur a similar but reduced risk. With improved methods of detection, the true incidence of the disease is becoming better understood, as well as the pathogenesis of deep vein thrombosis, including the time of initiation of thrombi and their location. Major predisposing factors remain: age (over 40), lower extremity surgery, immobilization, obesity, malignancy, prior venous surgery, prior thromboembolic disease, and venous disease. Those in the last three categories are very high-risk patients.

The peak incidence of clinically evident thromboembolism is between the seventh and fourteenth day postoperatively, but studies employing fibrinogen uptake have shown that most thrombi may be initiated within 48 hours after operation—some are present at the end of the operation. Because of the high incidence of venous thrombosis and pulmonary embolism, total hip replacement has presented an excellent opportunity to investigate the problem and seek the best method of prophylaxis. In the last decade, a large body of literature has emerged, which was derived from investigations into the scope of this grave problem and attempts at its solution.* The area has drawn interest particularly because of improved detection techniques such as venography,[46,65] ^{125}I-fibrinogen scan,[35] and autopsy studies to correlate clinical diagnosis and objective findings.[23,51-53,55,57]

The distinction between calf and thigh thrombi as potential sources of pulmonary emboli is more sharply defined by these diagnostic methods. It is now suggested that although calf thrombi develop frequently, they are not likely to cause embolization unless they extend proximally into the popliteal region and thigh. The major life-threatening emboli are generated in the thigh and pelvis (95% of all pulmonary emboli and 90% of all fatal pulmonary emboli), and detection of these "hazardous thrombi" is most important. However, it is thought that these thrombi are not primary lesions, and often they are extensions from a calf thrombus or arise in association with a discontinuous but concomitant calf thrombus. It is suggested that isolated thrombi in the ipsilateral thigh are common and account for at least 20% of all thrombi formed following total hip surgery.[12,15] Salzman[50] feels that this predilection for the operated or injured area is due to local trauma, and initiation of thrombi preferentially at this hazardous site is responsible for the unusually high risk of fatal pulmonary emboli following total hip surgery. On the other hand, in contrast, celiac and pelvic thrombi following hip surgery are rarely observed. In fact, only one was observed in over 400 roentgenographic studies following total hip surgery.[50]

Although venous thrombosis is the most common complication of adult hip surgery,† fatal pulmonary emboli, which occur in 0.5% to 2% of patients undergoing elective total hip surgery (according to different series), constitute the major concern. Because of this high death rate following total hip replacement, most investi-

gators cannot justify an untreated control group in an experiment to evaluate drug effectiveness or other methods of prophylaxis.[29,50] According to a comprehensive recent study by Salzman,[50] fatal pulmonary emboli occurred in 1.8% to 3.4% of patients after total hip replacement, and in 1.7% to 2.5% following cup arthroplasty and prosthetic replacement; however, after hip fractures the reported rate was 4% to 10% in the absence of preventive measures.

The postmortem examination perhaps is the ultimate objective method for determining the true incidence of the disease, as it is the end point of the process. However, reports of most series contain insufficient studies of the patient or incomplete autopsies; data related to the incidence of deep vein thrombosis also suffer considerably for the same reasons.

Given the frequency of venous thrombosis and the mortality rate with pulmonary emboli, prophylactic benefits must be judged against the danger of complications resulting from prophylaxis.[26,34] Crawford reports discontinuation of prophylaxis due to complications arising from the treatment itself. He and his co-workers[11] reported a study of 900 total hip arthroplasties in which half the patients received oral anticoagulants and half did not; the death rate in both groups was approximately the same: 2%. While deaths in the untreated group were due to fatal pulmonary embolism, deaths in the treated group were related to pulmonary emboli and gastrointestinal bleeding associated with the anticoagulents; there also was a considerably high (threefold) increase in the incidence of deep wound infection and an increased number of hemorrhagic complications in the treated group. As stated, the patients most susceptible to thromboemboli are those with a previous history of thromboembolic disease and a compromised venous system, with concomitant obesity and cardiopulmonary dysfunction. It has been clearly established that patients over 40 years of age are especially susceptible. In patients with a history of bleeding dyscrasias, melena, hematuria, cerebral hemorrhage, hypertension, and peptic ulcer, anticoagulation prophylaxis is generally contraindicated or used with extreme caution. Crawford's criticism of anticoagulation was not related to its *efficacy*— but rather focused on its bleeding complications. Oral anticoagulants such as warfarin (Coumadin) have been proven most effective in

---

*See references 9, 11, 17, 24-30, and 49-52.
†See references 19, 23, 25, 27, 29, 44, 51, 55, 57, and 60.

prophylaxis, but require careful control and immediate discontinuation should local or remote hemorrhage complications develop.

The statistical data of Coventry,[9] Crawford,[11] and Salzman[50] substantiate the efficacy of anticoagulation with warfarin in reducing fatal pulmonary embolism. Because of the high incidence of thromboembolic disease (up to 50% in the age group generally undergoing total hip replacement)—approximately 10% attributed to pulmonary embolism, 30% to 50% to deep vein thrombosis, and 2% to 4% to fatal pulmonary embolism—it is reasonable to assume that some form of prophylaxis should be considered. Clinical double-blind control studies may no longer be justifiable. Because each method of prophylaxis is accompanied by complications or disadvantages, the search still must continue for a method that is totally effective, universally applicable, and free of complications.

DIAGNOSIS OF THROMBOEMBOLIC DISEASE

As clearly pointed out by Harris, Salzman, and others,[29] clinical signs and symptoms of thromboembolic disease are grossly inadequate for diagnosis. Harris and his associates suggested that physical examination of the extremities fails to detect 50% to 90% of thrombi in deep venous systems. It has also been suggested that when the physical signs are interpreted as indicative of thrombosis, incorrect diagnoses may be made in as many as 34% to 50% of the cases.[31] These observations make it of paramount importance to diagnose deep vein thrombosis only after clinical suspicion is confirmed by objective evidence from newer methods of detection. The only study in the past involving thromboembolic disease using objective means of diagnosis was that of Sevitt and Gallagher,[56] in which the incidence of fatal pulmonary embolism in the patients studied was determined by autopsy. Fortunately, a considerably accurate diagnosis of deep venous thrombosis and pulmonary embolism is now possible in living patients. Objective diagnostic tests have radically changed our concepts of the detection, incidence, and prevention of thromboembolic disease. It has been suggested that more than 50% of thromboses are silent. This makes the clinical recognition of deep vein thrombosis exceptionally tenuous. Calf tenderness or Homan's sign are grossly inaccurate and inadequate when

making the diagnosis. In a recent study by Harris and associates[29] in 172 patients who underwent total hip replacement, none of the 52 patients with deep vein thrombosis complained of symptoms at the time the thrombi were first demonstrated by radioactive fibrinogen scan or phlebography, with the exception of two patients who had clinical evidence of a pulmonary embolism. Similarly, the clinical diagnosis of pulmonary embolism is unsubstantial; approximately 80% of the cases of pulmonary embolism are unsuspected. In a study of patients referred to the Medical Examiner's Office in Philadelphia, the true incidence of pulmonary embolism occurring following hip fractures was 38%. These figures compare dramatically with a similar population of patients in which only 2% of the cases had been diagnosed prior to death.[19] If one bases the diagnosis of pulmonary embolism on the clinical situation alone, one sees that pulmonary embolism may kill immediately in some instances. Consequently, we urgently need accurate, objective, repeated tests rather than inaccurate clinical evaluation to detect deep vein thrombosis and pulmonary embolism, and thereby guide prophylaxis and effective treatment of established thromboembolic disease. Two thirds of the patients with fatal pulmonary emboli die within 30 minutes of the event.[15] This statistic alone demonstrates that some form of routine effective prophylaxis must be instituted, as opposed to waiting for thromboembolic disease to occur, as recently suggested by some surgeons,[32] since once an embolism has occurred, a fatal outcome may be unavoidable.

DIAGNOSIS OF DEEP VEIN THROMBOSIS

The clinical diagnosis of deep venous thrombosis is based on the presence of several signs and symptoms, including lower extremity pain, tenderness, swelling, erythema, cord formation, increased skin temperature, distended superficial veins, calf fullness, induration, edema, and positive Homan's sign. More accurate, objective diagnostic tests include phlebiography, ^{125}I-fibrinogen scan, and ultrasonic plethysmographic techniques.

Phlebography

By conventional methods of phlebography (such as that described by Rabinov and Paulin[46]), the common femoral and iliac veins can

195

be adequately exposed to view in approximately 70% of the cases, and the muscular veins of the calf can be shown regularly in all cases. As suggested by Salzman,[50] this technique is without doubt the "diagnostic benchmark" of deep vein thrombosis in the living patient, and in the last analysis it is the final arbiter in areas of dispute. It should be recognized, however, that phlebography is not a routine procedure available to all patients, since a skilled radiology expert is required. Furthermore, phlebitis and other complications such as extravasation of the dye have been reported in approximately 3% of the cases. We feel that since phlebography is painful, not readily repeatable, and invasive, it should not be routinely used, but reserved for clinical problems when it would be of significant importance in the care of the patient.

[125]I-fibrinogen test and cuff-impedance phlebography

The ^{125}I-fibrinogen test has been extensively used experimentally in the past decade to detect deep vein thrombosis. It is based on the incorporation of radioactive fibrinogen into the fibrin clot. This technique is attractive because it is sensitive, accurate (approximately 90%), noninvasive, repeatable, and painless. In total hip replacement, however, it has been shown by Harris and his associates[28] to be inadequate in assessing the thigh and proximal limb for thrombus formation. This is because of the postoperative accumulation of fibrinogen in the wound, abrasion, and hematoma proximal to the knee—the area where thrombi-causing pulmonary emboli are usually generated. Harris has recently demonstrated that cuff-impedance phlebography is distinctly more accurate and suitable than the ^{125}I-fibrinogen scanning technique in the detection of major thrombi in the thigh following total hip replacement.[30] It must be pointed out that cuff-impedance phlebography is of no value in the detection of thrombi in the calf. However, as stated before and based on Kakkar's[35] observations, the thrombi formed in and limited to the calf are generally of no consequence and do not cause major pulmonary embolization. The clinical signs or symptoms of venous thrombosis were present in only two of 78 limbs examined, but many of these patients subsequently had clinical signs. The detection of major thrombi by cuff-impedance phlebography with accuracy prior to signs and symptoms

of deep vein thrombosis is extremely significant, since prophylaxis can thus be instituted early and exclusively in those with major thigh thrombi.

Plethysmography and ultrasound

Obstruction to venous flow can also be detected by pneumatic or hydraulic (impedance) plethysmography and Doppler ultrasound methods. Plethysmographic techniques are based either on electrical impedance or on physical volume changes in the blood content of the limb in response to respiration or application of a tourniquet (inflation and deflation). In some techniques it is supplemented by assessment of the effect of compression of the calf or the pumping effect of foot movement.[10,64] It is suggested that these methods are most accurate in the detection of occlusive thrombi in iliac, femoral, or popliteal veins, and are generally ineffective in the detection of calf thrombi. In a recent study by Hume and associates[32] of 140 total hip patients, both impedance plethysmography and ^{125}I-fibrinogen scanning of the lower extremities were used. It was demonstrated that half had no evidence of thrombosis, one-quarter had moderate or extensive thrombosis, and one-quarter had abnormal scans only. Those patients with "abnormal scans" appeared to resolve spontaneously. Impedance plethysmography differentiated between thrombi that would or would not resolve, and on this basis it was suggested that for some patients a monitoring regimen may be preferentially selected over routine prophylaxis.[32] If on further testing noninvasive methods prove adequate, they present great hope for early detection and treatment of thrombi—particularly those in the thigh—prior to embolization.

DIAGNOSIS OF PULMONARY EMBOLISM

The diagnosis of pulmonary embolism is clinically suggested by the presence of pleuritic chest pain, shortness of breath, tachycardia, hemoptysis, diaphoresis, pleuritic friction rub, increased temperature, an elevated erythrocyte sedimentation rate and white blood count. Arterial blood-gas change is a good gross scanning test; diagnosis of pulmonary embolism in a patient with P_{O_2} above 90 mm. Hg, breathing room air, is suspect. Abnormal electrocardiograms and consistent chest x-ray films are of diagnostic assistance but are generally nonspecific; a positive lung perfusion scan, pulmonary ventilation scan, and selective pulmonary angiography, on the other hand, are most specific for diagnosis but are not readily repeatable. Basing the diagnosis of pulmonary embolism on clinical signs and symptoms alone can be grossly inaccurate. Hemoptysis, for example, occurs in only 17% of the documented pulmonary emboli, and actually there must be an infarct present before hemoptysis is seen.[53,59] Salzman[50] states that the risks inherent in prolonged anticoagulation treatment of pulmonary embolism and the inaccuracies of clinical findings suggest that this diagnosis should not be accepted without objective confirmation. This is particularly true if there is a suggestion of recurrent embolization despite adequate anticoagulation, in which case one must consider vena cava ligation.

Patients receiving anticoagulation treatment must be observed for the clinical signs of hematoma, represented by local pain, swelling, fluctuation, warmth, falling hematocrit, temperature elevation, and occasional spontaneous drainage of dark blood from the wound. The patient's urine and stool are observed for evidence of gastrointestinal and genitourinary bleeding.

MODES OF PROPHYLAXIS

As stated previously, at the present time it is felt that some form of prophylaxis is necessary in view of the high incidence and suddenness of fatal pulmonary embolism in unprotected patients undergoing total hip replacement. One must consider the risk of thromboembolic disease, especially fatal pulmonary embolism, for each patient specifically. Specific contraindications to various anticoagulants, potential complications, and the efficacy of the prophylactic regime all must be balanced.

Prophylactic measures include mechanical methods such as external pneumatic compression of the calf and electrical stimulation during surgery (still in the experimental stage) as well as early ambulation, elastic stockings, elevation of the legs, passive flexion of the foot during surgery, and early range of motion of the joints of the extremity postoperatively. Antithrombotic drugs such as warfarin, low-dose heparin, dextran, aspirin, hydroxychloroquine, and sulfinpyrazone constitute the only proven form of prevention against thromboembolic disease. The methods, agents, and duration of antithrombo-

embolic therapy used in total hip arthroplasty have varied according to observed effectiveness in preventing thromboembolic disease. Associated complications have also been documented.[11,21]

There are several approaches to the prevention of thromboembolic disease following total hip replacement; the first is to wait for clinical evidence of embolism or phlebitis and then institute anticoagulation therapy. However, as stated previously, the fatal pulmonary embolism is often sudden and unheralded; clinical signs may not appear until it is too late. A second alternative is prophylactic anticoagulation in high-risk patients, for example, patients who have a history of prior thromboembolic disease, cardiac disease, vein surgery, or who show significant venous disease. A third approach is routine prophylactic anticoagulation in all patients unless contraindicated by hypertension, bleeding diathesis, liver disease, peptic ulcer, ulcerative colitis, and so on. The fourth—and perhaps most logical way—is to employ the newer objective noninvasive techniques such as ^{125}I-fibrinogen scanning and impedance plethysmography, switching from prophylactic anticoagulation to therapeutic anticoagulation if fresh thrombi are noted. Fifth, a combination of objective detection techniques and administration of aspirin (shown to be effective in reducing thromboembolic complications) can be used.

Warfarin

Warfarin has been proven effective in reducing the incidence of postoperative venous thrombi in a number of clinical investigations.* Indications and modes of administration have varied with investigators. Anticoagulation with sodium warfarin used at the Mayo Clinic after 1,900 total hip arthroplasties proved safe and effective in preventing fatal thromboembolic disease and was achieved by delayed administration of the drug—that is, anticoagulation did not begin before the fifth postoperative day.[9] Clinical diagnosis of thromboembolic disease was the main criterion used for this study. It is of special interest that 50% of all thromboembolic complications occurred during the first 5 days prior to anticoagulation. Sodium warfarin requires very careful monitoring if hemorrhagic complications are to be avoided, as there is a 10% to 20% risk

---

*See references 24, 27, 51, 54, and 60.

of bleeding with this drug. However, when carefully and effectively used, sodium warfarin is the best method available for reducing and treating thromboembolic conditions. Harris and associates[29] in a random prospective study demonstrated that there was no significant difference in the prophylactic efficacy of warfarin, dextran, and aspirin in reducing the number of patients with fresh thrombi, but warfarin and dextran were superior to aspirin in reducing the number of thrombi formed. There were, however, significantly fewer bleeding complications with the use of aspirin as compared with warfarin. Those investigators further concluded that prophylactic use of warfarin or aspirin, followed by warfarin therapy whenever a thrombus was detected by phlebography, provided effective protection against pulmonary embolism. They used phlebography to detect venous thrombosis of the lower extremities, since in their view the clinical diagnosis of venous thrombosis was grossly inaccurate.

Low-dose heparin

Although low-dose heparin has been found to be a dependable method of prophylaxis in general surgery, its use in orthopaedic surgery is now in dispute, and the bulk of evidence suggests that it is inadequate for patients undergoing major hip surgery.[18,20,22,29] On the other hand, several papers have appeared documenting the efficacy of low-dose heparin in cases of hip fracture and elective hip surgery;[13,37,48,52] 5,000 units of aqueous calcium heparin is injected subcutaneously 2 hours before surgery and then postoperatively every 8 hours during the next 10 days. Obviously, full therapeutic doses of heparin are not appropriate for prophylaxis since there is a considerable risk of associated bleeding following surgery.

Low molecular weight dextran

Some investigators have reported that low molecular weight dextran also reduces thromboembolic complications.* It is usually administered in the operating room at the beginning of surgery, and then on a schedule of 500 ml. daily for 3 days, followed by 500 ml. on alternate days until the patient is discharged from the hospital. However, although it is equally effective as oral anticoagulants, it is also equally

*See references 17, 27, 37, 38, 41, and 42.

198

likely to cause bleeding. Other possible complications are renal failure and anaphylaxis. Pulmonary edema is another deleterious side effect and may be caused by erroneous judgment in postoperative fluid therapy.[47] Since dextran must be administered intravenously, its main disadvantage is the potential to produce congestive heart failure by overhydration. Despite its efficacy, therefore, it has not gained wide acceptance as a prophylactic agent for routine administration because of its cost, frequent side effects, and the need for intravenous administration. At our institution, dextran was less than effective and was accompanied by serious complications.[47]

Combined low-dose heparin–warfarin prophylaxis

During the period from August 1972 to June 1976, 1,000 total hip replacements were performed at our institution, mainly using the Charnley low-friction arthroplasty method. The vast majority of these patients were operated on by one of two surgeons and were followed principally by one of two internists as well as the resident staff.[21] All patients were prophylactically anticoagulated, including those with chronic venous insufficiency and prior vein surgery, as well as those with a history of prior thromboembolic disease. The only patients excluded were those for whom the drugs were contraindicated (those with prior or current bleeding history). At 24 hours postoperatively —or at any time thereafter—when it was determined that Hemovac drainage was less than 100 ml./24 hr., and there was no evidence of excessive thigh swelling or pain suggestive of hemorrhage, anticoagulation was instituted. Each patient was placed on 2,500 units of heparin intravenously or deep subcutaneously every 6 hours (divided dosage to further lessen the risk of local hemorrhage) and begun on nightly warfarin, as ordered by the internist. When the daily prothrombin time reached 1½ times normal (usually 15 to 18 seconds), the heparin was discontinued; however, the heparin was reinstituted if the prothrombin time later fell below that effective prophylactic level. This regimen of anticoagulant administration was continued during the patient's entire hospital stay. Antiembolic stockings and elevation of the foot of the bed were utilized, and patients were encouraged to move their feet and ankles as soon as they had awakened from anesthesia. Quadriceps and buttocks sitting exercises were begun on the second postoperative day, and knee and hip active and passive range-of-motion exercises on the fourth postoperative day. Ambulation generally started between the fifth and seventh day postoperatively. Clinical examination was made daily by a member of the operating team and the internists; the final decision as to the occurrence of pulmonary embolism, deep venous thrombosis, or hemorrhage was made jointly by the operating team as well as the internist. In this study,[21] clinical signs and symptoms were the main criteria used for detection of thromboembolic disease, but in addition, a lowered P_{O_2}, abnormal ECG, consistent chest radiograph, and positive lung scan helped to confirm the diagnosis. When the diagnosis of deep venous thrombosis or pulmonary embolism was made, higher dosage therapeutic heparinization was instituted.

In this retrospective uncontrolled study, 796 patients satisfied the requirement of having been placed on the prophylactic anticoagulation treatment program during the first two postoperative days. (It should be noted that in this series 34% of the patients had evidence of prior venous disease or a history of prior thromboembolic disease.) The incidence of deep venous thombosis and pulmonary embolism in the entire group was 1.8% and 3%, respectively. For all patients without a prior history of thromboembolic disease and without venous disease the figures were 1.1% and 2.4%, respectively. The incidence of fatal pulmonary embolism was 0.1% for the total population on the study protocol; the single fatality occurred in a patient with a history of two prior episodes of phlebitis.* It was concluded, therefore, that this combined program of low-dose heparin–warfarin anticoagulation treatment was efficacious in preventing thromboembolic disease in the general population and in high-risk patients with prior thromboembolic disease and venous disease.

Complications occurring during the anticoagulation program in this study deserve special comment—13.1% of the patients in this study

developed a wound hematoma. For a better understanding of the scope of the problem, hematomas were divided into three categories: early (occurring during the first 3 days postoperatively), late minor, and late major. A 2% incidence of hematoma formation was found during the first three postoperative days and thought to be related to the surgery itself rather than to the complications inherent in prophylaxis.[21] However, hematomas developing after the third postoperative day were assumed to be secondary to anticoagulation, since postoperative hemostasis should have occurred by this time. Of all patients, 6% had minor bleeding during this period and responded in 1 to 3 days to local ice, bedrest, and suspension or discontinuation of the anticoagulation. On the other hand, 5% of the patients developed major hematomas. These hematomas were clinically significant and coincidental with a fall in the hematocrit or need for transfusion of two or more units of blood. It was rarely necessary for surgical evacuation of the hematoma followed by a primary closure. These 5% were considered a prime drawback to the anticoagulation protocol.

Based on this study by Goss and his associates,[21] low-dose heparin–warfarin prophylactic anticoagulation affords significant protection against fatal pulmonary embolism and reduces thromboembolic complications without the use of venography for all patients, including those with venous disease or a history of prior thromboembolic disease. It was felt that the 13.1% hematoma rate (5% major) was a small nonlethal and acceptable price to pay for this protection. It is noteworthy to recognize that one of the senior investigators in the study, Dr. Stuart W. Cosgriff, provided much of the absolutely essential medical follow-up in these cases and monitored the drug therapy enthusiastically without interruption.[21] Undoubtedly, such a successful outcome may not result unless careful monitoring of this combination anticoagulation regimen is performed.

Aspirin and other agents

Salzman and his associates[52] reported reduction of venous thromboembolism with prophylactic aspirin. This agent is attractive due to its ease of administration and management; 600 mg. is administered orally b.i.d. on the day before the operation, and postoperatively the patient is given 600 mg. orally twice a day or 1,200

---

*Those patients with venous disease had an incidence of deep vein thrombosis and pulmonary embolism of 2.0% and 4.1%, respectively; those with a history of thromboembolic disease had an incidence of 4.3% and 4.3%, respectively. The "prior thromboembolic disease" group had a fatal pulmonary embolism rate of 0.9%.

mg. twice a day rectally. As previously stated, Harris and his associates found warfarin and dextran superior to aspirin in reducing the number of thrombi formed. However, the three drugs were equally effective in reducing the prevalence of thrombi in the thigh. Also of note was the significantly lower rate of bleeding complications associated with aspirin as compared with the other two agents. Harris and associates[28,33] felt that aspirin may be the drug of choice in patients without prior thromboembolic disease or significant venous disease.

In reanalysis of further studies, Harris has suggested that aspirin may not be as effective in females as in male patients as a prophylactic against thromboembolic disease.

The use of other agents that alter platelet function (adhesiveness) in an attempt to prevent thromboembolic disease is under clinical trial. One is sulfinpyrazone; another is an antimalarial agent, hydroxychloroquine (Plaquenil). Chrisman and his associates[5] recently suggested the prophylactic effectiveness of this agent with regard to thromboembolism, but in total hip replacement its effectiveness has not been investigated. Charnley now uses hydroxychloroquine in preference to all other drugs at his clinic.

The prophylactic use of the vena caval umbrella is rarely indicated. One might consider its use in the case of a very high-risk patient for whom aspirin, warfarin, and dextran are contraindicated. There remains a need for further study of combinations of existing drugs.

SUMMARY OF ESSENTIALS

- Thromboembolic disease is considered the leading cause of death following total hip replacement. A death rate of 1% to 2% has been attributed to pulmonary embolism following total hip replacement.
- Increased elective surgery in older patients, the extent of surgery performed, underlying cardiovascular abnormalities, and immobilization following surgery all contribute to a higher incidence of recognized pulmonary embolism than in the past. Basically, three elements, stasis, hypercoagulability, and local trauma to the vessels, are predisposing factors that may occur during total hip replacement. Hypercoagulability is now clearly a definite factor, proven both clinically and experimentally, in patients developng thromboembolism.
- Of the modern techniques in diagnosing deep vein thrombosis roentgenographic phlebography, the labeled fibrinogen uptake test, impedance plethys-

mography, and augmented ultrasound techniques based on the Doppler effect have been most useful in early detection and proper management of this condition. In this regard total hip arthroplasty undoubtedly has offered an opportunity to study thromboembolic disease.

- There are numerous methods of prophylaxis against thromboembolic disease, each with a specific mechanism against this condition; heparin works by decreasing platelet adhesiveness and augmenting the effect of antithrombin 3 (heparin factor)—a potent naturally occurring inhibitor of activated factor X and thrombin. Coumadin interferes with the synthesis of clotting factors by depressing vitamin K activity. Dextran alters the function of platelets and also disturbs the structure of the fibrin clot formed in its presence.
- In addition to chemical agents, modalities such as external pneumatic compression, electrical stimulation of the calves during operation, and more recently, newer antithromboembolic agents such as aspirin and hydroxychloroquine (Plaquenil) have been introduced. The significance of the role played by these modalities awaits adequate clinical documentation.
- Regardless of the method of prophylaxis, the single most critical complication following anticoagulation treatment is hemorrhage at the surgical site or in a remote area. It is essential to minimize this complication by scrupulous patient selection for anticoagulation and a well-controlled and balanced management throughout the prophylactic period. It is also essential that one person be responsible for anticoagulation of each patient; the role played by the interested medical consultant is invaluable in this regard.
- The incidence of the thromboembolic condition in the literature has varied considerably, which reflects the efforts made on the part of the surgeons in detecting this condition. It is generally felt that the true picture is of a much greater magnitude than clinical diagnosis. It is now clearly evident that calf thrombi develop frequently but are not likely to cause embolization, unless they extend proximally into the popliteal region and thigh. The major life-threatening emboli are generated in the thigh and the pelvis, and the detection of these emboli is most important. However, it must be recognized that these thrombi are not primary lesions, and most often they are extensions from a calf thrombus or associated with a discontinued but concomitant calf thrombus.
- Because fatal pulmonary emboli may occur in 1% to 2% of patients in elective total hip surgery, early detection and prophylaxis are essential.
- There is now substantial evidence that heparin, warfarin, dextran, and aspirin are all effective in the prevention of the disease, but, most important-

ly, detection of major thigh and pelvic emboli seems essential in preventing a major pulmonary embolus.

- While the diagnosis of deep vein thrombosis by phlebography is most accurate, this diagnostic test carries considerable morbidity and should be considered invasive to deter its routine use in all cases. On the other hand, ^{125}I-fibrinogen test and calf-impedance ultrasound plethysmography are sufficiently accurate to consider them for routine use. The clinical diagnosis of deep vein thrombosis and pulmonary embolus is grossly inaccurate and an underestimation of the real state of affairs.

- The clinical diagnosis of pulmonary embolism can only be made if the surgeon suspects it and if the presence of symptoms such as pleuritic chest pain, shortness of breath, hemoptysis, diaphoresis, and pleuritic friction rub are not attributed to other conditions. A good monitoring test for the diagnosis of pulmonary embolism is arterial blood-gas changes. In addition to an abnormal ECG and consistent chest x-ray changes, a positive lung perfusion scan, pulmonary ventilation scan, and pulmonary angiography are most specific diagnoses. No diagnosis of pulmonary embolism should be accepted without objective confirmation.

- Because of the high incidence of fatal pulmonary embolism, some form of prophylaxis is necessary; this is a common feature on which most authorities agree. Several methods are available, including mechanical methods such as compression of the calf and electrical stimulation; antithrombotic drugs such as warfarin, heparin, dextran, aspirin, and other newer drugs; and early ambulation, antiembolic stockings, and elevation of the foot of the bed. The least invasive agents must be considered singly or in combination.

- At the present time a wide range of experiences suggests that although heparin and warfarin are effective and must be used in patients with a "prior history" of thromboembolic disease undergoing total hip replacement, perhaps for routine use an agent such as aspirin is the most practical and effective without serious side effects. On the other hand, dextran, although equally effective as oral anticoagulants is less advantageous than other drugs because of side effects and the need for intravenous administration.

- Based on recent reports, aspirin appears to be the drug of choice in patients without prior thromboembolic disease. Aspirin, cuff-impedance phlebography or ultrasound plethysmography (for early detection of thigh and pelvic thrombi), and proper management when thromboembolic disease is detected appear to comprise the method of choice. The use of other agents such as hydroxychloroquine and newer drugs awaits adequate clinical trials.

REFERENCES

1. Ahlgerg, A. K. E., Nylander, G., Robertson, B., Kornberg, S., and Neilson, I. M.: Dextran in prophylaxis of thrombosis in fractures of the hip, Acta Surg. Scand. [Suppl.] **387:**83-85, 1968.
2. Atik, M., Harkness, J. W., and Richmond, H.: Prevention of fatal pulmonary embolism, Surg. Gynecol. Obstet. **130:**403-413, 1970.
3. Carter, A. E., and Eban, R.: Prevention of postoperative deep venous thrombosis in legs by orally administered hydroxychloroquine sulphate, Br. Med. J. **3:**94-95, 1974.
4. Charnoff, J. G., Rosen, R. L., Sadler, A. H., and Ibarra, I. G. C.: Prevention of fatal pulmonary thromboembolism by heparin prophylaxis after surgery for hip fractures, J. Bone Joint Surg. **58A:**913-918, 1976.
5. Chrisman, O. D., Snook, G. A., and Wilson, T. C.: Prevention of venous thromboembolism by administration of hydroxychloroquine a preliminary report, J. Bone Joint Surg. **58A:**918-920, 1976.
6. Clagett, G. P., and Salzman, E. W.: Prevention of venous thromboembolism in surgical patients, N. Engl. J. Med. **290:**93-96, 1974.
7. Clagett, G. P., and Salzman, E. W.: Prevention of venous thromboembolism, Prog. Cardiovasc. Dis. **17:**345-366, 1975.
8. Clark, C., and Cotton, L. T.: Blood flow in deep veins of leg, recording technique and evaluation of methods to increase flow during operation, Br. J. Surg. **55:**211-214, 1968.
9. Coventry, M. B., Nolan, D. R., and Beckenbaugh, R. D.: "Delayed" prophylactic anticoagulation: a study of results and complications in 2,012 total hip arthroplasties, J. Bone Joint Surg. **55A:** 1487-92, 1973.
10. Cranley, J. J., Gay, A. Y., Grass, A. M., and Simeone, F. I.: A plethysomographic technique for the diagnosis of deep venous thrombosis of the lower extremities, Surg. Gynecol. Obstet. **136:**385-94, 1973.
11. Crawford, W. J., Hillman, F., and Charnley, J.: A clinical trial of prophylactic anticoagulant therapy in elective hip surgery, Internal Publication No. 14, Center for Hip Surgery, Wrightington Hospital, England, May, 1968.
12. Culver, D., Crawford, J. S., Gardiner, J. H., and Wiley, A. M.: Venous thrombosis after fractures of the upper end of the femur, a study of incidence and site, J. Bone Joint Surg. **52B:**61-69, 1970.
13. Dechavanne, M., Saudin, F., Viala, J. J., Kher, A., Bertrix, L., and De Mourgues, G.: Prevention des thromboses veineuses. Succès de l'héparine á fortes doses lors des coxarthroses, Nouv. Presse Med. **3:**1317-1319, 1974.
14. Delen, J. S., and Alpert, J. S.: Natural history of pulmonary embolism. In Sasahara, A. A., Sonne-

201

blick, E. H., and Lesch, M., editors: Pulmonary emboli, New York, 1975, Grune & Stratton, Inc., pp. 77-88.

15. Donaldson, G. A., Williams, C., Schnnell, J. G., and Shaw, R. S.: A reappraisal of the application of the Trendelenberg operation to massive fatal embolism. Report of a successful pulmonary artery thrombectomy using a cardiopulmonary bypass, N. Engl. J. Med. **268:**171-174, 1963.

16. Doran, F. S. A., Drury, M., and Sivyer, A.: A simple way to combat the venous stasis which occurs in the lower limbs during surgical operations, Br. J. Surg. **51:**486-492, 1964.

17. Evarts, C. M., and Feil, E. J.: Prevention of thromboembolic disease after elective surgery of the hip, J. Bone Joint Surg. **53A:**1271-1280, 1971.

18. Evarts, C. M., and Alfridi, R. J., Thromboembolism after total hip reconstruction. Failure of low doses of heparin in prevention, J.A.M.A. **225:**515-516, 1973.

19. Fitts, W. T., Jr., Lehr, H. B., Bitner, R. L., and Spelman, J. W.: An analysis of 950 fatal injuries, Surgery **56:**663-668, 1964.

20. Gallus, A. S., Hirsch, J., Tuttle, R. J., Trebilcock, R., O'Brien, S. E., Carroll, J. J., Minden, J. H., and Hudecki, S. M.: Small subcutaneous doses of heparin in prevention of venous thrombosis, N. Engl. J. Med. **288:**545-551, 1973.

21. Goss, T. T., Stinchfield, F. E., and Cosgriff, S. W.: The efficacy of heparin-warfarin anticoagulation prophylaxis after hip replacement. Arthroplasty. Unpublished data, 1977.

22. Hampson, W. G. J., Harris, F. C., Lucas, H. J., Roberts, P. H., Mcall, I. W., Jackson, P. C. Powell, N. L., and Staddon, G. E.: Failure of low dose heparin to prevent deep vein thrombosis after hip replacement arthroplasty, Lancet **2:**795-797, 1974.

23. Hampton, A. O., and Castleman, B.: Correlation of postmortem chest teleroentgenograms with autopsy findings with special reference to pulmonary embolism and infarction, Am. J. Roentgenol. Radium Ther. Nucl. Med. **43:**305-326, 1940.

24. Harris, W. H.: The incidence and prevention of thromboembolic disease. In American Adademy of Orthopaedic Surgeons: Instructional course lectures, vol. 19, St. Louis, 1970, The C. V. Mosby Co., pp. 36-40.

25. Harris, W. H.: Thromboembolic disease in elective reconstructive surgery in the adult hip. In American Academy of Orthopaedic Surgeons: Instructional course lectures, vol. 23, St. Louis, 1974, The C. V. Mosby Co., pp. 242-244.

26. Harris, W. H., Salzman, E. W., and DeSanctis, R. W.: The prevention of thromboembolic disease by prophylactic anticoagulation. A controlled

27. Harris, W. H., Salzman, E. W., DeSanctis, R. W., and Courtts, R. D.: Prevention of venous thromboembolism following total hip replacement: warfarin vs. dextran 40, J.A.M.A. **220:**1319-1322, 1972.

28. Harris, W. H., Anthansoulis, C., Waltman, A. C., and Salzman, E. W., Cuff-impedance phlebography and ¹²⁵I fibrinogen scanning vs. roentgenographic phlebography for the diagnosis of thrombophlebitis following hip surgery, a preliminary report, J. Bone Joint Surg. **58A:**939-944, 1976.

29. Harris, W. H., Salzman, E. W., Anthanasoulis, C., Waltman, A. C., Baum, S., and DeSanctis, R. W.: Comparison of warfarin, low-molecular-weight dextran, aspirin, and subcutaneous heparin in prevention of venous thromboembolism following total hip replacement, J. Bone Joint Surg. **56A:** 1552-1562, 1974.

30. Harris, W. H., Salzman, E. W., Athanasoulis, C., Waltman, A. DeSanctis, R. W., Potsaid, M. S., and Sise, H.: Comparison of ¹²⁵I fibrinogen count scanning with phlebography for detection of venous thrombi after elective surgery, N. Engl. J. Med. **292:**665-667, 1975.

31. Hull, R., Van Aken, W. G., Hirsh, J., Gallus, A. S., Hoicka, G., Turpie, A. G. G., Walker, I., and Gent, M.: Impedance plethysmography using the occlusive cuff technique in the diagnosis of venous thrombosis, Circulation **53:**696-700, 1976.

32. Hume, M., Turner, R. H., Kuriakose, T. X., and Suprenant, J.: Venous thrombosis after total hip replacement, J. Bone Joint Surg. **58A:**933-939, 1976.

33. Jennings, J. J., Harris, W. H., and Sarmiento, A.: A clinical evaluation of aspirin prophylaxis of thromboembolic disease after a total hip arthroplasty, J. Bone Joint Surg. **58A:**926-928, 1976.

34. Johnston, R. C., and Larson, C. B.: Results of treatment of hip disorders with cup arthroplasty, J. Bone Joint Surg. **51A:**1461-1479, 1969.

35. Kakkar, V. V.: The diagnosis of deep vein thrombosis using the ¹²⁵I fibrinogen test, Arch. Surg. **104:**152-159, 1972.

36. Kakkar, V. V., Field, E. S., Nicholaides, A. N., and Flute, P. T.: Low doses of heparin in prevention of deep-vein thrombosis, Lancet **2:**669-671, 1971.

37. Kakkar, V. V., Corrigan, T., Spindler, J., Fossard, D. P., Flute, P. T., Crellin, R. Q., Wessler, S., and Yin, E. T.: Efficacy of low doses of heparin in prevention of deep-vein thrombosis after major surgery, Lancet **2:**101-106, 1972.

38. Lazansky, M. G.: Complications revisited, Clin. Orthop. **95:**96-103, 1973.

39. Medical Research Council: Effect of aspirin on

postoperative venous thrombosis, Lancet **2:**441-444, 1972.

40. McLachlin, A. D., McLachlin, J. A., Jory, T. A., and Rawling, E. G.: Venous stasis in the lower extremities, Ann. Surg. **152:**678-685, 1960.
41. Morris, G. K., Henry, A. P. J., and Preston, B. J.: Prevention of deep-vein thrombosis by low-dose heparin in patients undergoing total hip replacement, Lancet **2:**797-799, 1974.
42. Multicentre Trial: Prevention of fatal postoperative pulmonary embolism by low doses of heparin, Lancet **2:**45-51, 1975.
43. Mustard, J. F., and Packham, M. A.: Factors influencing platelet function, adhesion release and aggregation, Pharmacol. Rev. **22:**97-187, 1970.
44. Neu, L. T., Jr., Waterfield, J. R., and Ash, C. J.: Prophylactic anticoagulant therapy in the orthopaedic patient, Ann. Intern. Med. **62:**463-467, 1965.
45. Nicolaides, A. N., Kakkar, V. V., Field, E. S., and Fish, P.: Venous stasis and deep-vein thrombosis, Br. J. Surg. **59:**713-717, 1972.
46. Rabinov, K., and Paulin, S.: Roentgen diagnosis of venous thrombosis in the leg, Arch. Surg. **104:**134-144, 1972.
47. Rothermel, J. E., Wessinger, J. B., and Stinchfield, F. E.: Dextran 40 and thromboembolism in total hip replacement surgery, Arch. Surg. **106:**135-137, 1973.
48. Sagar, S., Nairn, D., Stamakis, J. D., Maffei, F. H., Higgins, A. F., Thomas, D. P., and Kakkar, V. V.: Efficacy of low-dose heparin in prevention of extensive deep-vein thrombosis in patients undergoing total hip replacement, Lancet **1:**1151-1154, 1976.
49. Salzman, E. W.: Prevention of venous thromboembolism with drugs that alter platelet function. In Frantantoni, J., and Wessler, S., editors: Prophylactic therapy of deep vein thrombosis and pulmonary embolism, U.S. Department of Health, Education, and Welfare, Publication (NIH) No. 76-866, Washington, D.C., 1975, pp. 149-157.
50. Salzman, E. W., and Harris, W. H.: Prevention of venous thromboembolism in orthopaedic patients, J. Bone Joint Surg. **58A:**903-913, 1976.
51. Salzman, E. W., Harris, W. H., and DeSanctis, R. W.: Anticoagulation for prevention of thromboembolism following fractures of the hip, N. Engl. J. Med. **275:**122-130, 1966.
52. Salzman, E. W., Harris, W. H., and DeSanctis, R. W.: Reduction in venous thromboembolism by agents affecting platelet function, N. Engl. J. Med. **284:**1287-1292, 1971.
53. Sasahara, A. A.: The diagnosis of pulmonary embolism, current status. In Fratantoni, J., and Wessler, S., editors: Prophylactic therapy of deep vein thrombosis and pulmonary embolism, U.S. Department of Health, Education, and Welfare, Publication (NIH) No. 76-866, Washington, D.C., 1975, pp. 114-122.
54. Sevitt, S.: Venous thrombosis and pulmonary embolism—their prevention by oral anticoagulants, Am. J. Med. **33:**703-716, 1962.
55. Sevitt, S.: Venous thrombosis in injured patients (with some observations on pathogenesis). In Sherry, S., Brinkhaus, K. M., Genton, E., and Stengle, J. M., editors: Thrombosis, Washington, D.C., 1969, National Academy of Sciences, pp. 29-49.
56. Sevitt, S., and Gallagher, N. G.: Prevention of venous thrombosis and pulmonary embolism in injured patients, Lancet **2:**981-989, 1959.
57. Sevitt, S., and Gallagher, N.: Venous thrombosis and pulmonary embolism. A clinicopathological study in injured and burned patients, Br. J. Surg. **48:**475-489, 1961.
58. Sharnoff, J. G.: Results in the prophylaxis of postoperative thromboembolism, Surg. Gynecol. Obstet. **123:**303-307, 1966.
59. Szucs, M. M., Jr., Brooks, H. L., Grossman, W., Banas, G. S., Jr., Meister, S. G., Dexter, L., and Delen, J. E.: Diagnosis sensitivity of laboratory findings in acute pulmonary embolism, Ann. Intern. Med. **74:**161-166, 1971.
60. Tubiana, R., and DuParc, J.: Prevention of thromboembolic complications in orthopaedic and accident surgery, J. Bone Joint Surg. **43:**7-15, 1961.
61. Wessler, S.: Studies in intravascular coagulation. Part 3. The pathogenesis of serum induced venous thrombosis, J. Clin. Invest. **34:**647-651, 1955.
62. Wessler, S.: Venous thromboembolism, scope of the problem. In Frantantoni, J., and Wessler, S., editors: Prophylactic therapy of deep vein thrombosis and pulmonary embolism, U.S. Department of Health, Education and Welfare, Publication (NIH) No. 76-866, Washington, D.C., 1975, pp. 170.
63. Wessler, S., and Yin, E. T.: Theory and practice of minidose heparin in surgical patients. A status report (editorial), Circulation **47:**671-676, 1973.
64. Wheeler, H. B., O'Donnell, J. A., Henderson, F. A., Jr., and Bendict, K., Jr.: Occlusive impedance phlebography. A diagnostic procedure for venous thrombosis and pulmonary embolism. In Sasahara, A. A., Sonnedlick, E. H., and Lesch, M., editors: Pulmonary emboli, New York, 1975, Grune & Stratton, Inc., pp. 37-43.
65. Williams, W. J.: Venography, Circulation **47:**220-221, 1973.

PART THREE

PERIOPERATIVE MANAGEMENT

CHAPTER 8

Indications and contraindications for total hip replacement

. . . surgery should be performed, where the deformity or inconvenience is such as will induce the patient to endure the pain and incur the risks of an operation.

JOHN RHEA BARTON

. . . I offer the thought for consideration that, if the present popularity of total joint replacement goes into a future decline because its contributions to welfare become obscured by its contributions to misery, the failure will reside not in the biomechanical laboratories, but in failure to select patients properly.

SIR JOHN CHARNLEY

This is an area where the evils of the popular press in promoting the spectacular must be combatted by teaching this new science to clinicians so as to establish true perspectives.

SIR JOHN CHARNLEY

The ability of a surgeon to perform a given operation is not, in itself, an indication for that operation.

ROBERT B. SALTER

PHILOSOPHY AND GENERAL COMMENTS

The enormous extra work load imposed by total hip replacement in clinics and outpatient offices poses the problem of selectively choosing patients for this type of surgery. It has been suggested that if the present popularity of total hip replacement declines in the future because its contributions to the general well-being do not outweigh its contributions to misery, the failure will reside not in the biomechanical laboratories but in the failure of surgeons to select patients properly.[9] This is an area where the harm done by the popular press in "promoting the spectacular" must be neutralized by preparing competent clinicians so as to establish a balanced and reasonable perspective in selecting patients for this type of surgery.[28]

When a new surgical technique or a drug has reached a certain point in its development, it is essential to consider strict criteria for its use. Following the development of total hip replacement, considerable caution was exercised in advocating the new procedure over the time-tested, conventional operations.[10-12,18] Following failure of Teflon as material for arthroplasty, Charnley[9] emphasized the need for caution in using new materials (high-density polyethylene) in total arthroplasty of the hip. At the time of this writing, some 15 years following the first insertion of a total hip prosthesis utilizing acrylic cement and high-density polyethylene, it is generally agreed that the operation is suitable for adult patients with advanced degenerative arthritis and rheumatoid arthritis at any age after epiphy-

207

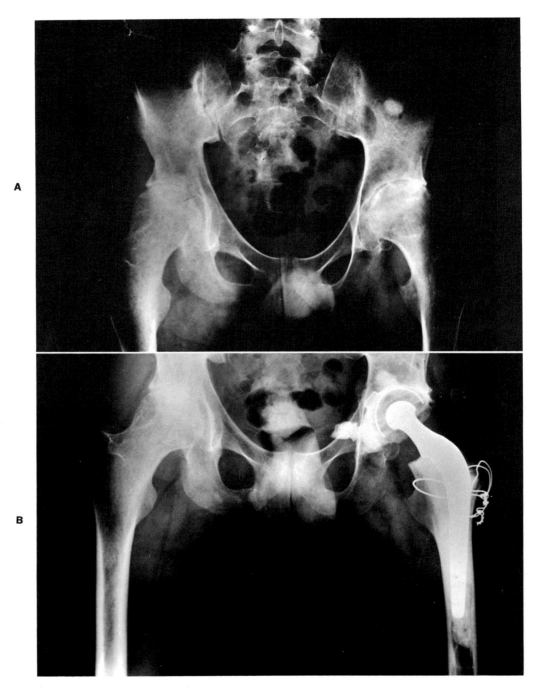

Fig. 8-1. A, Radiograph of 21-year-old male with rheumatoid arthritis of adolescent onset. His preoperative evaluation score was C-right 5,2,3 and C-left 3,2,5. Patient's rheumatoid arthritis was active and sedimentation rate was ranging from 50s to 80s. He was receiving corticosteroids as well as salicylates. **B,** Following left total hip replacement. Score 3 years following left total hip replacement is C-right 4,2,3 and C-left 6,2,5.

seal closure, or over 18 years of age. The procedure remains unchallenged because of the spectacular results of this operation, that is, relief of pain, increase and preservation of mobility, and above all, ease in rehabilitation without extensive physiotherapy. These features far surpass the results of conventional operations such as osteotomy or cup arthroplasty. The success rate of over 95% when this operation is properly performed bears witness to the superiority of the procedure. With certain provisions, total hip replacement may be indicated as the method of choice for all kinds of patients where both the acetabulum and the femoral surfaces are involved. It is ideally suited for rheumatoid hips, particularly because the prosthesis bonds to porotic bone with cement. In addition, the severe disability of polyarthritis shelters the artificial joint against heavy mechanical stress. It is ideally suitable for older patients for the same reason.

The most common application of total hip replacement (by statistical analysis) is in primary or secondary osteoarthritis caused by trauma, congenital dysplasia, or other conditions. As a general rule, total hip replacement should be reserved for patients over 60 years of age who are close to retirement or retired. However, under certain circumstances, a younger patient may be accepted, especially when there is a co-existing condition that leads to a shortened life expectancy. In patients with polyarthritis (rheumatoid or ankylosing spondylitis) this procedure can be performed at almost any age, especially if knees and ankles will remain a disabling factor following the hip operation (Fig. 8-1).

It is a well-known fact that the most spectacular results are achieved when surgery of both hips is performed. Patients with bilateral hip disease are usually handicapped because of lack of mobility in addition to the pain. Rehabilitation is long and tedious when conventional arthroplasties are employed and prolonged non-weight bearing is necessary,[3,14,30-32] but with total hip replacement, mobility is achieved rapidly and weight bearing is assumed early. Therefore this operation is ideally suited for bilateral hip conditions (Fig. 8-2), and based on these facts, it is appropriate to accept patients of almost any age with bilateral hip disease for total hip replacement if the disease is severe and advanced enough.

In planning bilateral surgery, the interval between the two operations should be less than 3 months, and in certain circumstances both hips may be done during the same hospitalization. It is my experience that in the absence of marked deformity, it is best to postpone operating on the less symptomatic side for reconsideration at a future date. In some instances following surgery the opposite hip will improve to the point where further operation will not be necessary. It should be noted that early radiological changes of the opposite hip without symptoms do not justify plans for surgery. The second hip may remain unchanged for many years or even indefinitely after arthroplasty of one hip (Fig. 8-3). However, there are three instances in which early surgery of both hips is advisable: (1) when treating bilateral disease in patients who are in their 70s, (2) when a severe fixed flexion deformity is present bilaterally, and (3) when a technical failure arises following arthroplasty and the second hip is also arthritic. In the first case, early surgery should be advised because of the possibility of medical complications developing should the patient wait too long for the operation.[18] If medical complications do arise, one would not want to risk operating on the second hip. In the second instance, a resistant fixed flexion deformity of the unoperated side would greatly interfere with hip mobility and postoperative rehabilitation (Fig. 8-4). In the third instance, if revision of a failed operation will require prolonged partial or non-weight bearing, operation on the second hip prior to the revision provides a sound extremity that will help with rehabilitation (Fig. 8-5).

In general, it is not a good idea to plan bilateral surgery for patients in their 80s. Although we no longer must maintain the ultraconservative attitude of accepting a chairbound existence for the very old patient, it is best to plan such surgery before a patient reaches this age. Pain as a result of osteoarthritis may be very intense. A low pain threshold in the aging may cause disability, and compounded by a narrowing socioeconomical horizon, may result in total confinement of these elderly patients. Seeing an elderly person who was suffering acute misery from arthritis of the hips totally free from pain and able to function in 2 to 3 weeks makes a profound impression (Fig. 8-6). He is gratified to know that his decision to operate on this patient is justified. Aged female patients are usually more durable after this operation than their male counterparts.

Text continued on p. 216.

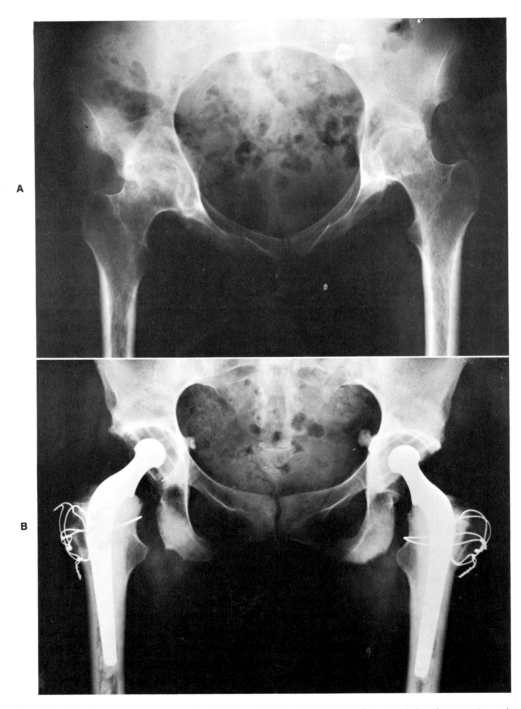

Fig. 8-2. This 31-year-old woman with history of bilateral painful hips of 5 years' duration was to undergo bilateral total hip replacement because of pain and stiffness (preoperative grading of the hips, B-right 3,3,3 and B-left 3,3,3). No conventional operation would be indicated here despite young age of patient for total hip replacement. Obliteration of sacroiliac joints is suggestive of diagnosis of ankylosing spondylitis, although spine and other joints are spared. **A,** Preoperative radiograph. **B,** Three-year postoperative radiograph.

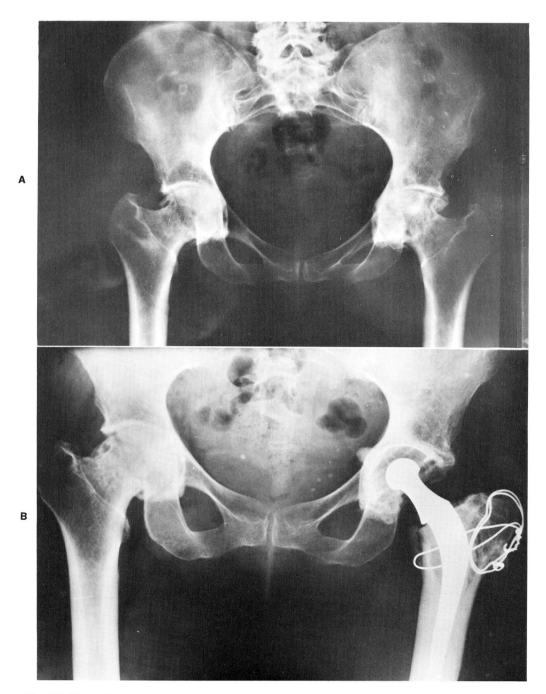

Fig. 8-3. Bilateral degenerative osteoarthrosis of hip in 56-year-old housewife. Patient had pain in left hip predominantly, limiting her daily living activities, such as shopping and cleaning. Right hip was somewhat painful, but she could cope well with it. Preoperative grading of hips was B-right 5,3,5 and B-left 3,3,2. **A,** Preoperative status of both hips in 1969. **B,** One year after left total hip replacement, 1970. **C,** Status of right hip in 1973. **D,** Status of both hips in 1976. It is of special interest that following total hip replacement of left hip pain from right hip has completely disappeared. There are no material radiological changes of right hip. Final grades B-right 6,6,6 and B-left 6,6,6. Whether this patient might require further surgery in the future on right hip cannot be ascertained, but it is now 7 years following surgery on left hip and she has no pain to justify recommending surgery on right hip. *Continued.*

211

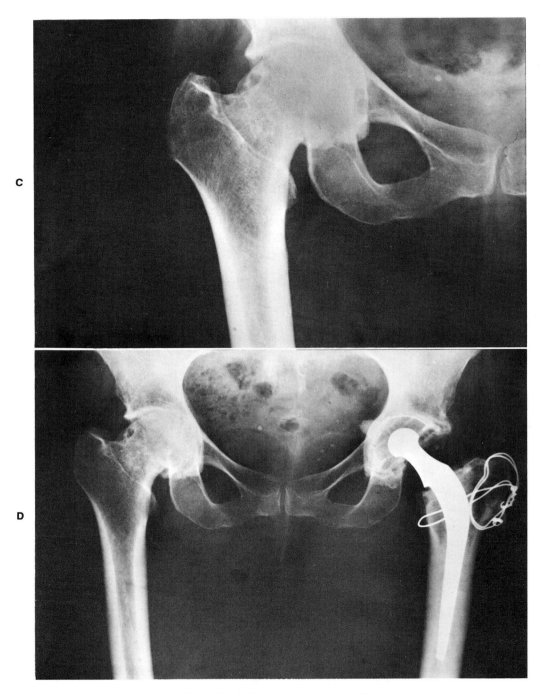

Fig. 8-3, cont'd. For legend see p. 211.

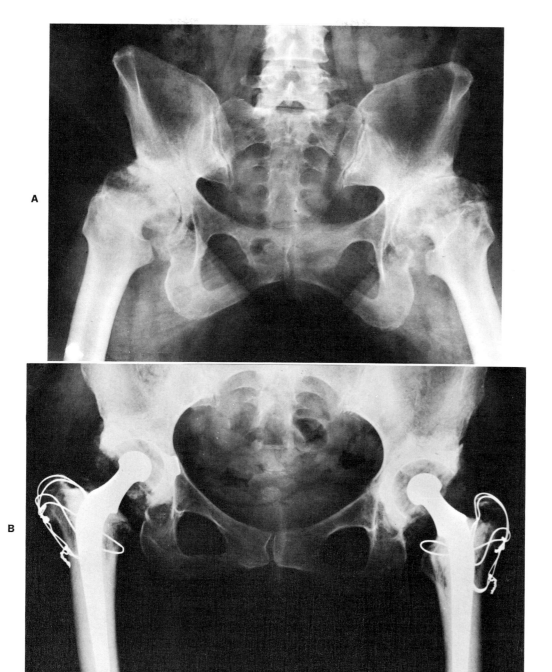

Fig. 8-4. A, Bilateral degenerative osteoarthrosis of hips in 55-year-old female who weighed 205 pounds and was only able to get about with aid of two crutches. She graded C-right 4,2,2 and C-left 4,2,2. NOTE: pelvis deformity as result of bilateral fixed flexion deformity of 65 degrees. Following weight reduction prior to surgery; at surgery weight was 180 pounds. **B,** Five years following surgery patient grades B-right 6,6,6 and B-left 6,6,6.

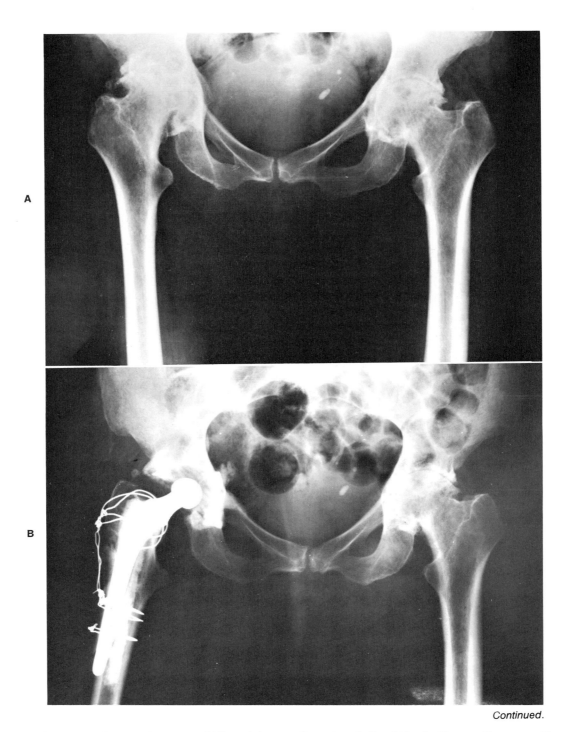

Continued.

Fig. 8-5. A, Preoperative status of bilateral degenerative osteoarthritis of hips in 66-year-old woman with marked stiffness of both hips. Hip grade B-right 4,3,1; B-left 4,3,1. **B,** Three months postoperative radiograph of patient with unfortunate complication of fracture of shaft of femur and circlàge wiring of upper femur to rectify problem at surgery. At this point patient was referred to us for treatment of defective surgery.

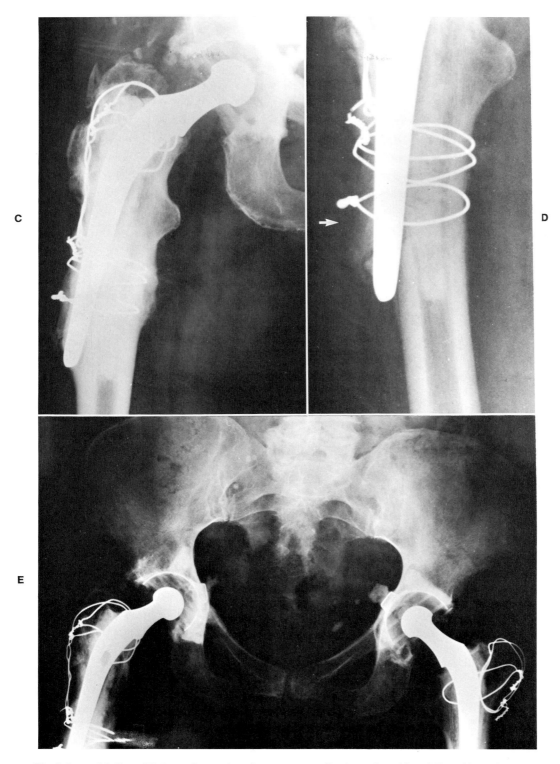

Fig. 8-5, cont'd. C, and **D,** Lateral extrusion of stem. NOTE: callus formation with stability achieved by "nature repair." In **D** arrow shows bone formation at stem tip level. **E,** Instead of revising right hip, it was decided to perform left total hip replacement to provide patient with good and sound weight-bearing joint. Following recovery of left total hip replacement, patient did exceptionally well while she remained non-weight bearing on right with gradual increased weight bearing as tolerated. By 6 months following second hip operation patient had no pain in right hip and became functionally satisfactory. Now 6 years following second hip operation, **E,** patient is totally asymptomatic despite precarious situation of right hip.

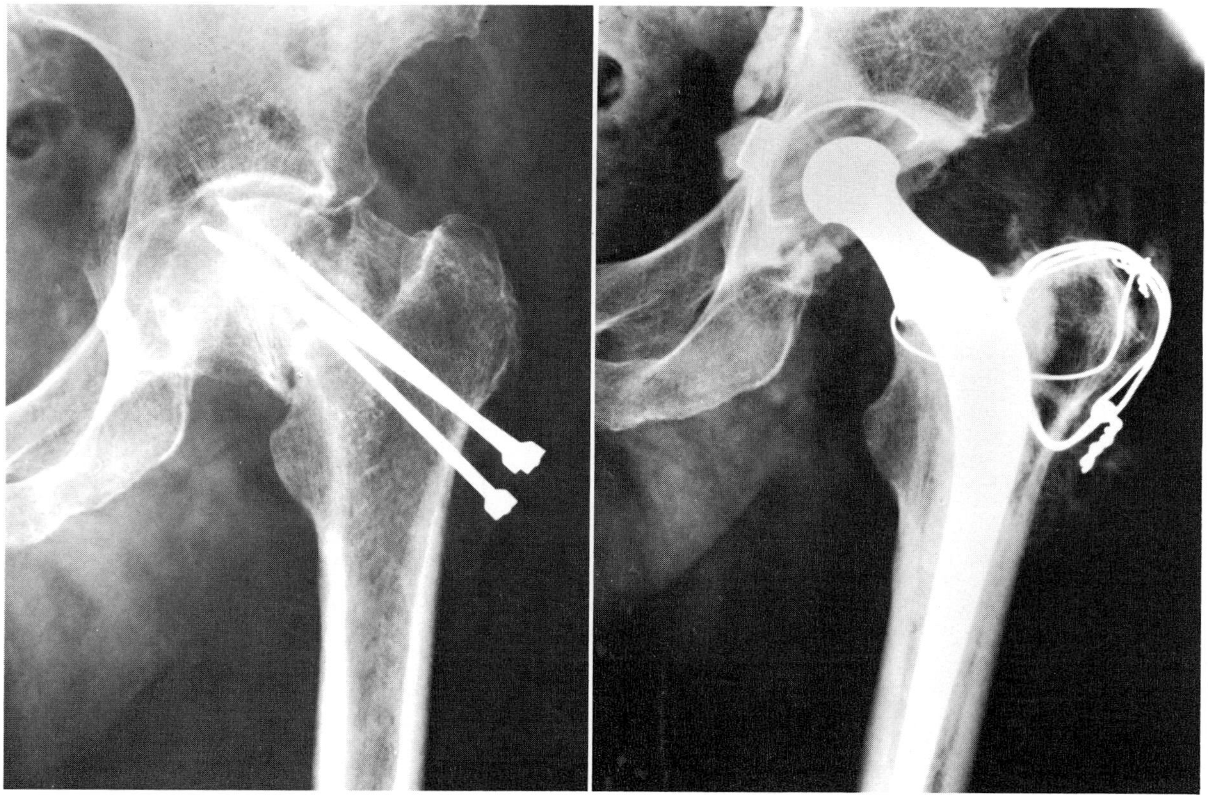

Fig. 8-6. Chronological age alone is not contraindication to total hip replacement. If patient's physiological age permits and systemic examination reveals no contraindication, total hip replacement will be great bonus to invalid aged person. **A,** Anteroposterior view of left hip in an 86-year-old woman who sustained fracture of hip followed by pinning and avascular necrosis and nonunion. Medial migration of pins additionally led to acetabular damage. Hip evaluation revealed A-left 3,3,2. Because of patient's desire despite age, total hip replacement was performed. **B,** Left hip 6 years following total hip arthroplasty. Now at age 92, patient is independent, walks without assistance, and is pleased with decision regarding surgery. She had been denied surgery by three other orthopaedic consultants because of her age.

A CASE FOR CONSERVATISM

As a note of caution when treating a younger patient, the possibility of introducing ultrafine particles of plastic into the tissue, and the consequences 10 or 20 years later, must never be underestimated. Therefore the patient and the surgeon both are faced with an exceedingly difficult decision: Should the patient who is presently handicapped wait for surgery another 5 or 10 years when long-term results will be available on those presently undergoing hip replacement surgery? Or is the physician to balance the present degree of disability against the worst that could happen if the total prosthesis failed and consider possible changes produced in the tissues as a result of implantation? Clearly, this demands careful clinical judgment, and the patient must be fully acquainted with all alternatives and participate in the decision-making process. Surgeons practicing total hip surgery will soon find themselves under enormous pressure to perform this operation from patients in whom the only indication is pain, unsupported by objective signs of crippling disability. As our experience develops, doubtless it will be justifiable to perform this major procedure, with all its theoretical hazards, when the precipitating factor is simply a low threshold for tolerating pain. But we must not forget that this operation is still a relatively recent development and we have not yet seen a 15 or 20 years' result in a large number of patients who are also active. Surgeons would be well advised to ascertain that they are operating for objective signs of disability. Patients will still be grateful for the surgeon's decision to postpone surgery based on

216

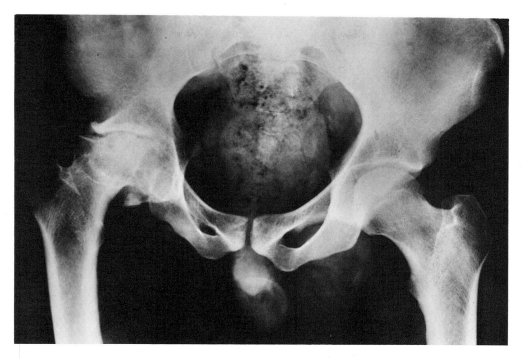

Fig. 8-7. Unilateral degenerative osteoarthritis secondary to childhood septic arthritis in 29-year-old lawyer. Despite extensive radiological changes and evidence of avascular necrosis of femoral head by radiography, patient has minimal discomfort, is able to work without taking medications, and has only minimal limp. Radiological changes alone are not indications for surgery in this patient.

logical grounds. This is elementary advice for experienced surgeons, but it is quite easy to forget when a patient has been intoxicated by news of spectacular results concerning this surgery.

An absolute indication for a total prosthetic replacement at any age is a case in which a Girdlestone pseudarthrosis would be beneficial.[9] This is frequently true when a prosthesis, cup, or osteotomy fails. Total hip replacement can be performed at any age as a salvage procedure to correct a previously unsuccessful operation. When total hip replacement is considered in such a case, the possibility of infection as the cause of failure must be ruled out prior to the procedure. If infection is present, then a special understanding must be reached between surgeon and patient regarding the magnitude of the problem and the possibility of failure.

While in the past great emphasis was placed on the inadvisability of total hip replacement arthroplasty in patients with previous infection, recent studies suggest that it is possible to consider this type of surgery in cases of low grade infection. It is generally a good policy to advise against total hip replacement in the following

conditions: (1) if there is a history or presence of osteomyelitis in the upper femur or radiological evidence of pyogenic infection in the hip joint with gram-negative organisms; (2) if a patient with unilateral hip disease is under 60 years of age and can continue to work without undue disability; (3) where the pain or disability is not sufficient to call for pain medications, and the patient's principal motivation is participation in sports activities; (4) obesity is a definite contraindication. Patients weighing over 200 pounds should not be accepted for surgery without a genuine effort to reduce weight. In addition to increased risks of thrombophlebitis, infection, and so on, surgical technique is more difficult and early mechanical failure may be anticipated. (See Chapters 3, 16, and 17.) Whenever possible, the patient's weight should be reduced to about 175 pounds prior to the planned surgery. Likewise, weight must be monitored postoperatively.

In general, skilled or unskilled manual laborers under 60 years of age who are still able to work should not undergo total hip replacement. The same applies to a retired 70-year-old person

217

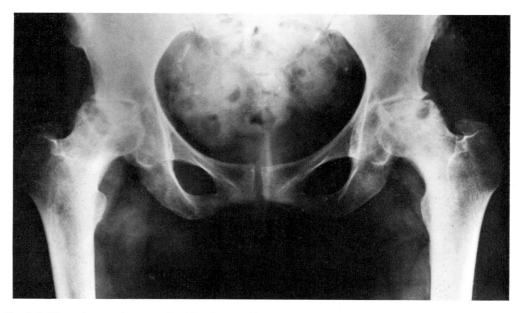

Fig. 8-8. Bilateral avascular necrosis with collapse of femoral head in 19-year-old female with lupus erythematosus. Currently she is taking 40 mg. prednisone and weighs 200 lbs. Despite radiological changes, she is able to get about without pain with assistance of cane. Because of history of kidney involvement and absence of pain, despite bilateral hip involvement, no surgery is contemplated particularly because of her weight and high steroid dosage (see text).

who is able to walk without a cane for unlimited distances. This type of patient is not a good candidate for total hip replacement. Radiological changes alone are never a sufficient criterion for patient selection (Figs. 8-7 and 8-8).

PATIENT INTERVIEW

The patient should be considered as a whole and not as a hip. Although referrals for total hip arthroplasty are from sources where the patient has been previously examined and he may be psychologically prepared to undergo surgery, I believe that the original interview by the surgeon contemplating total hip replacement is by far the most important means of evaluation. His decision must be completely independent of the recommendations and evaluations of his colleagues who originally referred the patient for consideration of total arthroplasty.

As a rule, one interview is adequate to make a decision as to whether or not total hip replacement is indicated. However, in considering a patient whose objective findings do not correspond with his subjective complaints, a second or third interview might be required, coupled with initial conservative management. Still, it is often the first interview and examination that will influence the surgeon's thinking and inspire the pa-

tient's confidence. Therefore it is of paramount importance that all questions be answered sincerely. Since it is often difficult to dissuade a patient from wanting to have the operation, it is essential to establish a good relationship with him during the original interview. Allow the patient to tell his own story in his own words. Listen attentively until he has finished speaking about his disability. It is best not to interrupt until some guidance or direction is required. When his complaints have been fully expressed, it is then best to direct questions toward the evaluation of the hip disability, based on the pain and functional activities. It is good to elicit the social and personal motivation behind the patient's consultation. Leading questions will help in formulating a correct opinion such as how limiting the hip disability is in work and social situations and whether continuation of certain hobbies and sports are the prime reason for correction. The amount of "pain medication" taken by the patient in 24 hours usually aids in determining the intensity of pain. Knowledge of the location and distribution of pain, as well as type and duration, and the need for medication, will give a better understanding of the problem. Often a polyarthritic patient may have more disability from related joints, such as the sacro-

218

iliac and lumbar spine, than the hip. It is not uncommon that abdominal or gynecological sources of pain are interpreted as hip pains. In such instances the pain may be referred and unrelated to the hip joint. It is also essential to consider the source of referral as a capital point in the overall evaluation. Many patients with mild hip disability will seek advice because they have read or seen spectacular results of such a procedure, or they ask for surgery under pressure from sympathetic friends or relatives.

PAIN—THE CARDINAL SIGN

The surest guide in determining the need for total hip replacement is the severity of the pain and its resultant disability. The pain may be described as fatigue, inability to stand on the leg, or inability to function or accommodate certain motions. It may be referred or radiating, confounding the patient's ability to explain it accurately, in the buttock, groin, or upper thigh, or completely in the knee. Often a patient's lack of anatomical knowledge may cause him to mistake the location of the hip, and the principal pain may not be related to the hip at all—patients will point to the greater trochanter or the crest of the ilium. What is more important, though, is the character of the pain, generally mechanical in nature, that is produced by walking, weight bearing, or other physical activities. Some patients with severe hip involvement and severe handicaps resulting from marked destructive changes in their hips have little or no complaint of "pain," but with questioning they reveal that their activities have been minimized. Indeed, some may have become housebound to avoid pain. This is best exemplified by the disappearance of discomfort when a patient is admitted to the hospital for surgery and after resting for a few days he wonders whether he requires surgery after all! There are other instances where the hip joint becomes insensitive, following marked absorption of the femoral head or expansion of the acetabulum with reduction of friction in the joint; ankylosis of the hip will occasionally reduce the pain at the cost of stiffness. Pain in the osteoarthritic hip is rarely spontaneous, and, when present at night, it usually appears after turning in bed. Pain in rheumatoid arthritis may be severe at times but rarely will be described as throbbing, burning, or stabbing. It is often coincidental with inflammatory exacerbation of the disease and is similar to the

pain of gouty arthritis. Pain is always elicited in the patient's joint with passive movement and is also produced with sharp internal or external rotation.

The location of the pain must be pinpointed from a careful history and physical examination based on normal functional anatomy. This is of the utmost importance (especially when examining a previously failed hip operation) in order to ascertain its origin. The following locations are used as a guide in determining the specific origin of pain about the hip joint: (1) groin pain, (2) gluteal pain, (3) trochanteric pain, (4) back pain, (5) knee pain, (6) anterior thigh pain, (7) sciatic pain, and (8) abdominal and deep groin pain.

The diffusion of pain about the hip stems from the fact that nerve fibers supplying the hip joint (derived from the femoral obturator and sciatic nerves) also innervate the skin, muscle, and bone in the region. The sympathetic nerve fibers that supply the joint supply the blood vessels and also produce pain. While mechanical arthritic pain is completely eliminated following total hip replacement, minor discomfort from scars of previous surgery or inflammatory response in soft tissue may persist and must be accepted. These responses are generally self-limiting, and the patient with previous surgery and a low pain threshold (especially one who obsessively speaks about his scar sensitivity or appearance) should be forewarned of their possibility.

If pain is in the gluteal region, it may originate in the area of the hamstrings or be related to the gluteal bursa. In the trochanteric region the greater trochanteric bursa may be responsible. Pain posterior and deep to the trochanter may originate from the piriformis bursa and occasionally may radiate to the buttock or midposterior thigh. Or the pain in this area may, indeed, be referred from the hip joint. Pain in the back is usually located in the area of the sacroiliac joint, especially when there is fixed deformity of the hip transmitting motion to this region. When the pain is in the knee, it may be related to the hamstring attachment, to the hip, or the innervation of the obturator along the adductor muscle. Irritation of the psoas muscle and its bursa may produce a pain radiating toward the inner abdominal region. If the patient has had previous reconstructive surgery of the hip, the pain may be diffused or it may be in more than one of the previously mentioned locations. The

219

patient with hip pain as the result of arthritis is often unable to bear weight fully, but there is no pain when at rest. An exception to this rule is pain resulting from avascular necrosis of the femoral head; this pain is intense and unrelated to motion. It is often disproportionate to radiological changes or the range of motion in the affected hip.

It is important to consider the cause of pain in the hip in terms of more remote areas; abdominal tumors, pelvic tumors, or adhesions and infections within the abdomen may refer pain to the region of the obturator nerve, causing pain in the groin. Degenerative disease of the low back or the sacroiliac joint may lead to pain referred to the hip area. Benign or malignant tumors in the hip region may produce hip pain; occasionally inflamed abdominal viscera, including bladder, bowel, rectal sigmoid colon, prostate, or the female genitourinary tract, may lead to radiating pain in the area of the hip.

When a hip is solidly fused, it is not painful, but often strain on the sacroiliac or lower lumbar spine will produce pain in the hip region. Thorough evaluation of the location and source of pain, therefore, is of paramount importance, especially when radiological changes of the hip are not consistent with the intensity and location of the pain as described by the patient. Examination of the hip to elicit painful points requires gentle expert handling. It is generally best to identify the landmarks on the unaffected or less symptomatic side just to assure the patient of the gentleness of the examination, and then move on to the affected hip. If the intensity of the pain cannot be determined, the patient can be asked to walk while the physician observes the gait. Many patients can better identify the source of pain produced by walking.[2]

SELECTION BY AGE ALONE

Because of the newness of this procedure, one of the considerations in selecting a candidate for total hip replacement is the patient's age. It is agreed that if the patient is close to retirement, 60 or 65 years old, then there will be less restriction in considering him for surgery. However, patients in their 40s and 50s still present the problem of possible mechanical failure and replacement in subsequent years. Another factor is the fear that one or more of the substances used in total hip arthroplasty may theoretically become carcinogenic, although no such

a case has ever been reported. The functional age of the patient and his general physical condition should be considered rather than chronological age alone. For instance, an otherwise healthy 55-year-old man with osteoarthrosis of the hip may impose greater strain on the hip joint than a 45-year-old man with rheumatoid arthritis in which the other joint involvement may prevent full activity. The 55-year-old, incidentally, may be an ex-tennis champion, looking forward to returning to the game.

Perhaps an even more important criterion for determining surgery at any age is the list of alternatives and their ramifications. Considering other methods and age alone, for example, a surgeon must recognize that he will never satisfy a 30-year-old man with cup arthroplasty. This is true in terms of rehabilitation required, economical implications, and physical demands on the hip itself. With bilateral arthritis, approximately 1 year of rehabilitation is needed. Often a patient may not be psychologically prepared to undergo surgery on the other side after one operation. A similar problem may be posed in performing an arthrodesis on an osteoarthritic hip in an otherwise healthy 50-year-old man who is holding an important job that provides him and his family upper-class status. Would osteotomy, with its unpredictable character, satisfy a 45-year-old woman, or would cup arthroplasty in an attractive 35-year-old housewife accommodate her in all of her activities? Obviously, this question must be balanced against the worst possible outcomes and potential risks involved and the theoretical objections to total hip arthroplasty in a young person. Although we are enjoying an astonishing absence of late defects in surgeries performed 10 or 11 years ago, we must still consider possible mechanical failure in the future and the risk of sepsis at present. Furthermore, based on statistics of the more successful series, no more than 95% of the operations would be successful; 1 in 20 will fail, and this should be kept in mind when recommending total hip replacement.

Only a surgeon who has acquired sound surgical skill and who keeps abreast of new revision techniques should select younger patients for total hip arthroplasty. I believe that when a surgeon selects a young patient for surgery, he must acknowledge a threefold responsibility: first, advising the patient of the potential risks involved including further intervention, if need be; second, accepting the responsibility of performing a technically perfect operation; and third, accepting the moral responsibility of an unwritten contract to provide future service should it become necessary. Therefore he must follow up each patient for as long as he and the patient believe necessary to determine whether any technical problems arise and rectify them accordingly. Ability to recognize the need for revision arthroplasty plays a vital role in the surgeon's decision to concentrate exclusively on this type of practice. It is mandatory that a surgeon involved in total hip arthroplasty commit himself to providing "maintenance operations" as needed.[9-13]

PATIENT'S DEMANDS AND PSYCHOLOGY

When a younger patient consults us about total hip replacement surgery, it is important to elicit the reasons for the consultation. Is it because of anxiety and fear of progressive disability, or is the existing problem sufficient to justify the present consultation? Often it turns out that the patient has observed a friend or heard of a person who became chairbound a few years after becoming arthritic. Clearly, many patients consult us because they have heard that the condition becomes so severe that nothing can be done about it, and they want surgery done now to preserve hip mobility. Patients in their 40s and 50s who are very active socially and demonstrate a limp, but have no severe pain, also seek surgery.

In cautioning against total hip replacement, the surgeon's reasons for refusing to operate at the time are often challenged by the patients. Considering only statistics, there is approximately a 1% to 2% death rate from this type of surgery. Mechanical failure occurs in perhaps no more than 2% (in the first 10 years) and infection in not more than 1% of the cases. Therefore the 95% success rate is a good estimate. Of course, these figures are based on results in older patients whose activities are limited, and we cannot be sure if they would apply to younger persons with more active lives. So far there is no suggestion of significant wear or tissue reaction to the prosthetic materials. Revisions of the prostheses are a possibility if excessive wear takes place. Perhaps in the next 5 to 10 years greater relaxation of the criteria for total hip replacement will be indicated and justifiable; let us bear in mind that as recently as 1967 this

operation was not recommended for anyone under 65 years of age, and we now routinely accept any patient over the age of 60 if his pain is genuine and his disability severe.

While awaiting the long-term results, within the next few years it is advisable to delay operating on active and vigorous patients who can tolerate the delay. Surgeons frequently have difficulty dissuading these patients who pressure them to go ahead with surgery, but a very candid conversation should be held citing all the potential risks and complications, including the 1% to 2% death rate. This occasionally dissuades them from insisting on surgery. Furthermore, if the patient understands the philosophy behind the postponement, and the fact that the operation may be done just as well or with better results in the future, and that techniques and materials could be improved in the meantime, he may decide to wait. To temporize with a conventional operation such as osteotomy or cup arthroplasty and then proceed with total hip replacement at a later date is a policy that is not advocated. As a rule, these patients are dissatisfied with a temporizing operation, and then we are forced to perform a total hip replacement sooner than previously anticipated (Fig. 8-9).

Another consideration in advising total hip replacement is the patient's attitude of cooperation following surgery. One of the greatest advantages of total hip arthroplasty is that only a minimum amount of cooperation from the patient is required during recovery. Nevertheless, willingness to maintain optimal body weight and avoid athletic activities may dictate the long-term survival of the artificial joint. A patient with a history of drug addiction and alcoholic avascular necrosis accompanied by obesity is socially maladjusted and not a suitable candidate for total hip replacement. These individuals are prone to falls and infection leading to failure and might best be treated by a psychiatrist prior to contemplating hip replacement. We can accept borderline psychotic or neurotic patients and have as good results as in emotionally stable patients. In the past, hysterical or neurotic patients were failures in standard operations because the procedures often required their extensive cooperation and never entirely relieved their pain. However, because it is so successful in eradicating pain, total hip replacement alters the patient's attitude remarkably, and the result is similar to that seen in a nonhysterical patient. Similarly,

221

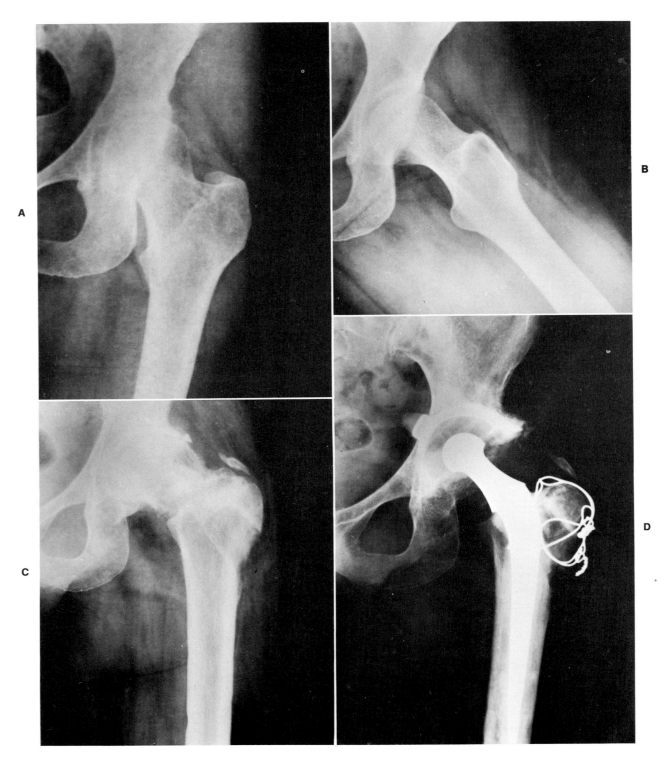

Fig. 8-9. This 34-year-old nurse was subjected to osteotomy of left hip (in another institution) for early signs of degenerative joint disease. At time of osteotomy her range of motion was good and she had only minimum discomfort necessitating occasional aspirin. **A** and **B,** Anteroposterior and lateral views of hip prior to osteotomy. Osteotomy had been performed to prevent further progression of osteoarthritis and to achieve better coverage of femoral head. **C,** Same hip 1 year after osteotomy with progression of osteoarthritis despite osteotomy. Patient indeed was worse after osteotomy, which had been done to prevent progression of osteoarthritis. Internal fixation device was removed. **D,** Because of persistent pain and inability to walk patient was forced to have total hip replacement, which successfully relieved her pain (4-year follow-up radiograph after replacement). Patient could have been well treated by conservative treatment originally and perhaps total hip replacement at her age would have not been needed.

in senile patients with borderline "senile psychosis" and a low threshold of pain, this operation remarkably improves their attitude and often prevents confinement.

TOTAL HIP REPLACEMENT IN VERY YOUNG PATIENTS

Patients under 30 years of age constitute the most difficult group in which total hip replacement is considered in view of their age and potential use of the artificial device. In this group we are not including juvenile and other types of rheumatic disease, where a built-in restriction such as a short life expectancy precludes excessive or prolonged use of the artificial device. In younger patients with traumatic unilateral disease or a unilateral slipped capital femoral epiphysis with degenerative osteoarthritis, arthrodesis is still an accepted procedure. In such an instance we must be certain that the ipsilateral knee, back, and opposite hip are unequivocally normal. In our view, mold arthroplasty or osteotomy has an extremely limited place in these cases because of the long rehabilitation required in the former and the unpredictable results in the latter. In most cases, because of severe anatomical changes, they are not applicable. There are a few rare cases of vascular necrosis without any degree of collapse of the femoral head in which prosthetic replacement may be appropriate. However, temporization and procrastination are quite possible for many of these younger patients who have a limp but not sufficient pain to justify surgical intervention. Therefore the majority of patients under age 30 with hip disability may be able to get along well with analgesics and the use of a cane for long-distance walking, although the majority must eliminate sports activities. However, because of their critical age, especially in females, the psychological pressure put on us for surgical intervention is considerable. At times, pain or deformity will be a determining factor in proceeding with surgery, especially where the patient has had one or more previous unsuccessful operations of the hip. Generally, patients with other than rheumatic conditions fall into the categories of degenerative osteoarthritis secondary to slipped femoral epiphysis, traumatic arthritis, or congenital subluxation or dislocation, leading to early degenerative osteoarthritis. An aseptic necrosis of the femoral head as a result of previous treatment or systemic conditions such as Gaucher's disease, childhood sepsis in the hip, or, as stated before, failure of previous operations, accounts for a large portion of this group.

It cannot be overemphasized that at this time total hip replacement is not a procedure to be considered for patients under 30 years of age in lieu of conventional operations. It is here that the so-called Girdlestone pseudarthrosis test is applicable; that is, if the patient is sufficiently disabled, a Girdlestone procedure might help. In such a case we might consider total hip replacement. It is extremely important that all potential risks and complications are fully discussed with the patient and his family and that the decision for surgery is shared and agreed upon. In those patients who must have something done because of severe hip disease (with little likelihood that any other type of procedure will succeed), total hip replacement may be considered, especially since repeated operations on the hip will increase the chances for sepsis and may prevent a total hip replacement at a later date. If a patient in this age group has bilateral hip disease, it is advisable to operate on one hip and postpone surgery on the opposite hip as long as possible. A combination of arthrodesis (one side) and total arthroplasty is not a good policy.

In patients between 20 and 30 years of age with local hip conditions and no systemic disease, indications for total hip replacement are extremely difficult to define at the present time. The commonest examples in this group are congenital dysplasia of the hip joint and delayed results of traumatic accidents. There is no restriction of activities in these young patients, and artificial joints would be faced with perhaps 30 to 40 years of violent trauma prior to imposition of physiological restrictions of aging. With such prolonged intense use we could not expect success comparable to that we have had with elderly patients. In these cases it is essential to consider "pseudarthrosis tests," and if resection of the neck and the head would be the only solution, then one may consider a total replacement. If, on the other hand, one would not consider a pseudarthrosis procedure, total hip replacement is not indicated. In this context, a temporizing operation that would not satisfy the patient (such as cup arthroplasty or osteotomy) might result in a premature decision for total hip replacement; whereas without surgery he

223

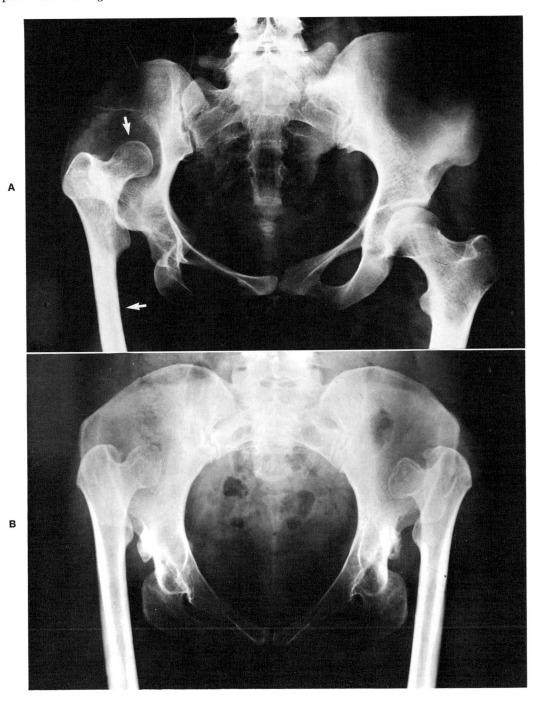

Fig. 8-10. A, Unilateral congenital hip dislocation in 26-year-old graduating medical student who has no pain and can cope well with her disability. She has no pain except for fatigue in hip and mild low back discomfort. No arthritis can be demonstrated by x-ray film (top arrow). Three-inch lift is required to compensate for short extremity. Patient is of Mediterranean extraction and an attractive young woman who wishes improvement in her appearance more than relief of pain. Because of extreme dysplasia of hip (lower arrow), especially medullary canal of femur, at her active age operation is not performed. **B,** Bilateral congenital dislocations in 32-year-old female who has no leg length discrepancy with excellent range of motion in both hips. She walks unlimited but with bilateral, symmetrical, weak gluteal lurch; she can cope well with daily living activities and is fully gainfully employed as secretary. This clinical picture is contraindication for total hip replacement at this time. Hip grades, B-right 5,5,6 and B-left 5,5,6.

224

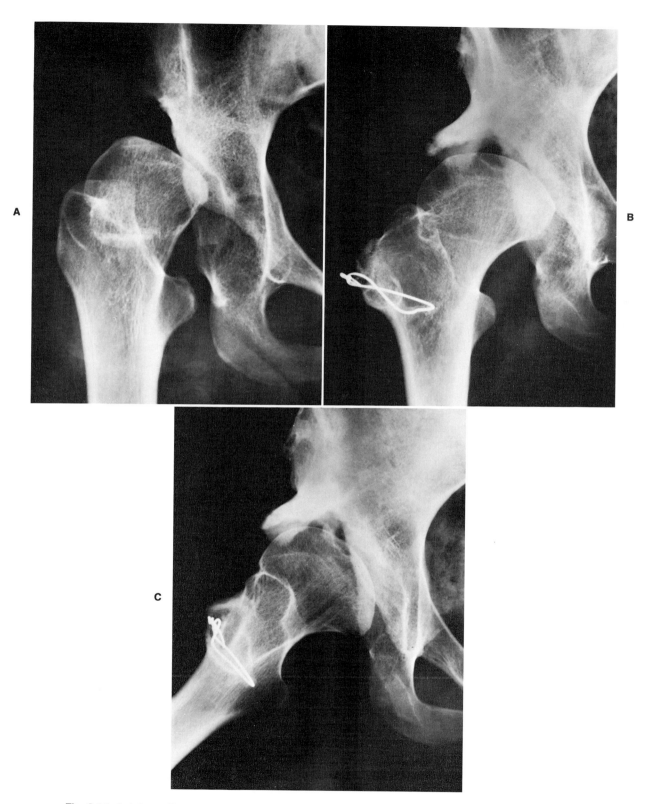

Fig. 8-11. A, Intermediate congenital dislocation in 18-year-old female with marked dysplasia in addition to low back pain, fatigue, and hip pain. Because of back pain and ipsilateral valgus knee, fusion of hip joint is not indicated. **B,** Four years following shelf procedure. **C,** Lateral view of same hip showing amount of coverage of femoral head following shelf procedure in addition to transfer of abductor muscles. Six months following surgery patient's pain had completely resolved, limp had diminished, and patient at present is very pleased with result. Hip joint has become stable and functional.

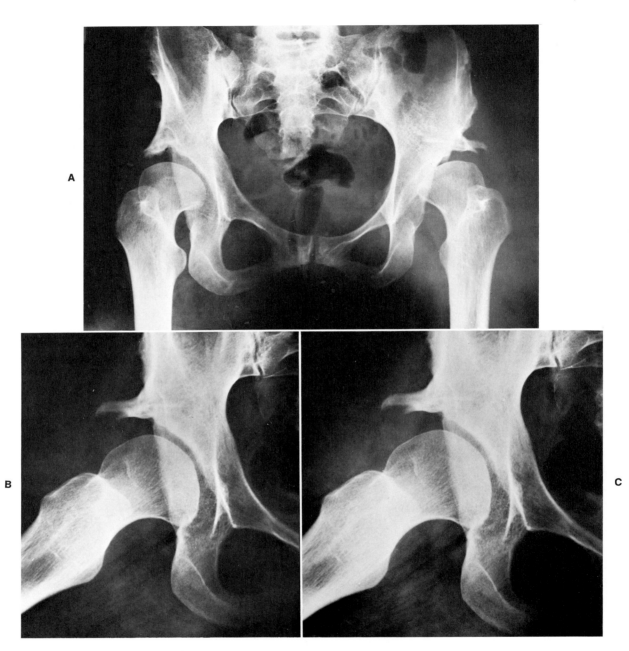

Fig. 8-12, A, Postoperative shelf procedure in 38-year-old school teacher who had her operation at age 28. Now 10 years following bilateral shelf operation, she has only minimal discomfort in hips. She has full range of motion and walks without assistance but with minor bilateral gluteus medius gait. Operation definitely reduced her symptoms and discomfort, especially in reference to fatigue and obviously development of degenerative joint disease. **B,** Lateral view of right hip. **C,** Lateral view of left hip.

could perhaps tolerate the delay until more is known about the procedure.

We hope that someday we will be able to replace hip joints in young females whose main concern is appearance rather than pain (Fig. 8-10). Patients in their teens and twenties with severe dysplasia are helped considerably by pelvic osteotomy or a shelf procedure as a temporizing measure (Figs. 8-11 and 8-12). It definitely reduces the symptoms of pain and fatigue and provides a better bony stock for subsequent replacement. Similar results may be obtained by a Chiari or Salter type pelvic osteotomy. However, it must be fully conceded that none of these procedures is definitive.

SPECIFIC CONSIDERATIONS IN TOTAL HIP REPLACEMENT
Total hip replacement in bilateral hip disease

Bilateral disability is usually more than double that from one hip; obversely, following successful unilateral surgery, many patients improve by more than 50%. A patient with one arthritic hip can frequently cope with the stiffness and pain by conservative means such as a cane and analgesics. While a single compromised hip improved with orthodox surgical methods may be entirely satisfactory, involvement of both hips makes the compromise intolerable. All activities with which one can cope with one normal hip are now curtailed, and the patient is unable to get about without crutches or two canes. At this point he usually is unable to travel to work and becomes housebound. Resting, sitting, and sleeping become difficult because any motion in one extremity affects the other. It is a well-known fact that the results of any surgical reconstructive method other than total hip replacement are poor when both hips are diseased.[30-32] Therefore treatment of bilateral hip disability is exigent. Alleviation of the affliction and confinement from two arthritic hips is one of the most challenging experiences for the hip surgeon, and the operative state must always be deliberated—not against the successful outcome, but against the patient's plight if failure occurs. Since loss of motion or fixed deformity may be of more concern than pain per se, *total disability* must be considered in advising surgery, even in patients in their 40s and 50s. Patients with some deformity of one or both hips have complaints of low back pain and frequently

knee pain as well. Although established deformity of the spine and knee from osteoarthritis is not always present, the patient's main complaint commonly is "low back pain." Extreme lumbar lordosis and marked degenerative changes in the lumbar region are often found. In females, bilateral adaption deformity interferes with perineal hygiene and sexual function. It is not uncommon for one hip to assume abduction and the other adduction. Frequent falls are a common occurrence in these patients, as they are unable to balance themselves when walking.

Bilateral surgery is performed most frequently in the following conditions:
1. Primary (idiopathic) bilateral monoarticular osteoarthritis
2. Primary generalized osteoarthritis
3. Late results of ischemic necrosis of the femoral head with secondary acetabular changes
4. Late involvement of the second hip
5. Secondary degenerative osteoarthritis of congenital dysplasia

The plan for bilateral total arthroplasty is a clinical decision not a radiological one. When the patient has symmetrically advanced degenerative changes with bilateral hip disease, it is only natural to assume that both hips may require surgery. However, as borne out by statistics, only about 25% of the patients who have this condition will need bilateral hip surgery within the first 5 years (Fig. 8-13). Consequently, it is advisable to ignore the radiological changes of the hip and recommend bilateral hip surgery only if these conditions coexist:
1. Severe flexion deformity (more than 30 degrees) of the hips
2. One hip in fixed adduction, the opposite in abduction
3. Marked shortening or severe lumbar spine deformity with degenerative changes
4. Bilateral hip disease in older patients (usually over the age of 70)
5. Progressive acetabular protrusion—especially in rheumatoid arthritis
6. Severe loss of motion as a result of ectopic bone formation following total hip replacement on the operated side
7. Correction of fixed deformity, even if the hip has been arthrodesed or is relatively pain free

227

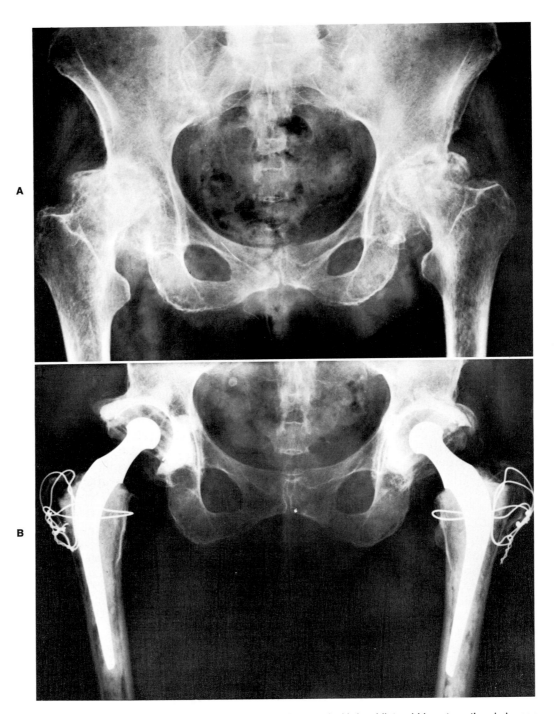

Fig. 8-13. A, This 68-year-old female retired pharmacist coped with her bilateral hip osteoarthrosis by continuous intake of steroids to alleviate pain. Preoperative grades of hip were B-right 2,3,4 and B-left 3,3,4. **B,** Following accepting surgery, two hip operations were performed within 2 weeks apart. Right hip (more symptomatic hip) was done first. Postoperative grading at 1 year following surgery was 6,6,6 on right and 6,6,6 on left.

8. Contemplated bilateral knee surgery
9. Ankylosing spondylitis, with any degree of flexion deformity
10. Low back pain and advanced degenerative osteoarthritis of the lumbar spine

If both hips have been immobile for a long time, a good range of motion may not be achieved following the first operation. It is our policy, therefore, to do the second hip operation at the same stage or soon thereafter, as the first operation may not bring about sufficient recovery of the unoperated hip, which acts as a splinting medium of the operated hip. The same policy applies to revision of a failed total hip replacement following severe ectopic bone formation.

The sequence of bilateral hip operating

In most cases one hip is less symptomatic than the other, and there is no apparent fixed deformity that might have been a determining factor for surgical intervention. So as a rule, the decision to operate on the opposite hip is postponed. On the other hand, if both hips are equally involved and painful, plans must be made for bilateral simultaneous operation or sequential operation during the same hospitalization. Barring complications, rehabilitation and recovery from one hip operation is from 10 to 14 days. On the other hand, we must bear in mind that general recovery is never complete in 2 weeks, and physical strain on the patient would be less if he were discharged and readmitted 3 to 6 months later for surgery of the opposite hip. It is psychologically stressful to the patient who has recovered from one operation to undergo a second one soon afterwards, and we have often observed the effects of this stress during the second recovery. Of course the second operation is no longer optional if the unoperated hip is a handicap following surgery.

Bilateral operation during the same anesthesia is a practical possibility, but recommended only in well-organized centers where surgical and anesthesia teams are expertly geared to deal with multitudinous operations of this type. An excellent example is the Centre for Hip Surgery at Wrightington, England, where bilateral operations are repeatedly performed during the same anesthesia. Although there are definite advantages to bilateral operations during the same anesthesia, this approach must be cautiously considered in teaching institutions and reserved for specialized centers.

In a study of bilateral low-friction arthroplasty done at Wrightington as a single operation, the duration of hospitalization for patients was 30.3 days, a few days longer than the average stay for a patient undergoing unilateral low-friction arthroplasty. It was considerably shorter than the established duration for patients undergoing bilateral hip surgery in most other institutions (including our own) in which the operations are performed as separate unilateral surgeries. The duration of hospitalization at our hospital has been approximately 5 weeks, with the second operation performed at the end of the second week. In their series, Jaffe and Charnley[27] found that there was minimal risk to the patient, and the results were very good. Nevertheless, it must be emphasized that the minimal risk to the patient is largely due to the efficient surgical team developed at a center specializing in this particular type of hip arthroplasty. At the Centre for Hip Surgery over 1,000 low-friction arthroplasties are done per year; 10% of these are bilateral and done in a single operative session, with two surgical teams often operating on the same patient successively. The rapidity of surgery, conservation of time, and minimization of blood loss cannot be realistically duplicated in a general teaching hospital. In Jaffe and Charnley's series, the remarkably good results in the 50 cases of bilateral simultaneous surgery are not surprising. The patients chosen for this procedure expect to get better since they are generally stronger, younger, and better motivated than the average patient. The patients responded well to early ambulation when the opposite hip was not slowing them down. An added benefit of the single anesthesia operations is that theoretically the patient is exposed to less risk than he would be with repeated anesthetization.

As stated before, two operations may be planned during the same hospitalization and performed with a 2-week intervention period. As a rule, the more symptomatic hip is done first (Fig. 8-13). In bilateral fixed deformity, one in adduction and one in abduction, the abducted hip must be done first. If postoperative complications arise and the second operation cannot be realized, recurrence of fixed adduction deformity of the operated hip will have been avoided. Progressive destructive hip changes in rheumatoid conditions such as protrusio acetabuli must be treated early and without undue conservatism in hopes of stopping these changes

229

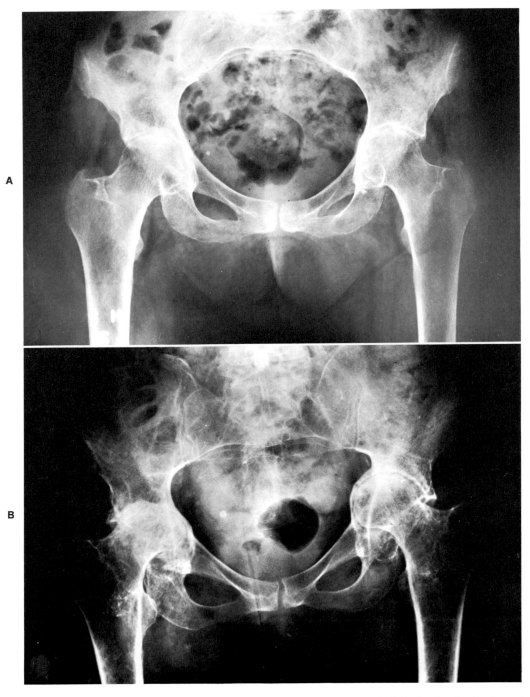

Fig. 8-14. A, Patient with rheumatoid arthritis and bilateral hip involvement. Left hip is already showing evidence of protrusio. **B,** Rapid progression of protrusio acetabuli during period between 1974 and 1975, just prior to surgery. Hip surgery was procrastinated until 1975.

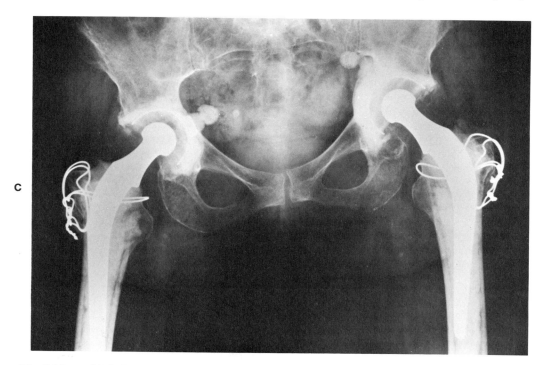

Fig. 8-14, cont'd. C, Preoperative evaluation indicated hip grading C-right 3,2,2 and C-left 3,2,2. Postoperative evaluation 1 year following surgery grading is C-right 6,4,6 and C-left 6,4,6.

(Fig. 8-14). It is important that both hips are considered for early treatment to allow preservation of muscle strength while sparing other joints. This approach also permits a lower maintenance dose of cortisone in patients undergoing steroid therapy because two major sources of inflammation (the hips) are now eliminated.

In general, when a hip is arthrodesed and in good position, it must be left alone unless disability of the low back or the ipsilateral knee forces us to "take it down." (See Chapter 14 and "Hip Stiffness and Total Hip Replacement," p. 252.)

Total hip replacement in congenital dysplasia and dislocation

Because of its largely predictable successful results, total hip replacement has been extended to the treatment of secondary osteoarthritis resulting from congenital dysplasia and dislocation of the hip. There is no treatment that can compare with a normally developed hip; but early recognition of congenital dysplasia with dislocation and efforts toward treatment and restoration during childhood present distinct advantages. Unrecognized early childhood dys-

plasia will continue to be a common cause of degenerative osteoarthritis of the hip,[22,23,41] and a large percentage of so-called idiopathic degenerative osteoarthritis may be due to insidious dysplasia hidden until much later in life. Therefore only thorough treatment of congenital dislocation of the hip in the newborn is likely to render the hip functional and prevent degenerative osteoarthritis. Even if treatment in childhood fails to achieve "perfect results," we feel that attempts should be made to reduce and locate completely dislocated hips. This is true even in older children, 8 or 9 years of age, when bilateral hip disease is present. A compromised result with a stiff hip(s) as the result of late treatment (6 to 8 years) is far better than a completely dislocated hip to manage by total hip replacement later in life when the magnitude of technical difficulties is far greater (Figs. 8-15 and 8-20).

Many young patients in their teens and twenties suffer from a limp and fatigue following activity. These patients usually do not have a true painful limp but rather a weak abductor lurch. On radiographs they may show nothing more than moderate to severe dysplasia of the

231

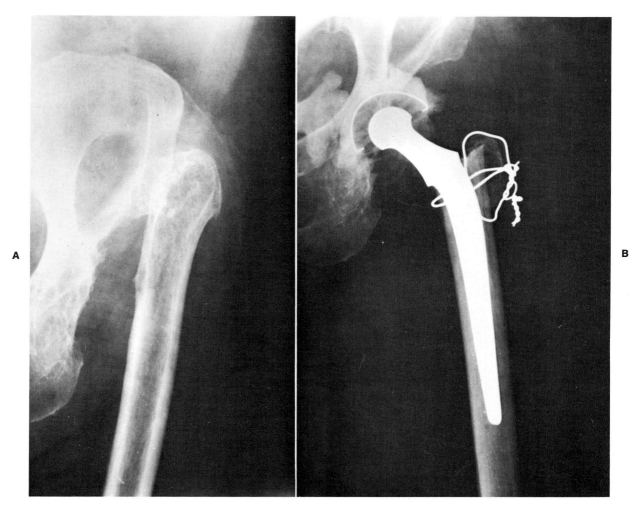

Fig. 8-15. Complete and unreduced congenital dislocation of hip without reconstructive procedures of acetabulum is relative contraindication for surgery. **A,** Unilateral dislocation in 69-year-old female with congenital dislocation of left hip. Hip graded 3,3,5 prior to surgery and patient had moderate low back pain. **B,** Immediate replacement in which portion of acetabular component was not well seated and remained uncovered because of inadequate bony roof. (Bone graft would have been beneficial.)

hip related to unrecognized congenital dysplasia of childhood or a hip inadequately treated during the developmental stage of the acetabulum and upper femur. These patients are extremely young for consideration of total hip replacement, but some form of treatment seems justifiable to temporize the situation until a total hip replacement is performed at a later date. A Salter osteotomy, Chiari osteotomy of the pelvis, or an upper femoral varus derotation osteotomy may be indicated based on the principal anatomical pathology. A number of reports have appeared in the literature suggesting that these procedures are valuable in reducing the symptoms and providing patients several years of comfort,

but with no guarantee of permanent effects. The operation we favor and have performed on a number of occasions is a shelf procedure, which is a less radical approach than the Chiari or other types of osteotomy; we have found it very effective in reducing the symptoms of discomfort and fatigue in these young patients (Figs. 8-11 and 8-12). Rehabilitation is generally quick, and the early results have been most rewarding.

When there is good functioning, radiological evidence of dysplasia (even with minor to moderate osteoarthritis) does not necessarily indicate surgery. These patients should be encouraged to delay surgery until their disability becomes

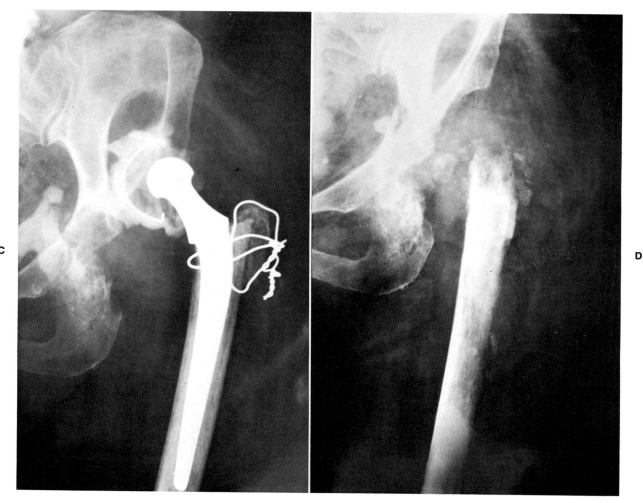

Fig. 8-15, cont'd. C, Spontaneous detachment of acetabular component 2 months following surgery. **D,** Hip was converted to Girdlestone pseudarthrosis after removal of artificial device.

more severe. This applies specifically to young patients who wish to be active but are hampered by the precarious hip. With dysplasia, on the other hand, there is no disagreement that congenital subluxation and dysplastic hips with degenerative osteoarthritis should be treated as general indications for total hip replacement. Generally, intermediate and high dislocations technically lend themselves well to hip replacement (Fig. 8-16), and where severe disability exists, surgery is indicated. However, reconstruction may be formidable or impossible on completely dislocated, unreduced hips without evidence of any development of the acetabulum and with marked dysplasia. Even where a new acetabulum could be created and inserted, it remains doubtful whether the shortened abductor

muscles would allow downward displacement of the abductor mechanism. It is fortunate that the contact between the upper end of the femur and the acetabulum has been minimal throughout life in these patients, and there is no true "constrainment osteoarthritis" with a main complaint of shortening and a gross limp. When hips have been bilaterally dislocated throughout life and no false acetabulum has formed, leg length is equal and back pain usually is not significant. Like Charnley, we feel that this type of patient should be discouraged from having surgery because of the obvious technical problems and because they may be subjected to a dangerous operation without improvement of the basic problem, that is, the limp, which is generally related to underdeveloped adductor muscles.

233

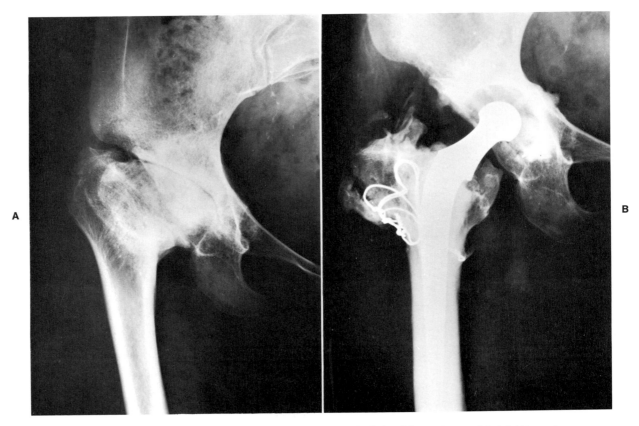

Fig. 8-16. Generally, intermediate and high dislocations technically lend themselves well to total hip replacement despite shallow socket; floor permits adequate deepening allowing insertion of prosthesis. **A,** Unilateral congenital subluxation of hip with high-riding greater trochanter. **B,** Postoperative view of same patient 5 years following total hip replacement with excellent recovery. Preoperative grading of hip, A-3,4,3; postoperatively, A-6,6,6. NOTE: marked improvement of cortex as result of excellent function.

Harris[23] and Tronzo[43] have attempted reconstruction in cases of untreated complete dislocation of the hips with early success. In our experience, a completely dislocated hip (usually a unilateral condition where marked leg discrepancy exists) is a problem, especially when a very young woman (usually in her 20s) or an older person (60 or 70) seeks advice and demands surgery. The young woman, usually unmarried, finds her hip a serious cosmetic as well as physical handicap; the older person suffers from degenerative arthritis elsewhere (for example, contralateral knee or spinal deformity with osteoarthritis). Both patients present serious implications; the former is excessively active, and the latter may not be able to withstand a major reconstructive procedure involving bone grafting, delayed ambulation, and so on.

Reconstructive surgery in congenital dislocation and dysplasia is not difficult, but it requires special attention and experience with total hip replacement technique. Surgeons should postpone the decision to perform this operation until they are altogether familiar with its details, usually not before considerable experience in total hip surgery.

At present we can categorically state that arthrodesis, osteotomy, and arthroplasty are not suitable alternatives to total hip replacement. Arthrodesis in women is undesirable, and a varus or displaced osteotomy may aggravate an already significantly shortened extremity. Mold arthroplasty results are not satisfactory because of the lack of bony stock in the acetabulum and excessive anteversion of the femoral neck. In the past such operations yielded poorer results than total hip replacement in younger individuals. Early results of total hip replacement for congenital subluxation and dislocation have been extremely encouraging. Nonetheless,

234

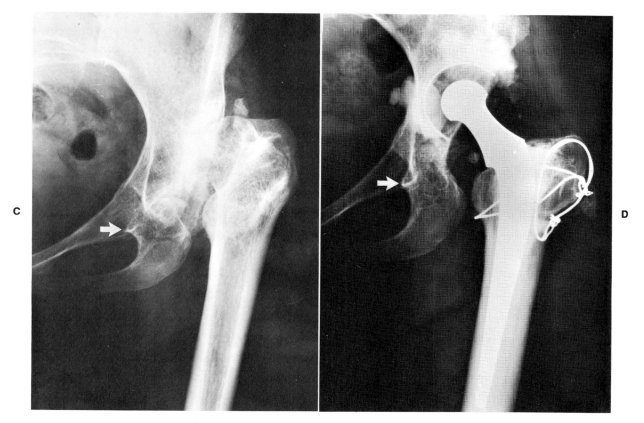

Fig. 8-16, cont'd. C, Preoperative radiograph of unilateral hip dysplasia with marked dysplasia of socket but good bone stock at floor of acetabulum. Arrow points to inner wall of pelvis (teardrop and thickened floor). **D,** Same hip as in **C,** with optimum deepening and seating of acetabulum, component in slightly higher position as compared with **A** and **B** (see Chapter 13). Preoperative grading, A-4,4,3; postoperatively, A-6,6,5.

selection of patients must be done with special care because of the age factor and the possibility of a persisting defective abductor mechanism and a permanent limp. The 22-mm. Charnley femoral head has proven superior to others for this particular purpose, but there is no warranty of lifelong fixation of the socket, especially if it is subjected to vigorous physical activity. Further technical and mechanical complications must always be borne in mind, considering the degree of disability in this particular group of patients.

Chronic suppurative and tuberculous arthritis

As stated elsewhere (see Chapter 6), osteomyelitis is a contraindication to total hip replacement. An exception to this rule may be considered if the infection occurred in childhood or adolescence with complete resolution without evidence of local or systemic recurrence. In this regard old pyogenic arthritis is manifested radiologically as primary osteoarthritis, and only occasionally is there a scar or adherent sinus formation about the hip indicating an early life problem. As a general rule, we maximize "once the bone has been infected, always infected" and select these cases for surgery with caution. This is particularly true in the case of a previously tuberculous hip that has been quiescent for many years. It is justifiable to treat these patients prophylactically with antibiotics and consider prolonged postoperative coverage with antituberculosis drugs (Fig. 8-17). We have performed hip replacements in many patients with a previous history of childhood or adolescent infections with no subsequent reactivation of infection following replacement surgery (Figs. 8-18 and 8-19).

235

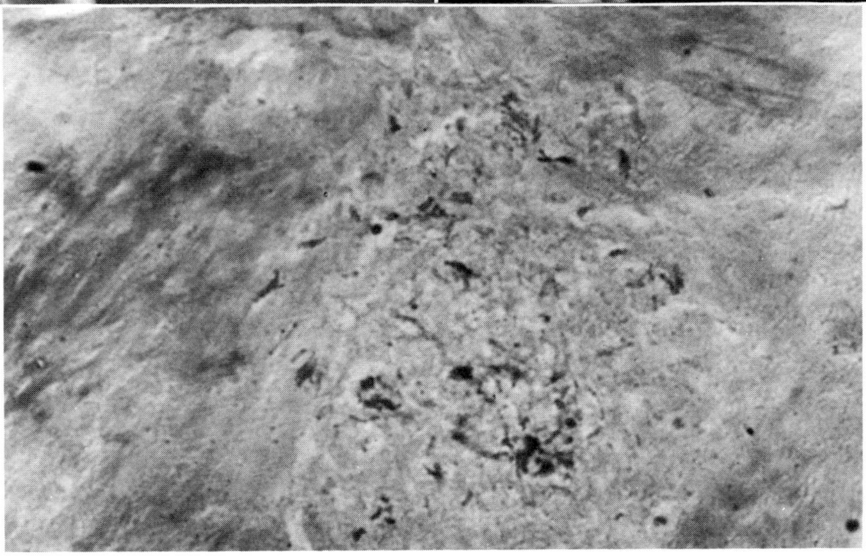

Fig. 8-17. Preoperative, **A,** and 4-year postoperative, **B,** radiographs of 65-year-old woman whose hip was fused at age 15. Fifty years after hip fusion because of low back pain and ipsilateral knee pain with valgus deformity, it was necessary to convert hip fusion to total hip replacement. Original hip fusion had been performed for tuberculosis. Following total arthroplasty pain from back was relieved and knee condition improved, but finally knee arthrodesis was indicated. It is of special interest that 50 years after hip fusion for tuberculosis acid-fast bacillus was recovered from hip, **C.**

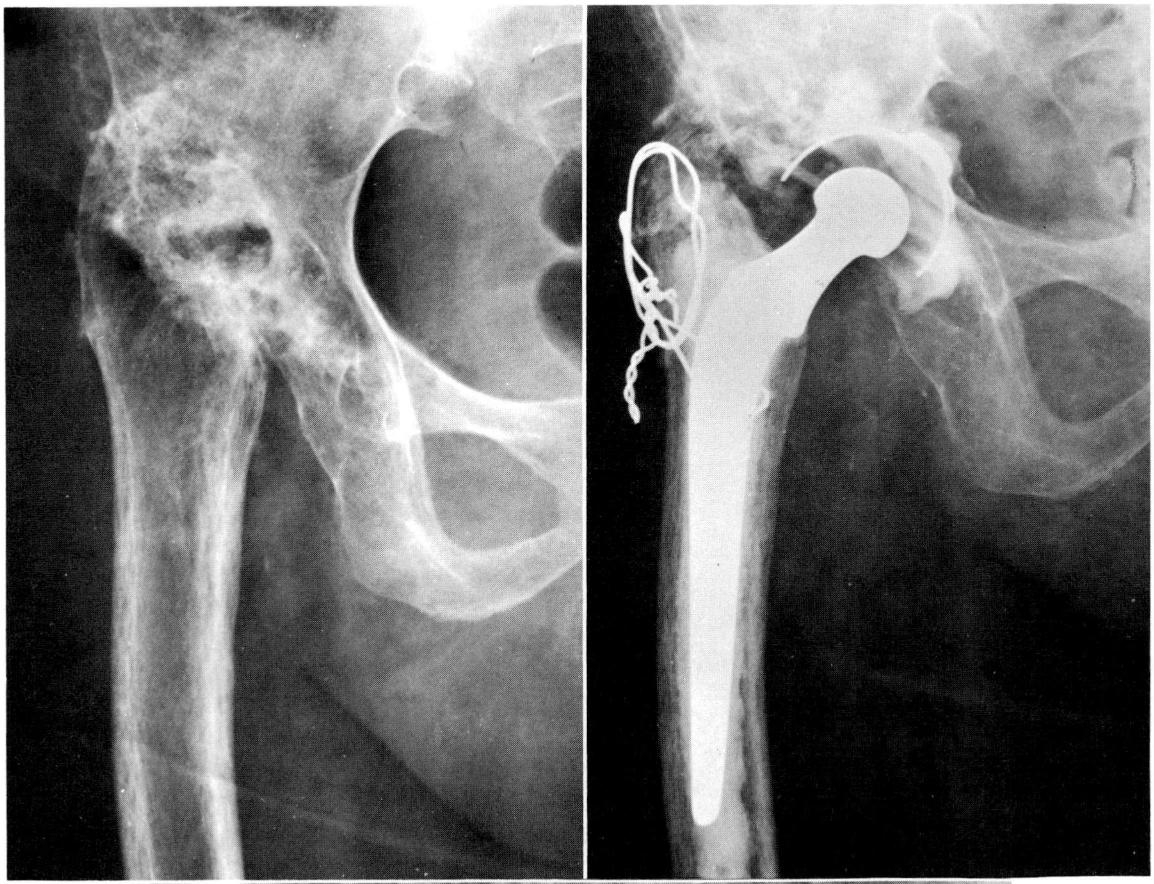

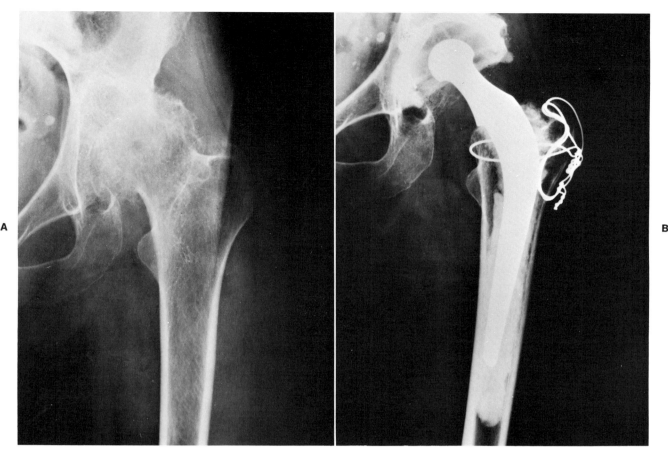

Fig. 8-18. A, Preoperative radiograph of 48-year-old woman with septic hip at age 12. Original infective organism was staphlococci and several scarred chronic sites of drainage from hip were present. Sedimentation rate was within normal range, and there was no evidence of infection for over 36 years. Preoperative grading of the hip was A-3,4,2. **B,** Five-year postoperative radiographic improvement was A-6,6,6. Patient received prophylactic antibiotics during surgery and 3 months postoperatively. No organism was cultured from hip following surgery.

Scoliosis and total hip replacement

In many instances total hip replacement may become necessary in an arthritic hip accompanying an old unrecognized or untreated scoliosis in the lumbar or lumbosacral spine. The preexisting scoliosis usually leads to pelvic obliquity, often exaggerating the limp and causing deformity and complete decompensation. Usually the hip disease in these individuals is unilateral. The affected hip is on the concave side of the lumbar or lumbosacral curve and higher than the opposite side. The hip on the convex side is well located (in abduction); the affected hip consequently assumes the position of adduction with marked subluxation. Treatment is particularly indicated in these individuals because

of extreme shortening produced by the fixed adduction deformity, which cannot be compensated because the lumbar spine is fixed by secondary osteoarthritis. Early surgery may be indicated because of difficulty in walking and/or extreme stress and strain in the lumbosacral region contributing to severe back pain. It is best to consider replacement without any aim toward equalization, since deformity of the spine is often fixed and further elongation of the limb may place further strain on the lumbar area leading to further decompensation. When the accompanying spinal deformity is equally painful to the patient, spinal arthrodesis prior to hip surgery may be suggested. On the other hand, we often consider surgery of the hip the

237

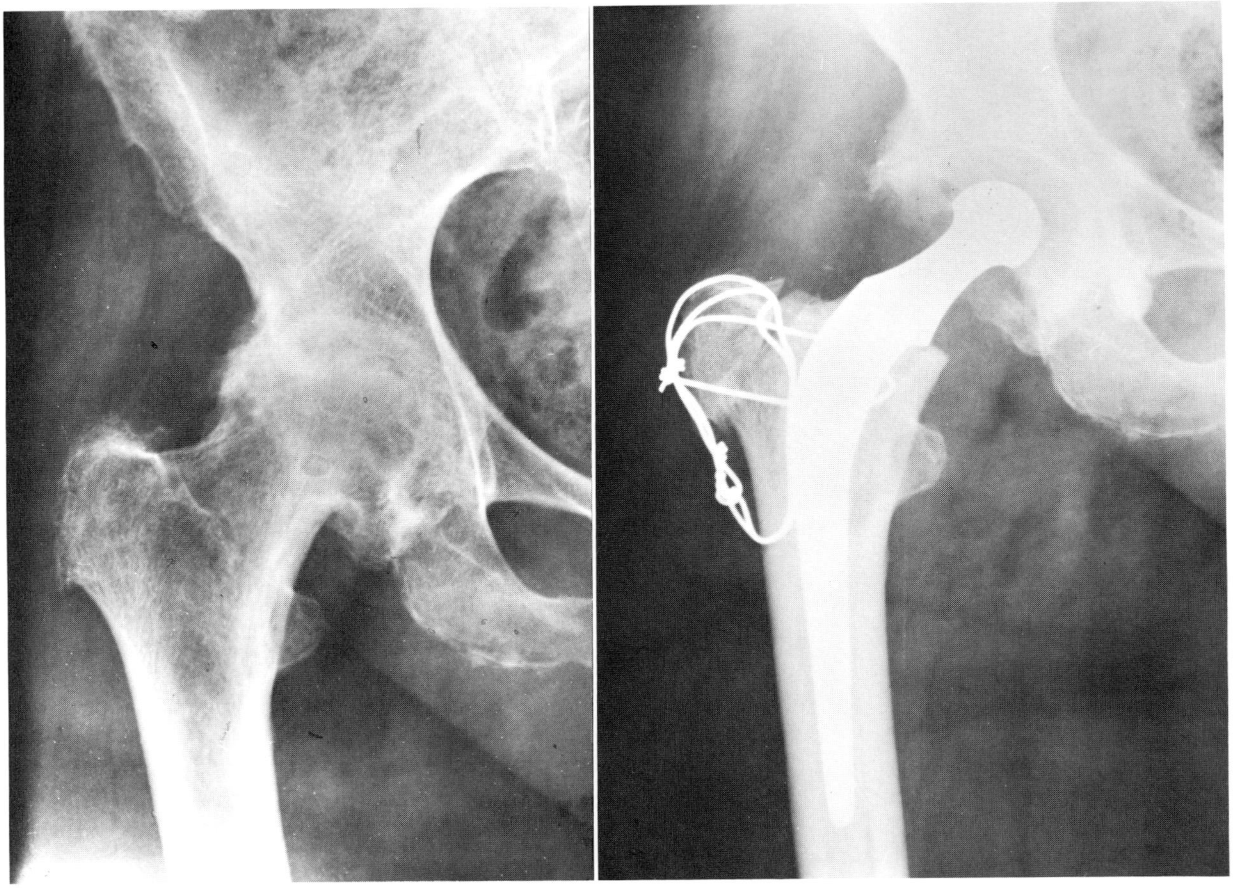

Fig. 8-19. There should be no concern in performing total hip replacement in cases of hematogenous child-hood infections. In this 55-year-old woman with drainage at age 2, only small old scar was present postero-lateral to greater trochanter. Sedimentation rate was normal without any history of drainage since childhood. **A,** Preoperative radiograph of right hip shows it to be completely ankylosed. Grading A-5,3,1. **B,** Three-year postoperative grading, right hip 6,5,6.

ultimate solution where spinal strain will be alleviated following total hip replacement.

Systemic disease and total hip replacement

In many conditions such as sickle cell disease, lupus erythematosus, Gaucher's disease, and disseminated avascular necrosis of the bone, the general systemic disease leads to destructive changes of the hip necessitating mechanical replacement. Because in most instances life expectancy is shorter than normal, age is not a factor in patient selection. However, the outcome of total hip replacement might be somewhat in jeopardy because of abnormal bone (Fig. 8-20), and progressive loosening or per-

sistent pain might occur despite total hip arthroplasty. True indications for surgical procedure are derived from weighing the disability of the patient against the systemic conditions leading to impairment of the hip (Fig. 8-21).

Rare congenital and developmental conditions

A number of congenital and developmental conditions such as multiple epiphyseal dysplasia, coxa vara, and osteopetrosis may eventually require mechanical replacement because of secondary arthritic changes in the hip. These conditions are rare but may present idiosyncratic anatomical changes requiring specific preparation and handling at surgery. For example, a

238

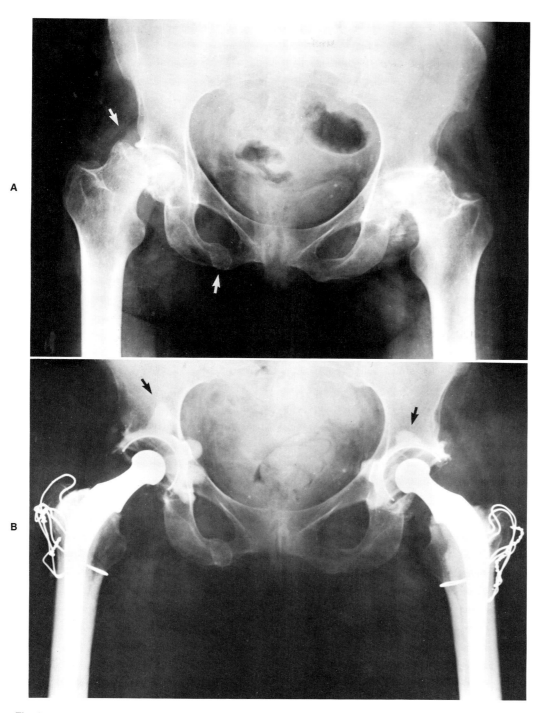

Fig. 8-20. A, Preoperative radiograph of hips in 26-year-old female with sickle cell disease. Patient was chairbound at time of surgery in view of spontaneous fracture of femoral neck. Top arrow shows acute fracture of head. Bottom arrow shows fracture through ilioischial ramus. **B,** Postoperative radiograph showing satisfactory clinical results of arthroplasty despite patient's complaint of pain in both hips. Sedimentation rate was within normal limit and patient had no indication of infection. It is possible that bone infarction within region of hip and spontaneous microfractures in area of pelvis are responsible for cause of pain. Preoperative grades of hip were C-right 1,2,2 and C-left 1,2,2; postoperative assessment, C-right 4,4,6 and C-left 4,4,6.

239

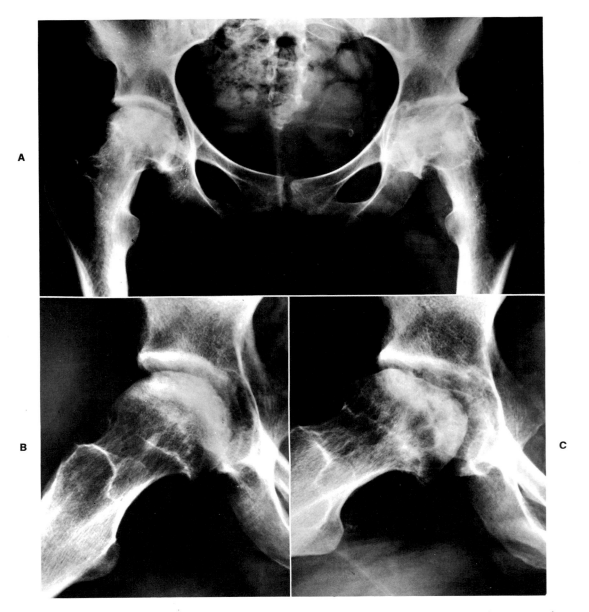

Fig. 8-21. Cortisone-induced bilateral avascular necrosis in 21-year-old female who received short course of high-dose cortisone for cerebral hemorrhage. At present time patient is fully functional, has only minimum discomfort in hips, and is happily married. Despite extensive radiological changes, no surgical intervention is being contemplated. Grading of hips is B-5,5,5 bilaterally. **A,** Anteroposterior view of hips. **B,** Lateral view of right hip. **C,** Lateral view of left hip.

patient with coxa vara may present technical problems similar to congenital dysplasia: a shortened femur neck and high-riding of the upper femur. In those instances where multiple joints are involved, the perspective of total function and the patient's activities must also be considered.

Hemophilia and total hip replacement

Because of recent advances in the management of hemophilia, surgery with acceptable risk has become a reality for these patients.[16] As cited in the discussion of perioperative management in Chapters 9 and 11, proper indication and care of these individuals must be coordinated with an interested hematologist who can determine the degree of severity and the risks involved. Reported extensive experiences with hemophiliac patients undergoing total hip replacement from Oxford, England and other centers are most encouraging.[16]

Charcot's joint of tabes dorsalis

The neurological imbalance and lack of sensitivity of these patients make total arthroplasty unsuitable to perform. Frequent complications such as dislocation make this operation contraindicated in neurotrophic joints. Isolated reports of replacement with subsequent dislocation support this conclusion.[9] Because of lack of pain, patients with Charcot's joint may be treated conservatively in most instances; in fractures of the hip, a simple prosthetic replacement is advantageous and preferable to total replacement.

Neurovascular conditions and total hip replacement

At times a difficult decision must be reached as to whether a patient with an osteoarthritic hip with vascular compromise of the lower extremity should have a total hip replacement or not. There are two main concerns: (1) If the patient subsequently becomes more active, the severity of vascular compromise will be enhanced (in effect, removal of the safety valve), and claudication and vascular compromise will prevent use of the corrected hip. (2) If the vascular condition of the extremity would be further jeopardized, ischemia may develop and result in loss of the limb. It is of paramount importance that a vascular surgeon be consulted in these situations and a mature decision reached after complete evaluation of potentials and vascular re-

serve of the limb. If, indeed, claudication is present despite limited activities, total hip replacement is contraindicated since improved activities would only deteriorate the vascular compromise of the limb. If arteriosclerotic disease of the extremity is well tolerated despite absent dorsalis pedis pulse (but with good posterior tibialis pulse) without dystrophy of the skin of the toes, total hip replacement may be considered. At times, vascular repair such as arterial bypass may be performed prior to the contemplated surgery (Fig. 8-22). Venous flow and venous stasis may present difficulties following total hip replacement, especially in older people with diabetes. This unfortunate situation can compromise the results of arthroplasty because of persistent trophic ulcers of the lower leg following surgery.

Paralytic neurological conditions in an extremity should be carefully evaluated and no replacement surgery contemplated if there are imbalanced muscles or atonia about the hip. A case in point would be a long-standing palsied hip in which the flexors and adductors are overacting against weak abductors and extensors. Obviously in these situations instability of the hip and dislocation may be anticipated. In contrast to neurological imbalance of the ipsilateral limb, an affected contralateral hip or knee is no contraindication for hip surgery. Patients with prior poliomyelitis or other peripheral neuropathies may be extremely benefitted by total replacement of the opposite hip. However, it must be recognized that the involved opposite hip will place a considerable burden on the operated side (Fig. 8-23), and it might be a good idea to suggest continued use of a walking aid for these patients.

Bone tumors, tumorous conditions, and total hip replacement

A considerable number of primary and metastatic lesions may involve the hip joint, and part or all of the joint may be replaced following elimination of the tumorous condition. The goal here is to eradicate the tumor and cure the patient, then consider hip joint reconstruction for improved function. The former is a lifesaving procedure, and the latter is obviously secondary to the primary goal. In the past, lack of interest in replacing the upper femur was related to difficulty in securing prosthetic components to the pelvis and femur. But because of advances in

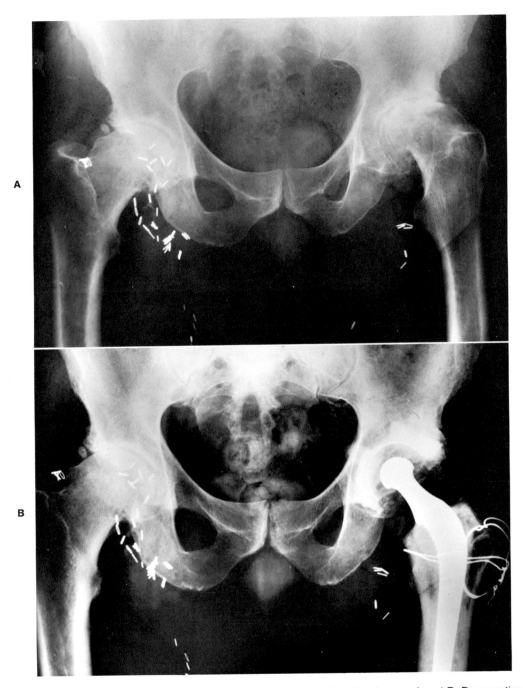

Fig. 8-22. Examples of arterial disease accompanied by degenerative joint disease. **A** and **B,** Preoperative and postoperative radiographs of 64-year-old man with bilateral degenerative osteoarthrosis. When patient was originally seen, he demonstrated bilateral claudication as result of arteriosclerosis and compromise of blood supply to lower extremities. Following bilateral arterial bypass 1 year later, left total hip replacement was performed, which was uneventful postoperatively.

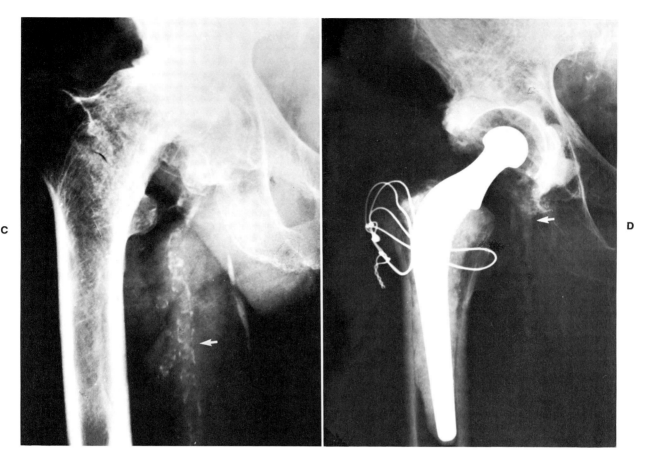

Fig. 8-22, cont'd. C, Preoperative radiograph of hip in 74-year-old mildly hypertensive patient with extensive atheroma (arrow). **D,** Three-year postoperative radiograph of same patient. Presence of atheroma on radiograph is not contraindication for surgery.

total hip surgery, several attempts have been made to reconstruct the pelvis or upper femur following segmental resection of bone and soft tissue in this area.[36,38] En bloc resection of a tumor depends on the aggressiveness of the tumor, the patient's age, and the feasibility of resection; obviously, radical resection or amputation must not be compromised because of advances in total hip replacement and feasibility of such a procedure. An occasional metastatic lesion of the upper femur may be satisfactorily replaced by total hip arthroplasty, but again, the alternate modes of treatment must be considered before advising a major undertaking such as reconstruction of the upper femur and the hip with total hip replacement. Periosteal osteogenic sarcoma and low-grade, primary malignant bone tumors (for example, giant cell tumors) may be considered for en bloc resection. Improvement in function makes total arthroplasty an attrac-

tive mode of treatment, especially because of quick recovery and rehabilitation following this procedure. Nonetheless, there are numerous surgical technical considerations that make replacement less than optimal in all cases.[36,38] (For details of technique for hip replacement in tumorous conditions, see Chapter 13.)

Avascular necrosis and total hip replacement

Osteonecrosis of the femoral head as a result of traumatic conditions, such as fracture of the neck of the femur or dislocation of the hip, is a well-known problem that is observed in many older patients as well as young persons following traumatic conditions of the hip.

The patients with nontraumatic avascular necrosis are usually young and suffer from bilateral hip disease. Often an underlying cause for avascular necrosis may be determined, such

243

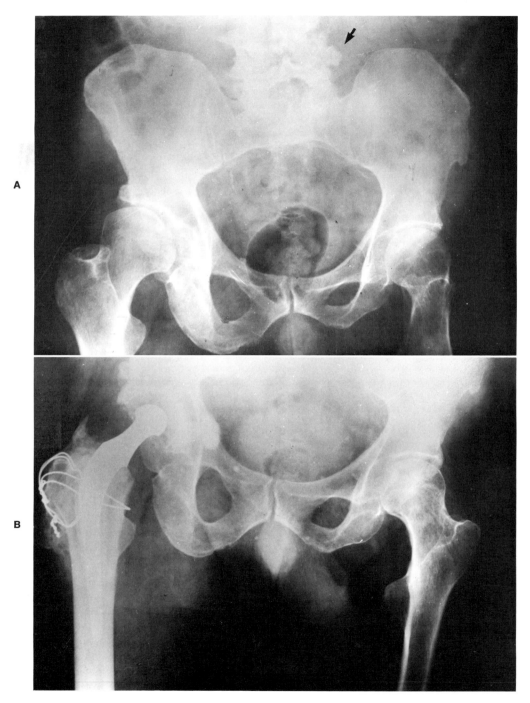

Fig. 8-23. Fifty-six–year-old male with long-standing postpolio paralysis of left lower extremity and marked atrophy. **A,** He developed severe pain in left hip and lumbar spine due to scoliosis and degenerative arthritis (arrow). Preoperative grading of hips on right was C-3,3,4 but left was C-6,3,6. Two inches of shortening were present on left side. **B,** Following total hip replacement patient continued to use cane, but pain was relieved both from hip and back. Postoperative grading was C-6,4,5.

as alcoholism, steroid medications, and blood dyscrasia, and patients with renal transplants receiving immunosuppressive drugs are seen with increasing frequency in orthopaedic practice. The so-called idiopathic avascular necrosis, usually presenting itself as a unilateral hip condition with ultimate bilateral involvement, may be seen in very young patients. In the routine practice of a hip surgeon a startling number of patients are seen without any evidence of joint narrowing on radiographs and only minimal or no changes of the femoral head as evidenced by increased radiodensity of the femoral head, but extreme degrees of pain are sustained by the patient during rest as well as with activity. The problem is often compounded by the lack of underlying conditions and the young age of the person subjected to the treatment, especially when augmented by the absence of symptoms of the opposite hip and an unknown fate regarding development of avascular necrosis of the opposite hip.

When patients are seen early, prevention of subchondral fracture with collapse of the head leading to osteoarthrosis is the prime goal, particularly in young patients. In past attempts conservative management, including weight reduction by crutches, has rarely been successful. Treatment by surgical intervention, bone grafting, or osteotomy has remained controversial. It is now commonly agreed that if subchondral fracture is evident and the sphericity of the head is lost, there is no point in attempting bone grafting or osteotomy. On the other hand, in very early stages (stage 1 or 2), especially in very young patients, bone grafting or osteotomy might be of some value.[5-7,35,39] However, with subchondral bone fracture or any evidence (radiological changes) of collapse of the femoral head, a total arthroplasty is indicated. The major question often confronting us is whether one should replace the femoral head alone by hemiarthroplasty, such as insertion of a femoral head prosthesis, or whether a total hip replacement should be performed. To verify this question we must address ourselves to the question of indications of hemiarthroplasty at the present time. Then, by exclusion of hemiarthroplasty, bone grafting, and osteotomy, indications for total hip replacement become clear.

Hemiarthroplasty vs. total arthroplasty.[18a] At the present time, it is commonly agreed by most surgeons that hemiarthroplasty must be re-

served for treating femoral neck fractures in older persons where the acetabulum is normal. The traumatic conditions such as fracture dislocation of the femoral neck, comminuted fractures that cannot be reduced, pathological fractures, fractures poorly reduced at surgery, Pauwell type III (vertical) fractures, fractures whose treatment was delayed for several days, and fractures not suitably fixed by nailing or that fell apart after nailing must be considered for prosthetic replacement of the femoral head. Most surgeons now accept patients whose average age is 75 years for replacement of the femoral head alone. In addition to the traumatic conditions listed, patients with Parkinson's disease or severe osteoporosis and patients with a limited life expectancy may be considered for prosthetic replacement. There are some orthopaedic surgeons who have advocated treating all fractures of the femoral neck in patients past the age of 65. The reason is the high incidence of nonunion and avascular necrosis that often results in these patients when the fragments are fixed internally by nailing. While it is true that fracture of the neck of the femur is usually prone to such complications as nonunion and avascular necrosis, especially when there is displacement, the fact remains that in a good many of these cases there is successful union after internal fixation and that avascular necrosis does not develop. Nor can the fact be overlooked that no prosthetic replacement can ever be as good as the patient's own femoral head.

In this context, Boyd and Salvatore[7a] for more than a year followed 160 patients with acute displaced fractures of the femoral neck. These patients had sustained fractures (Pauwell types II and III) and were treated by nailing. Ideal results—sound union without avascular necrosis—were obtained in 56% of the cases. In only 18% was a second operation necessary, and in nearly all instances it entailed the insertion of a prosthesis. If these results may be taken as being at all representative, the routine treatment of all femoral neck fractures by prosthetic replacement would certainly sacrifice the 56% of the cases that could be successfully resolved by internal fixation.

The argument for the routine use of the prosthetic replacement is weakened even more when the results of primary and secondary procedures utilizing the prostheses are compared. The Campbell Clinic has reported 85% good-to-

245

excellent results in the use of primary prosthetic replacement in femoral neck fractures[7a]; Moore[33] and Stinchfield and co-workers[42] have reported similar results. In patients who were treated secondarily by a prosthetic replacement at the Campbell Clinic, 71% had good-to-excellent results in cases of nonunion, and 79.5% had good-to-excellent results in cases of avascular necrosis.[7a] The wide difference in the results between the primary and secondary patients, therefore, does not seem to justify the routine use of a prosthesis in preference to nailing.

From our own experiences, we believe that prosthetic replacement of the femoral head must be reserved for those patients whose fractures cannot be reduced, who have conditions that may limit ambulation, or who will not be satisfactorily handled by internal fixation of their fractures. The prosthesis may be used when a fracture is more than 1 week old or in cases of subcapital fractures in aged patients. On occasion, when closed reduction is not possible, it is advisable to use an open reduction and nailing in a very young and active patient and prosthetic replacement in a less active individual. We believe that fractures of the femoral neck or head associated with dislocation always deserve primary prosthetic replacement. Naturally, with any degree of acetabular damage associated with these injuries, total hip arthroplasty must be considered; however, there is no place for the routine use of total hip replacement in treatment of fractures of the femoral neck.

Hip fractures and total hip replacement

Total hip arthroplasty has a very limited place at the present time in the treatment of fresh femoral neck fractures. It may be considered

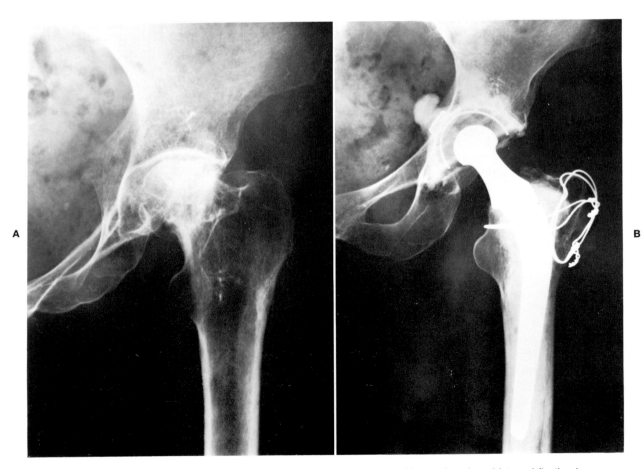

Fig. 8-24. A, Avascular necrosis of femoral head following fracture of femoral neck and internal fixation in 73-year-old female. Nail had been previously removed. **B,** Postoperative status following total hip replacement. NOTE: femoral head collapse but only minor acetabular changes. Hemiarthroplasty is contraindicated in this situation. Preoperative grade was A-3,3,4; postoperative, A-6,6,6.

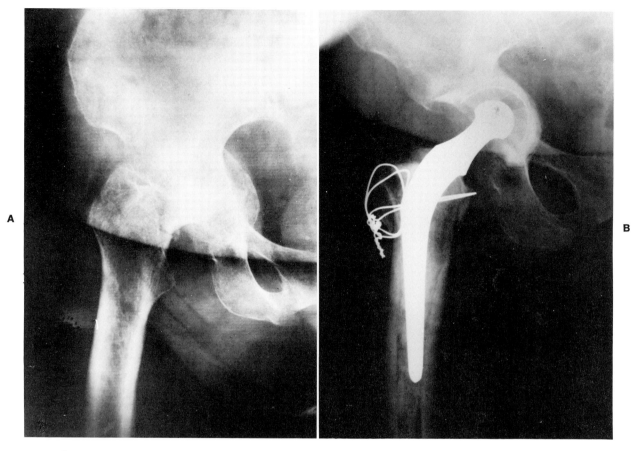

Fig. 8-25. A, Fractured neck of femur in 64-year-old woman with rheumatoid arthritis and severe protrusio acetabuli. **B,** Primary total hip replacement was performed in view of preexisting arthritis in hip joint.

only in the following situations:

1. When the acetabular lesion is present either as the result of primary treatment or collapse of the femoral head following avascular necrosis with acetabular involvement (Fig. 8-24)
2. A hip fracture in patients with rheumatoid arthritis (Fig. 8-25)
3. Existing osteoarthritis of the hip
4. Pathological conditions such as Paget's disease
5. Systemic conditions, such as lupus erythematosus complicated by fracture (Fig. 8-20)
6. Porosis of the acetabulum as the result of prolonged non-weight bearing (Figs. 8-26 and 8-27)

Let us now consider the interesting, and yet provocative, issue of simple femoral head replacement vs. total replacement in treating cases of fractures of the femoral neck. In about 20% to 30% of fractures treated by replacement of the femoral head, there is pain caused by proximal migration of the prosthesis. Therefore it is argued that if the migration of the prosthesis is to be prevented, it is necessary to eliminate the involvement of the acetabulum by cementing a socket into the acetabulum prophylactically; this has been advocated by some surgeons in preference to hemiarthroplasty for the fracture of the femoral neck. Their argument is that with total hip replacement a good result can be anticipated in better than 95% of the cases, while with the simple femoral head replacement a good result can be anticipated in no more than 70% to 80% of the cases. They further argue that the life expectancy of total hip replacements is now clearly within the range of 10 to 15 years (for an older person), whereas the length of time that one can expect good per-

247

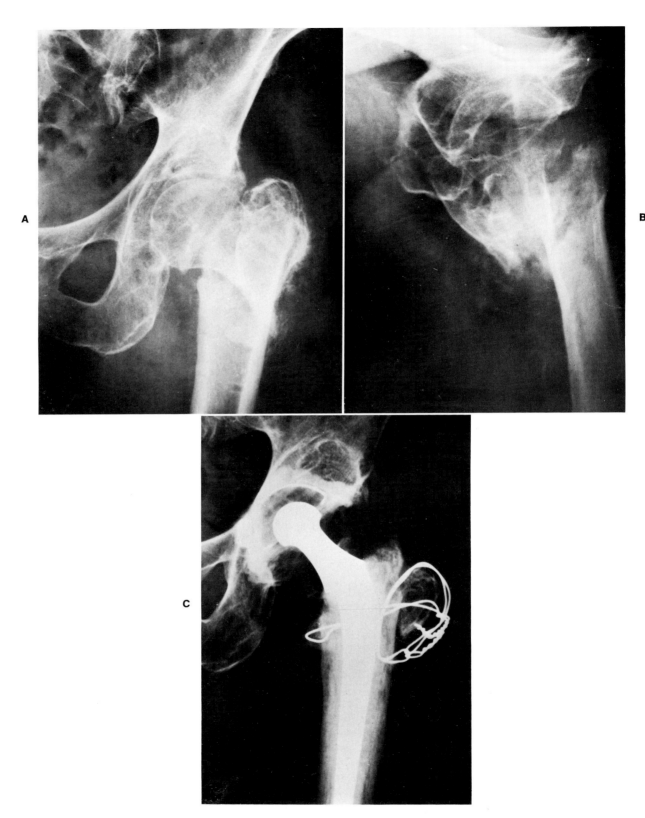

Fig. 8-26. A, Intertrochanteric fracture of neck of femur extending to shaft has been treated elsewhere by internal fixation and its subsequent removal. Patient had been kept non-weight bearing for approximately 6 months following removal of plate. **B,** Amount of displacement of fracture but no evidence of union at fracture site. Hemiarthroplasty is contraindicated because of severe osteoporosis, and lack of articular cartilage nourishment during non-weight-bearing period. **C,** Postoperative total hip replacement.

248

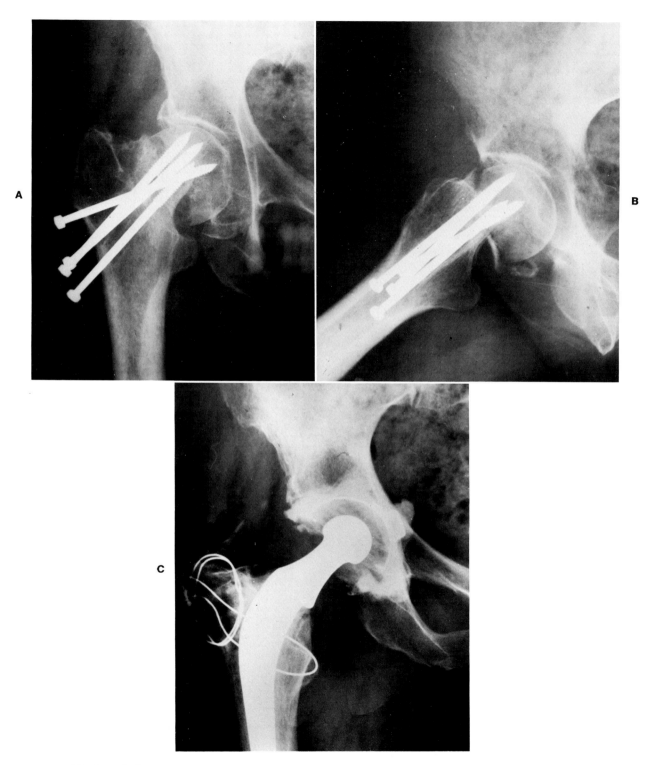

Fig. 8-27. A, Anteroposterior view. **B,** Lateral view of 63-year-old female 15 months following fracture fixation. NOTE: good joint space but severe osteoporosis (see text). **C,** Six years following total hip arthroplasty for nonunion of neck of femur.

formance from a femoral head replacement is not clearly known.

Despite this argument, we believe that while there is a definite place for primary total hip replacement in femoral neck fractures with certain provisions, there is, as yet, no justification for the universal and routine application of this particular method in view of the following reasons:

1. The fate of materials and methods of application in this rather extensive procedure in patients who may live longer is not clearly known.

2. Adequate organization to undertake such a major procedure in large volume does not exist at the present time.

3. Routine application of the procedure would require specially equipped centers and trained personnel to cope with the number of fractures that would have to be treated.

4. Considering the incidence of fractures of the neck of the femur in New York City alone, perhaps several specialized centers would be needed in one city alone to cope with fractures requiring total hip replacement.

5. Inherent complications of total hip replacement should not be taken lightly, particularly in the very debilitated, elderly patient sustaining these fractures.

6. The implants available for total hip replacement are usually too large in size to be accommodated in a healthy acetabulum. It is a fortunate coincidence that in arthritic hips the acetabulum is larger than in normal, nonarthritic cases.

7. If we can reduce and treat a femoral neck fracture by the simple method of nailing, most fractures of the hips are amenable to this much simpler treatment; healing will ensue without incident, and a normal hip joint will result.

There are situations where total hip replacement may be recommended as a primary procedure. However, the indications are limited to the following: extreme osteoporosis of the acetabulum as the result of unrecognized fracture and/or displaced femoral head or where weight bearing has not taken place for some time.

In treating common fractures, such as femoral neck fractures, and in reviewing available information on the overall management, I can only conclude that there is agreement that there is no complete substitute for the normal, natural femoral head; that prosthetic replacement procedure of any kind, whether hemiarthroplasty or total arthroplasty, is, as Ghormley[19] pointed out nearly two decades ago, at best only a "compromise procedure."

Idiopathic avascular necrosis

With regard to bilateral so-called idiopathic avascular necrosis, there are a variety of procedures available in the management of this condition, including femoral head replacement, but none offers a more definite and superior result than total hip arthroplasty. In the early stage of the disease, when there are only minimum radiological changes and the patient has no symptoms whatsoever and complete sphericity of the femoral head, a bone graft procedure might be indicated. On the other hand in the disease process the femoral head softens and the subchondral bone no longer transmits the load to the acetabular weight-bearing zone, causing gradual malnutrition of the cartilage locally in the acetabulum; thus fibrillation will in turn jeopardize the result of arthroplasty by femoral head replacement. In selecting patients for simple femoral head replacement, one should be extremely cautious of the fact that acetabular disease is often present at the time of the femoral head replacement.

Osteonecrosis and renal transplantation

One of the common complications of renal transplantation is avascular necrosis of the femoral head as the result of long-term or lifelong chemical immunosuppression in the form of daily steroids and/or azathioprine (Imuran) to prevent allograft rejection (Fig. 8-28). Patients who continue to receive these drugs are prone to the development of multiple avascular necroses, commonly in the hips. These patients are also usually prone to orthopaedic complications of chronic hemodialysis,[20] including osteoporosis, osteomalacia, secondary hyperparathyroidism, and peripheral neuropathies. They may also suffer steroid myopathy and pathological fractures. There are many reports indicating that total hip replacement is ideally suited for patients with relatively short life expectancies with dramatic improvement of their condition. It must be recognized, however, that this population of patients presents a relatively high risk of infection because of systemic immunosuppressive drugs that they receive and will continue to receive postoperatively, and in most cases indefinitely. From the standpoint of anesthesia and postoperative morbidity, one should also consider these cases as potentially more at risk,

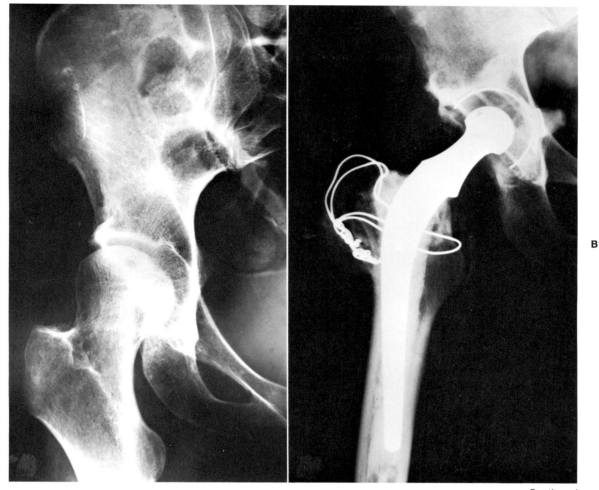

Continued.

Fig. 8-28. Avascular necrosis of femoral head following kidney transplant and immunosuppressive drugs is now best treated by total hip replacement. **A,** Status of hip in 28-year-old female 6 years following cadaveric kidney transplant. One year, **B,** and 6 years, **C,** following total hip replacement with excellent clinical result. Preoperative grading of hip is C-2,3,4; postoperative grade, C-6,6,6. NOTE: hypertrophy (arrow) of femoral shaft at level of tip of prosthesis.

especially with reference to urinary tract infections and kidney problems. In many of these patients, chronic renal disease may be responsible for fluid and electrolyte retention as well as hypertension. Usually these patients are especially young, many of them under the age of 50, but fully active. Therefore they impose considerable stress on an artificial joint while their bones might not be adequately supportive of a prosthesis, thus inviting the problem of loosening and perhaps fracture of the prosthesis because of vigorous activities.[29] It is now the consensus of those with vast experience[15,20,29,34] that total hip replacement can be safely performed in this high-risk population of patients

with the expectancy of good early results. It must be recognized, however, that no long-term results of a sizable series are available to make a final judgment in treating this particular condition.

Infected opposite hip and total hip replacement[*]

Total hip replacement may be done with post-surgical infection existing in the opposite hip. In a report of 14 instances where this was done, all had an uneventful recovery. In all but three of those infected hips, the prosthesis was still in

---

[*]For a discussion of infected previous surgery and total hip replacement, see Chapter 16.

251

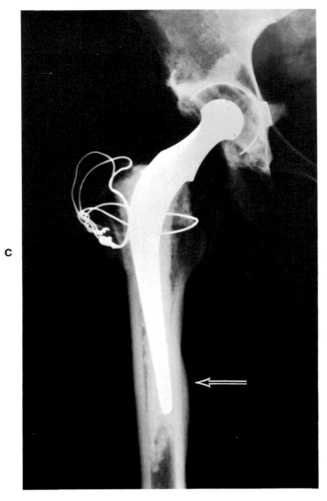

c

Fig. 8-28, cont'd. For legend see p. 251.

throsis following complete recovery of the new hip replacement. I planned such a combined program in four patients whose first hip was infected at the time the second hip was operated on. None of the four developed further infection; in three, more than 3 years have passed since their surgery.

Hip stiffness and total hip replacement

Occasionally we are confronted with indications for total hip replacement where there is no pain, but advanced stiffness is present. To achieve an adequate range of mobility in hips that have been completely ankylosed for many years (Fig. 8-29) a bilateral operation is often needed. This is especially true when the lumbar spine is painful or the patient has another distal joint disability such as a knee problem. It may also be a problem in young females whose hip joint arthritis has progressed to a stage where it has produced sexual difficulties. No measure of a guarantee can be offered for gain in mobility following surgery. This is especially true if the patient has a very stiff hip preoperatively or has a tendency to form bone (as the result of previous surgery). Total hip replacement complicated by heterotopic bone may be treated by "revision" surgery, especially if bilateral ankylosis is present or the stiff hip is in an unacceptable position. (See Chapters 14 and 16.)

Paget's disease and total hip replacement

Total hip replacement is indicated in Paget's fracture; hemiarthroplasty is contraindicated. It has been said (following total hip replacement) that the pain of Paget's disease may be only partially relieved by total hip replacement in view of the pathological condition of the bone itself. This is in contrast with our experiences in hips with Paget's pelvis, femur, or both, where total hip replacement has proven highly successful in relieving pain (Fig. 8-30). In fact, our experiences indicate that surgical results can be as good as those in simple so-called idiopathic osteoarthritis of the hip joint. Because of the gradual process of bone deformity and rapid rate of bone absorption and formation in this disease, it remains to be seen whether or not these results are maintained; the ultimate rate of long-term "loosening" is unknown. Because of deformity and abnormal bone texture and consistency, simple prosthetic replacement of the femoral

place when the operation of the opposite hip was performed.[13] One may conclude that the decision to go ahead with surgery of the second hip was an excellent one, since the combination of pseudarthrosis and bilateral hip disease is extremely incapacitating. It is unnecessary to deny a patient the second hip operation for fear of bloodborne infection, since this eventuality has not been reported in patients with similar complications. This is not a matter of academic interest alone. It is a remarkable practical solution to the problem of a patient who, already having had an infected hip, is now suffering from a painful nonoperated hip and naturally afraid that it too will become infected. Clearly the patient must be protected with appropriate and adequate antibiotics during and after surgery. The infected side should be converted to a pseudar-

252

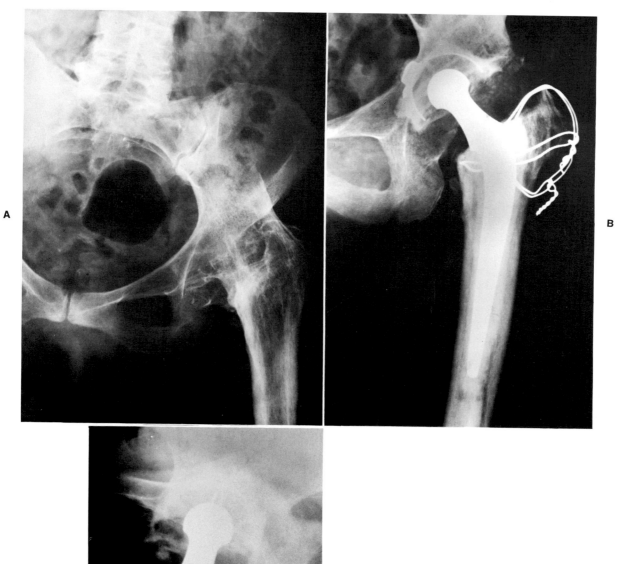

Fig. 8-29. Seventy-three–year-old woman (M.D.) with history of long-standing low back pain and left hip pain. Hip had been fused at age 30 for tuberculosis. Because of severe intractable back and ipsilateral knee pain, surgical intervention was necessary. **A,** Hip grade C-6,3,1. **B,** and **C,** Postoperative grade C-6,5,5.

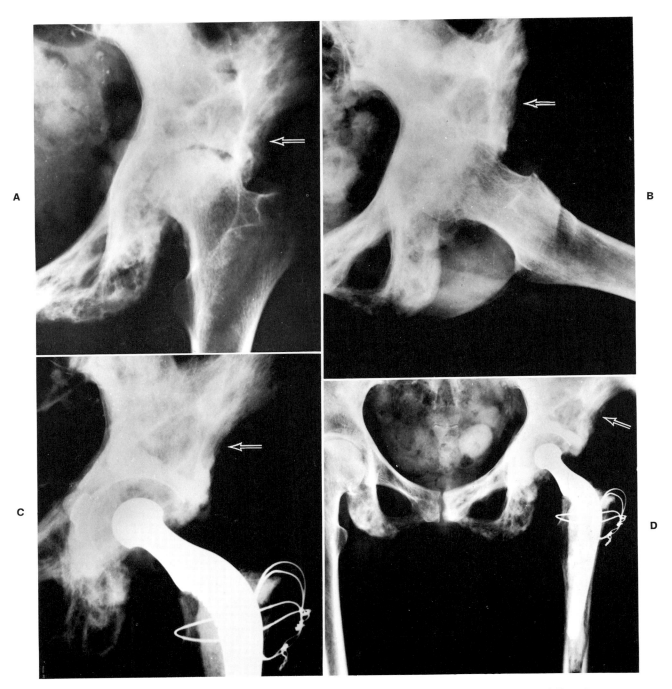

Fig. 8-30. Preoperative anteroposterior, **A,** and lateral, **B,** view of left hip in 62-year-old female with Paget's disease. Grade A-3,3,3. **C** and **D,** six months and 4½ years, respectively, following low-friction arthroplasty. NOTE: large cyst (arrows) (supra-acetabular region) has remained unaltered. Grade A-6,6,6.

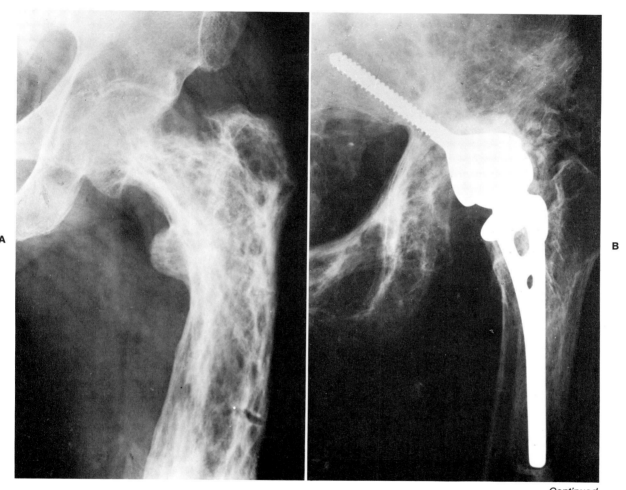

Continued.

Fig. 8-31. A, Paget's disease and degenerative osteoarthrosis of left hip in 54-year-old man. **B,** Two years following Ring total hip replacement. NOTE: marked loosening of both components and proximal migration as evidenced by sclerosis of weight-bearing portion of acetabulum. **C,** Hip was converted to low-friction arthroplasty. **D,** Two years following replacement with good functional results. Preoperative grade following Ring prosthesis (inserted elsewhere) was 2,2,2; postoperative result 2 years following surgery is 6,5,5.

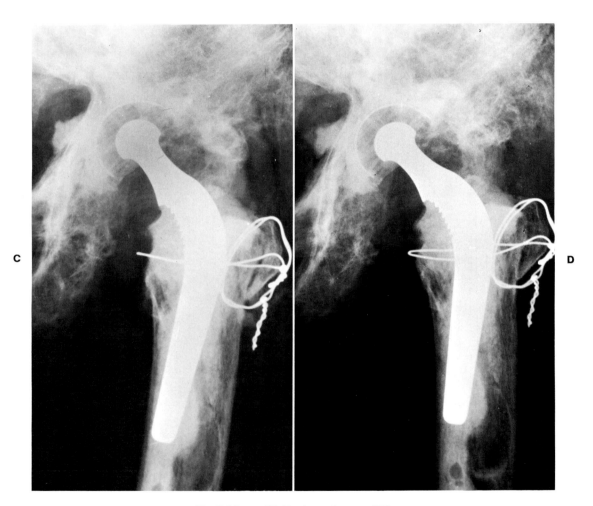

C

D

Fig. 8-31, cont'd. For legend see p. 255.

head is not indicated, even where the acetabulum appears normal. Fractures of the femoral neck are known for a notoriously slow rate of healing. Furthermore, because of changes in the bone with Paget's disease of the upper femur, prosthetic fixation without cement is not successful (Fig. 8-31).

Other results of total hip arthroplasty concur with our observations of a high success yield following total hip replacement in Paget's disease.[26,40] Medical treatment by diphosphonates, calcitonin-salmon or other drugs is entirely independent of mechanical treatment of the diseased hip joint. If sufficient disturbance and pain exist, then mechanical treatment by total hip replacement should precede treatment by medications. Spontaneous and severe "rest pain" unrelated to activity must be considered suspicious of sarcomatous changes of Paget's disease.

SUMMARY OF ESSENTIALS

- One of the most difficult aspects of total hip arthroplasty is the selection of patients for this procedure. It is not generally realized that radiological manifestation by itself is not an indication for hip replacement. As time passes and progress evolves in this field, indications may be altered and selection criteria for patients may be modified.
- At the time of this writing, now some 15 years following the first total hip replacement utilizing acrylic cement and high-density polyethylene (HDP), it is agreed that the operation is suitable for aged patients with degenerative arthritis or rheumatoid conditions. The operation remains unchallenged because of spectacular results such as relief of pain, increased mobility, or preservation of mobility without extensive physiotherapeutic management.
- When possible, the operation must be reserved for patients with osteoarthritis over 60 years of age or those who are close to retirement; it may be considered in younger patients who are affected by systemic conditions leading to a shortened life expectancy.
- In patients with rheumatoid or ankylosing polyarthritis, surgery may be performed at almost any age when other joints remain a disabling factor.
- In bilateral hip disease, however, patients in a younger age group may be accepted despite lack of other disabling factors.
- In planning bilateral hip surgery, it usually is advisable to operate on the more symptomatic hip, observe the results, and project surgery of the second hip for a later date. Exceptions to this rule include patients who are in their 70s, those with severe fixed deformity, and those who already have

a failed operation on one hip with the second hip becoming symptomatic.

- Bilateral hip replacement during the same anesthesia is an advisable procedure, but it should be performed only in a highly organized center for this type of operation and with a first-class operating team in order to minimize the morbidity of such an undertaking.
- Total hip arthroplasty is relatively contraindicated if there is a history or presence of infection in the upper femur or hip joint, if the patient has unilateral hip disease and is under 60 years of age, or where pain and disability do not require pain medications or support with a cane.
- Obesity is a contraindication for surgery. Both surgeon and patient are advised to postpone a decision regarding surgery until weight reduction to an optimal level is achieved.
- Pain is the cardinal sign and the major determining factor in advising total hip replacement. The source of pain and the motivation of the patient in seeking advice should be clarified prior to any decision for surgery. For the next decade, at least, surgeons are well advised to be certain they are operating for objective signs and symptoms. No patient should be considered for surgery if his present condition would be exacerbated should complications arise necessitating removal of the prosthetic device (Girdlestone pseudarthrosis test).
- Patients in their 40s and 50s still present a difficult problem when severe disability is present. These patients may be cautiously selected for total hip arthroplasty if they understand that further surgery may be necessary if or when mechanical failure develops. In a teenager or young adult with unilateral hip disease of traumatic origin, arthrodesis is the best solution.
- While awaiting the long-term results of total hip arthroplasty, it is advisable to delay operating on active and vigorous patients who can tolerate the delay. Surgery based purely on the patient's demand should be refused, especially when objective disability is not present. This is particularly true in patients who are too young, too obese, or whose subjective complaint does not correlate with objective findings.
- Any surgeon undertaking the technique of total hip arthroplasty must have an unwritten contract with the patient to look after him as long as both live. It cannot be overemphasized that any surgeon who recommends surgery of this type to his patient has to be able to solve all the complications by himself, a task that is much more exacting than the primary operation.
- Hopefully, one day we will be able to replace hip joints in young females whose main concern is not so much pain but appearance. This is especially relevant to congenital dysplasia of the hip

joint, which constitutes the most difficult and challenging problem. The young age and potential vigor of these patients would subject the arthroplasty to enormous strain and wear, and they should be encouraged to delay the decision for surgery as long as possible.

■ One of the most rewarding aspects of total hip surgery comes from patients with bilateral hip disability, which is generally more than double that from one hip. The more symptomatic hip should be treated first.

■ Detailed consideration must be given to patient selection and the sequence of bilateral hip operations. Hip surgery may be particularly indicated to promote mobility when bilateral hip disease is present.

■ The details of patient selection and contraindications are presented in order to formulate a guideline rather than as a "code of practice." The selection of patients is a complex matter that must be done on an individual basis while keeping all the facts in perspective.

REFERENCES

1. Amstutz, H. C., Christie, J., and Mensch, J. S., Treatment of osteonecrosis of the hip. In The Hip Society: Proceedings of the third open scientific meeting of The Hip Society, 1975, St. Louis, 1975, The C. V. Mosby Co., pp. 19-34.
2. Aufranc, O. E.: Constructive hip surgery with the Vitallium mold, J. Bone Joint Surg. **39A:**237-248, 1957.
3. Aufranc, O. E., and Sweet, E. B.: Study of patients with hip arthroplasty at Massachusetts General Hospital, J.A.M.A. **170:**507-515, 1959.
4. Bisla, R. S., Ranawat, C. S., and Inglis, A. E., Total hip replacement in patients with ankylosing spondylitis with involvement of the hip, J. Bone Joint Surg. **58A:**233-238, 1976.
5. Bonfiglio, M.: Aseptic necrosis of femoral head in dogs, Surg. Gynecol. Obstet. **98:**591-599, 1954.
6. Bonfiglio, M., and Bardenstein, M. B.: Treatment by bone-grafting of aseptic necrosis of the femoral head and non-union of the femoral neck (Phemister Technique), J. Bone Joint Surg. **40A:**1329-1346, 1958.
7. Bonfiglio, M., and Voke, E. M.: Aseptic necrosis of the femoral head and non-union of the femoral neck, J. Bone Joint Surg. **50A:**48-66, 1968.
7a. Boyd, J. B., and Salvatore, A.: Acute displaced fracture of the femoral neck, J. Bone Joint Surg. **46A:**1066-1068, 1964.
8. Chandler, H. P., and Dickson, D. B.: Total hip replacement in the young patient. In American Academy of Orthopaedic Surgeons: Instructional course lectures, vol. 23, St. Louis, 1974, The C. V. Mosby Co., pp. 184-198.
9. Charnley, J.: Personal communications.
10. Charnley, J.: Total prosthetic replacement of the hip joint using a socket of high-density polythylene, Internal Publication, Centre for Hip Surgery, Wrightington Hospital, England, 1966.
11. Charnley, J.: Total prosthetic replacement for advanced coxarthrosis, Internal Publication No. "0", Centre for Hip Surgery, Wrightington Hospital, England, 1967.
12. Charnley, J.: Present status of total hip replacement, Ann. Rheum. Dis. **30:**560-564, 1971.
13. Charnley, J.: Total hip replacement following infection in the opposite hip, Internal Publication No. 48, Centre for hip surgery, Wrightington Hospital, England, 1974.
14. Coventry, M. B.: Selection of patients for total hip arthroplasty. In American Academy of Orthopaedic Surgeons: Instructional course lectures, vol. 23, St. Louis, 1974, The C. V. Mosby Co., pp. 136-142.
15. Cruess, R. L., Blennerhassett, M., MacDonald, F. R., Maclean, L. D., and Dosetor, J.: Aseptic necrosis following renal transplantation, J. Bone Joint Surg. **50A:**1577-1590, 1968.
16. Dinley, J., and Duthie, R. U. B.: Hip surgery in hemophiliacs. In The Hip Society: The hip, proceedings of the fourth open scientific meeting of the Hip Society, 1976, St. Louis, 1976, The C. V. Mosby Co., pp. 143-160.
17. Dunn, H. K., and Hess, W. E.: Total hip reconstruction in chronically dislocated hip, J. Bone Joint Surg. **58A:**838-845, 1976.
18. Eftekhar, N. S.: Low-friction arthroplasty, indications, contraindications, and complications, J.A.M.A. **218:**705-710, 1971.
18a. Eftekhar, N. S.: Status of femoral head replacement in treating fractures of femoral neck; Parts I and II, Orthop. Rev. **2**(6):15-23; **2**(8):19-30, 1973.
19. Ghormley, R. K.: A review of the pertinent current literature on prostheses of the hip. In American Academy Orthopaedic Surgeons: Instructional course lectures, vol. 15, Ann Arbor, 1958, J. W. Edwards, pp. 4-14.
20. Harrington, K. D., Murray, W. R., Kountz, S. L., and Bleezer, F. O.: Avascular necrosis of bone after renal transplantation, J. Bone Joint Surg. **53A:**203-215, 1971.
21. Harris, W. H.: Traumatic arthritis of the hip after dislocation and acetabular fractures: treatment by mold arthroplasties; an end result study using a new method of result evaluation, J. Bone and Joint Surg. **51A:**737-755, 1969.
22. Harris, W. H.: Indications for major elective reconstructive surgery of the hip in the adult. In American Academy of Orthopaedic Surgeons: Instructional course lectures, vol. 23, St. Louis, 1974, The C. V. Mosby Co., pp. 143-149.
23. Harris, W. H.: Total hip replacement for con-

genital dysplasia of hip: technique. In The Hip Society: Proceedings of the second open scientific meeting of The Hip Society, 1974, St. Louis, 1974, The C. V. Mosby Co., pp. 251-264.

24. Hohl, J. C., editor: Symposium on metabolic bone disease, Orthop. Clin. North Am. **3:**3, 1972.

25. Ivins, J. C., Benson, W. F., Bickel, W. H., and Nelson, J. W.: Arthroplasty of the hip for idiopathic degenerative joint disease, Surg. Gynecol. Obstet. **125:**1281-1284, 1967.

26. Jackson, C. T.: The results of low-friction arthroplasty of the hip performed in Paget's disease, Internal Publication No. 47, Centre for Hip Surgery, Wrightington Hospital, England, January, 1974.

27. Jaffe, W. L., and Charnley, J.: Bilateral Charnley low friction arthroplasty as a single operative procedure, Bull. Hosp. Joint Dis. **32:**198-214, October, 1971.

28. Jayson, M.: Total hip replacement (Forward by J. Charnley), Philadelphia, 1971, J. B. Lippincott Co.

29. Kenzora, J. E., and Sledge, C. B.: Hip arthroplasty and the renal transplantation. In The Hip Society: The hip, proceedings of the third open scientific meeting of The Hip Society, 1975, St. Louis, 1975, The C. V. Mosby Co., pp. 35-59.

30. Lazansky, M. G.: A study of bilateral low friction arthroplasty, Internal Publication No. 3, Centre for hip surgery, Wrightington Hospital, England, 1967.

31. Lazansky, M. G.: Total hip replacement in patients with bilateral disease. In American Academy of Orthopaedic Surgeons: Instructional course lectures, vol. 23, St. Louis, 1974, The C. V. Mosby Co., pp. 150-154.

32. Lipscomb, P. R.: Reconstructive surgery for bilateral hip joint disease in the adult, J. Bone Joint Surg. **47A:**1-30, 1965.

33. Moore, A. T.: The Moore self-locking Vitallium prosthesis in fresh femoral neck fractures. In American Academy of Orthopaedic Surgeons: Instructional course lectures, vol. 16, St. Louis, 1959, The C. V. Mosby Co., pp. 309-321.

34. Murray, W. R.: Hip problems associated with organ transplants, Clin. Orthop. **90:**57-69, 1973.

35. Phemister, D. B.: Treatment of necrotic head of femur in adults, J. Bone Joint Surg. **31A:**55-66, 1949.

36. Scales, J. T. Massive bone and joint replacement involving the upper femur, Acetabulum and iliac bone. In The Hip Society: The hip, the proceedings of the third open scientific meeting of The Hip Society, 1975, St. Louis, 1975, The C. V. Mosby Co., pp. 245-275.

37. Shepherd, M. M.: A review of 650 arthroplasty operations, J. Bone Joint Surg. **36B:**567-577, 1954.

38. Sim, F. H., Chao, E. Y., and Peterson, L. F. A.: Reconstruction following segmental resection of primary bone tumors of the hip. In The Hip Society: The hip, proceedings of the third open scientific meeting of The Hip Society, St. Louis, 1975, The C. V. Mosby Co., pp. 302-324.

39. Springfield, E. S., and Ennecking, W. F.: Role of bone grafting in idiopathic aseptic necrosis of the femoral head. In The Hip Society: The hip, proceedings of the third open scientific meeting of The Hip Society, 1975, St. Louis, 1975, The C. V. Mosby Co., pp. 3-18.

40. Stauffer, R. N., and Sim, F. H.: Total hip arthroplasty in Paget's disease of the hip, J. Bone Joint Surg. **58A:**476-478, 1976.

41. Staulberg, S. D., Cordell, L. D., Harris, W. H., Ramsey, P. L., and MacEwen, G. D.: Unrecognized childhood hip disease; a major cause of idiopathic osteoarthritis of the hip. In The Hip Society: The hip, proceedings of the third open scientific meeting of The Hip Society, 1975, St. Louis, 1975, The C. V. Mosby Co., pp. 212-228.

42. Stinchfield, F. E., Cooperman, B., and Shea, C. E.: Replacement of the femoral head by Judet or Austin Moore prosthesis, J. Bone Joint Surg. **39A:**1043-1058, 1957.

43. Tronzo, R. G., and Okin, E. M., Anatomic restoration of congenital hip dysplasia in adulthood by total hip displacement, Clin. Orthop. **106:**94-101, 1975.

CHAPTER 9

General workup and methods of assessment

One should hesitate to judge the effect of a surgical procedure, even in a large series of cases, when 'any attempt to compare accurately the patient's condition before the operation with that after the operation was actually impossible.'

OTTO E. AUFRANC

An impersonal method of assessment that is comprehensive, generally applicable and reliable, is essential.

MARGARET M. SHEPHERD

Perioperative management includes: (1) preoperative evaluation and recording, (2) preparation for surgery, and (3) postoperative management. This chapter is intended to assist in selecting patients, standardizing perioperative management, and assessing the quality of results following surgery. Information regarding operative preparation will establish guidelines that may be modified according to the surgeon's preference and experience.

PREOPERATIVE EVALUATION AND RECORDING

Thorough preoperative evaluation is of primary importance for patients about to undergo major elective surgery. Each patient is admitted to the hospital at least 2 or 3 days prior to the proposed surgery. A detailed history and physical examination are done by a member of the house staff. Ideally, the resident who sees the patient preoperatively follows him through the postoperative period. Medical consultation is always obtained. In our institution an internist sees the patient preoperatively and then follows him through the postoperative period. Close follow-up by the internist further secures the patient's confidence and enhances his care if medical complications should occur.

A complete systematic examination is a basic requirement for any surgical procedure. However, because age per se is not a contraindication for total hip replacement (many patients over age 65 are now considered for this major elective surgery), it is essential to carefully assess a patient's health before accepting him for surgery, as a large proportion of geriatric patients over 55 years of age have coexisting diseases.[27,49] Some of these complicating factors can be identified and corrected prior to surgery given sufficient time. Therefore it is essential to arrange preadmission internist evaluation for patients with an involved medical background.[13,14,39,46] In dealing with older patients, special consideration should be given to incipient diabetes, electrolyte balance (especially in patients on hypertension medications), physical and mental attitude, and alertness.

Separate records for hip patients may be used in addition to the routine hospital documents kept on all patients. We have adopted a separate record in order to have access to these records without chance of their being misplaced in the hospital record room. They constitute six sheets that deal with different aspects of patient management.[16] Some features of the patient's history are of special importance such as personal or family history of bleeding, phlebitis, gastrointestinal anomalies, and urinary and cardiopulmonary symptoms. The importance of medical assistance in the evaluation and management of the patient cannot be overemphasized; we rely heavily on the internists who have a special

The Presbyterian Hospital in the City of New York   Form #1: History
Orthopaedic Surgery Service
Columbia–Presbyterian Medical Center

Preoperative and Postoperative Assessment for HIP SURGERY

Name _____ Unit # _____ Date _____ Location _____

Age _____ Sex: M _____ F _____ Race: C _____ E _____ Weight _____ lbs

Chief complaint: 1.
with duration   2.
since onset   3.
                         4.

History of complaint:
with mode of onset
and duration

Previous treatment:
nonsurgical

Previous treatment: 1. Type:
surgical   2. Duration since operation:

Relevant additional   1. Medical:
medical and social   2. Occupational:
data   3. Home circumstances:
                         4. Hobbies/sports:
                         5. Other:

What patient expects   1. Freedom from pain:
as the result of   2. Better mobility:
treatment   3. Better function:
                         4. Other:
                         5. Other:

Motivation: 1. Excellent:
                         2. Good:
                         3. Average:
                         4. Below:
                         5. Poor:

Comments

Fig. 9-1. Preoperative and postoperative assessment form for hip surgery: history.

261

interest in the perioperative care of the total hip patient. Hypertension, diabetes, gout, and cardiac insufficiency increase the risk of complications in both surgery and anticoagulation treatment. (A narrative history is recorded on Form 1 of the hip assessment record, Fig. 9-1.)

A relevant laboratory examination should include a complete blood count, erythrocyte sedimentation rate, SMA 12, electrolyte measurement, and urinalysis. In addition, we obtain clotting and prothrombin times, stool hematest, and a platelet count. Baseline arterial blood gases and pulmonary function studies are essential for patients with preexisting pulmonary dysfunction. A chest radiograph and electrocardiogram are obvious prerequisites for general anesthesia. If any abnormalities are found, further consultation and/or laboratory studies are made, especially relative to the urinary tract, as this is a frequent site of postoperative problems. A thorough orthopaedic evaluation is obviously very important. X-ray films of both hips, femurs, knees, and lumbosacral spine are obtained. In our experience, approximately one out of ten patients admitted for total hip surgery reveals unexpected medical or surgical findings necessitating postponement.

The physical therapy staff works closely with each patient throughout his hospital stay. Prior to surgery, the therapist evaluates the patient to anticipate potential problems during the postoperative rehabilitation phase—deep breathing, coughing, ankle and quadriceps exercises, and positioning are taught preoperatively—and male patients are urged to practice urination in the supine position.[16]

CARDIOVASCULAR AND PULMONARY SYSTEMS

Increased morbidity and mortality rates in older patients are attributed to hypertensive cardiovascular disease and arteriosclerotic heart diseases, as well as kidney and brain changes. History of coronary artery disease, cardiac arrhythmia, or extensive hypertension must be evaluated and managed. Cardiac arrhythmias in particular present a high risk for elective surgery. Evidence of cardiovascular decompensation and generalized arteriosclerosis, abdominal aneurysms, peripheral vascular insufficiency, and carotid artery insufficiencies must be sought; a carotid endarterectomy or repair of an abdominal aorta aneurysm may take precedence over elective surgery of the hip.

Patients with severe hypertension must not be deprived of their medications before surgery. If alterations in medication are planned, they should be done by an internist familiar with the patient and they must be brought to the attention of the anesthetist before surgery. Occasionally, prophylactic digitalization is considered in view of potential perioperative stress caused by fever, volume shifts, anemia, and so on. ECG abnormalities such as "T" wave changes are frequent and should be carefully interpreted. Insertion of an indwelling urinary catheter in a patient with borderline cardiovascular compensation is advisable as a good method for monitoring blood volume during and immediately following surgery.

Denial of total hip replacement because of a complicated medical history must be based on objective and unbiased scientific facts. In their final years of life, many patients are desperate to have the hip surgery to alleviate pain and disability; they are willing to accept some added calculated risk as long as it is not formidable. A good example is a patient with a low-grade malignancy or borderline cardiovascular compensation in addition to painful arthritis of the hip. The patient may express a wish for death rather than continued existence in his present state, and in this case, obviously the degree of disability and the patient's attitude may counterbalance the risk involved. In this context, the judgment of an internist familiar with morbidity and mortality following total hip replacement surgery is invaluable in arriving at a decision.

Pulmonary complications in older people also contribute to a high mortality rate. Fortunately, because rehabilitation following total hip replacement is early, these complications are relatively rare. Pulmonary function must be evaluated by determining arterial blood gases, spirometry, and other routine studies. Pulmonary toilet care and breathing exercises may significantly diminish the risks of postoperative complications.[1,36,47,49] Regional anesthesia may be preferentially selected for patients with chronic pulmonary disease.

GENITOURINARY AND GASTROINTESTINAL SYSTEMS

Of special concern to us are patients with urological symptoms, generally manifested in males by obstruction secondary to prostate hypertrophy and in females by urinary incontinence and asymptomatic infection. Also of special concern is silent prostate adenocarcinoma in older men. Impaired renal function must also be evaluated preoperatively; obstructive conditions should be rectified prior to surgery to avoid the possibility of chronic urinary tract infections leading to postoperative complications, specifically, hematogenous infections. Elective pre- or postoperative catheterization must be considered in patients who have shown symptoms of urinary tract obstruction, and urological consultation should be sought.

Because of the prevalence of postoperative thromboembolic complications, requiring the use of anticoagulants, a history of peptic ulcer or danger of stress reactivation of a past peptic ulcer, mandates a thorough evaluation of the gastrointestinal system. This should include a rectal examination, stool examination for blood, and proctoscopy as indicated. Patients with previous corticosteroid therapy also have a higher tendency for postoperative bleeding and hematoma. Salicylates, used for control of pain or prophylaxis against thromboembolism, may risk a gastric/peptic ulcer in addition to their effect on platelet function.

SKIN AND OTHER SOURCES OF INFECTION

All total hip replacement candidates must have a thorough search for potential infection sites, some of which may be incipient and/or asymptomatic. Several authors specify possible implications of a remote infection following total hip arthroplasty.[6] Skin must be considered a potential source of wound contamination and infection; infected traumatic lesions, insect bites, rashes, and the like are all sufficient cause to postpone surgery. Chronic dental abscess or periodontal pyogenic lesions of the mouth require specific attention. If dental extraction is required, it must be completed prior to surgery.

The sources for hematogenous infection seeded in the hip joint must be sought, especially where there have been previous operations. Often this is verifiable by careful x-ray examination and repeated erythrocyte sedimentation rate, as well as aspiration of the joint. If the joint is aspirated, a culture should be made for aerobic and anaerobic organisms as well as acid-fast bacteria and fungi. For details see Chapters 6 and 16 on infection and Chapter 14 on revision of previous surgery.

CHOICE OF PROSTHESES AND INSTRUMENTATION

Special reference must be made to Chapter 3, "Biomechanics and Biomaterials," concerning choice of a prosthesis. The surgeon must be thoroughly acquainted with one system of instrumentation and its underlying principles. It is disadvantageous to use more than one system

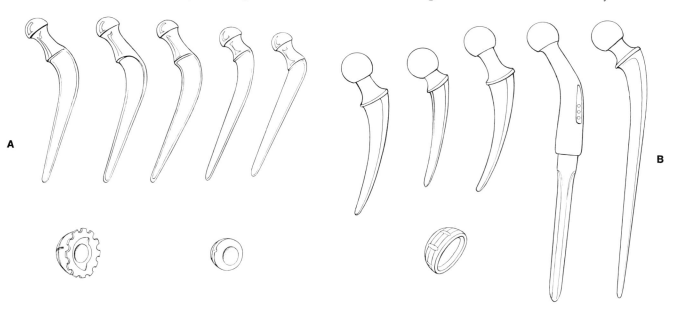

A

B

Fig. 9-2. Examples of available total hip prostheses. **A,** Charnley series (incomplete) with 22-mm. head diameter. **B,** Müller series (incomplete) with 32-mm. head diameter. Configuration of sockets is shown in lower part of each series.

because mixed experience reduces one's expertise with a particular system of instrumentation and approach. The principles applied in instrumentation for a given prosthesis are specific, and one should not interchange prostheses and different techniques. For example, a 22-mm. Charnley–type femoral head prosthesis should be used with the transtrochanteric approach and Charnley's technique. With this method, for example, the capsule of the joint is preserved. Attempting to use this prosthesis without the removal of the greater trochanter may result in considerable difficulty in the placement of the components and added risk of dislocation. The system of instrumentation one chooses must be versatile and allow perfect implantation of the prosthesis and correction of deformity. For complications such as loosening or fatigue fracture of the femoral stem, the surgeon must be able to select a prosthesis that is adequately strong as well as adaptable to a specific anatomical situation. For example, it is useless to consider a heavy-stem prosthesis for a situation that would require extreme reaming of the medullary canal, which may damage the shaft or reduce the amount of cement for fixation should such a prosthesis be used. During the past 10 years we have used Charnley's system with only minor modifications and have found his instrumentation and the 22–mm. head prosthesis most satisfactory for all patients. The rationale for this choice has been documented in Chapters 2 and 3. Müller's modification of the Charnley prosthesis (with a 32-mm. diameter head) has also been used at our institution, but only for demonstration and teaching of the technique of total hip replacement without removing the greater trochanter. This latter technique and prosthesis are recommended in situations where surgical technique includes a capsulectomy of the hip joint. The available prostheses, including Charnley's 22-mm. head and Müller's 32-mm. head, are illustrated in Fig. 9-2. The illustrations represent examples of these prostheses in 22- and 32-mm. sizes. For details the reader must consult commercial literature on these prostheses.*

In performing total hip replacement with un-

---

*Charnley prostheses and instruments are manufactured by Chas. F. Thackary, Ltd., England and distributed exclusively in the United States by Cintor division of Codman & Shurtleff, Inc. M. E. Müller prosthesis is manufactured by Protek, Ltd., Switzerland and distributed in the United States by De Puy, Inc.

usual anatomical situations (such as failure of previous surgery), one must anticipate likely problems at surgery. The special prosthesis must be available to accommodate the specific situation such as a prosthesis with an extra long neck or stem, with or without undersized dimensions. While it is often possible to resect the bone to accommodate the prosthesis, it is more advantageous to use the prosthesis that is most suitable without sacrificing the bony stock. At times, a special prosthesis may have to be manufactured in advance to meet the demand of a certain anatomical situation (for example, juvenile rheumatoid arthritis with small pelvic and femoral dimensions).

SELECTION OF ANESTHESIA

In selecting anesthesia the safety of the patient is the prime consideration.[41,48] In most of our cases, general anesthesia (normotensive) and endotracheal intubation are recommended by the anesthesia team after reviewing the patient. An expert anesthesia team is invaluable in dealing with older patients who, at times, may have minor cardiopulmonary compromise. There are basically three ways to approach the problem of anesthesia for patients undergoing total hip replacement: (1) normotensive standard techniques, (2) hypotensive anesthesia, and (3) regional anesthesia.

Normotensive anesthesia

When general anesthesia is considered, endotracheal intubation is used, and careful monitoring of the patient should include continuous ECG observation, central venous and arterial blood pressure monitoring as indicated, and continuous monitoring of heart beat and breath sounds with an esophageal stethoscope. The patient's temperature is monitored with an esophageal probe, and arterial blood gases are measured as required. This method is frequently used and provides safe and reliable anesthesia with a great deal of flexibility. After induction with a barbiturate, diazepam, or ketamine, anesthesia is maintained with nitrous oxide (N_2O) in combination with narcotics, neuroleptics, or halogenated inhalation agents as well as muscle relaxants. Precise attention to blood and fluid replacement is essential. The method and details of anesthesia are selected by the anesthetist according to the patient's individual history and physical examination.

Hypotensive anesthesia

Since its inception, controlled hypotensive anesthesia has been a controversial issue. It was accompanied by considerable increased morbidity in its developmental years,[2,3,12] but in subsequent studies Bodman[3] and Larson[30] concluded that most of the complications were not inherent in the technique, but rather were the results of technical flaws of the anesthesia. In their technique, Davis and associates[11] used pentolinium tartrate to lower the systolic blood pressure to 65 to 75 mm. Hg, a method previously used by others.[19,20,21,23] Controlled hypotensive anesthesia has recently been enthusiastically accepted at several centers. Although it had been accepted in such areas as neurosurgery, plastic surgery, and general surgical procedures where copious blood loss is anticipated, it is only recently that it has been used in orthopaedic surgery, particularly total hip replacement. There are several reports supporting its validity and advantages, including decreased blood loss and consequently decreased blood replacement, as well as improved operative technique and decreased operative time, and some claim improved wound healing.[13,23,27,33]

Charnley[7] has used hypotensive anesthesia extensively at Wrightington Hospital with remarkable success and minimal morbidity. Mallory[35] and Harris[25] have also used it with success and encountered no major complications. There are some patients, however, who do not qualify for deliberate hypotensive anesthesia such as those with severe hypertension, obstructive pulmonary disease, cerebrovascular disease, a history of arteriosclerotic heart disease, or a history of renal conditions. Mallory and his associates did not exclude patients with a history of myocardial infarction, providing there was no history of coronary ischemia within 6 months prior to the time of anesthesia. They explicitly emphasized careful patient selection for success with this method, considering the fact that the decision to accept a candidate should be mutually agreed upon between anesthesiologist and internist. In their series, 80% of the patients qualified. Successful anesthesia with minimum morbidity and reduction in the operative blood loss and need for subsequent blood replacement was observed in all cases, along with reduced operative time. Balanced anesthesia was used in conjunction with trimethaphan camphorsulfonate (Arfonad).[35]

In a study of 253 total hip replacement patients anesthetized by induced hypotensive anesthesia, no lasting complications could be attributed to the technique. As in prior studies, blood loss was considerably reduced, and procedures were done more easily than under normotensive anesthesia. However, the technique is considered demanding, requiring a highly competent anesthesia staff.

In summary, while induced hypotension during anesthesia has been recommended in orthopaedic surgery, in-depth study of its usefulness and related morbidity is lacking. Its proper place under general circumstances, without an intent and skillfully trained team of anesthesiologists, is not well defined. The best overall method of lowering the blood pressure during anesthesia is also disputed. The recent use of nitroprusside to produce hypotension seems to offer some advantages, but it is our feeling that unless the anesthesia team is prepared to accept full responsibility for the selection of patients as well as precise monitoring during surgery, this type of anesthesia should not be used, despite unquestionably important dividends attributed to it in total hip replacement surgery.

Regional anesthesia—spinal

Spinal anesthesia has been accepted in general surgery and in urological and gynecological procedures, resulting in a decrease in operative blood loss and cardiopulmonary complications. A smoother postoperative course also has been attributed to it.[5,15,29,34]

In a study of 234 total hip replacements (in 199 patients) performed by one surgeon, Sculco and Ranawat[42] compared the effect of spinal versus general anesthesia. Thiopental sodium (Pentothal sodium) was used for the induction of all patients undergoing general anesthesia, maintained with N_2O (nitrous oxide in combination with fentanyl, thiopental sodium, or droperidol O fentanyl citrate [Innovar] or nitrous oxide in combination with halothane). Spinal anesthesia was performed with 10 to 15 mg. of 0.5% tetracaine injected in the interspace of the third and fourth lumbar vertabrae, achieving anesthesia below the tenth thoracic vertebra. In addition, most patients were sedated with diazepam (Valium) during the procedure. Blood loss was reduced by an average of 600 ml. In these patients the amount of blood loss during postoperative suction was also reduced significantly. It was concluded that there were fewer postoperative complications in the spinal anesthesia group, thus spinal anesthesia was deemed preferable. This view is supported by my own experience: spinal anesthesia, when indicated, seems to be superior to normotensive general anesthesia in performing total hip replacement. Practical difficulties encountered in our experience include: (1) difficulty in positioning the patient on the table because of fixed deformities and painful hips, (2) a combination of arthritis and arthritis of the lower lumbar spine present in most patients with arthritic hips, and (3) difficulty in achieving a satisfactory spinal tap. We have also found that epidural anesthesia is quite satisfactory for total hip replacement. Epidural or spinal anesthetics may be given by a catheter with continuous medication as needed to prolong anesthesia.

Corticosteroid coverage

Many patients who undergo total hip arthroplasty have been treated previously with corticosteroids. Prior multiple intra-articular injections usually do not call for a regimen of preoperative treatment by corticosteroids; however, if patients have been on corticosteroids for at least 4 to 5 years, regardless of the dose, they require parenteral steroid coverage during surgery. Normally, surgical shock and stress are coped with successfully by a considerable increase in the corticosteroid output of the adrenal glands. However, prolonged corticosteroid treatment can result in depression of the normal output by the glands, leading to dysfunction and atrophy. To cope with a stressful condition such as major surgery, supplementary corticosteroid coverage during the preoperative course is required. It has been suggested that approximately three to four times the normal daily dose of corticosteroids should be administered to patients who have received corticosteroids prior to the time of surgery. As a general rule, the preoperative dosage should not determine the amount given during surgery; the extent of surgery and operative complications must also be weighed. Corticosteroids should begin at least 12 hours before surgery, for example, cortisone acetate administered 6 P.M. the night before surgery; 50 to 75 mg. is given by intramuscular injection every 6 hours until the patient goes to the operating room. Hydrocortisone succinate (Solu-cortef) (water-soluble preparation) 100 mg./L.

of intravenous fluid is administered intraoperatively. This immediately provides and maintains a sufficient level of steroids for the duration of surgery without any need for mobilization of Depo forms, even in the presence of hypotension. Fluids lost and replaced carry adequate corticosteroids until the patient's return to the recovery room.

When the patient is brought to the recovery room, 75 mg. cortisone acetate is injected intramuscularly and then given every 8 hours postoperatively. Including preoperative medication and intraoperative hydrocortisone succinate (Solu-cortef), at least 250 to 300 mg. cortisone is given on day of the operation. During the first postoperative day the patient should receive 75 mg. of cortisone acetate every 8 hours—total 225 mg. The subsequent day 50 mg. should be given every 8 hours for a total of 150 mg., and then 25 mg. every 12 hours for a total of 50 mg., and lastly, a single injection of 25 mg., after which the recommended dose of prednisone should be the equivalent of 5 mg. per day. It must be noted, however, that the tapering schedule should stabilize when one reaches a daily dose equivalent to the preoperative prednisone or other steroid preparations and should subsequently be kept at that level. No attempt should be made at this point to diminish the dosage below the preoperative steroid dose equivalent.

Changing from parenteral to oral forms of steroids should occur only when dependable gastrointestinal function has returned. The preceding schedule of tapering should be modified as required by the patient's postoperative course to provide higher levels for a longer period of time if required. Steroids should be given intravenously instead of intramuscularly if shock, relative hypertension, hypotension, or cardiac decompensation ensues. Careful ongoing evaluation should focus on the short-term side effects of steroids, including hypokalemia, alkalosis, hyperglycemia, salt and fluid retention, or psychosis. The schedule presented here is basically a guideline and must be individualized for each case, weighing the preoperative steroid dosage, the nature of the illness that is being treated with steroids and its activity at the time of surgery, the extent of the surgical procedure contemplated, the relative ease or difficulty in the postoperative course, the complications, the patient's nutritional status, and the postoperative wound-healing process.[4]

BLOOD TRANSFUSIONS IN TOTAL HIP SURGERY

The average patient undergoing total hip replacement with normotensive anesthesia requires 2 to 3 units of blood during and/or after surgery. This usually can be reduced by one-half if a hypotensive anesthesia is used. When operative time is increased as in revision surgery or with difficult technical problems, more blood transfusions may be anticipated. Conventional bank blood is used in most hospitals. However, this method of transfusion has carried a high incidence of serum hepatitis. In our series this complication has been noted in approximately 2% to 3% of the cases, although in many instances a nonicteric hepatitis may escape diagnosis, and the patient may suffer only from minor symptoms such as anorexia or slight chemical changes manifested by serial SMA 12 examinations. Therefore it must be recognized that transfusions with homologous blood expose the patient to an appreciable risk. If hypotensive anesthesia is available and the patient might require only 1 unit of blood, the transfusion should be avoided if the patient can tolerate the mild degree of anemia. On the other hand, if blood has to be transfused, the ideal blood is banked autologous blood. In addition to serum hepatitis, dangers inherent in transfusion are mismatched blood, clerical errors, and immunological reactions to blood proteins.

According to some studies as many as 5% of patients receiving homogolous blood transfusion may have some type of serious reaction. Problems of blood reactions, in particular, serum hepatitis, are a greater problem in large cities, where considerable numbers of unrecognized addicts participate in blood donor pools. It has been estimated that for each unit of blood the risk for transmitting hepatitis is approximately 6% to 8%. The advantages of autologous banked blood have been pointed out by Grant,[24] Milles and co-workers,[37] and Newman and co-workers.[38]

Complete cooperation among the surgeon, patient, and the blood bank is essential if autologous banked blood is to be used. The technique involved in phlebotomy prior to surgery has been described by Polesky.[40] The patient must be referred to the blood bank for evaluation approximately 3 weeks prior to the planned surgery. One unit of blood is drawn every 5 days and stored. A hemoglobin and hematocrit examination prior to each phlebotomy is essential, and the patient must immediately be placed on iron therapy. Both osteoarthritic and rheumatoid patients are good candidates for this type of blood transfusion.

The surgeon faced with the problem of transfusion of 3 to 4 units of blood or more for elective surgery must consider the risks involved and the benefits gained by banked autologous blood. Most blood banks are reluctant to perform this service owing to work overload and the special screening necessary for these patients. However, the benefits from this method fully compensate for inconvenience to the patient and the blood bank. In my personal experience with this method, no adverse reactions have been observed, and no special problem related to hemoglobin-hematocrit level has occurred.

We strongly advise against transfusion of a single unit of blood postoperatively; if the patient needs as little as 1 unit, he may well forego it *and* the attendant risk of transfusion complications. Older patients usually do not tolerate a low hemoglobin-hematocrit level postoperatively. If they are showing any evidence of restlessness, agitation, or psychosis, they should be transfused with packed cells in adequate amounts to avoid overloading their cardiovascular system. Since with blood-freezing techniques blood may be drawn several weeks before surgery and stored, it is possible for the patient to have a normal hemoglobin-hematocrit level on admission to the hospital for the planned surgery. As a prophylactic means against serum hepatitis, patients receiving a homologous blood transfusion are given 10 ml. gamma globulin on the fifth and tenth days postoperatively.

METHODS OF ASSESSMENT

The importance of identical preoperative and postoperative evaluation in orthopaedic surgery needs little emphasis. An impersonal method of assessment that is comprehensive, reliable, and generally applicable is essential. As Aufranc stated, "One should hesitate to judge the effect of a surgical procedure, even in a large series of cases, when any attempt to compare accurately the patient's condition before the operation with that of after the operation was actually impossible.'"

At the New York Orthopaedic Hospital, a separate "Hip Assessment Record" has been developed for all total hip replacement candidates.

Text continued on p. 274.

The Presbyterian Hospital in the City of New York | Form #3: Radiological
Orthopaedic Surgery Service | A: Diagnostic
Columbia–Presbyterian Medical Center

Preoperative and Postoperative Assessment for HIP SURGERY

Name _____ Unit # _____ Hip Serial # _____ Date _____

1. Osteoarthritis (Primary) Monoarticular (unilateral) _____ (bilateral) _____
    Poliarticular (G O A) _____

2. Osteoarthritis (Secondary) Perthes disease
    Congenital subluxation
    Congenital dislocation
    Slipped epiphysis
    Fracture femoral neck
    Fracture acetabulum
    Traumatic dislocation
    Fracture dislocation
    Paget disease
    Other

3. Rheumatoid arthritis
4. Ankylosing spondylitis
5. Psoriatic arthritis
6. Protrusio acetabuli
7. Spontaneous ischemic necrosis
8. Congenital subluxation) without arthritis
9. Congenital dislocation)
10. Nonunion femoral neck without arthritis
11. Coxa vara (cervical)
12. Coxa vara (subcapital, i e, slipped epiphysis)
13. Paget disease without arthritis
14. Tuberculosis
15. Pyogenic arthritis
16. Sepsis following surgery
17. Pyogenic arthritis
18. Failure previous surgery: specify:

19. Other: specify:

            Unilateral _____ Bilateral _____

Patient's complaint

Radiological appearance

Fig. 9-3. Roentgenographical analysis forms.

Findings (side #2)

Form #3: Radiological
B: Morphology

Congruity				Nonunion			Subchondral line of cortical bone	
none (dislocated)				Neck	Intertrochanteric area		Head	Acetabulum
minimal (marked subluxation)				present	present		normal	normal
poor				absent	absent		reduced	reduced
fair				Shenton line	Dysplasia of socket		very thin	very thin
good				broken	none		absent	absent
normal				intact	mild		irregular	irregular

Joint space	Avascular necrosis		Protrusion	Coxa magna	Periosteal new bone along neck
none	none			moderate	
very thin	mild		Protrusion	Coxa magna	none
reduced	moderate		none	none	minimal
normal	severe		mild	mild	moderate

Joint space / Avascular necrosis
- none — none
- very thin — mild
- reduced — moderate
- normal — severe

Protrusion / Coxa magna
- none — none
- mild — mild
- moderate — moderate
- — severe

Periosteal new bone along neck
- none
- minimal
- moderate
- marked

Cyst formation

Head	Acetabulum
none	none
mild	mild
moderate	moderate
severe	severe

Myositis ossificans

Volume	Restriction
none	none
mild	mild
moderate	moderate
severe	severe

Slipped epiphysis
- none
- mild
- moderate
- severe

Collapse of head
- none
- mild
- moderate
- severe

Implant / Osteopenia
- nail — none
- nail plate — mild
- pins — moderate
- prosthesis — severe
- cup
- total replacement
- spline
- other
- none

Head/Neck angle
- normal
- varus
- valgus
- degrees _____
- other (specify) _____

Loss of sphericity of head
- none
- minimal
- moderate
- severe

Osteophyte formation

Head	Acetabulum
none	none
mild	mild
moderate	moderate
severe	severe

Sclerosis of acetabulum
- none
- mild
- moderate
- severe

Descriptive Morphology of Chronic Arthritis of the Hip (without reference to underlying pathology)

	Right	Left		Right	Left
Normal joint			Destructive head type		
Incipient arthritis (minimal changes)			Destructive acetabulum type		
Upper pole type (minimal to moderate, intact Shenton line)			Destructive tuberculous type, both acetabulum and head		
Upper pole severe (broken Shenton line)			Quadrantic head necrosis		
Medial pole type (without protrusio)			Subluxation type		
Protrusio type			Dislocation type		
Concentric type (i e, polyarthritis)			Septic type		
			Postoperative		
			Other (specify)		
			More than one type		

Fig. 9-3, cont'd. Roentgenographical analysis forms.

The Presbyterian Hospital in the City of New York   Form #4: Operation
Orthopaedic Surgery Service
Columbia-Presbyterian Medical Center
Details of Operation in TOTAL HIP REPLACEMENT
Name _____ Unit # _____ Hip Serial # _____ Time _____
Date _____ Location _____
Type operation: L F A _____ McKee-Farrar _____ Other _____
Indication for operation _____
Revision arthroplasty for _____
Surgeon _____ Assistants _____ OR Nurse _____
Side: R _____ L _____ Bilateral (specify which side first) _____
Skin preparation: Phisohex _____ Iodine _____ Stockinette _____ Plastic drape ____
          Other _____ Other _____
Prophylactic antibiotics: yes _____ no _____
Prophylactic anticoagulants: yes _____ no _____
Special precautions: sealed doors _____ number persons in OR _____ observers _____
          comment on OR traffic _____ nurses _____
          double gloves _____ apron: yes _____ no _____
Range in motion under anesthesia: flexion _____ abduction/adduction _____
          internal/external rotation _____
Exposure: incision: straight _____ T _____ other _____
          skin towel: yes _____ no _____
Quality of muscle: excellent _____ no comment _____ flabby _____
Greater trochanter detached: yes _____ no _____
Greater trochanter elevated with: Gigli saw _____ osteotome _____ power saw ____
Dislocation: easy _____ difficult _____
Removal hardware: easy _____ difficult _____
Femoral neck divided and head extracted retrograde: _____
Psoas tendon divided: _____
Capsule: normal _____ thickened _____ ectopic bone _____
Acetabulum: exposure: excellent _____ adequate _____ inadequate _____
  Osteophytes: present _____ absent _____ removed _____ remain _____
  Size: shallow _____ very shallow _____ average _____ deep _____
  Quality of bone: very soft _____ normal _____ very hard _____
  Preparation: reamed to 2 inches _____ not reamed _____ curetted only _____
  Acetabular rim: defective _____ anteriorly _____ posteriorly _____
          superiorly _____
  After reaming: floor depth _____ inches membrane thin _____
          irregular soft bone _____ gross defect _____
Additional anchor holes: _____ number and size _____
Type of cement: C M W _____ Simplex _____ other _____
Socket: Charnley _____ McKee-Farrar _____ other _____
Orientation: _____ special device _____
Projection of rim of socket lateral to rim of acetabulum: yes _____ no _____
          amount _____

Fig. 9-4. Details of total hip replacement surgery form.

(side #2)   Form #4: Operation

Femur: extent of periosteal stripping under calcar _____ inches

  Preparation of canal: easy _____ difficult _____

  Drilling jig used to find canal: yes _____ no _____

  Power driven reamer: yes _____ no _____

  Canal curetted: yes _____ no _____

  Femoral shaft split: yes _____ no _____ perforation: yes _____

                                                                      no _____

  Type of prosthesis: Charnley _____ revision pattern _____ chrome cobalt _____

  Type of cement: C M W _____ Simplex _____ other _____

  Prosthesis driven by: hand pressure _____ slight hammering _____ heavy hammering _____

  Unstable reduction: traction pulls surfaces apart _____ inches _____

                      position which dislocation occurs _____

  Stable reduction: degrees adduction producing dislocation _____

                      degrees flexion producing dislocation _____

Greater Trochanter:

  Rotators released: yes _____ no _____

  Quality of trochanter: sound bone _____ soft _____ very soft _____ fragmented _____

  Adductors resutured with: _____ material; no _____

  Trochanter attached: crosswires _____ stainless steel _____

  Position: original _____ halfway _____ outside shaft _____

  Adductors divided: yes _____ no _____ during operation _____ end operation _____

Wound Closure: Assessment of thickness of fat layer _____ inches

  Antibiotics in wound: yes _____ no _____ type _____

  Suction drainage: into joint _____ under fascia _____ into fat _____

  Deep fascia: interrupted _____ continuous material _____

  Fat layer: interrupted _____ continuous material _____

  Pull-out stitches to fat: yes _____ no _____

  Skin closure: material _____ type of closure _____

Total duration of operation: _____ minutes

Surgeons gloves known to be punctured: yes _____ no _____

X-ray seen: yes _____ no _____ cement _____

Postoperative splinting: 1 week _____ 2 weeks _____ 3 weeks _____

Pathological material sent to laboratory (specify): _____

_____

Special comments:

Fig. 9-4, cont'd. Details of total hip replacement surgery form.

271

The Presbyterian Hospital in the City of New York   Form #5: Complication
Orthopaedic Surgery Service
Columbia–Presbyterian Medical Center
_____

HIP SURGERY
_____

A. GENERAL   No complication
                     Pleurisy
                     Pneumonia or bronchopneumonia
                     Cardiac failure
                     Pulmonary embolus
                     Coronary occlusion
                     Fat embolus
                     Paralytic ileus
                     Urinary retention
                     Urinary infection
                     Other (specify)

B. LOCAL   No complication
                     Hematoma
                     Superficial wound infection
                     Deep wound infection
                     Dislocation
                     Deep vein thrombosis (ipsilateral)
                     Deep vein thrombosis (contralateral)
                     Drop foot

Prophylactic antibiotics   yes ____   no ____

Prophylactic anticoagulants   yes ____   no ____

Comments
_____

Fig. 9-5. Postoperative hip surgery complications form.

The Presbyterian Hospital in the City of New York
Orthopaedic Surgery Service
Columbia–Presbyterian Medical Center

Form #6: Therapy

Routine Physiotherapy Progress Note   (to be completed by therapist)

Name _____   Unit # _____   Location _____

Date	Date Operated	Condition of Wound	Abduction Pillow	S L R		Knee Flexion		Hip Flexion		Aids	Comments
				R	L	R	L	R	L		

Fig. 9-6. Routine physiotherapy progress form.

This record is initiated preoperatively and includes history, physical examination, and results of hip examination (Fig. 9-1). Other areas recorded are roentgenographic analysis (Fig. 9-3), details of operative procedure (Fig. 9-4), postoperative complications (Fig. 9-5), and follow-up evaluation (Fig. 9-6). Additional records are adapted to study other parameters of the patient's care and management such as anticoagulation, antibiotics, and postoperative physiotherapy.

METHODS OF GRADING AND THEIR LIMITATIONS

Various scales for rating hip disability have been attempted to help compare preoperative and postoperative results of different types of procedures.* They are mainly aimed at comparing the preoperative and postoperative status of the patient in regard to pain, function, and mobility. Despite all efforts to maintain objectivity, it is interesting to note that in many instances an overrating by the surgeon may be found on comparison with the therapist's assessment, based on the same scale system.[18]

Larson[31] suggested a scoring system based on a 100-point scale to evaluate cup arthroplasty. In addition to scoring functional ability, including pain and gait, he considered anatomical assessment such as range of motion and deformity, for example, shortening of the limb. These factors were weighed with 35 points for pain, 35 for function, 10 for gait, 10 for absence of deformity, and 10 for motion. Harris proposed a 100-point scale giving 44 points for pain, 47 for function, 5 for range of motion, and 4 for absence of deformity. Obviously, both systems involve an arbitrary loading, which defies the advantage of presenting the patient in one numerical scale. Shepherd[43] further modified the Larson method as an improved means of evaluating hip disability. She suggested that the variables be incorporated in a way that would make them equally applicable to different problems and methods of treatment. Shepherd's system can be criticized because it does not integrate function with motion and lacks a single overall value for all ratings.

Shepherd, in attempting to compare the results of cup arthroplasty with osteotomy or arthrodesis, uses the Gade[22] index, whereby

---

*See references 8, 10, 18, 26, 28, 31, 32, and 43-45.

more than 45 degrees flexion is given fewer points than flexion less than 45 degrees. The purpose of Shepherd's approach is to evaluate the benefit derived from an operation, the results of which cannot be compared to a normal hip joint. This approach, although somewhat more comprehensive, is rather complicated and subject to the same criticism for loading as the other systems. This is an especially important point since results of total hip arthroplasty should approximate a normal hip condition, and full-scale points should be given to mobility.

The first objective method was suggested by D'Aubigne and Postel in 1954;[10] they used three units: one for pain, one for function, and one for mobility. Each unit ranged from 1 to 6, with 1 representing complete disability and 6 representing normality. D'Aubigne and Judet further evolved one digit to describe the patient's "amelioration factors."[28]

Lazansky adopted 26 separate items of clinical information (the "Green Card" used at Wrightington Centre for Hip Surgery) in an attempt to arrive at an objective system representing the patient by a single digit. His method was largely derived from those of Shepherd, the Judets, D'Aubigne, and Postel. Although Lazansky's grading system expresses the condition of the entire patient rather than the hip (whether unilateral or bilateral), it is subject to the same criticism as the other systems, that is, a rather complex "loading" in scoring, and the total score weighed to emphasize mobility.

Charnley[8] modified the D'Aubigne and Postel numerical classification. We[16,17] adopted this modified 6-6-6 grading system, which is popular in Great Britain and continental Europe, at the New York Orthopaedic Hospital at the beginning of the total hip replacement program there in 1969. The advantage of this method is its simplicity; the reviewer can quickly and separately evaluate the three parameters of hip disability: pain, function, and mobility. In addition, the results can be directly compared with a larger series such as Charnley's. The assignment into one of three groups makes it possible to describe the patient as a whole rather than as a hip. The first, group A, includes those patients with unilateral hip disease; group B consists of patients with bilateral hip disease without other restraining factors; and group C is comprised of those patients with either unilateral or bilateral hip disease who also have systemic

THE PRESBYTERIAN HOSPITAL
in the City of New York
Department of Orthopaedic Surgery
Columbia—Presbyterian Medical Center

Preoperative and Postoperative Assessment for Hip Surgery

Form #2 Assessment

Hosp. No.

Type operation: _____

Date operation: _____

Work: _____

Last Name		First Name	M.I.	Age	Weight

Type and Number of Pain Tablets/day

Spontaneous Pain at Night YES ☐ NO ☐

PAIN

BEDRIDDEN OR CHAIR LIFE	TWO CRUTCHES	TWO STICKS	ONE STICK ALWAYS	ONE STICK OUTSIDE	NO STICKS
1 Severe Spontaneous	**2** Severe on attempting to walk Prevents all activity	**3** Pain tolerable permitting limited activity	**4** Pain only after some activity; disappears quickly with rest	**5** Slight or intermittent. Pain on starting to walk but getting less with normal activity	**6** No pain
R L	R L	R L	R L	R L	R L

FUNCTION

1 Bedridden or few yards; two sticks or crutches	**2** Time and distance very limited with or without sticks	**3** Limited with one stick (less than one hour) Difficult without stick. Able to stand long periods	**4** Long distances with one stick; limited without a stick	**5** No stick but a limp	**6** Normal
R L	R L	R L	R L	R L	R L
GAIT WITHOUT STICKS — Cannot walk	Just able to walk	Walks but with gross limp	Walks with moderate limp	Slight limp	Normal gait

Gait (Describe)

Limp   Short leg limp YES ☐ NO ☐   Hip limp YES ☐ NO ☐

Trendelenburg: Positive   R: L   ;   Negative   R: L

Length of stride: (estimated by sight)

Dresses self	With Difficulty YES ☐ NO ☐	Can climb stairs	With Difficulty YES ☐ NO ☐
Puts on stockings	With Difficulty YES ☐ NO ☐	— with banister	With Difficulty YES ☐ NO ☐
Ties shoes	With Difficulty YES ☐ NO ☐	— one at time	With Difficulty YES ☐ NO ☐
Walks outside	With Difficulty YES ☐ NO ☐	Cuts toenails	With Difficulty YES ☐ NO ☐
Bathing self	With Difficulty YES ☐ NO ☐	Drives car	With Difficulty YES ☐ NO ☐
Regular toilet	With Difficulty YES ☐ NO ☐	Sits comfortably	With Difficulty YES ☐ NO ☐
Public transportation	With Difficulty YES ☐ NO ☐	— only high chair ½ Hr.	With Difficulty YES ☐ NO ☐

CATEGORICAL CLASSIFICATION FOR FUNCTION

A) Unilateral hip: no other functional disability
B) Bilateral hip; no other functional disability
C) Unilateral or bilateral WITH other joints or medical condition affecting function

COMMENTS:

Category 'C' Cases
☐ CVS
☐ RS
☐ CNS
☐ Senility
☐ Obesity
☐ Psychiatric
☐ Other

☐ orthopaedics

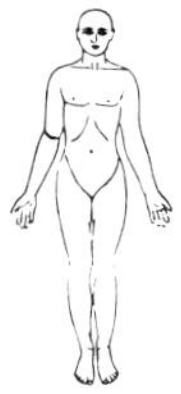

Fig. 9-7. Hip evaluation form used at New York Orthopaedic Hospital.

Continued.

275

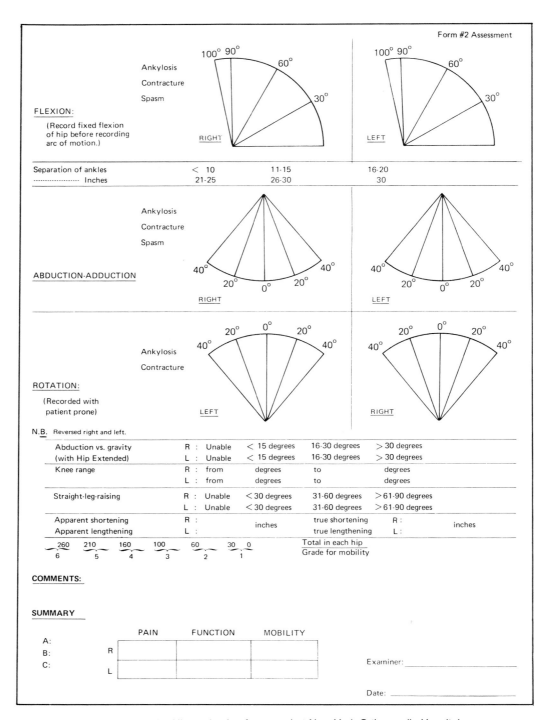

Fig. 9-7, cont'd. Hip evaluation form used at New York Orthopaedic Hospital.

or other conditions that restrict their function. For example, a rheumatoid arthritis patient with multiple joint involvement and one with excessive obesity would both be placed in group C if their overall function were limited by those conditions. This division is extremely valuable when assessing the results of arthroplasty as a surgical procedure (the hip), and the overall performance of function (the patient). Fig. 9-7 represents the "Hip Evaluation Form" used at the New York Orthopaedic Hospital and contains 54 items as part of the permanent evaluation of a patient's preoperative status. A similar postoperative evaluation sheet is completed at each subsequent hospital or office visit.

SUMMARY OF ESSENTIALS

- For the most part the success of total hip replacement depends on not only a sound technical surgical operation, but on overall management, which would include preoperative evaluation and recording, preparation for surgery, and sound postoperative management of the patient.

- Ideally, the patient should be admitted to the hospital 2 to 3 days prior to proposed surgery for a careful detailed history and physical examination, not only by a member of the house staff, but also by an interested internist who will also follow the patient closely during the postoperative period.

- A complete systemic examination is a basic requirement for any surgical procedure. This is particularly applicable to total hip replacement because it is a major elective operation. A review of systems is most important to ensure a safe and uncomplicated postoperative recovery.

- In dealing with older patient's, special consideration should be given to incipient diabetes, electrolyte imbalance, physical and mental attitude and alertness, hypertension, cardiac insufficiency, and the need for anticoagulation prophylaxis during the postoperative course.

- Relevant laboratory examinations should include a complete blood count, erythrocyte sedimentation rate, SMA 12, electrolyte evaluation, urinalysis, clotting profile, stool hematest, baseline arterial blood gases, and pulmonary function studies. In addition, a routine chest radiograph and an electrocardiogram are basic requirements for general anesthesia. In case of any abnormalities, further consultations and/or laboratory studies are essential.

- Of those patients admitted for total hip replacement 10% to 20% may not qualify for surgery immediately because of poor health. To reduce morbidity these individuals must be singled out before operation.

- Systemic review of the patient to rule out or disclose cardiac arrhythmias, extensive hypertension, evidence of cardiac decompensation, severe and advanced generalized arteriosclerosis, abdominal aneurysm, and carotid artery insufficiencies must be sought. In most instances the general condition of the patient may be improved by treatment of these conditions prior to the contemplated hip surgery.

- Patients with severe hypertension must not be deprived of their medications before surgery, but alterations in medications and close attention by an internist as well as the anesthesiologist may provide a safe procedure for these individuals.

- Denial of total hip replacement in elderly patients suffering from painful arthritis of the hip in their final years must be based on objective and unbiased scientific facts. The degree of disability and the patient's attitude toward that disability may counterbalance the added risks involved. In this context the judgment of an internist familiar with morbidity and mortality following total hip replacement is invaluable in arriving at a decision.

- Pulmonary complications in older patients contributing to a high degree of morbidity can be lessened in most instances by pulmonary toilet care and breathing exercises, which diminish these risks. An expert anesthetist and the choice of the method of anesthesia may reduce the risk.

- Review of genitourinary and gastrointestinal systems is essential. The former may lead to postoperative infection if a dormant chronic infection of the genitourinary system remains undiagnosed. An unrecognized gastrointestinal bleeding source may require avoidance of the use of anticoagulant drugs, with an adverse effect on the prevention or treatment of pulmonary embolism or deep vein thrombosis.

- All sources of potential and real remote infections must be sought. In this context the skin must always be considered as a potential source of wound contamination. Infected traumatic lesions, insect bites, rashes, and the like are sufficient cause to postpone surgery.

- The role of the physiotherapist to include close working relations with the patient cannot be overly emphasized. When patients are seen preoperatively by the therapist who will treat them postoperatively, better cooperation regarding deep breathing, coughing, ankle and quadriceps exercises, as well as ambulation using walking assistance is afforded.

- The choice of prostheses and surgical approach must be carefully thought out based on the surgeon's experience and his background training. It is disadvantageous to use more than one system of instruments and surgical approach because mixed experiences reduce one's expertise with a particular system of instrumentation and operation.

277

- The system of instrumentation must be versatile; it must allow a perfect implantation of the prosthesis and fully correct the deformity. The prosthesis must possess adequate strength and afford adaptability to specific anatomical situations. Specific prostheses must be available to the surgeon according to the preoperative appraisal of the anatomical situation.
- Normotensive, hypotensive, and regional (spinal) anesthesia may be used. While hypotensive and regional anesthesia have considerable advantages over normotensive conventional anesthesia, the selection of anesthesia must be left to an interested anesthesiologist and internist to recommend the anesthesia of choice for each individual. Undoubtedly, with more experience, hypotensive anesthesia ultimately will replace other types of anesthesia in most instances in performing total hip replacement.
- An average patient undergoing a total hip replacement with normotensive anesthesia would require 1,000 to 1,500 ml. blood during and/or after operation. This can be reduced by one-half if a hypotensive anesthesia is used.
- Conventional blood bank blood used in most hospitals carries a high incidence of serum hepatitis. Autologous banked blood is ideal to eliminate the danger of serum hepatitis and inherent transfusion problems such as mismatched blood, clerical errors, and immunological reactions to blood proteins.
- Transfusion of a single unit of blood postoperatively is not recommended. However, older patients usually do not tolerate low hemoglobin-hematocrit levels postoperatively. With any signs of restlessness, agitation, or psychosis accompanied by anemia postoperatively, transfusion is essential. With blood-freezing techniques, blood may be drawn several weeks before surgery from the patient and stored for transfusion at the time of operation or postoperatively. As a prophylactic means against serum hepatitis, patients receiving homologous blood transfusions are given gamma globulin on the fifth and tenth day postoperatively.
- Those interested in performing arthroplasty of the hip joint, regardless of the method used, must be able to form an impersonal method of assessment that is comprehensive, reliable, and generally applicable in all cases.
- Methods of making assessment records are suggested, not only for clinical use, but also for future research work as well. In particular, late complications can only be properly evaluated if adequate preoperative data is at hand.
- There are numerous methods of rating for comparison of preoperative and postoperative results in different types of arthroplasty of the hip joint. Among these, Larson's Judet's, D'Aubigne's, Lazansky's, Gade's, and Charnley's modification of D'Aubigne's and Postel's as well as Harris's are worth noting. The best method is one free of "loading," giving equal points for pain, function, and mobility—it is also one that represents the patient as a whole. The use of a modified 6-6-6 grading system with additional preface A, B, and C used by Charnley has proved to be satisfactory in this regard.

REFERENCES

1. Aufranc, O. E.: Preoperative and postoperative treatment of patients with reconstructive surgery of the hip, Clin. Orthop. **38:**40-44, 1965.
2. Bodman, R. I.: Death after anaesthetic with hypotension, Lancet **11:**1085, 1952.
3. Bodman, R. I.: Controlled hypotension, Int. Anesthesiol. Clin. **5:**90, 1967.
4. Blume, R.: Personal communications.
5. Bond, A. G.: Conduction anesthesia, blood pressure and haemorrhage, Br. J. Anaesth. **41:**942-946, 1969.
6. Burton, D. S., and Schurman, D. J.: Hematogenous infection in bilateral total hip arthroplasty, J. Bone Joint Surg. **57A:**1004-1005, 1975.
7. Charnley, J.: Personal communications.
8. Charnley, J.: The numerical grading of hips. Internal Publication No. 20, Centre for Hip Surgery, Wrightington Hospital, England, December, 1968.
9. Charnley, J.: Postoperative management of total hip reconstruction by low friction method, Internal Publication No. 27, Centre for Hip Surgery, Wrightington Hospital, England, November, 1970.
10. D'Aubigne, R. M., and Postel, M.: Functional results of hip arthroplasty with acrylic prosthesis, J. Bone Joint Surg. **36A:**451-475, 1954.
11. Davis, N. J., Jennings, J. J., and Harris, W. H.: Induced hypotensive anesthesia for total hip replacement, Clin. Orthop. **101:**93-98, 1974.
12. Davison, M. H. A.: Pentamethonium iodide in anaesthesia, Lancet **1:**252-253, 1950.
13. Ditzler, J. E., and Eckenoff, J. E.: Comparison of blood loss and operative time in certain surgical procedures completed with and without controlled hypotension, Ann. Surg. **143:**289-293, 1956.
14. Dolkart, R. E.: Medical considerations of orthopedic surgery in the elderly patient, J. Bone Joint Surg. **47A:**1041-1042, 1965.
15. Donald, J. R.: The effect of anesthesia, hypotension, and epidural anesthesia on blood loss in surgery for pelvic floor repair, Br. J. Anaesth. **41:**155-166, 1969.
16. Eftekhar, N. S., Bush, D. C., Freeman, A. R., and Stinchfield, F. E.: Perioperative management of

total hip replacement, Orthop. Rev. **3**(1):17-27, 1974.

17. Eftekhar, N. S., and Stinchfield, F. E.: Experience with low friction arthroplasty: a statistical review of early results and complications, Clin. Orthop. **95:**60-68, 1973.

18. Ehrlich, G. E., editor: Total management of the arthritic patient, Philadelphia 1973, J. B. Lippincott Co.

19. Enderby, G. E. H.: Controlled circulation with hypotensive drugs and posture to reduce bleeding in surgery, Lancet **1:**1145, 1950.

20. Enderby, G. E. H.: Pentolinium tartrate in controlled hypotension, Lancet **11:**1097-1098, 1954.

21. Enderby, G. E. H.: A report on mortality and morbidity following 9,107 hypotensive anesthetics, Br. J. Anaesth. **33:**109-113, 1961.

22. Gade, H. G.: A contribution to the surgical treatment of osteoarthritis of the hip joint, Acta Chrirg. Scand. **95:**[Suppl. 120] 1-290, 1947.

23. Gardner, W. J.: The control of bleeding during operation by induced hypotension, J.A.M.A. **132:** 572-574, 1946.

24. Grant, F. C.: Autotransfusion, Ann. Surg. **74:** 253-254, 1971.

25. Harris, W.: Personal communications.

26. Harris, W. H.: Traumatic arthritis of the hip after dislocation and acetabular fractures; treatment by mold arthroplasty, J. Bone Joint Surg. **51A:**737-755, 1969.

27. Janecki, C. J., DeHaven, K. E., and Benton, J. W.: Preoperative and postoperative management in total hip reconstruction, Orthop. Clin. North Am. **4:**(2)523-531, 1973.

28. Judet, J., and Judet, R.: Technique and results with the acrylic femoral head prosthesis, J. Bone Joint Surg. **34B:**173-180, 1952.

29. Kallos, T., and Smith, T. C.: Continuous spinal anesthesia with hypobaric tetracaine for hip surgery in lateral decubitus, Anesth. Analg. **51:**766-773, 1972.

30. Larson, A. G.: Deliberate hypotension, Anesthesiology **25:**682-706, 1964.

31. Larson, C. B.: Rating scale for hip disabilities, Clin. Orthop. **31:**85-92, 1963.

32. Lazansky, M. G.: A method for grading hips, J. Bone Joint Surg. **49B:**644-651, 1967.

33. Little, D. M.: Induced hypotension during anesthesia and surgery, anesthesiology **16:**320-332, 1955.

34. Madsen, R. E., and Madsen, P. O.: Influence of anesthesia form on blood loss in transurethral prostatectomy, Anesth. Analg. **46:**330-332, 1967.

35. Mallory, T. H.: Hypotensive anesthesia in total hip replacement, Orthop. Rev. **4:**(8)21-30, 1975.

36. Matheson, N. A., and Diomi, P.: Renal failure after administration of dextran 40, Surg. Gynecol. Obstet. **131:**661-668, 1970.

37. Milles, G., Langston, H., and Dalessandro, W.: Experiences with autotransfusions, Surg. Gynecol. Obstet. **116:**689-694, 1962.

38. Newman, M. M., Hamstra, R., and Block, M.: Use of banked autologous blood in elective surgery, J.A.M.A. **218:**861-863, 1971.

39. Nicholson, J. T.: Symposium: surgical care of the elderly patient is different. General remarks and the importance of good nursing care and early rehabilitation, J. Bone Joint Surg. **47A:**1035-1040, 1965.

40. Polesky, H. S.: Autologous transfusion, Lab. Med. **5:**37-40, 1974.

41. Scott, D. L.: Anaesthetic experiences in 1300 major geriatric operations, Br. J. Anaesth. **33:** 354-370, 1961.

42. Sculco, T. P., and Ranawat, C.: The use of spinal anesthesia for total hip replacement arthroplasty, J. Bone Joint Surg. **57A:**173-177, 1975.

43. Shepherd, M. M.: Assessment of function after arthroplasty of the hip. J. Bone Joint Surg. **36B:** 354-363, 1954.

44. Shepherd, M. M.: A review of 650 hip arthroplasty operations, J. Bone Joint Surg. **36B:**567-577, 1954.

45. Shepherd, M. M.: A further review of the results of operations on the hip joint, J. Bone Joint Surg. **42B:**177-204, 1960.

46. Stahlgren, L. H.: An analysis of factors which influence mortality following extensive abdominal operation upon geriatric patients, Surg. Gynecol. Obstet. **113:**283-292, 1961.

47. Thomas, W. H.: Postoperative program for patients having cup arthroplasty, Surg. Clin. North Am. **49:**779-786, 1969.

48. Viikari, S. J., and Vaalasti, T.: Surgery in aged persons, Ann. Chir. Gynaecol. Fenn. **48:**19-30, 1959.

49. Wilder, R. J., and Fishbein, R. H.: Operative experience with patients over 80 years of age, Surg. Gynecol. Obstet. **113:**205-212, 1961.

CHAPTER 10

Radiological studies

When schemes are laid in advance, it is surprising how often circumstances fit in with them.

SIR WILLIAM OSLER

RADIOLOGICAL MORPHOLOGY
General comments

A careful review of preoperative radiographs and recording of the radiological morphology is essential in order to appreciate the diagnostic and technical aspects of total hip arthroplasty. In this context the study of radiographs is as essential to the surgeon as analysis of blueprints is to the engineer and builder.

1. Generally, distinction between osteoarthritis, rheumatoid arthritis, or a septic hip can be made. Although diagnosis is not always possible by radiographs alone, telltale signs and clinical symptoms of these conditions may be established through radiological study.

2. Conditions such as suppurative arthritis or tuberculosis may be screened out.

3. Difficult anatomical situations may be verified and technical problems anticipated so that appropriate measures may be taken during surgery. An outstanding example is equalization of leg length following replacement of one or both hips. Conditions such as fusion of the hip, ectopic bone, protrusio acetabuli, or severe osteoporosis are all indications for special technical requirements.

4. Hardware from previous surgery may be identified as to type so that its removal at surgery can be anticipated and special instruments or prostheses made available when necessary.

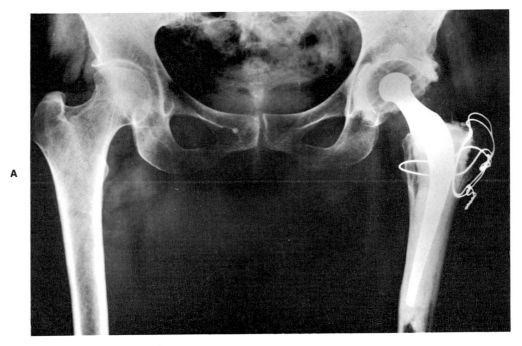

Fig. 10-1. Good quality radiographs that include upper third of femurs and isthmus of femur are essential. Anteroposterior view must include both hips and upper third of femurs. **A.** Manfredi lateral, **B** and **C,** (shoot-through) is preferrable since frogleg lateral position is not usually possible because of stiffness of hip in arthritic conditions.

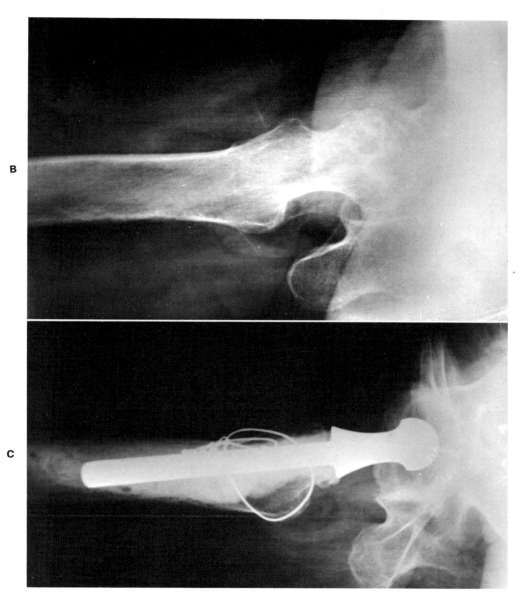

Fig. 10-1, cont'd. For legend see opposite page.

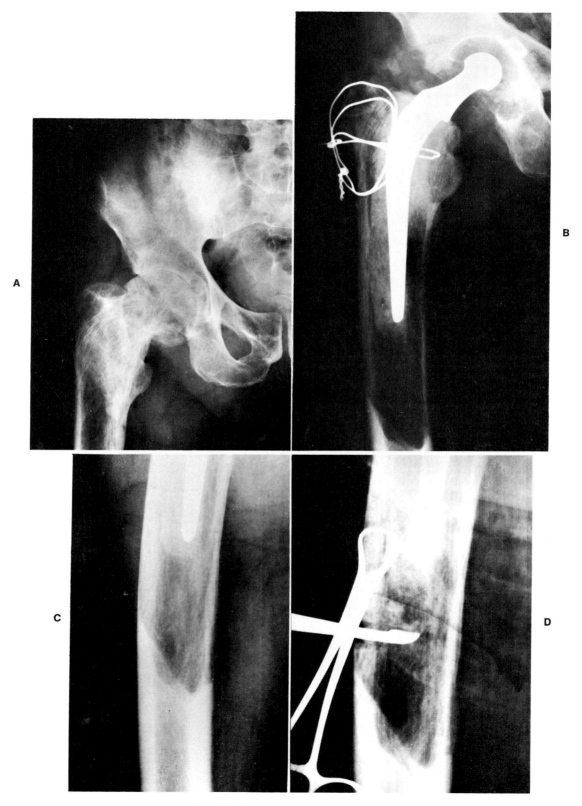

Fig. 10-2. For legend see opposite page.

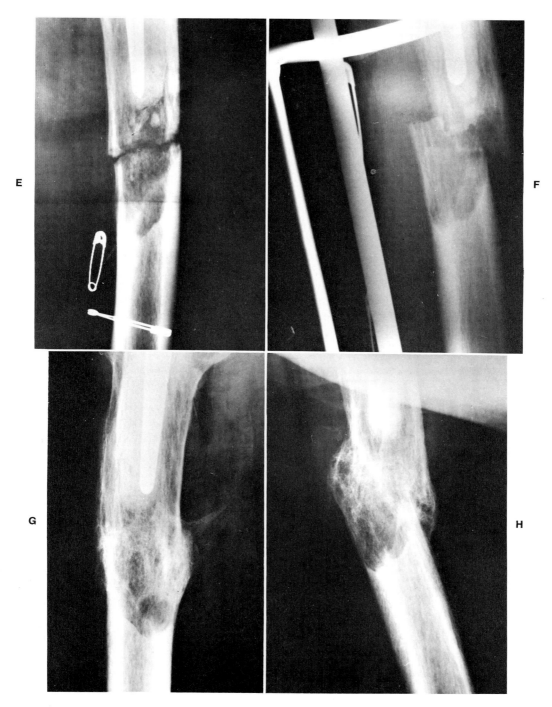

Fig. 10-2. Films not adequately including entire hip joint and upper third of femur may lead to unrecognized pathology at surgery. **A,** Degenerative osteoarthrosis in 54-year-old man with Paget's disease of bone. NOTE: this preoperative x-ray film, which was only available radiograph at surgery, was inadequate. It did not include upper third of femur. **B,** Immediate postoperative x-ray film revealed large area of radiolucency (osteoporosis circumscripta), which had not been recognized prior to surgery. **C,** This localized film was taken following surgery to show defect. **D,** Because of fear of sarcomatous changes of this lesion, which was painful following surgery, biopsy was performed; intraoperative radiograph shows lesion. **E,** Two months following discharge, patient fractured femur at level of weakened bone. **F,** Limb suspended in balanced suspension traction apparatus with fracture aligned. **G** and **H,** Anteroposterior and lateral view of femur fracture healed 9 months following original surgery. This complication could have been prevented by appropriate radiographs, preoperatively, assessing lesion, obtaining biopsy at original operation, and use of long-stem prosthesis to bypass weakened area of femur.

283

5. Mechanical failure often can be distinguished from infection only by examination of serial radiographs.

An aware and interested radiologist familiar with specific problems of total hip replacement is invaluable in performing certain diagnostic procedures or establishing a correct diagnosis.

Generally, an anteroposterior view of both hips and the upper third of both femurs is obtained on a single film. Although on one film, radiographs cannot be centered on both hip joints, such a film provides details adequate for diagnostic purposes.

A standard x-ray table with a Potter-Bucky diaphragm is used. For a standard image, the distance of tube to film is 42 inches, which usually produces a 1.2 times magnification of the bone and prosthesis. For example, the over-

all image of a Charnley prosthesis will measure 18.5 to 19.5 cm. Attention to the details of radiographic magnification is essential, particularly for assessing the width of the femoral canal.

A lateral view of the hip is helpful for comparison of cortical changes of the bone with postoperative films, that is, to verify the possibility of infection or loosening. A Manfredi lateral (shoot-through) view of both hips is preferable since a "frogleg" lateral position is not suitable. (External rotation on abduction often is painful or impossible in patients with arthritis.) (Fig. 10-1.) Good quality radiographs that include the upper third of the femurs and the isthmus of the femur are essential. Films not adequately visualizing the upper femur may result in unrecognized pathology, as in Fig. 10-2, which illustrates a patient with Paget's disease. Another ex-

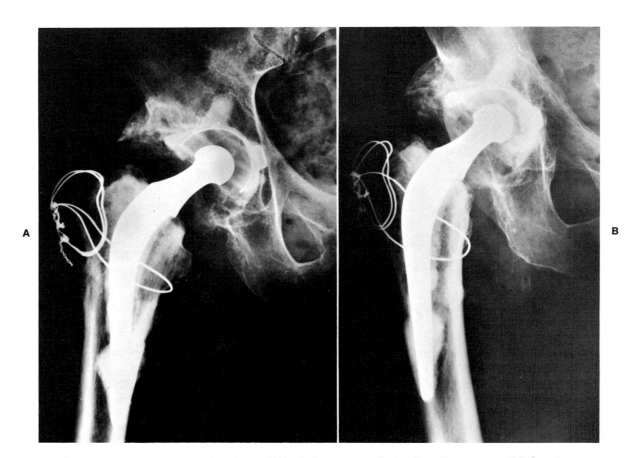

Fig. 10-3. To locate actual location of stem within shaft, two perpendicular plane films are essential. On anteroposterior view, hip must be in neutral rotation and shoot-through lateral view to include upper third of femur must also be obtained. **A,** Postoperative x-ray film of low-friction arthroplasty in 61-year-old man, suggestive of femoral stem penetration through medial cortex. **B,** With internal rotation stem looks as if it has penetrated through lateral cortex.

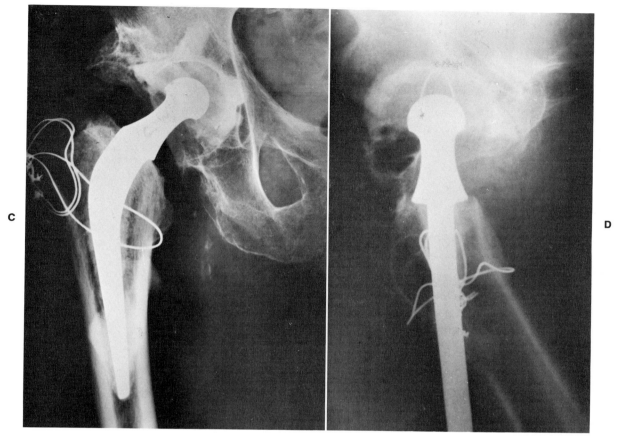

Fig. 10-3, cont'd. C, Hip in neutral rotation; stem is within shaft of femur. **D,** Situation was not well appraised until lateral view was obtained (Manfredi lateral) where actual penetration was discovered to be posterior.

ample is a case where the stem of a previous prosthesis extends from the femoral shaft and is not recognized in the anteroposterior view (Fig. 10-3).

A film of the pertinent areas does not reveal potential problems of technique at surgery, such as a narrow isthmus, but comparison of both hips on a single plate, 17 × 14 inch film, is helpful for evaluation of any fixed pelvic deformity with compensatory scoliotic changes in the lumbosacral spine. The surgeon will be alerted by such a film when positioning the acetabular component in the pelvis.

Documentation of the details of x-ray films in the evaluation record is an effective teaching tool and insurance against loss of the radiographs, since the descriptive details become a permanent record in the patient's chart. (See Chapter 9.) (Fig. 9-3 represents Form No. 3, used for recording the radiological morphology

of the hip.) In addition to routine preoperative radiographs, similar x-ray studies are carried out immediately after surgery, 6 days later (at the start of rehabilitation), then at 6 weeks, and annually thereafter.

Special radiological studies

Laminagrams, magnified views, arthrograms, bone scans, arteriographs, and cystograms all have their specific indications. These radiological tests are necessary in the study of complications following replacement. Special contrast studies (Fig. 10-4), cineradiography, as well as special views, may help to define certain abnormal situations.

Arthrography. Salvati and associates[31] advocated arthrography to detect loosening in total hip replacement. This technique was developed at the Hospital for Special Surgery in New York to verify the cause of complications following

285

Fig. 10-4. Special studies using contrast media may be useful in elaborating certain conditions of hip. Attempts for arthrograms may reveal soft tissue collection of pus or infective cavities about hip joint. **A,** Preoperative radiograph of 56-year-old accountant without history of tuberculosis but radiological appearance of hip tuberculosis and calcific area within vicinity of hip joint. **B,** Postoperative x-ray film of hip arthroplasty performed in another institution with early successful results.

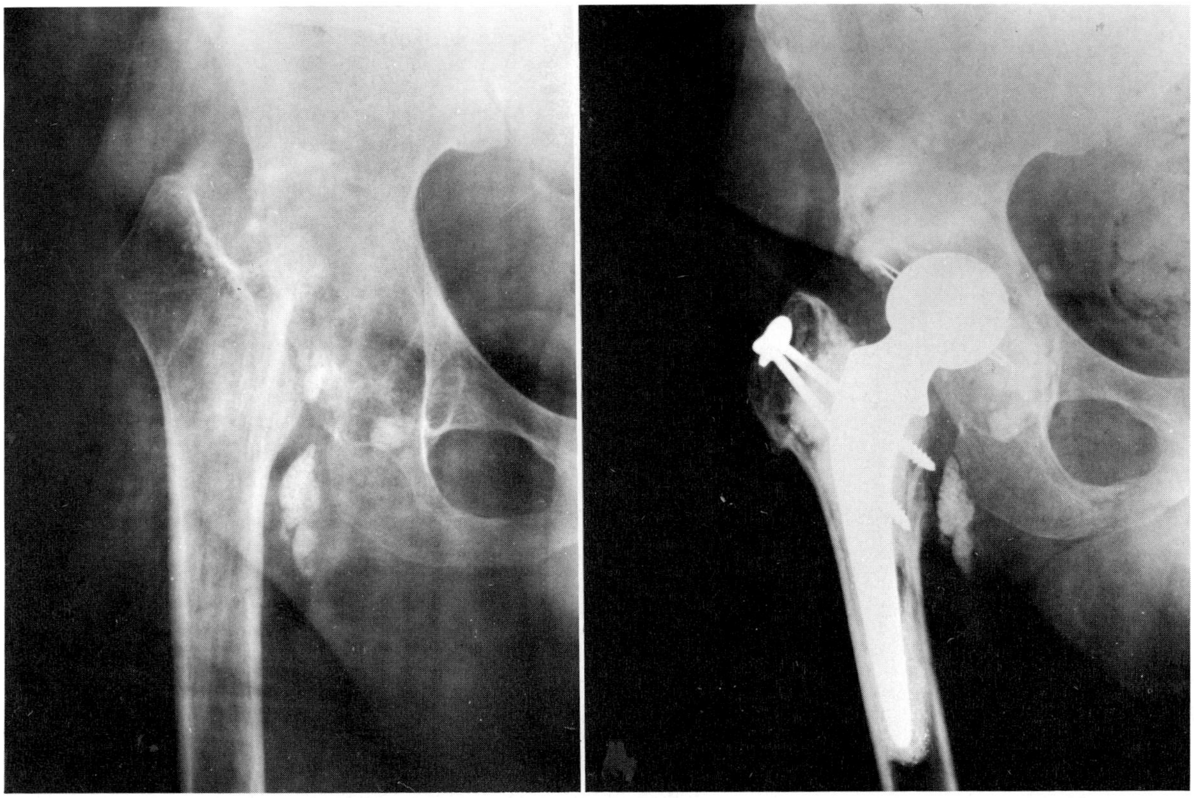

total hip replacement and to differentiate between loosening and low-grade infection. It includes aspiration of the hip under fluoroscopy using a spinal needle (20 to 22 gauge) and injection of 60% meglumine diatrizoate sodium (Renografin 60). Because of difficulty in interpreting arthrograms when radiopaque cement had been used in surgery, a subtraction technique[18] (used commonly in neuroradiology) was recommended.[33] When the prosthesis is loose, plane radiographs invariably depict a radiolucent zone between cement and bone. However, because this radiolucent zone is commonly seen in postoperative routine radiographs without any clinical significance, injected contrast media will penetrate between cement and bone, and this establishes the diagnosis of loosening through differentiation between injected contrast media and opaque cement.[31] Salvati and associates[33] state that this method affords a reliable diagno-

sis of loosening, providing details of the technique are observed. For example, the patient must be absolutely immobile during x-ray examination to avoid producing false images when the radiographs obtained before and after injection are superimposed.

My experience with arthrography has been unsatisfactory because the correlations between the positive arthrograms and findings at surgery have been insignificant. (See Chapter 14.) Others have expressed similar concerns regarding interpretation of arthrograms. In a prospective study of 25 painful hips in 21 patients following total hip arthroplasty and in 53 asymptomatic hips in 42 patients after total hip arthroplasty, it was found that arthrographic evidence of loosening was not always associated with pain. More than one fifth of the patients without pain had arthrographic proof of loosening. Also, loosening was not confirmed in all patients who

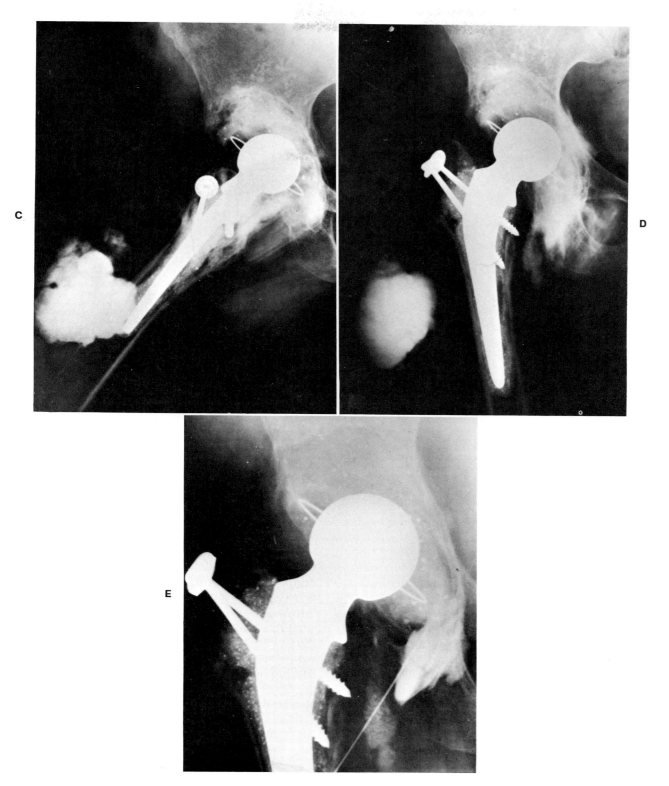

Fig. 10-4, cont'd. C, One year following surgery, hip was painful and swelling appeared in lateral aspect of thigh. **D,** Contrast media, 20 ml., was injected into soft tissue located at level of tip of prosthesis. No communication was observed between soft tissue abscess and bone. **E,** Subsequently, needle was also inserted into hip joint to obtain arthrogram in addition to injection of contrast media at interface between cement and bone. No communication was detected between soft tissue abscess and hip joint. *Continued.*

287

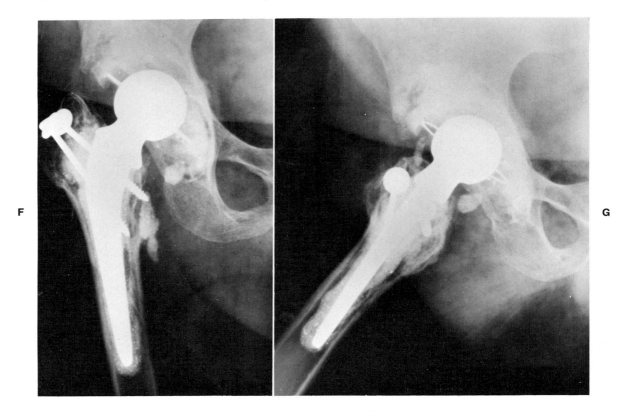

Fig. 10-4, cont'd. F and **G,** Three years following removal of soft tissue abscess and exploration of joint, which confirmed original impression of diagnosis of tuberculous abscess and extension to hip joint. Artificial hip joint was not disturbed because of good mechanical fixation; patient who had not originally received chemoprophylaxis for tuberculosis was placed on antituberculous drugs for 2 years.

had a positive arthrogram. Loosening was confirmed only in 7 of 12 hips explored. All 12 had a positive arthrogram for loosening. There was no apparent relationship between arthrographic loosening and the presence of Trendelenburg's sign. This study concluded that doubt exists concerning the value of an arthrogram in diagnosing the cause of a painful total hip.[27]

Arteriographic evaluation. Arteriography has been used for both diagnosis and treatment of hemorrhagic conditions accompanied by pelvic trauma.[30] Development of false aneurysm of the femoral artery following total hip surgery and arteriographic management of postoperative bleeding following removal of a total hip device have also been reported.[10,28] Obviously, when one is confronted with the possibility of excessive trauma to the pelvis at surgery or following total hip replacement, awareness of arterial complications and arteriography in consultation with the vascular surgical team is the only lifesaving procedure.

Cystograms. Retrograde cystograms may be a useful means of verifying bladder injury after total hip replacement, especially following revision of a complicated total hip prosthesis or undue trauma to the pelvis (Fig. 10-5). If infection is present and there is evidence of a sinus formation with a communicating tract, then a sinogram may reveal the dye in the bladder. On the other hand, a retrograde cystogram may verify communication between the bladder and the hip joint. A thermal injury by self-curing acrylic cement leading to a bladder fistula must also be considered.[24]

Bone scanning. As an aid to diagnosis in painful total hip replacement, bone scanning has been used with success. However, it must be recognized that at the present time specific indications for this technique are not clearly identified. Technetium 99–stannous phosphate scanning comparing the patterns with those of a normal pain-free hip replacement has been attempted. A characteristic pattern of increased

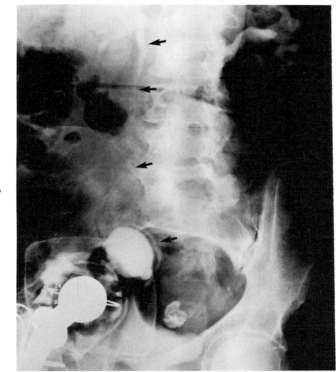

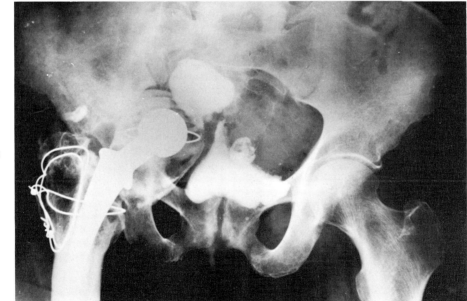

Fig. 10-5. Intravenous pyelogram or retrograde cystogram may be of great assistance in locating prosthetic components in relation to genitourinary tract when failure has resulted in severe protrusion of components into pelvis. **A,** Sixty-two–year-old woman with severe protrusion of prosthetic component. Intravenous pyelogram demonstrated location of ureter (arrows) in relation to bolus of cement within pelvis. **B,** Cystogram shows approximation of protruded mass of cement and inner wall of acetabulum in relation to bladder.

289

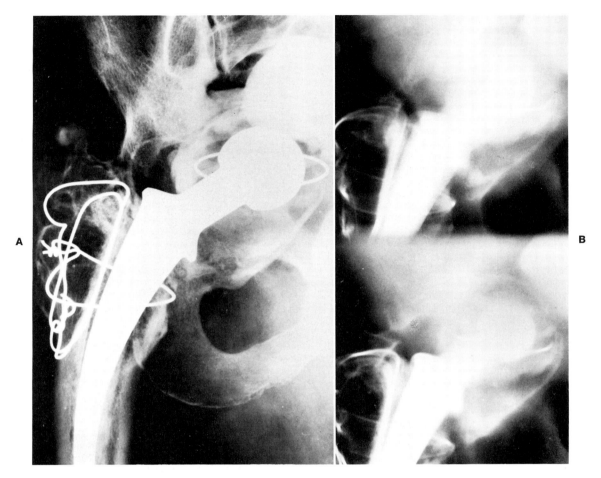

Fig. 10-6. Laminagram may be helpful in demonstrating presence or absence of bone where surgical intervention is contemplated and presence or absence of bone cannot be fully determined. **A,** Standard anteroposterior view of hip in failed total hip prosthesis; 0.5 cm. cuts, **B** to **F,** illustrate presence of bone as continuous membrane (shell) throughout most of area of protruded acetabulum.

isotope uptake was found when the prosthesis was loose and there was infection, ectopic bone formation, trochanteric nonunion, or trochanteric bursitis. It is suggested that in many cases the abnormal pattern develops before other clinical signs are present, thus its early use in evaluating a painful postoperative hip may lead to an earlier and more accurate diagnosis.[25] The use of strontium radionuclide scintimetry in infected total hip arthroplasty has been reported with success.[2] From our own experience we feel that bone scanning with light radioactive isotopes is relatively nonspecific and is of limited value. However, we recognize that when the details of this method are verified and better understood, it may find an established place in the diagnosis of complications of total hip replacement.

Laminagrams and magnified views. We have frequently used a laminagram prior to surgery, or with a painful total hip, to clarify details of the bone that might not appear on a regular x-ray film. This method has been particularly helpful when femoral head collapse in avascular necrosis has been in question or compression (stress) fractures were suspected. It has also been valuable in certain cases of loosening of the femur shaft in revealing the entrapped column of cement at the site of loosening. An interpositioned fragment of cement between the acetabular cup and femoral head can also be verified by a laminagram, which otherwise may be represented by an explained subluxation of the hip prosthesis on the plane films. Likewise, magnified views of the hip using standard mag-

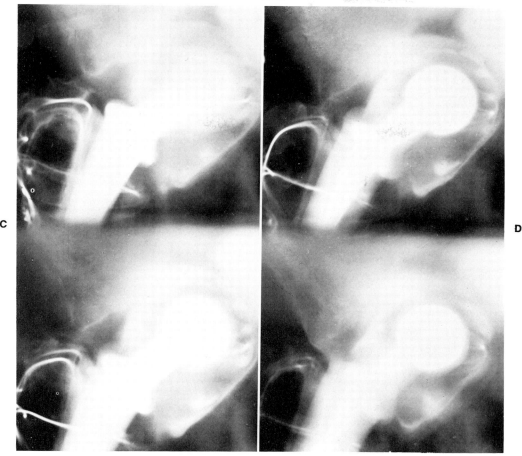

Fig. 10-6, cont'd. For legend see opposite page.

Continued.

nification techniques have been helpful in verifying the details of bone, which could not otherwise have been observed by routine x-ray films (Fig. 10-6).

RADIOLOGICAL MORPHOLOGY OF OSTEOARTHRITIS

Osteoarthritis may be present in a number of radiological features that vary, or it may resemble almost any condition of the hip ranging from rheumatoid or septic arthritis to Charcot's joint. However, preoperative diagnosis may be made in a typical case solely on the basis of radiological changes. Osteoarthritis can generally be divided into two types, migratory and nonmigratory,[5] which vary with changes of time, severity, and progression of the disease. However, there are intermediate and combined features that may not fall into either distinct diagnostic group. Descriptive terminology is help-

ful in assessing these variations of radiological morphology of the osteoarthritic hip.[12]

Nonmigratory

Incipient arthritis. The early phase of osteoarthrosis is characterized by slight osteophytic formations and very slight narrowing of the joint space. At this stage osteoarthritis may appear as a concentric, upper pole or quadratic head necrosis without collapse (Fig. 10-7).

Concentric type. The concentric type may resemble early polyarthritis, such as rheumatoid arthritis or spondylitis, with narrowing of the joint space. The head of the femur remains intact and spherical, and there is no evidence of osteophytic change. Narrowing of the joint space is uniform, but secondary sclerosis may be seen. In the early phase of this type of arthritis, the joint space may be preserved, and only sequential radiographs will reveal its gradual narrow-

291

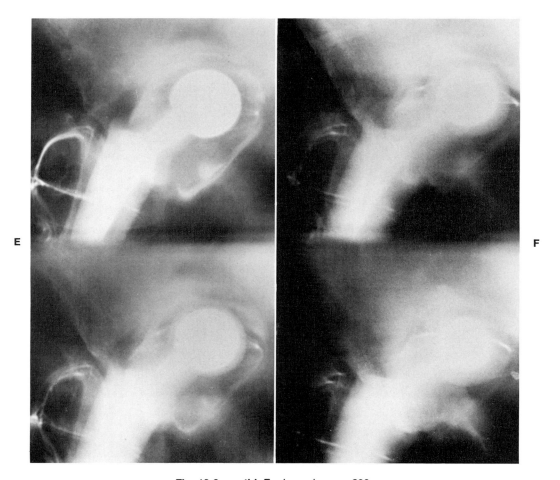

E

F

Fig. 10-6, cont'd. For legend see p. 290.

ing and eventual obliteration, without protrusion of the head into the floor of the acetabulum. When observed at surgery, concentric involvement of the head and acetabulum is impressive, the ligamentum teres is usually absent, and, as a rule, the acetabular size has remained relatively small without expansion (Fig. 10-8).

Upper pole. This type of deformity usually is recognized in three grades. In grade 1, the joint space is narrowed or absent at the upper pole of the head (the weight-bearing zone), and the femoral head has remained spherical or become only slightly flattened. Small osteophyte(s) may be present, but there is no evidence of proximal migration. In grade 2, the head is considerably flattened on the top. Usually a moderate-sized inferior acetabular osteophyte is present, and the head is slightly subluxated laterally out of the socket. Shenton's line is still intact. In grade 3, the disease is usually advanced as marked by

complete loss of the head substance and flattening of the acetabular roof; the head is subluxed proximally and laterally with gross inferior osteophytosis. Shenton's line is broken (Figs. 10-9 and 10-10).

Head collapse. A small portion of the head may be collapsed, as evidenced by osteosclerosis and avascular necrosis. At times, a major portion of the head has a good bony texture and may show minor cystic changes. Shenton's line is intact and there is no migration of the head out of the acetabulum (Fig. 10-7). On radiographs the acetabulum appears normal.

Quadrantic head necrosis. Quadrantic head necrosis presents a classic rectangular-shaped radiodensity at the weight-bearing zone as evidence of avascular necrosis. Without collapse at this stage, the head and the acetabulum maintain their normal size. There may or may not be evidence of any collapse in the early stages,

292

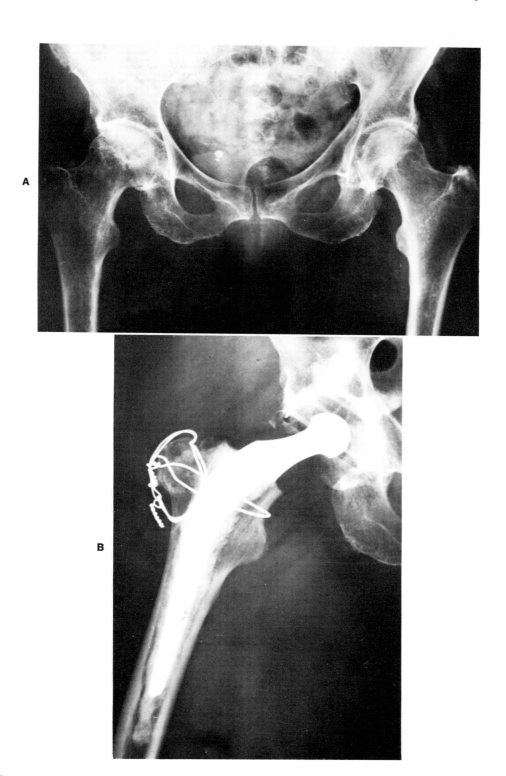

Fig. 10-7. A, Early phase of osteoarthritis is usually characterized by slight osteophytic formation and slight narrowing of joint space (left hip). This is regarded as "incipient form" of arthritis. Osteoarthritis at times may show only minimum joint space narrowing, but main feature may be resembling that of "quadrantic head necrosis" without collapse (right hip). **B,** Postoperative low-friction arthroplasty performed on right side.

293

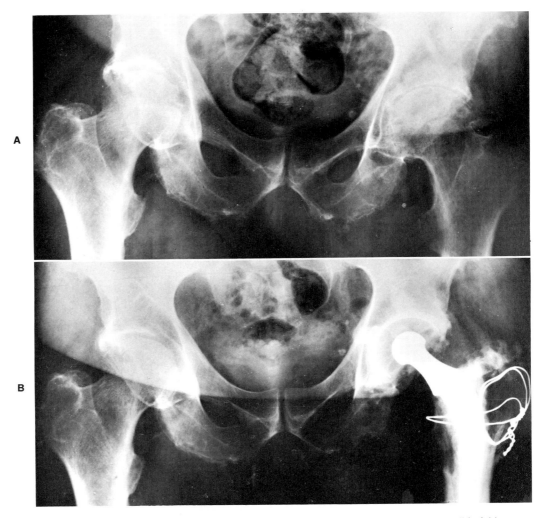

Fig. 10-8. A, Another example of nonmigratory-type osteoarthritis known as "concentric type." Left hip: narrowing of joint space is uniform but secondary sclerosis may be seen. Right hip: evidence of similar changes but predominantly at this stage over medial pole. **B,** Postoperative low-friction arthroplasty performed for same.

despite the fact that the patient is symptomatic usually in disproportion to radiographical changes. With proximal migration of the head and disruption of Shenton's line, the condition becomes obvious. The head of the femur assumes a "bell shape" following its collapse, and there is loss of sphericity in the weight-bearing portion. A large marginal osteophyte is a usual and striking feature in this type of arthritis (Fig. 10-11).

Of the 34% of all cases representing nonmigratory types in one series, 12% were concentric, 20% were superior, and 2% were bell-shaped.[5]

Medial pole arthritis. With medial pole arthritis good joint space is evident at upper pole but narrow or absent medially. There is no bulging of the pelvic aspect of the acetabulum (Fig. 10-12).

Central protrusion type. Generally, a thinning of the floor of the acetabulum is present with central protrusion type and may range from minor thinning to complete central displacement of the head into the pelvis with severe "bulge-in" effect of the floor. In such a case usually the medial aspect of the greater trochanter reaches the acetabular margin. Anatomical pathology of osteoarthritic protrusion is differ-

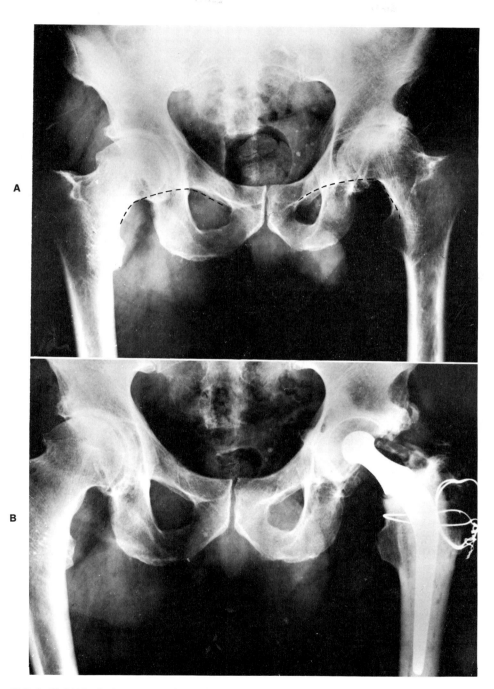

Fig. 10-9. A, Right hip depicts upper pole grade 1, in which joint space is narrowed at level of upper pole of femoral head. Here femoral head is remaining more or less spherical. Small osteophyte is present, but there is no evidence of proximal migration of head. Left hip depicts grade 2 upper pole; head is flattened on top and moderate-sized inferior acetabular osteophyte is present, although head is slightly subluxated out of socket. Shenton's line is still intact. **B,** Postoperative low-friction arthroplasty performed on left hip.

295

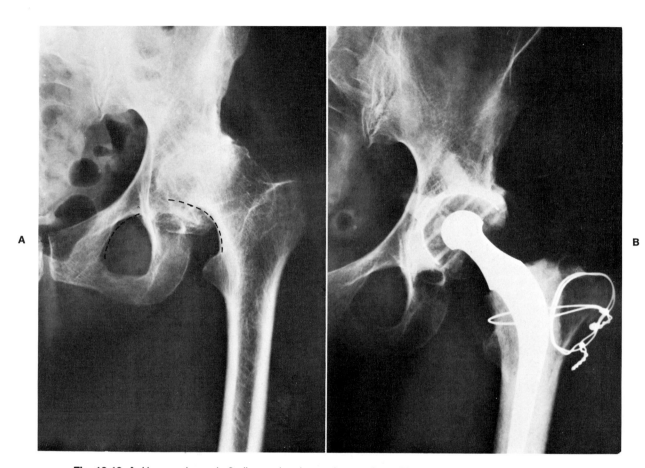

Fig. 10-10. A, Upper pole grade 3, disease is advanced. NOTE: loss of head substance and flattening of acetabular roof. Head is subluxated proximally. Large inferior osteophyte is also present. Shenton's line is broken. **B,** Postoperative low-friction arthroplasty for same.

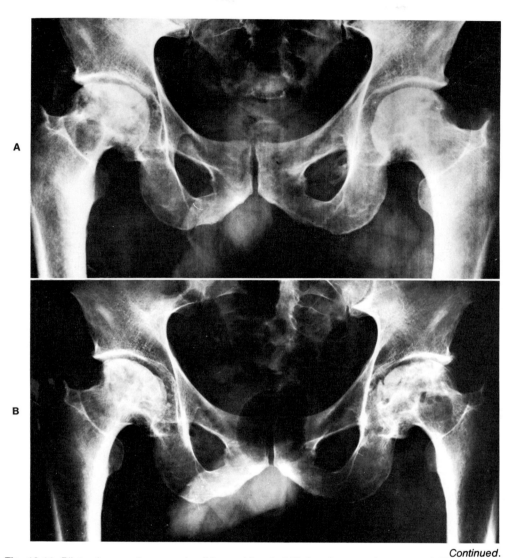

Continued.

Fig. 10-11. Bilateral avascular necrosis of femoral heads initiating degenerative osteoarthritis in otherwise healthy person. There was no history of alcoholism or systemic condition to explain presence of avascular necrosis. With proximal migration of head and disruption of Shenton's line, condition becomes obvious. **A,** Bilateral changes more severe on right with some flattening of head as result of collapse. Although acetabulum appears normal, even at this stage, acetabular cartilage involvement is inevitable. **B,** Within 6-month interval, further collapse of head on left as well as on right is observed. **C,** Postoperative insertion of cemented endoprosthesis, 2 years following surgery, shows evidence of proximal migration of prosthesis and clinical evidence of failure because of acetabular cartilage wear. Absence of acetabular changes by radiograph does not necessarily indicate healthy acetabular cartilage, therefore, hemiarthroplasty is not indicated (see text Chapter 8).

297

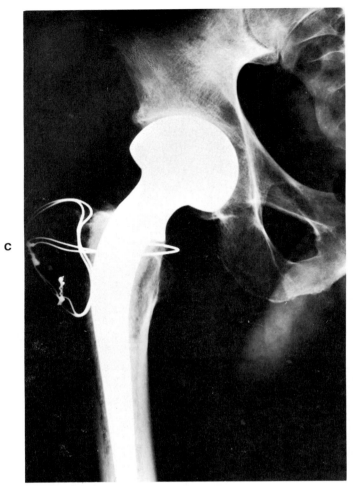

c

Fig. 10-11, cont'd. For legend see p. 297.

ent from that of rheumatoid protrusion. In the former, as a rule, there is a sclerotic layer of cortical bone present, whereas in the latter the floor may be defective (Figs. 10-13 and 10-14).

In the anteroposterior view of the pelvic film, the so-called teardrop formed laterally by the acetabular floor and medially by the pelvic wall can be taken as a point of reference to determine the degree of medial protrusion. This is an easily recognized landmark, and the crossing of this anatomical feature by the femoral head may be taken as a sign of central migration of the head. This can best be assessed in the anteroposterior view of both hips on the same plate with the tube centered at the midpoint between the hips.

It has been suggested that patients with protrusion of the acetabulum tend to have a varus neck of the femur with a decreased neck shaft angle, but it was not possible to determine from these studies the degree of varus deformity of the neck. Increased varus may produce a medial and downward force that enables the femoral head to protrude to the pelvis. Further details of protrusion of the acetabulum in osteoarthrosis will be discussed in Chapter 13.*

Migratory

This type constitutes 66% of all osteoarthritic hips, making it the most common type of osteoarthrosis. Approximately 40% of the cases show upward and lateral displacement of the head, and 20% show downward and medial displacement. Only 6% show central migration of the head in the acetabulum. From early stages of

---

*For a detailed discussion on this subject, see references 1, 4, 8, 15, 16, 23, 26, 29, and 34.

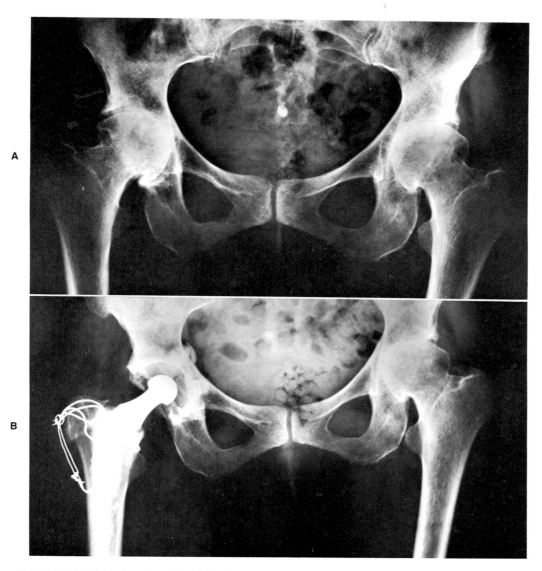

Fig. 10-12. A, Bilateral medial pole arthritis in 65-year-old female. **B,** Postoperative replacement of same on right hip.

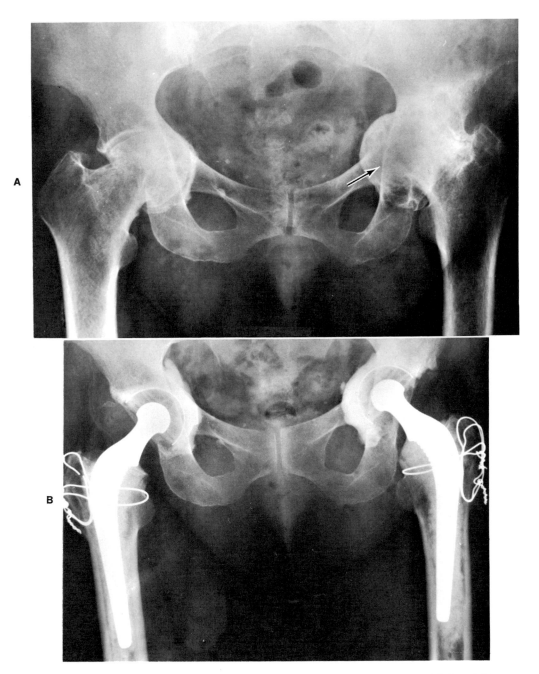

Fig. 10-13. A, Bilateral protrusion of acetabulum in 58-year-old female, more severe on left than right. NOTE: so-called teardrop formed laterally by acetabular floor and medially by pelvic wall can be taken as point of reference to determine degree of medial protrusion. **B,** Postoperative radiographs of same following bilateral low-friction arthroplasty procedure.

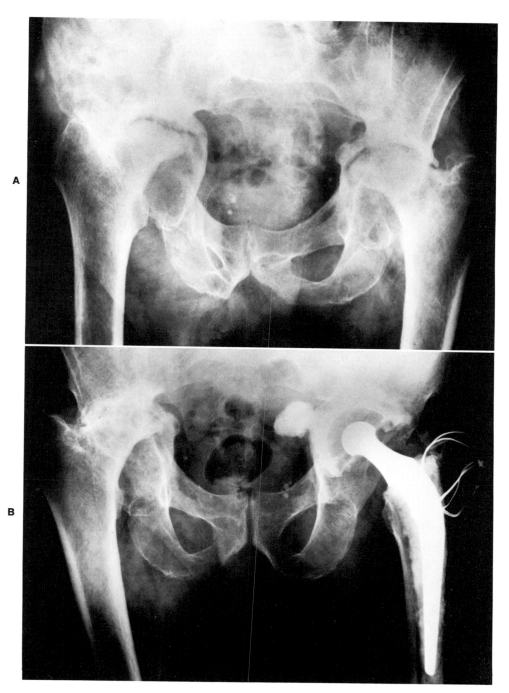

Fig. 10-14. A, Bilateral protrusio acetabuli in 68-year-old man with clinical diagnosis of osteoarthrosis. NOTE: head collapse as well as "wandering acetabulum." Protrusion is not only medial but proximal as well. **B,** Post-operative radiograph of replacement of left hip 6 years following surgery. This patient became active and symptoms of right hip did not require surgical intervention.

301

migration, the direction of the femoral head is determined and the acetabulum presents its normal configuration.[5] These changes are not related to dysplasia of the acetabulum but are primary changes of osteoarthrosis. In primary acetabular dysplasia the head of the femur is nonspherical and usually irregular and large before significant degenerative changes have taken place.

In addition to distortion of the "teardrop" pattern, the degree of protrusion may also be estimated by measurement of the center edge angle of Wiberg.[36] (The angle is between the perpendicular, through the midpoint of the femoral head and the upper and outer margin of the acetabulum.) Although measurement of this angle has been used in the assessment of abnormally shallow or deep acetabula, it may not provide an accurate and consistent basis for diagnosing alterations of the acetabular floor.[19]

Severe lumbar lordosis owing to flexion deformity of both hips usually accompanies the protrusion of the acetabulum, leading to the exaggerated position of the obturator foramina and changes in the relationship of the coccyx to the symphysis pubis.

Breaking of the Y cartilage with a normal teardrop as seen in adolescent acetabular deformity is not seen in adult protrusion.[1,4]

RADIOLOGICAL MORPHOLOGY OF RHEUMATOID ARTHRITIS

Approximately 10% of rheumatoid arthritic cases develop hip changes.[3,13,14] Radiological changes of affected hips occur in females earlier than in males. Kellgren[21] noted that the frequency of hip involvement is related to the duration of the disease and that the 10% hip involvement in his series is expected to increase to 50% if rheumatoid arthritis is of longer standing. (See Chapter 8.)

Early radiological changes of rheumatoid arthritis are minimal when the hip is involved; if joint distention is present, soft tissue and early erosive changes may occur in the early stages but generally take place prior to the time consultation is sought.

Osteoporosis involving both the pelvis and the upper femur is common in rheumatoid arthritis. In some cases it may be localized, limited only to a juxta-articular level. Asymmetrical osteoporosis is generally indicative of unilateral hip involvement, but it may be present bilaterally in bedridden patients. Radiologically, the appearance of the joint in advanced rheumatoid arthritis may present a variety of morphological characteristics and in some cases simulate those of osteoarthritis. Indeed, in some instances the characteristic x-ray changes may suggest osteoarthritis if other stigmata of rheumatoid change are absent. Narrowing of the joint space is common since the primary lesion is intra-articular and destructive. A slight sinking of the femoral head, with a wedge-shaped joint space, is a common early change. The joint space may also be narrowed medially without protrusion, similar to that found in osteoarthritis. In some cases, almost total obliteration of the joint space and complete ankylosis may occur. It is rare, however, to find a completely fused hip in rheumatoid arthritis. Should it occur, ankylosing spondylitis must be suspected. Osteophytic changes are also rare, but erosive changes, cystic formation, and concentric and symmetrical involvement are not (Fig. 10-15).

Compared to osteoarthritis, there is considerably less eburnation and osteophytic formation of the acetabulum in rheumatoid arthritis. However, a fully active patient with long-standing rheumatoid arthritis may develop secondary osteoarthritis with *reactive* changes on the femoral head and the acetabulum. Superimposed *reactive* changes of infection must also be sought in the rheumatoid patient whose x-ray films manifest marked sclerosis and reactive bone. In advanced cases, deformity of the head approaching complete disappearance may be observed with resolution of most of the joint or complete destruction of the head and portion of the neck. At times, a false acetabulum may be formed superiorly at the site of migration of the upper femur and resemble a destructive head type or destructive acetabular type, the former resembling a Charcot-type joint[14] (Fig. 10-16). An upward subluxation with destruction of the acetabulum and the appearance of a "bell clapper" is seen at times.

The medial protrusion of the femoral head into the acetabulum characterized by protrusio acetabuli is common in advanced stages of rheumatoid disease.[17] This is usually accompanied by severe osteoporosis and at times partial head collapse. The head and neck often appear cylindrical, and the neck shows some degree of varus deformity. There may be actual fractures on the acetabular floor or stress fractures on the femor-

Text continued on p. 308.

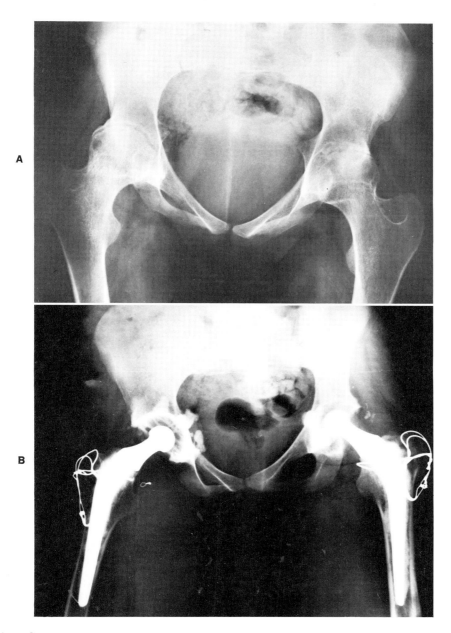

Fig. 10-15. Severe osteoporosis, microcystic changes, and symmetrical involvement of hips is common in rheumatoid arthritis. **A,** Twenty-two–year-old female affected by rheumatoid arthritis at age 18 with rapid progression. NOTE: symmetrical hip involvement. **B,** Postoperative radiograph following bilateral low-friction arthroplasty 4 years following surgery.

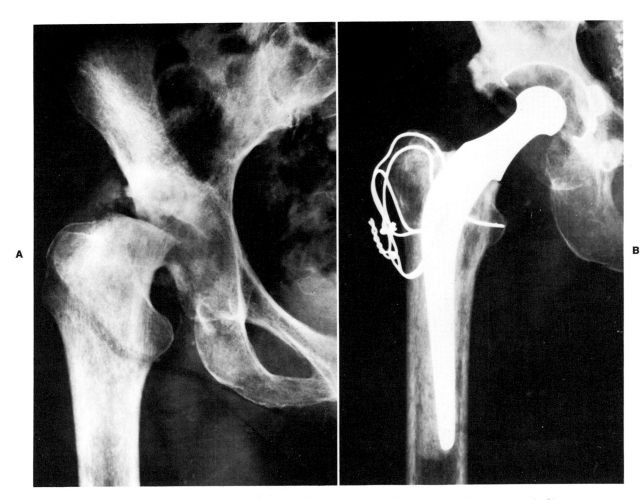

Fig. 10-16. A, Upward subluxation and collapse in hip of 52-year-old female gives impression of "Charcot-type" or infection. Patient also has received steroids for many years. **B,** Postoperative radiograph of **A** 8 years following replacement. Cultures were negative for aspirate and biopsy material.

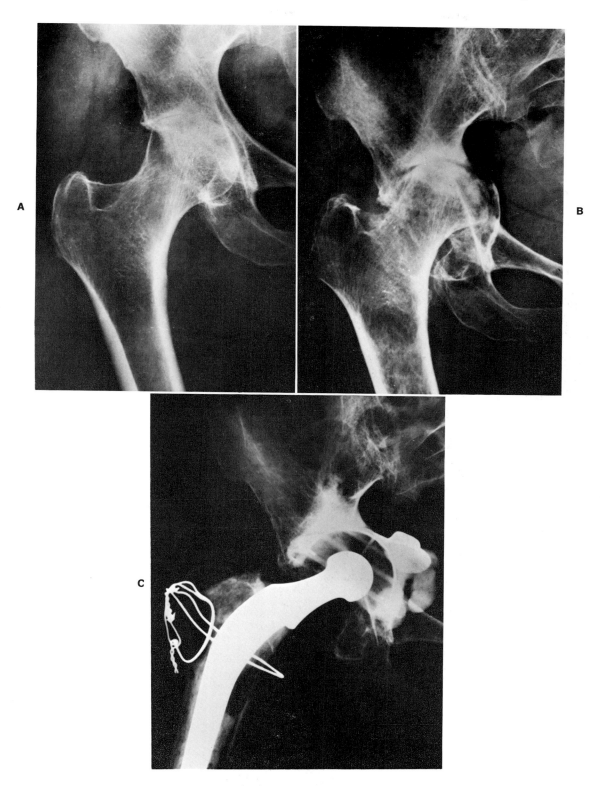

Fig. 10-17. A, Classic appearance of early involvement of rheumatoid hip. **B,** Rapid and progressive protrusion of femoral head into pelvis and defective floor created within only 2 years from onset of disease in hip. **C,** Following arthroplasty, note defective floor has led to escape of cement restrictor into pelvis.

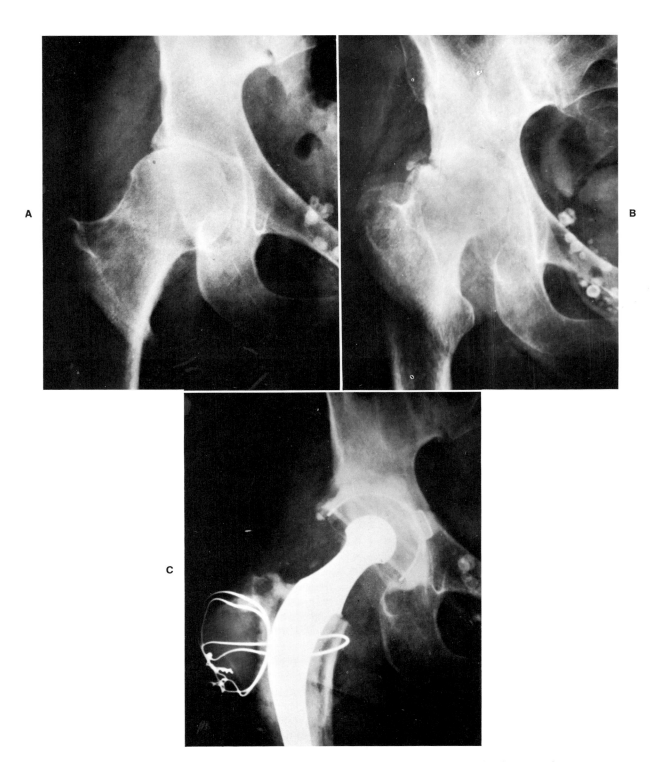

Fig. 10-18. Avascular necrosis of femoral head may only be recognized following development of osteo-arthritis in hip. Collapse of femoral head subsequently may clarify diagnosis. **A,** Preoperative radiograph of right hip in 54-year-old female suffering from Cushing's disease treated by corticosteroids. NOTE: joint narrowing but no evidence of avascular necrosis of head at this stage. **B,** One year following onset of hip pain, femoral head collapse is obvious. **C,** Postoperative radiograph following hip replacement.

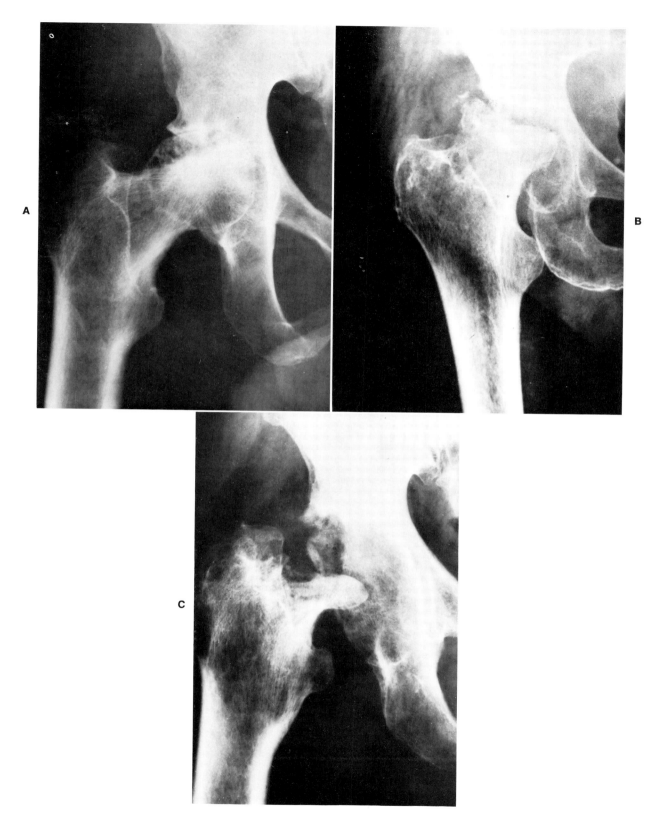

Fig. 10-19. A, Avascular necrosis of femoral head in 44-year-old male; rheumatoid disease is shown. Concentric involvement of hip and microcystic changes with secondary sclerosis are main features. **B,** Six months later, head collapse and upward migration of femoral head can be seen. **C,** Further dissolution of femoral head giving radiological pattern similar to Charcot-like joint.

307

al neck or acetabulum (Fig. 10-17). Often in rheumatoid arthritis a membranous floor may be found at the end stage.

The most severe and advanced protrusion is associated with long-term steroid therapy. Further protrusion of the acetabulum and medial shift of the prosthetic cup can occur in rheumatoid arthritis after surgery independent of faulty *technique*.[32]

Avascular necrosis of the femoral head may be associated with steroid treatment (Fig. 10-18). In the early stages there may be only minimal involvement of the acetabulum, but secondary *changes* in the cartilage lead to destructive *changes* similar to those of rheumatoid arthritis superimposed by osteoarthritic damage.

As in osteoarthrosis, radiological manifestations in both articular surfaces in rheumatoid arthritis vary from incipient and minor (stemming from the arthritic process) to extremely destructive (tuberculous). They may appear only in the upper pole of the femoral head, with its gradual upward migration or represent primarily a "medial pole" type of arthritis or protrusion of the acetabulum. There may be only a concentric involvement of the head without protrusion. The destructive head type or the acetabulum type is a common last stage of rheumatoid arthritis.

A *"quadrantic" head necrosis* may at times represent the early stage of a rheumatoid arthritic hip. Osteonecrosis accompanied by osteolysis may follow in rheumatoid arthritis. This pattern is radiologically similar to a Charcot-like neuroarthropathy pattern. There should be no concern regarding the lysis of the bone since this type responds satisfactorily to total hip replacement[22] (Fig. 10-19). In a recent study of protrusio acetabuli in rheumatoid arthritis following x-ray examination of 694 patients, 250 (36%) had clinical or radiological evidence of hip involvement; 36 (5.2%) showed evidence of protrusio acetabuli; 19 had unilateral hip involvement; and 17 had bilateral hip involvement.[5,20]

Acetabular protrusion is progressive in the rheumatoid hip. The femoral head migrates inward as the result of upward movement of the acetabular roof and the collapse of the femoral head. It has been suggested that corticosteroids may play a part in producing protrusio acetabuli in patients with rheumatoid arthritis. Progression following total hip replacement may continue leading to failure of fixation.[11,32] (See Chapters 8 and 13.)

RADIOLOGICAL CHANGES OF POSTOPERATIVE TOTAL HIP REPLACEMENT

In addition to general alignment, orientation, and relationship of the two components, the fixation and orientation of each separate component must be considered. Furthermore, cement fixation and its relation to the bone and the quality of the bone and the cement/bone interface must be specifically examined. While the changes might be evident on one radiograph, usually they are more significantly revealed on the serial, periodic films.

The acetabular component of the Charnley low-friction prosthesis is oriented 45 degrees to the long axis of the body as well as to the transaxis of the pelvis. This orientation is irrespective of the cavity that has been prepared to accommodate the prosthesis, which usually is more horizontal, that is *20 or 0 degrees* to the transaxis of the pelvis. The centering pilot hole obliterated by the cement restrictor usually is lower than the dome of the acetabular component because the prepared socket is lower than the original acetabulum (Fig. 10-1, C). A thin layer of cement is usually present between the cup and the bone, and the radiographical marker fixed to the outer aspect of the cup is oriented so that the full thickness of the cup is visible between the wire and the metal femoral component. Usually, a wedge-shaped segment (crescent) of cement is present in the superior aspect of the acetabulum, and the anchoring holes made in the pelvis in the direction of the ilium, ischium, and occasionally pubis are filled with cement. When the prosthesis has been placed in the acetabulum, the superior acetabulum completely covers the cup (the edge of the cup is slightly medial to the outer edge of the acetabulum), and the integrity of the pelvis wall is preserved without extravasation of the cement into the inner pelvis. Ideally, bone is maximally conserved, but subchondral bone and cartilage are removed from the acetabular area; thus in immediate postoperative x-ray films there should be no space between the cement and bone. A small line of radiolucency appearing later denotes a fibrous interface that is usually smooth and nonprogressive (in 60% of cases with a 10-year follow-up).[9] Progression or irregularity of this zone denotes loosening.

A Manfredi lateral view of the hip should reveal no anteversion or retroversion. Likewise, the femoral component must be anteverted no more than 5 degrees. In Müller's modification of Charnley's technique, 15 degrees anteversion is allowed in the acetabular and femoral components.

The orientation of the femoral component, especially its relation to the shaft and in reference to valgus orientation and the wedge-shaped cement at the concave side of the prosthesis, is best viewed with an anteroposterior view of the pelvis and upper third of the femur with the leg in neutral rotation. Without abduction and adduction, the femoral prosthesis is well seated in the acetabulum and completely covered by the plastic socket in Charnley's prosthesis.

Cement must also be present in a thick layer in the distal portion between the stem and the outer cortex of the femur. Cement must reach the tip of the prosthesis for maximum support. Texture of the bone at the region of the calcar femoralis is important since this area provides maximum support for the femoral component and compressive forces. Texture of the bone cortices, outline of the cement/bone junction, periosteal and extraosseous bone formation, cortical thickening of the femur by quality and quantity, cortical bone absorption, and changes of orientation of the femoral component all must be considered in reviewing postoperative radiographs. Presence of radiolucencies and/or punched-out lesions of the cortex must be evaluated both in anteroposterior and lateral projections.

It must be distinguished from the erratic appearance of sclerosis on one cortex alone. In a study of 190 femurs in 174 patients, in whom acrylic cement had been used in a medullary cavity in conjunction with the prosthesis for an average period of 4 years, Charnley and associates[7] concluded that bone remained radiologically normal in 81% of the cases. In 2.6% there was an increased thickness from preexisting atrophy. There was evidence of atrophy after insertion of the cement in 4.7% of the cases (greater than 10% in two cases). These patients all originally had severe osteoporotic bone. A fusiform hypertrophy of the femoral cortex was found in 9.4% of the cases; this was considered to be physiological, as a result of activities, a normal response to weight bearing and transmission of load. Charnley and associates[7] also found 2.2% changes that they attributed to "nonsuppurative" osteitis, although infection was not proven in these cases. Of the cases 44.8% showed a line of condensation in the cancellous bone demarcating the outer limit of the cement, which was considered physiological. Also 37.2% evidenced resorption at the cut surface of the calcar femoralis, considered to be related to the changes in the pattern of load transfer through the upper femur and physiological bone response to stress according to Wolff's law.

Presence or absence of cement around the femoral component of the prosthesis must be noted. An x-ray film indicating fracture of the acrylic cement column may be observed. In a study of 6,649 patients, 1½% of the radiographs showed a fracture related to the cement column, which was considered to be associated with sub-

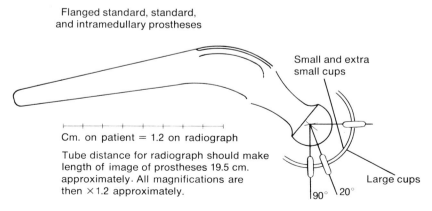

Flanged standard, standard, and intramedullary prostheses

Small and extra small cups

Cm. on patient = 1.2 on radiograph

Tube distance for radiograph should make length of image of prostheses 19.5 cm. approximately. All magnifications are then ×1.2 approximately.

Large cups

90° 20°

Fig. 10-20. Radiographic template can be used to judge prosthesis suitable for given bone size in addition to orientation of components within acetabulum and femur. (See text for instructions regarding use of radiographic template.) (Courtesy Chas. F. Thackary, Ltd., England.)

309

sidence of the prosthesis.[35] The significance of a fractured stem in relation to the failure of cement fixation will be discussed in Chapter 17. The subsidence of the prosthesis in the bed of cement appears to be favorable because the new position will stabilize the prosthesis. However, with progressive subsidence of more than 4 mm. separation at the fracture site, the prognosis may be doubtful and a chronic deep infection might be suspected. In radiological evaluation the length of the cement column, the time of fracture of the column, presence or absence of subsidence of the femoral prosthesis, separation of the fracture line, and attitude of the femoral prosthesis in the femur all must be observed during serial postoperative radiographs.

Use of radiographic templates

A radiographic template (Fig. 10-20)* can be used to judge the prosthesis suitable for a given bone size. However, Charnley has been concerned not only with the size of the components but also with their orientation within the acetabulum and femur and the socket location. Thus the object of the low-friction arthroplasty radiographic template is to help estimate the level at which the prosthetic socket should be implanted in the acetabulum in relation to the long axis of the body and adjusting the leg length by cutting the femurs at the precisely appropriate level.

---

*The instructions for this radiographic template are provided by Thackray Ltd. of England[6] for use with Charnley low-friction arthroplasty prostheses. The following is the method recommended by this manufacturer for the use of the template. The preoperative radiograph must be made with film-patient-tube distance such that the image of the femoral prosthesis measures between 18.5 and 19.5 cm. The template is centered with the outline of the stem of the femoral prosthesis over the medullary cavity of the femur. If the cavity is wide, it will permit a varus position tilted into valgus. The template should be adjusted to the exact level of the section of the neck of the femur; this level can be marked on the radiograph with a pencil through the slot in the template.

The subsequent procedure concerns the level of the upper limit of the exterior of the socket in relation to the level of the roof of the acetabulum. These two levels must be compared in a longitudinal direction, ignoring the fact that they will be displaced from each other in a transverse direction. Location of the exterior of the socket in relation to the roof of the acetabulum alerts the surgeon regarding the preparation of the socket, thus avoiding the possibility of a loose reduction if the socket were to be placed close under the roof of the acetabulum or overlengthening if the exterior of the socket is lowered excessively in relation to the acetabulum.[6]

SUMMARY OF ESSENTIALS

- A careful preoperative and postoperative radiological evaluation is an important and essential part of diagnosis and applied surgical techniques in total hip arthroplasty. Basically the surgeon must rely not only on a very informed radiologist but on his own skill in interpreting the radiographs.

- In general, distinction between osteoarthritis and rheumatoid arthritis and its differentiation from septic arthritis is possible by radiological examination alone. However, diagnostic features of postoperative septic hip may not be easily differentiated from mechanical loosening.

- Mechanical loosening and/or infection may only be diagnosed if serial radiographs of the hips are made periodically and compared for such a diagnosis.

- The most suitable radiological examination is an anteroposterior view of the pelvis to include both hips and the upper one third of the femurs. The overall image in such a film is approximately 1.2 magnification of the bone and the prosthesis. The lateral views are obtained to provide comparison for possible cortical changes of infection and/or mechanical loosenings.

- Special radiological studies such as laminagrams, magnified views, arthrograms, bone scans, arteriograms, and cystograms have their specific indications to assist in identifying certain technical and clinical problems related to total hip arthroplasty. While sinograms and arthrograms are helpful in the diagnosis of soft tissue infections, they are limited in differentiating between mechanical loosening and infection. Laminagrams and magnified views, on the other hand, may assist in verifying the details of the interface.

- Radiological morphology of osteoarthritis may be considered as migratory and nonmigratory; the nonmigratory appearance may be the incipient, concentric, upper pole, head-collapse type, quadrantic head necrosis, medial pole, or protrusion type. The migratory type constitutes the most common types of radiological morphology in osteoarthritis representing the distortion of the teardrop pattern and/or changes in the center edge angle as well as a broken Shenton's line.

- Although 10% of all rheumatoid arthritic patients develop hip changes, approximately 50% of those with long-standing disease develop severe hip involvement. While early radiological changes may be minimal, a rapid change of protrusion of the acetabulum is an alarming sign and early total hip replacement may be indicated.

- Concentric involvement of the hip in rheumatoid arthritis and involvement of the other joints make the clinical diagnosis possible in most instances. However, differentiation of a septic hip joint from that of rheumatoid arthritis may be difficult. The degrees of bone demineralization and osteoporosis accompanying rheumatoid arthritis with the loss of bone substance must be especially regarded as a cause for caution in technical aspects of total hip arthroplasty.

■ Postoperative serial radiographs not only reveal the orientation and relationships of the two components, but they also reveal the quality of the bone and cement interface, which identifies the cause of failure in most instances.

■ The use of a radiographic template is helpful to determine the size and location of the prosthesis in relation to the pelvis and femur.

■ Punched-out lesions, local radiolucencies, local densities, and cavitations must be regarded as abnormal. Likewise, the presence or absence of cement around the femoral component of the prosthesis, fractures of the stem or cement, search for changes in orientation of the prosthesis and cement, or progressive subsidence of the prosthesis should forewarn the surgeon of the complications. The use of a radiographic template has been discussed.

■ The use of radiopaque cement has made the standard radiograph an invaluable tool in diagnosis of defective results following total hip replacement.

REFERENCES

1. Alexander, C.: The aetiology of primary protrusion acetabuli, Br. J. Radiol. **38:**567-580, 1965.
2. Bauer, G. C. H., Lindberg, L., Naversten, Y., and Sjostrand, L. O.: 85 Sr radionuclide scintimetry in infected total hip arthroplasty, Acta Orthop. Scand. **44:**439-450, 1973.
3. Berens, D. L., Lin, R. K., and Lockie, L. M.: Roentgen diagnosis of rheumatoid arthritis, Springfield, Ill., 1969, Charles C Thomas, Publisher.
4. Brailsford, J. F.: Bilateral protrusio acetabuli: a progressive deformity from infancy, J. Int. Coll. Surg. **19:**555-567, 1953.
5. Cameron, H. U., and Macnab, I.: Observations on osteoarthritis of the hip joint, Clin. Orthop. **108:**31-40, 1975.
6. Charnley, J.: L.F.A. radiographic template. Chas. F. Thackray Ltd., P.O. Box 171, Park Street, Leeds L57 7RG.
7. Charnley, J., Follacci, F. M., and Hammond, B. T.: The long-term reaction of bone to self-curing acrylic cement, J. Bone Joint Surg. **50B:**822-829, 1968.
8. Crichton, D., and Curlewis, C.: Bilateral protrusio acetabuli, Br. J. Obstet. Gynaecol. **69:**47-51, 1962.
9. DeLee, J. G., and Charnley, J.: Radiological demarcation of cemented sockets in total hip replacement, Clin. Orthop. **121:**20-32, 1976.
10. Dorr, L. D., Conaty, J. P., Kohl, R., and Harvey, J. P., Jr.: False aneurysm of the femoral artery following total hip surgery, J. Bone Joint Surg. **56A:**1059-1062, 1974.
11. Eftekhar, N. S.: Charnley "low-friction torque" arthroplasty, Clin. Orthop. **81:**93-104, 1971.
12. Ferguson, A. B., Jr.: The pathological changes in degenerative arthritis of the hip and treatment by rotational osteotomy, J. Bone Joint Surg. **46A:**1337-1352, September, 1964.
13. Forestier, J.: Herberden oration: three French pioneers in rheumatology, Ann. Rheum. Dis. **22:**63-70, 1962.
14. Forestier, J.: The hip: radiological aspects of rheumatoid arthritis, International Congress Series, No. 61. Exerpta Medica Foundation, pp. 295-300, 1963.
15. Francis, H. H.: The etiology, development, and the effect upon pregnancy of protrusio acetabuli, Surg. Gynecol. Obstet. **109:**295-308, 1959.
16. Friedenberg, Z. B.: Protrusio acetabuli, Am. J. Surg. **85:**764-770, 1953.
17. Hastings, D. E., and Parker, S. M.: Protrusio acetabuli in rheumatoid arthritis, Clin. Orthop. **108:**76-83, 1975.
18. Hehman, K.: Subtraction in cerebral angiography, Semin. Roentgenol. **6:**14-16, 1971.
19. Hooper, J. C., and Jones, E. W.: Primary protrusion of the acetabulum, J. Bone Joint Surg. **53B:**23-29, 1971.
20. Hubbard, M. J. S.: The measurement of progression in protrusio acetabuli, Am. J. Roentgenol. **106:**506-508, 1969.
21. Kellgren, J. H.: The hip joint, radiological aspects of rheumatoid arthritis, International Congress Series No. 61, Exerpta Medica Foundation, pp. 301-306, 1963.
22. Kennedy, W. R., Johnston, A. D., and Becker, A.: Massive articular osteolysis in rheumatoid arthritis, treated by total hip replacement. Case report and review of literature, Clin. Orthop. **90:**161-173, 1973.
23. Lloyds-Roberts, G. C.: Osteoarthritis of the hip, J. Bone Joint Surg. **37B:**8-47, 1955.
24. Lowell, J. D., Davies, J. A. K., and Bennett, A. H.: Bladder fistula following total hip replacement using self-curing acrylic, Clin. Orthop. **111:**131-133, 1975.
25. Lynch, J. A.: Bone scanning—an aid to diagnosis in the painful total hip replacement, J. Bone Joint Surg. **57A:**1024, 1975.
26. MacDonald, D.: Primary protrusio acetabuli, J. Bone Joint Surg. **53B:**30-36, 1971.
27. Murray, W. R., and Rodrigo, J. J.: Arthrography for the assessment of pain after total hip replacement, J. Bone Joint Surg. **57A:**1060-1065, 1975.
28. Oppenheim, W. L., Harley, J. D., and Lippert, F. G.: Artheriographic management of postoperative bleeding following major hip surgery, J. Bone Joint Surg. **57A:**127-128, 1975.

311

29. Rechtman, A. M.: Etiology of deep acetabulum and intrapelvic protrusion, Arch. Surg. **33:**122-137, 1936.

30. Ring, E. J., Athanasoulis, C., Waltman, A. C., Margolies, M. N., and Baum, S.: Arteriographic management of hemorrhage following pelvic fracture, Radiology **109:**65-70, 1973.

31. Salvati, E. A., Freiberger, R. H., and Wilson, P. D., Jr.: Arthrography for complications of total hip replacement, J. Bone Joint Surg. **53A:**701-709, 1971.

32. Salvati, E. A., Bullough, P., and Wilson, P. D., Jr.: Intrapelvic protrusion of the acetabular component following total hip replacement, Clin. Orthop. **111:**212-227, 1975.

33. Salvati, E. A., Ghelman, B., McLaren, T., and Wilson, P. D., Jr.: Subtraction technique in arthrography for complication of total hip replacement fixed with radiopaque cement, Clin. Orthop. **101:**105-109, 1974.

34. Schaap, C.: Intrapelvic protrusion of the acetabulum, J. Bone Joint Surg. **16:**811-815, 1934.

35. Weber, F. A., and Charnley, J.: A radiological study of fractures of acrylic cement in relation to the stem of a femoral head prosthesis, J. Bone Joint Surg. **57B:**297-301, 1975.

36. Wiberg, G.: Studies on dysplastic acetabula and congenital subluxation of the hip joint, Acta Chir. Scand. [Suppl.]**83:**58, 1939.

CHAPTER 11

Postoperative management

Many hands must work together.

OTTO E. AUFRANC

This is the greatest error in the treatment of human sickness, that there are physicians for the body and physicians for the soul, yet the two are one indivisible.

PLATO

Postoperative care is a team approach of combined orthopaedic, medical, and physical therapy care. Specific problems should be discussed in detail with the patient preoperatively so that he knows what is expected of him after surgery.[2,3,10-12] Patients are also supplied with a booklet describing the procedure and steps to be taken during the postoperative course. This booklet also has a list of "do's" and "don't's," which can be used at home as an instructional reminder. (The postoperative details of anticoagulation and antibiotics are covered in Chapters 6 and 7.)

ABDUCTION SPLINTING

Immediately after the dressing is applied, the antiembolic stocking or elastic bandages are applied to both extremities, and the patient is placed in the abduction splint (Fig. 11-1). A specially designed abduction splint shown in Fig. 11-1, C,* is conveniently applied and used routinely in all cases at the termination of surgery. This splint has the advantage of ease of application and removal. It is well padded to prevent pressure necrosis, and the foam padding is replaceable for maintenance purposes.[7,9]

The abduction splint must be placed proximal to the malleoli. The amount of abduction achieved is governed by the mobility of the hip and the height of the patient. Two sizes of abduction splints have been found to be adequate for all patients, that is, small and large; the size is dependent upon the degree of bimalleolar separation. An excessively large abduction splint

*Abduction splint designed by author and supplied by Richards Manufacturing Co., Memphis, Tennessee.

for a patient with bilateral hip disease causes undue discomfort in the unoperated hip. An excessively small abduction splint in a tall patient with unilateral hip disease and good range of motion may not provide adequate abduction.

PATIENT TRANSFER PROCEDURE

The surgeon must supervise the transfer procedure. A draw sheet under the hips and buttocks to lift the patient is dangerous and should never be used because this by itself may dislocate the head out of the socket. Additionally, removal of a draw sheet by inexperienced individuals may lead to skin injuries similar to first- and second-degree burns. The patient is directly transferred from the operating table to his bed, obviating the need for further transfer, which is commonly practiced in conventional operations.

The patient is transferred to the bed by lifting the lower lumbar spine while an additional helper holds the legs and another holds the shoulders. The anesthetist supports the head and neck during transfer.

RECOVERY ROOM PROCEDURES

In the recovery room the Hemovac tubes must be connected to the wall suction immediately; the amount of blood in the Hemovac bottle is periodically marked on the bottle as opposed to repeated evacuation of these bottles, which increases the chance for contamination.

A hematocrit is obtained when the patient arrives in the recovery room and is repeated daily for 5 days. Frequently a postoperative transfusion is needed. It has been our practice to keep the hematocrit above 30% in all patients,

313

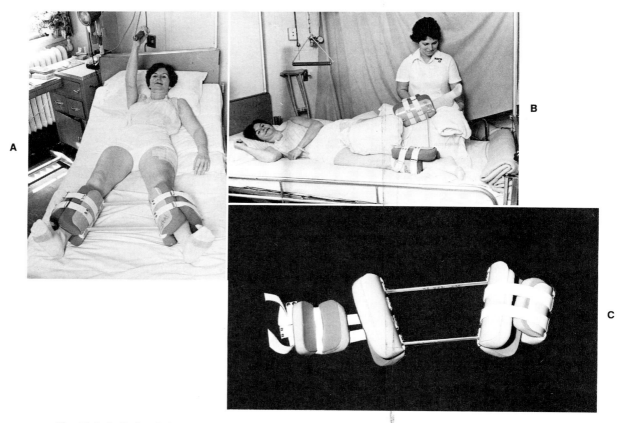

Fig. 11-1. A, Patient in bed wearing abduction splint. **B,** Position of legs in abduction splint with patient on side. Patient is propped on pillows to maintain lateral position. Splint allows frequent turning of patient with minimal risk of accidental adduction. Lateral positioning of patient requires support by two or three regular pillows placed along patient's back and legs to maintain this position. **C,** Abduction splint.

and above 35% in high-risk patients with a history of coronary or cerebrovascular disease.

Supportive measures including blood and fluid replacement as well as close monitoring of the patient are conducted by the anesthesia team in the recovery room, and the patient remains there until he is completely stabilized and has regained consciousness.

Postoperative x-ray evaluation has been discussed elsewhere. A radiograph should be taken before the patient leaves the recovery room to ensure the satisfactory position of the components, since during the transfer of the patient from the operating table to the bed, the prosthesis may dislocate.

OTHER POSTOPERATIVE PROCEDURES

An electrocardiogram is obtained on the first postoperative day and provides an evaluation of unrecognized surgical ischemia as well as a baseline should further complications arise.

Laboratory studies relative to anticoagulation are obtained as indicated. An SMA 12 is repeated prior to discharge.[3]

Because the initial dressing applied in the operating room remains undisturbed during the first five postoperative days, it is essential to check the fullness of the thigh daily. If the patient complains of undue or sudden onset of pain following anticoagulation, the dressing may be removed to search for a hematoma. This is a common complaint and should be diagnosed, with anticoagulation therapy reversed if necessary. As previously stated, it is not our policy to drain or aspirate hematomas at the bedside. For the most part they resolve spontaneously, but if evacuation is necessary, it is carried out under sterile conditions in the operating room. If for any other reason the dressing is changed within the first 5 days, the patient must be taken to a treatment room and the procedure done under sterile conditions.

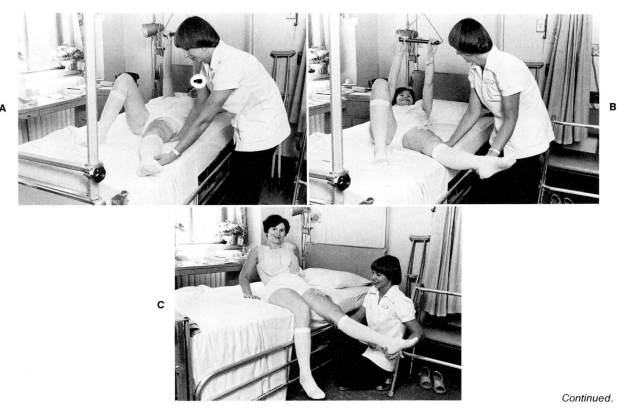

Continued.

Fig. 11-2. A, Ambulation is initiated with removal of abduction splint, assisted by patient using trapeze and by therapist to maintain operated hip in abduction, while unoperated extremity of patient is flexed to raise buttocks and move toward edge of bed. **B,** Same as **A** in more advanced stage. NOTE: therapist supporting operated extremity while patient turns in bed; in horizontal plane hip is maintained in extended position. **C,** Patient has assumed semisitting position with hip in only slight flexion and stabilized by upper extremities; position is maintained by therapist. **D,** Patient's main weight is supported by unoperated hip (right) and two arms leaning back onto bed. In this position patient momentarily rests and overcomes dizziness or apprehension during first day "out of bed." **E,** Walker may be used for start of ambulation. It is appropriately adjusted to patient's height and placed properly in relation to position of standing. NOTE: operated hip (left) is still in extension. Main weight is to be transferred onto unoperated side (right hip). **F,** Standing is assumed. Maximum support is obtained by pushing on bed while standing; unoperated leg (right leg) lifts patient off bed. **G,** Standing is assumed. Standing is encouraged with weight equally distributed on both hips.

The wound is usually inspected by the fifth postoperative day and a fresh dressing applied.

AMBULATION

Early ambulation is essential and depends on the patient's recovery from surgery. Many patients are very ill from surgical trauma, and premature ambulation can be very discouraging. There is no achievement in early ambulation when the patient is not physiologically or psychologically ready for it. Patients usually have considerable incisional pain during the first 2 or 3 days after surgery, but normally by the third or fourth day they are ready to stand up and take a few steps. Ambulation is begun with the attempt to stand, aided by the physical therapist.

The out-of-bed period the first day may be limited to two 10-to-15-minute sessions. This is increased to a longer time as tolerated by the patient, and further ambulation during the second and third week is attempted without the therapist when the patient masters the technique of transfer from the bed to standing and walking.

The patient has been previously instructed in methods of transfer from the bed to the standing position. The hip is kept in maximum extension while getting out of bed, and the knees are kept apart to maintain abduction at the hip. The patient uses the trapeze for turning toward the

315

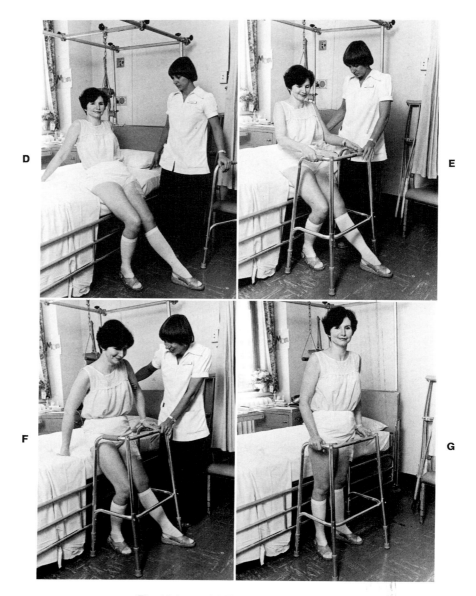

Fig. 11-2, cont'd. For legend see p. 315.

edge of the bed (Fig. 11-2, *A* and *B*). This maneuver can be done in two stages: (1) flexing the knee of the nonoperated side and using the trapeze to turn 90 degrees to the edge of the bed and then (2) assuming a semisitting posture at the edge of the bed (Fig. 11-2, *C* and *D*). For a tall person, the bed must be raised from the floor. Slippers are adequate for first day ambulation, but shoes are preferred for walking. A slippery floor or unsuitable bed may cause insecurity or falls and should be avoided. The first one or two ambulatory attempts may be limited to standing,

especially when there is light-headedness owing to orthostatic hypotension commonly found in these patients. The physiotherapist may initiate ambulation with a walker or crutches at his or her discretion (Fig. 11-2, *E* to *G*). Patients are encouraged to attempt to bear weight fully on the operated extremity from the first day of ambulation. There is a tendency to keep the operated hip in abduction during walking, which need not be discouraged at first, but a more normal gait should be expected after a week of ambulation (Fig. 11-3).

316

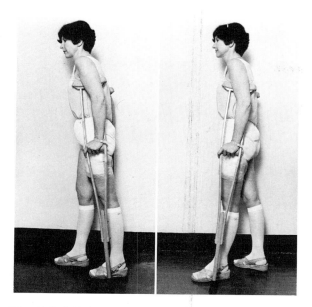

Fig. 11-3. Initiation of walking with crutches is by forward placement of nonoperated extremity and support by crutch from operated side. (See text.)

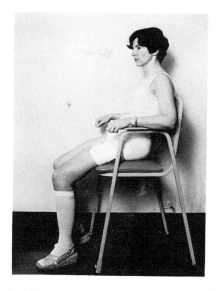

Fig. 11-4. After ambulation has begun and patient has achieved approximately 50 to 60 degrees of range of flexion, she/he may then be allowed to sit on high, raised chair.

Ambulation with crutches is to be encouraged in all patients. The continuous use of a walker may be limited to a very old and debilitated patient. The crutch walking is basically a two-point gait, with the crutch on the operated side synchronized with the unoperated extremity. With the next step the crutch on the nonoperated side will support the operated hip and so on.

SITTING OUT OF BED

Contrary to the patient's expectations, ambulation does not begin with sitting. In fact, the patient should be walking about a week prior to being allowed to sit in a chair. The abduction splint, replaced while the patient is in bed, may be removed after the first week, and the head of the bed may be raised 45 degrees for reading, eating, and the like. At no time does the patient sit straight up in bed or on the edge of the bed. If this is attempted, it should be discouraged. While sitting in bed, even at a 45-degree angle, the knees should be extended to stabilize the hip. The abduction splint may be discarded during the resting period after 1 week. However, it should be replaced if the patient is lying on his side. After ambulation is begun and the patient has achieved approximately 50 to 60 degrees range of motion, he may then be allowed to sit

on a high raised chair (Fig. 11-4) or a chair with two pillows in order to avoid excessive flexion at the hip. A high armchair with a firm seat is very helpful for all patients. While the patient is sitting on the chair, the knee remains extended. We recommend a raised toilet seat, which may be used as soon as the patient is allowed to sit out of bed. Prior to the use of the raised toilet seat and ambulation, a flat orthopedic bedpan is used. The use of the trapeze is essential in raising the pelvis onto the bedpan. The unoperated hip and knee are flexed to assist placement of the bedpan. The operated hip and leg need not be removed from the brace (Fig. 11-5). At the end of the second week or just before discharge, a second radiograph is obtained to verify the details of arthroplasty and trochanteric fixation. A good anteroposterior film includes both hips and the upper third of the femurs. The radiograph prior to discharge must be of good quality, since it is the only documentation prior to the patient's discharge from the hospital.

Patients are reminded to avoid extreme flexion such as sitting on a low chair or trying to put on their own stockings. Adduction by crossing the legs also should be avoided.

The use of crutches for 6 weeks following the operation is encouraged, after which the patient

317

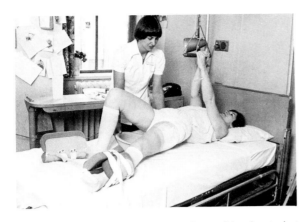

Fig. 11-5. In using bedpan, trapeze is used to elevate buttocks. Operated hip may remain in brace while unoperated hip is flexed and knee is bent to 90 degrees. By assistance of arms and by applying pressure on unoperated extremity, buttock is raised, thus allowing placement of bedpan.

may progress to one cane. He may ride in a car but should not drive for at least 3 weeks after his first postoperative outpatient visit (9 weeks following surgery).

PHYSICAL THERAPY MANAGEMENT
Preoperative

Every patient admitted to the hospital for total hip replacement is referred to the Physical Therapy Department at least 1 day before the scheduled surgery. The preoperative treatment program includes the following:

1. Instruction and practice in deep breathing and coughing
2. Active ankle exercises—especially plantar flexion and dorsiflexion
3. Instruction in postoperative bed-to-standing transfer, avoiding hip flexion and adduction of the operated hip
4. Instruction on crutch walking
5. Explanation of the physical therapy program to be used during the recovery period

The preoperative visit enables the physical therapist to establish a good working relationship at a time when the patient is best able to comprehend instructions. It also allows the therapist to clarify any questions the patient may have regarding the role of physical therapy.

Preoperative instruction is also given to the patient by the nursing staff. The nurses cover postoperative bed positioning and motion and use of the bedpan, and they also reinforce the physical therapist's instructions on deep breathing and coughing.

Postoperative

Some patients are overly anxious about returning to normal activities. They should be encouraged to proceed slowly. In the postoperative period the psychological aspects of rehabilitation are probably as important as the physical.[4] The physical therapist usually has more time than other medical staff to spend with the patient, and his sensitivity to psychological and physical handicaps could be instrumental in the patient's overall assessment and management.

The physical therapist must be fully acquainted with the rate of progression of the hip. His role is to guide the patient in a relaxed manner through activities that are now possible because of the new pain-free hip joint. However, the patient should be reminded that the muscles require time to be reeducated and strengthened. At the same time the physical therapist must reinforce the idea that there is no set timetable and that each patient is expected to progress at his own rate. This is particularly needed if two patients recovering from this type of surgery are in the same room, and one is not able to do certain active exercises, such as straight leg raising, as well as the other.

It is essential to adapt to the patient's temperament and individual needs concerning restrictions or additional exercises. For example, if a patient does not wish to do stair climbing (because there is no need to climb stairs at home), it should be eliminated from his individual program.

First postoperative week. Following surgery, the physical therapist sees the patient immediately on his return to the recovery room. For the first two postoperative days the physical therapy program consists of deep breathing and coughing and bilateral active ankle exercises. Isometric contraction of the quadriceps muscles is initiated following removal of the wound drains, usually on the second or third postoperative day. Active assisted hip and knee flexion and straight leg raising with the abduction splint removed only during the exercise period commences on the fourth postoperative day. For most patients this is the first experience of pain-free motion after several years of hip disability. The hip feels mobile ("lubricated"), and there is only incisional discomfort at the site of the wound. Passive hip flexion is to be avoided, thus limiting elevation of the head of the bed to no more than 45 degrees. During this period the nursing staff turns the patient on his unoperated side, with the abduction splint in place and with the side-lying position maintained with several regular bed pillows. The "bed-to-standing" transfer is executed by the patient without sitting on the edge of the bed and with the therapist assisting in the maintenance of the hip in abduction position. Full weight bearing is encouraged on ambulation with a walker or crutches (Figs. 11-2 and 11-3).

Second postoperative week. During the second postoperative week physical therapy continues with active assisted hip and knee flexion, straight leg-raising exercises, and the gait-training program. In most instances the patient is now able to walk with crutches in a three-point gait. Should the patient have pain and limitation in the unoperated hip, he is instructed in a four-point gait. Sitting is avoided until the end of the second postoperative week or until the patient has at least 55 degrees of hip flexion (Fig. 11-4).

When the physical therapist is sure that the patient is able to transfer from the bed to the standing position and walk independently, he is allowed out of bed as desired. An armchair with a pillow on the seat to avoid extreme flexion of the hip is used when sitting is permitted. Instructions in stair climbing are given toward the end of the second week.

Third postoperative week. Abduction on a powder board may be added to the exercise program during the third postoperative week. Instruction in stair climbing with crutches is also begun at this time. If necessary, the patient is referred to the occupational therapist for instruction in dressing techniques involving the lower extremities. Many patients are discharged from the hospital during this period, usually the first or second day of the third postoperative week. Thus this portion of the program is aborted in patients who can walk independently and climb stairs.

The patient may go home in his own car (but not a sports car with bucket seats), using a pillow to raise the height of the seat and with the knee and hip extended as much as possible. There is no need for an ambulance. If the patient has stairs to climb at home, this exercise should have been included in the postoperative course of therapeutic management prior to discharge.

Specific place and means of physiotherapy

Routine management requires little or no specific training; with attention to the details of postoperative routine, personnel could be trained to assist the therapist or to take the place of the physiotherapists after the first week. Personnel instructed in assisting the patient out of bed and walking with him could in fact alleviate demands on the nursing staff as well. They could serve in the capacity of technicians, assistant nursing staff, or nurses aides. These trainees would also be available to the patient over the weekend, when other trained staff is normally not available. Daily ambulation must not be disrupted, and it is essential that these patients continue their activities during the weekend.

On the other hand, for patients with polyarticular involvement as in rheumatoid arthritis, an expert physiotherapist is invaluable. He is instrumental in rectifying postoperative rehabilitation problems, including splinting of the lower or upper extremities, special modification of walking aids, and lifts when required. The problems of these patients should be discussed with the surgeon in charge, plotting a sensible and individualized rehabilitation approach. Often, whirlpool or other hydrotherapy is beneficial in polyarticular rheumatoid conditions.

Since psychological aspects of rehabilitation are as important as the physical, a therapist who is able to answer questions with intelligence and concern transfers a cheerful confidence to the patient and is indispensable during the rehabilitation course.

Gain in range of motion and management of fixed deformity

If there is considerable restriction of the range of motion prior to surgery, some postoperative restriction should be expected. Usually about 75% to 80% of the total range to be gained is achieved within the first 3 weeks after arthroplasty. A patient's mobility occasionally improves up to a year or more. It must be emphasized that the design of the artificial joint permits a range of only 90 degrees flexion. When accompanied by a few degrees of abduction, it may flex as much as 110 to 120 degrees. In a patient with a good preoperative range of motion, active and passive flexion of about 90 to 100 degrees will probably take place without any physiotherapeutic effort. This has been seen even in patients who were put in plaster following total

319

hip surgery and achieved similar ranges of motion. It seems that the soft tissue about the hip largely determines the range of motion, and perhaps other factors not yet fully understood may also contribute to this phenomena. A 90-degree flexion range is quite adequate for most daily functional activities, and it is suggested that forceful passive manipulation beyond that may jeopardize the hip joint. Gain in mobility does not seem to be related to degrees of exercises to promote mobility.[8]

Recovering the range of motion from a fixed adduction deformity is really a matter of its surgical correction. A flexion deformity corrected at surgery is usually eliminated postoperatively providing: (1) the patient remains flat on his back during recovery and (2) the opposite hip does not have a severe flexion deformity leading to lumbar lordosis, and thus resumption of the flexion deformity of the operated hip. If severe flexion deformity exists in both hips and both operations are planned within 2 to 3 weeks, it is advantageous to keep the operated hip in extension by supporting the opposite hip in a flexion position, that is, propped over several pillows, in order to keep the lumbar spine flat and avoid recurrence of flexion deformity. As an alternative method, if the patient has had release of flexion contracture deformity, he may be placed prone during recovery as opposed to the supine position.

The problem of fixed adduction deformity is a *serious* one, commonly found in combination with a short lower extremity. After adductor tenotomy surgery and complete mobilization of the medial aspect of the hip joint augmented by transfer of the abductor muscles to a new position, care must be taken by the therapist to maintain abduction postoperatively, especially by passive and active development of abduction

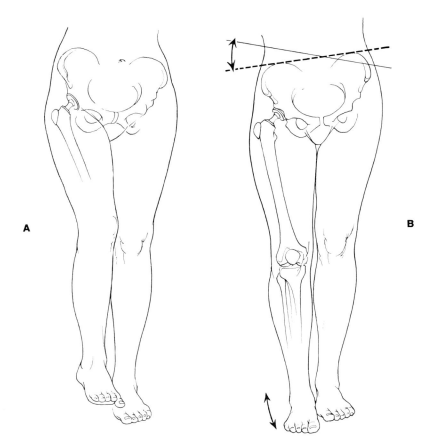

Fig. 11-6. "Pelvic shrug" excercise in which patient is taught to hike pelvis alternately by lengthening, **B,** and shortening, **A,** limb while in supine position. Opposite hip must be normal in order to accomplish this excercise. NOTE: effect of lengthening and shortening is producing abduction of "adducted hip."

power. Special emphasis on pelvic tilt exercises is necessary to overcome recurrence of this deformity.

To achieve abduction the patient is taught to shrug the pelvis—hiking by alternately lengthening and shortening the limbs.[1,5,9] The patient, in effect, abducts the previously adducted hip to a more favorable position. The opposite hip must be normal for this exercise (Fig. 11-6). A program of active "abduction exercises," instituted early during the postoperative course, is especially needed in patients with a tendency to develop adduction deformity (Fig. 11-7). Fixed external rotation deformity is also a serious problem that, like the flexion deformity, must be completely corrected during surgery. Occasionally, the lower extremity will resume external rotation despite correction. Insertion of a tibial pin postoperatively may correct severe external rotation (more than 30 to 40 degrees) deformities.[5,6] The therapist can keep the hip in internal rotation during exercise, and with effort

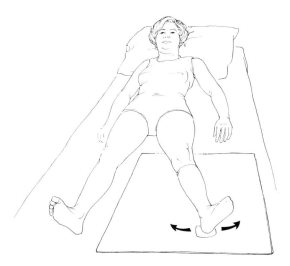

Fig. 11-7. Active program of "abduction excercises" is especially needed in patients with tendency to develop adduction deformity. Powdered board and rolled stockinette (or a roller skate) may be used to provide low-friction apparatus and prevent heel irritation while doing this excercise.

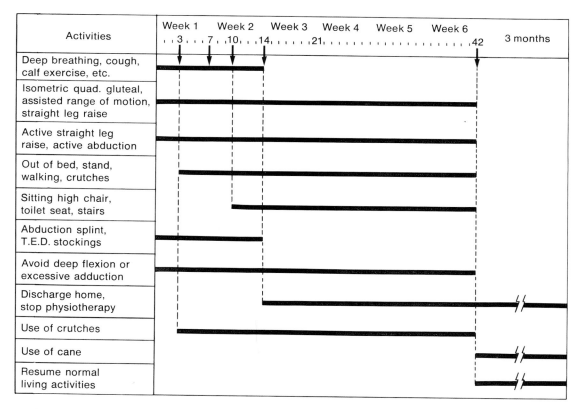

Fig. 11-8. Summary of beginning and end of excercises during postoperative course. NOTE: most restrictions and therapeutic modalities are stopped at end of 6 weeks following surgery. In routine case, by 3 months patient may resume all routine daily living activities but is discouraged from engaging in strenuous sports such as skiing or tennis.

321

the patient can learn to practice active internal rotation during walking to overcome resistant external rotation deformity during the postoperative course.

Fig. 11-8 summarizes the timetable for different activities following total hip replacement.

PATIENT INSTRUCTIONS

Many patients request instructions on discharge. These instructions should be uncomplicated and basically include all the activities that the patient has been doing while in the hospital. The patient should be encouraged to walk a lot, since this will improve the hip more than any other specific exercise. On discharge the patient may be instructed to avoid bathing in a tub but encouraged to shower, if possible. He may start swimming after the 6-week postoperative visit. Sexual intercourse can be commenced about 2 to 3 months after surgery. It must be frankly discussed, with specific instructions in reference to positioning. Excessive flexion or adduction at sexual engagement must be avoided. The patient may drive a car after the 3-week postoperative visit if permitted. Normal activities may be resumed as the patient feels able. A list of "do's" and "don't's" should be given to patients who specifically wish to have written instructions.[5]

Do's

Take your Ace bandages or thromboembolic disease (TED) stockings with you and wear them during walking periods; you may remove them while resting and at bedtime.

Have someone assist you with your shoelaces and toenails until adequate mobility in the hip is obtained.

Take an occasional aspirin, Bufferin, or other mild analgesic, if necessary, for mild aches or muscle spasm. It is not expected that you will have much pain upon departure from the hospital. The incisional discomfort should disappear gradually. Strong medications are not needed.

Follow the instructions regarding anticoagulation regimen and contact your physician as you have been instructed.

Call your surgeon if you have any severe pain in the hip area or undue swelling of the ankle and leg.

Continue the activities you were engaging in in the hospital, particularly walking within your tolerance ability. This is your principal exercise.

No physical therapy is needed. Walk as long and as far as you want using two crutches. Use two crutches for 6 weeks and then a cane for another 4 to 6 weeks.

A straight, high chair with arms to facilitate getting out of the chair should be used. Avoid the use of a sofa.

Women may wear a soft girdle when home, if so desired. Shower and wash hair as necessary.

Don't's

Don't cross your legs for 6 weeks.

Don't lie on your operated side; when lying on the other side, don't permit the operated leg to cross over. Place a pillow between your knees as a precaution.

Don't sit on a low sofa or chair for 6 weeks.

Don't bend down to pick up objects, bending your hips in excess.

Don't worry about range of motion of your hips. This usually will improve within 1 year after operation. Remember that the hip gets better with passage of time; let time take care of walking and strengthening.

Don't adduct your hips excessively.

You may *never* engage in activities that involve:

1. Placing heavy loading forces upon the hip joint—that is, running, jumping, carrying heavy loads
2. Placing excessive bending and twisting stresses upon the hip joint—that is, lifting, shoveling, forceful turning

MODIFICATION OF ROUTINE

The surgeon may prescribe a specific modification of the postoperative regimen according to the special conditions encountered at the time of surgery; similarly, certain pathological conditions may necessitate modification of basic routine in postoperative management. There are generally three situations where slow rehabilitation is recommended.

1. Extreme osteoporosis with fragmentation of the trochanter at surgery or inability to achieve any perfect fixation of the trochanter at the time of surgery (A slow rehabilitation is recommended because of fear of further separation of the trochanter or the possibility of postoperative dislocation.)

2. Instability at surgery, especially in revision operations where extensive soft tissue releases are necessary and the tension of the tissue

across the hip joint is inadequate to produce a stable reduction

3. Fracture of shaft or acetabulum during preparation or cementing technique

In addition to these conditions, a precautious gain in mobility should be advocated in certain situations, that is, where extreme ranges of motion were present preoperatively or if an overly enthusiastic patient initiates enormous range of motion within the first week. (This must also be modified and guarded against possible dislocation and subluxation of the hip joint.) It may be necessary, if dislocation or trochanteric problems exist at surgery, to apply a hip spica cast or to treat the patient in a balanced suspension apparatus. The total immobilization period required need not exceed 3 weeks (in the conditions of failure of the fixation of the trochanter or instability). Another situation that requires drastic modification of postoperative management is when a fracture of the shaft of the femur is sustained during operation. It would be best to fix these fractures immediately at surgery (Chapter 17) and then to place the patient in a balanced suspension apparatus for comfort. Depending on the severity of the fracture—or the method of fixation at surgery—a hip spica cast may be applied within 2 weeks following surgery upon removal of the sutures. The patient may resume walking (with the cast) if the fracture has been securely fixed, and partial weight bearing may be resumed within 2 to 3 months following surgery. It must be recognized that the combination of a fracture of the shaft of the femur and total hip arthroplasty requires diligent observation concerning the status of the fracture healing before authorizing weight bearing and independent walking. (See Chapter 17.)

Many surgeons and therapists claim successful results in patients who achieve early and spectacular ranges of motion within the first 2 weeks during recovery. We, however, consider this effort ineffective because most patients will gain the same range of motion without jeopardy to the hip joint within 3 to 6 months. Extreme ranges of motion may be damaging to the artificial hip joint and should not be encouraged at any time. Nature is the greatest guide in attempting and achieving range of motion in most instances. Passive forceful range of motion directed by a therapist must be avoided; it is for this reason that no physiotherapeutic modality should be prescribed for the patient when he leaves the hospital.

In contrast to range of flexion, gain in abduction postoperatively is essential and fundamental to a successful total hip arthroplasty. If an adduction deformity is not corrected during surgery or if patients develop adduction contractures, this must be specifically attended by a therapist (in order to overcome such a fixed deformity with consequential pelvic obliquity). Fixed adduction deformities must be corrected by "powdered" board exercises coupled with "pelvic-shrugging exercises."[1,4,9]

Another aspect of a modified program for total hip arthroplasty is related to patients with rheumatoid arthritis and multiple joint involvement. In rheumatoid conditions the patient is affected not only by the hip but also by the knees and the ankles—as well as the joints of the upper extremities. Modification of crutches and assistive devices must be individualized in these patients. More assistive support is necessary in these individuals during the first few days of rehabilitation; a modification of a program of early sitting for these individuals may be necessary as opposed to extensive walking prior to allowing them out of bed. Longer postoperative recuperation and rehabilitation periods must be sought for these patients. Specific therapies —including hydrotherapy—are essential for many of the severely handicapped rheumatoid patients (in addition to the splinting of the lower extremities as needed during their ambulation period).

Other modifications of the program may include the number and duration of patient's exercises. For example, patients with borderline cardiac problems are advised to be out of bed once a day only—as opposed to twice daily in routine cases. The postoperative standing in younger patients may be modified to the second or third day postoperatively—as opposed to the routine fourth day. The earlier the patient can stand and walk, the better the chance for prevention of thromboembolic disease.

While the routine postoperative course calls for full weight bearing as soon as it can be tolerated on the operated extremity, partial weight bearing may be required in patients with additional bone graft procedures or precarious anatomical defects based on observation at surgery. Patients showing signs of being overactive (reaching a range of motion of 80 to 90 degrees within the first 10 days following surgery) should be restricted and reminded of the conse-

323

quences of possible dislocation and/or trochanteric problems. It is essential to inhibit further exercises and disallow the patient's sitting in bed with the knees flexed or on a low chair leaning forward. If recovery of postoperative range is slow and the patient is not gaining a range of motion by the second week, then the patient should be instructed to sit at more of a "right angle" (against conventional advice) and range of motion, including flexion, should be encouraged.

While the straight leg-raising exercise is routinely encouraged, patients who fail to perform the straight leg-raising must be psychologically supported, and the surgeon must insist on their continuing an attempt to do the exercise. The degree of rehabilitation is not related to the ability to do straight leg-raising prior to ambulation.

As stated elsewhere, we consider crutch walking (6 weeks) and use of a cane (6 weeks) for a total of 3 months following surgery advisable. On the other hand, if after 3 months following surgery there is a pronounced limp and the gluteal muscles have not recovered fully, we then encourage a continuance of walking with a cane for a total of 6 to 12 months, in those elderly patients who are not steady, we encourage them to use the cane permanently if they wish. It is essential to transmit cheerful confidence during the patient's recovery period—with emphasis on using "nature" as a guideline rather than a comparison of their ability to perform as other patients who have undergone the same procedure.[9]

POSTOPERATIVE LEG LENGTH DISCREPANCY AND SHOE LIFT

Recommendations regarding leg length discrepancies—often a source of complaint from the patient—must be attended no earlier than 3 months following surgery. This lapse of time between surgery and a complete evaluation of leg length discrepancy is necessary in order to allow the spine to adjust to the new position of the hip joint (thus allowing correction of pelvic tilt resulting from an arthritic condition). In general, the lengthening of an extremity as the result of surgery (an unfortunate complication) is quite disturbing to the patient, but, again, it is possible to rectify this situation if time is allowed for pelvic level adjustment. We have found a small insole lift (¼ inch) and a small heel lift (¼ inch) to be quite adequate for minor adjustments, but

this is rarely necessary if 3 to 6 months are allowed for the lumbar spine to adjust to the leg length following arthroplasty. Patients who have been told of the possibility of the need for a shoe lift prior to surgery accept this recommendation postoperatively without disappointment.

REMOTE INFECTION AND ANTIBIOTIC COVERAGE

Instructions regarding the use of prophylactic antibiotic coverage for patients who may develop a source of infection elsewhere is necessary. Because of the importance related to the possibility of infection of the total hip secondary to a remote source, patients should be advised to remain in touch with their surgeon at any time they may run a risk of bacterial infection or surgical manipulation. They are advised to suggest to their family physician (or other medical professionals) that in the event of developing any infectious lesions, that is, dental, skin, genitourinary, and so on, they should receive prophylactic antibiotics; depending on the source of infection and the type of organism, specific prophylactic antibiotics covering a broad spectrum for both gram-positive and gram-negative organisms have been recommended. During surgery and for genitourinary infections or dental manipulations, patients must receive the appropriate antibiotics in large doses to combat possible bacteremia and unfortunate seeding of these organisms into the artificial hip joint. (See Chapter 6.)

SUMMARY OF ESSENTIALS

- The overall postoperative management of the patient is a combined approach headed by the surgeon; of equal importance are the roles of the medical consultants, physiotherapists, and the nursing staff. An informed patient (who is instructed properly preoperatively) facilitates the postoperative rehabilitation and recovery program, thereby minimizing the complications.
- The initial dressing applied at surgery should remain undisturbed for the first 4 or 5 days. Wounds are not repeatedly examined, and hematomas are not drained at the bedside. Postoperative x-ray evaluation is essential in the recovery room as well as at the time of the patient's discharge from the hospital. The role of early ambulation in prevention of thromboembolic disease and other complications cannot be overly emphasized.
- Supportive measures such as blood transfusions, anticoagulation regimens, and handling of medical

complications should be coordinated with the surgeon and not left to the discretion of the most junior members of the staff. A standard policy for the management of most complications will only evolve in an organized center handling a large number of operations of this type.

■ While early ambulation is essential, many patients are too ill from surgical trauma to ambulate the first or second day following surgery. However, on the third or fourth day postoperatively most patients can begin ambulation. The details of nursing and therapeutic management are vital in the prevention of postoperative complications. The rehabilitation program must be coordinated by a physiotherapist according to the patient's degree of performance and ability rather than a standard formula applied to all patients.

■ It is essential that crutch walking, bed-chair transfer, and walking are rehearsed with the patient prior to surgery in order to facilitate the postoperative recovery. Contrary to the patient's expectations, ambulation does not begin with sitting out of bed. Walking experiences precede (by at least 1 week) allowing the patient to sit out of bed.

■ A high, raised chair, avoidance of sitting in bed, and avoidance of passive flexion of the hip are all directed toward the goals of developing a capsule around the artificial joint and future stability of the hip joint. Excessive early motion within the first 2 weeks is discouraged, but patients who are too slow in gaining motion are to be encouraged in the gain of mobility.

■ Specific physiotherapeutic management includes instruction in deep breathing and coughing, active ankle exercises, instructions regarding bed-to-standing transfer, crutch walking, and abductor strengthening exercises. During the first postoperative week, isometric exercises including quadriceps and an attempt for straight leg raising are encouraged. While most patients' ambulation begins with crutches on the third or fourth postoperative day, an older patient may ambulate with a walker. Weight bearing is assumed as soon as it can be tolerated.

■ During the second postoperative week, further muscle strengthening exercises (isometric) in addition to a gait-training program are encouraged. During the second week, the patient is able to sit out of bed using an elevated seat (to avoid extreme flexion of the hip). Stair climbing may begin toward the end of the second week.

■ Hospitalization for the third postoperative week is required only of those patients who have not achieved complete independence in their rehabilitation and have not demonstrated a total independent transfer from the bed to a standing position and a satisfactory gait. During this period, besides additional gait training and stair climbing, and the like, an exercise program that includes "powdered" board abduction exercises is incorporated.

■ At discharge, a list of do's and don'ts are given to the patient—with emphasis. Basically, the patient will be discharged with a similar program of activities that was engaged in during the second and third week of his hospital stay.

■ The physiotherapy role in total hip replacement is as much one of psychological as physical support (efforts directed toward transferring cheerful confidence to the patient—and reinforcement). A knowledgeable physiotherapist is indispensable in supervising the patient's activities in addition to providing answers to questions that often worry the patient. For those patients who request instructions on discharge, a typewritten sheet or instruction booklet that includes a list of do's and don'ts is useful; this will serve simply as a reminder for patients who wish to have instructions.

■ One of the specific areas in which the physiotherapist is concerned with the management of patients following total hip replacement is in the care of rheumatoid arthritic patients who have multiple joint involvement requiring physical modalities for their joint disabilities other than the hip. Fixed deformities usually need specific attention similar to that of those with severe upper extremity involvement.

■ One of the most difficult aspects of handling total hip replacement is the psychological outlook of the therapist and the patient toward improved range of flexion following total hip arthroplasty. Contrary to most conventional arthroplasties—that is, cup arthroplasty and Moore self-locking prosthesis—patients with total hip replacement gain range of motion that is generally related to the preoperative range of motion. Most patients achieve a 90-degree flexion, which is quite adequate for most daily functional activities, regardless of a regimented exercise program. Early gain in range of flexion to this degree (within the first week) must be avoided; this would simply invite complications such as detachment of the greater trochanter or dislocation. Fixed adduction and external rotation deformity requires special attention (specific exercises and management.)

■ Because of technical, surgical complications—that is, fragmentation of the greater trochanter, instability noted at surgery, and the like—modification of the routine postoperative course must be considered; likewise, the method of rehabilitation must be adjusted to the patient's needs and ability with respect to his physiological state.

REFERENCES

1. Aufranc, O. E.: Constructive surgery of the hip, St. Louis, 1962, The C. V. Mosby Co.

2. Aufranc, O. E.: Preoperative and postoperative treatment of the patient with reconstructive surgery of the hip, Clin. Orthop. **38:**40-44, 1965.

3. Blume, R.: Personal communications.

4. Charnley, J.: Total prosthetic replacement of the hip in relation to physiotherapy. The Founder's Lecture. Annual Congress, Chartered Society of Physiotherapy, Sheffield, England, September, 1968.

5. Charnley, J.: Postoperative management of total hip reconstruction by low friction method, Internal Publication No. 27, Centre for Hip Surgery, Wrightington Hospital, England, November, 1970.

6. Charnley, J.: Personal communications.

7. Eftekhar, N. S.: Abduction splint for hip surgery, Orthop. Rev. **3:**51-52, 1974.

8. Eftekhar, N. S., and Stinchfield, F. E.: Experience with low friction arthroplasty, a statistical review of early results and complications, Clin. Orthop. **95:**60-68, 1973.

9. Eftekhar, N. S., Bush, D. C., Freeman, A. R., and Stinchfield, F. E.: Perioperative management of total hip replacement, Orthop. Rev. **3**(1):17-27, 1974.

10. Ehrlich, G. E., editor: Total management of the arthritic patient, Philadelphia, 1973, J. B. Lippincott Co.

11. Janecki, C. J., DeHaven, K. E., and Benton, J. W.: Preoperative and postoperative management in total hip reconstruction, Orthop. Clin. North Am. **4**(2):523-531, 1973.

12. Thomas, W. H.: Postoperative program for patients having cup arthroplasty, Surg. Clin. North Am. **49:**779-786, 1969.

PART FOUR

OPERATIVE TECHNIQUE

CHAPTER 12

Standard surgical technique

ROUTINE TROCHANTERIC OSTEOTOMY*

This is an operation of many details, every and all of which must be respected. Modifications are justifiable only if they can objectively improve the quality of the results.

A perfect cement technique is the sine qua non of a successful total hip arthroplasty.

The operation will be described in seven phases, each of which relates to a specific series of maneuvers and related instrumentation. It is designed so that a multiple tray system is used, with the instruments required in each specific phase presented in sequence. This method provides an organizational aid; since the trays are delivered to the surgeon in order, no part of the operation can be erroneously bypassed. The technique described here is adapted from Charnley with only minor modifications.[1-3] The instruments and prosthesis under discussion are those of Charnley.†

PHASE I: PREPARATION AND DRAPING OF THE SURGICAL FIELD
Requirements

Preferably, the operation should be performed in a clean air enclosure. We have used a vertical flow–type enclosure ("greenhouse"), but as stated elsewhere, a horizontal clean air room is equally satisfactory. (See Chapter 6.) This description of draping and preparation is designed to assist those performing surgery outside specialized centers and without the assistance of regular personnel who are fully acquainted with the surgical procedure.

An induction room for anesthetization and washup adjacent to the O.R.‡ (operating room) is essential. The O.R. should preferably be enclosed and equipped with ultra-filtration equipment. If it is not enclosed, the colony count must be low and traffic kept to a minimum (see Chapters 5 and 6). The surgeon and team, when available, should wear special masks and gowns with exhaust systems. A standard operating table with an x-ray cassette holder and a special "arm holder" for positioning of the upper extremities is used. A good adjustable light is of paramount importance to allow complete illumination both horizontally and vertically; it should also have a focal length that will

---

*It is recommended that the reader review Chapters 1 to 4. Review of Chapter 17 should help prevent complications at surgery, and review of Chapters 9 to 11 should assist in the preparation of the patient for surgery and aftercare. Surgeons who prefer to perform total hip replacement without trochanteric osteotomy[4] are advised to review Chapter 2; the technical principles involved in the preparation of bone, the orientation of prosthetic components, and fixation are the same for both of these techniques.

†Courtesy Chas. F. Thackary, Ltd., England, and Cintor Division of Codman & Shurtleff in the United States.

‡The term "O.R." used in this chapter applies to the operating room proper or the enclosure when it is used.

provide the deepest possible view of the wound and the acetabulum. If special suction masks and gowns are worn, they may also include a communication system.

Induction room. A trained technician or nurse and the most junior member of the team prepare the patient in the induction room under the supervision of the surgeon. The patient is anesthetized and placed on the operating table with the ipsilateral arm (or both arms if the frame is so designed) directly over his shoulder(s); the arm is held with the shoulder at 90 degrees flexion (Fig. 12-1).

The endotracheal tube must be secured before the arm is placed in the holder (this same arm usually carries the blood pressure cuff and the pulse stethoscope). The elbow is flexed to 90 degrees and well-padded to avoid pressure over the ulnar nerve. Stretching of the brachial plexus by shoulder hyperabduction must be avoided. If this positioning of the arm is not possible because of rheumatoid arthritis or other conditions, improvisation is necessary. The surgeon is responsible for proper positioning and

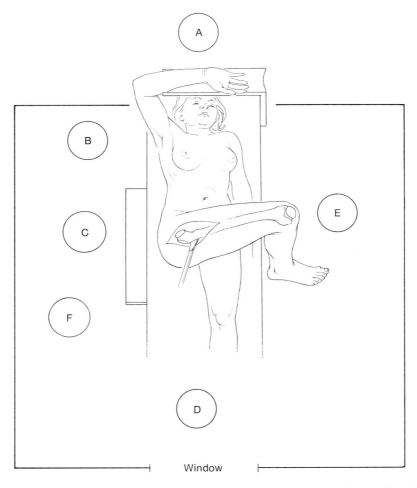

Fig. 12-1. General view of enclosure (solid lines), position of patient, operating table, position of personnel, and their relationship to operating and instrument tables. *A,* Anesthetist; *B,* first assistant; *C,* surgeon; *D,* nurse; *E,* second assistant; and *F,* second assistant may move to position *F* following application of self-retaining retractors to observe operation. Rectangular-shaped space attached to operating table in front of surgeon, *C,* is surgeon's instrument table. This table is used to place instrument trays as they arrive in enclosure.

must remain aware of the fact that carelessness can result in partial brachial and ulnar nerve palsy. This complication is the result of hyperabduction of the shoulder during surgery or direct pressure from poor positioning of the arm.

To position the patient on the operating table, the following steps are taken:

1. The feet are brought to the end of the table and the hip brought to the edge of the table so that the level of the greater trochanter and the table edge is the same.
2. An electric cautery (Bovie) plate is placed under the patient (chest region).
3. A Foley catheter is inserted (optional).

Side table and perineal adhesive sheet. The instrument side table is attached to the O.R. table so that the greater trochanter is located equidistant from either end (all subsequent draping will cover it). An 8 × 16 inch design is quite adequate; a larger table would prohibit free access to the field, as would placement excessively distal from the center of the wound (Fig. 12-1).

In both male and female patients with arthritic hips and limited range of motion a complete preparation of the perineum may be difficult; it is therefore advisable to isolate the perineum from the surgical field prior to skin preparation. Assisted by a technician, the surgeon positions an adhesive sterile sheet at the periphery of the perineum (Fig. 12-2). The adhesive sterile sheet must be applied so that it will remain fixed to the skin throughout the operation and isolate the perineum from the surgical field. If an indwelling catheter is to be inserted, it should be done prior to application of the adhesive sheet. Both legs are abducted maximally and flexed to about 45 degrees, exposing the perineum. The sheet is then applied, running from the abdomen to the perineum, avoiding the adductor region on the medial ipsilateral thigh, and extending onto the medial ipsilateral buttock, thereby walling off the genitalia and the anal region. The site of insertion of the adductor longus tendon to the pubic rumus must not be covered in case adductor tenotomy is necessary during surgery. In this way no preparation or washup of the contralateral thigh is necessary, and the genitalia and anus are isolated from the surgical field.

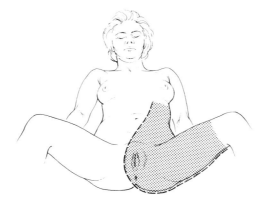

Fig. 12-2. Adhesive sheet is applied to isolate perineum. Both legs are abducted maximally and flexed to about 45 degrees to expose perineum. Sheet is then applied starting from abdomen to genitalia to perineum, avoiding adductor region on medial side of ipsilateral thigh, extending on to buttock at level of gluteal fold (at this point adhering to inner side of gluteal fold of ipsilateral side). It should then extend on to buttock of other side. Site of insertion of adductor longus to pubis must not be covered in case adductor tenotomy becomes necessary during surgery. In this way no preparation or washup of contralateral medial thigh is necessary (in this case left medial thigh). Genitalia and anus are isolated from surgical field.

Washup and skin prep

Any remaining hair is clipped or shaved prior to washup, then the second assistant or a trained technician, gloved but not gowned, prepares the surgical site with a 5-minute washup using surgical soap—povidone-iodine (Betadine) or hexachlorophene (pHisoHex). (If a surgical "prep team" is available in the hospital, the practice of induction room washup is unnecessary since the surgical field can be prepared prior to arrival and wrapped in sterile towels, so that the patient can be brought to the O.R. following anesthetic induction, positioning, and removal of the wrapping.) Prior to washup, a sterile impermeable plastic or paper sheet (3 feet by 4 feet) is positioned by the second assistant under the buttock area while the hip is maximally adducted (Fig. 12-3). The wash is from the nipple line to the toes on the affected side and from the anterior midline to the posterior midline. Utilizing two bath sponges and soap, the wash first extends down to the ankle while the technician holds the patient's foot and flexes the hip to about 45 degrees; the technician then holds the calf with a folded sterile towel, while the assistant finishes the wash by scrubbing the foot. The patient is finally moved into the surgical area in this position for the final preparation.

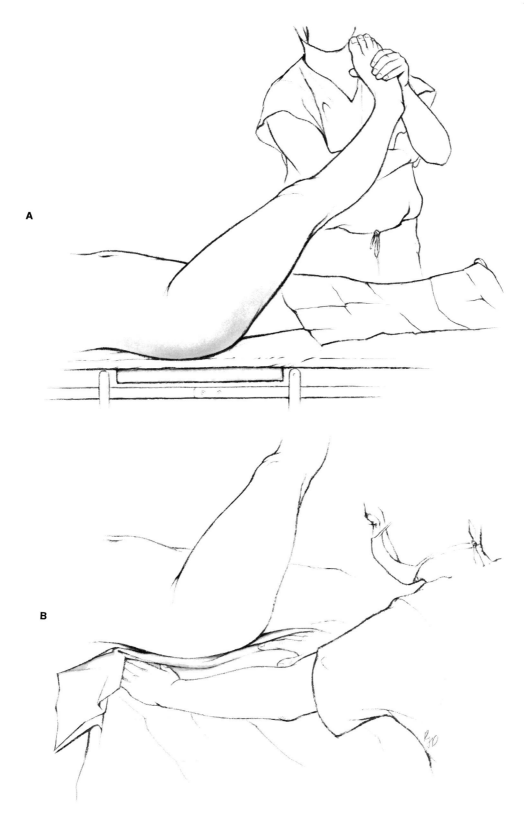

Fig. 12-3. A, Patient is positioned on operating table in supine position. X-ray cassette holder is positioned and centered under hip with tray instrument table also being centered at that position. Pelvis is flat on operating table without any sandbags. **B,** Orderly places hip in flexion and maximum adduction in order to elevate buttock for placement of impermeable sterile sheet by second assistant who prepares patient's lower extremity. Orderly need not wear sterile garments or gloves.

Application of antiseptic solution and draping

Requirements

8 Standard towel clips
1 Impermeable sterile sheet (70 in. × 40 in.)
1 Double-thickness sheet (for covering the end of the table) (52 in. × 47 in.)
1 Special double-thickness lateral sheet (72 in. × 45 in.)
1 Special double-thickness medial sheet (72 in. × 45 in.)

1 Double-thickness bottom sheet (104 in. × 94 in.)
1 Double-thickness top sheet
2 Side sheets (104 in. × 94 in.)
1 Double-thickness bag (for covering surgeon's sitting stool)
1 Large fenestrated sheet (98 in. × 180 in.) (18 in. long fenestration)

2 Rolled stockinettes (6 in. and 8 in. wide)
1 Adhesive plastic drape (optional)
Solutions: surgical alcohol, Freon or ether, tincture of iodine, 2%, in 70% alcohol
18 Moynihan clamps
2 Turkish skin towels (24 in. × 18 in.)

All sheets utilized for draping must be of double thickness; if this type is not available, doubling of the single sheets is required or disposable impermeable draping material is a good alternative. Spreading sheets over the bottom and top of the table requires assistance to avoid contamination. If there is an enclosure, the entrance is sealed off by special curtains, and the window (instrument hatch) and instrument table are draped with special sterile sheets by the scrub nurse. Gowns are prewrapped and handed to personnel as they arrive in the O.R. Completion of gowning is assisted by an ancillary nurse who is allowed to enter the enclosure. If special masks or gowns are used, the headpiece is worn by the surgical team prior to washup. The second assistant dons his headgear following the preparation of the limb.

The scrub nurse stays behind or at the side of the instrument table organizing the trays, handing out the sheets as needed during draping, cutting suture material, and so on, although no instrument table is required if prewrapped instruments are used because they are passed through the window of the enclosure during the operation. The double-glove technique is used for *all* personnel. If impermeable gowns are not available, an impermeable jacket is worn on top of the regular gown.

When the operating table arrives in the O.R., a double-thickness sheet is placed over the foot of the table as an added precaution against contamination. The table is not fully inserted into the O.R. at this point, so the nurse may continue setting up the instrument table and draping the instrument window (when an enclosure is used). The surgeon remains on the operative side as the first assistant prepares the foot and ankle by removing the soap with alcohol, defatting the skin with ether or Freon, and finally painting the area with 2% tincture of iodine. The foot is then held by the second assistant with a double rolled-up stockinette, while the surgeon completes the prep of the hip region and lateral thigh and the first assistant prepares the medial thigh and calf, using the same solutions in the same sequence.

Draping. A sterile towel is placed over the medial aspect of the opposite thigh and the perineum (Fig. 12-4); the hip can then be adducted and flexed, raising the ipsilateral buttock off the table without contaminating the inner thigh or groin. With the patient rolled toward the opposite side, the prep solutions are applied to the hip up to the costal margin and posteriorly to the sacrum.

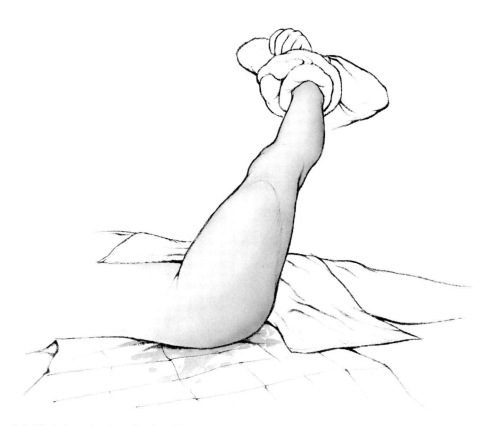

Fig. 12-4. Hip is flexed and maximally adducted by second assistant holding foot by double stockinette coverage at completion of washup of lower extremity so that prep solution can be applied by surgeon and first assistant. Sterile towel is placed over medial aspect of opposite thigh to prevent contamination by maximal adduction of ipsilateral thigh. NOTE: original sterile sheet applied in induction room is still in place.

335

The first impermeable posterior sheet is exchanged for a new one and it, in turn, is covered by double-thickness sheet No. 1 (Fig. 12-5, *A*). Particular care must be taken so that the initial posterior impermeable sheet used for washup does not come in contact with the surgical site as it is removed. The bottom of the table is now covered with double-thickness sheet No. 2, which is placed across the table only to the level of the perineum (Fig. 12-5, *B*).

Fig. 12-5. A, By maximal adduction of hip while buttock is raised following completion of application of prep solution to posterior trochanteric region, sterile impermeable sheet inserted in induction room is now removed and replaced by similar sheet by surgeon. It is then covered by sheet No. *1* (lateral sheet). **B,** Sheet No. *2* (bottom sheet) is applied. It is placed across end of table under lower extremity as second assistant holds hip in flexed position. This sheet is brought to level of perineum covering small towel (medial thigh towel) and lower portion of lateral sheet (sheet No. *1*). NOTE: stockinettes are now being unrolled on limb toward hip region.

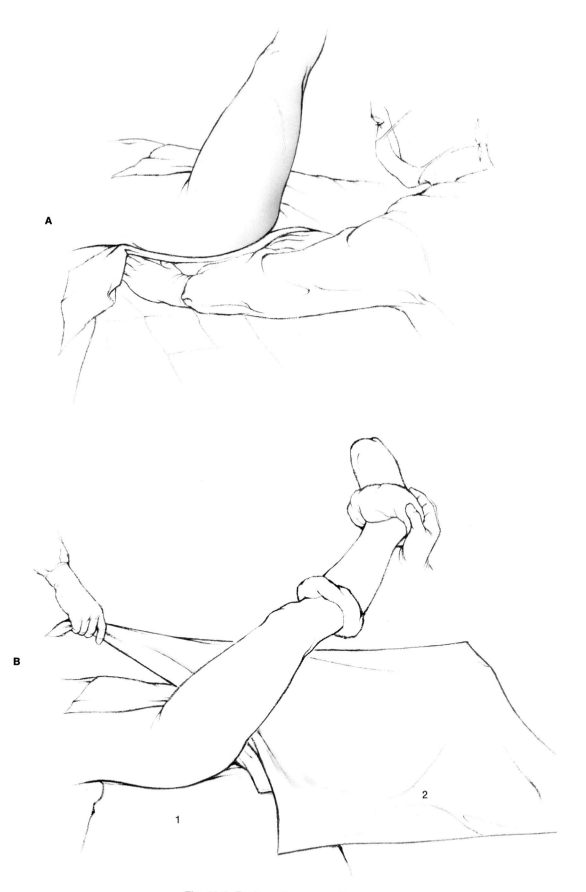

A

B

1

2

Fig. 12-5. For legend see opposite page.

The stockinettes are then unrolled toward the hip, the small stockinette to the knee level only. Unrolling the large stockinette requires some adduction of the limb so that it can be applied to the buttock area and held firmly against the rib cage. It is stretched taut over the crest of the ilium (Fig. 12-6, *A*), while the third sheet (special medial sheet, No. 3) is applied. The top (upper) sheet (No. 4) is now lowered and fastened along with the third sheet and the unrolled top to the stockinette over the patient's abdominal wall (Fig. 12-6, *B*).

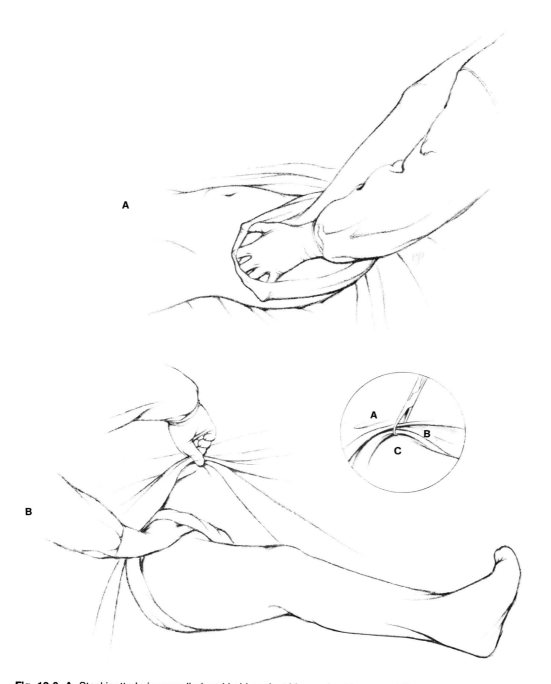

Fig. 12-6. A, Stockinette being unrolled and held against hip proximal to crest of ilium by surgeon. **B,** Application of medial and top sheets, Nos. 3 and 4, onto opening of stockinette as stockinette is being held unrolled toward patient's abdomen. Inset illustrates application of first towel clip to include medial sheet, *B,* top sheet, *A,* and unrolled stockinette, *C,* clipped together onto patient's abdominal wall. Site of application of first towel clip should be approximately 2 inches proximal and 2 inches medial to anterosuperior spine.

339

Four standard towel clips are used to anchor the draping: the first is placed approximately 2 inches medial to the anterosuperior spine, fastening the medial sheet, the top sheet (Nos. 3 and 4), and the unrolled stockinette together over the abdominal wall as described. With the hip flexed to 90 degrees the medial sheet (No. 3) is brought tightly across the medial thigh over the stockinette and fastened onto the midbuttock region with the second clip (Fig. 12-7, *A*). The assistant then adducts the hip, rolling the patient to the opposite side so that the buttock is slightly raised off the table and the surgeon is able to anchor the top sheet (No. 4), the stockinette, and the medial sheet (No. 3) to the skin 3 or 4 inches from the level of the greater trochanter (Fig. 12-7, *B*). It is essential to provide the maximum amount of space proximal to the level of the greater trochanter to allow adequate operative exposure and prevent cramping of the wound. The third clip must anchor the medial and top sheets tautly, encompassing the unrolled stockinette. It should be noted that the sheets are applied counterclockwise for the right hip and clockwise for the left hip.

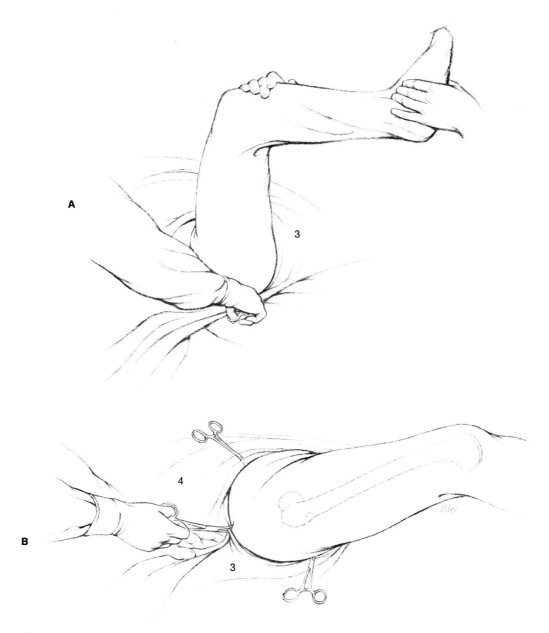

Fig. 12-7. A, Medial sheet (No. *3*) is brought on to medial thigh and gluteal fold of buttock and fastened onto midbuttock region with second towel clip. **B,** By adducting hip and rolling patient to opposite side, buttock is slightly raised off table, while surgeon anchors top sheet (No. *4*) and medial sheet (No. *3*) onto skin 3 or 4 inches proximal to level of greater trochanter.

Operative technique

A large, fenestrated sheet is now applied, stretched toward the head of the table and anchored proximally with the fourth towel clip to eliminate slack in the aperture (Fig. 12-8, *A*), while taking care, however, not to limit the exposure. An opening is cut in the stockinette over the greater trochanter, and extended 3 inches proximally and 6 inches distally; the rolled sheet of adhesive plastic Steri-drape is then applied to the skin (Fig. 12-8, *B*).

This is best done with the hip flexed about 30 degrees and adducted about 20 degrees by the second assistant. The first assistant opens a slit in the stockinette without touching the "painted skin." The corners of the Steri-drape are held by the first and second assistants (one each) and the backing peeled from the adhesive surface by the surgeon. This drape further isolates the operative field from its surroundings. An alternative technique involves the application of an adhesive solution (that is, acrylic base spray) to the skin, causing the stockinette to adhere; in this way the stockinette is incised together with the skin, and the need for the adhesive plastic drape is eliminated.

The surgical team, now gowned and gloved,* guides the table into position well inside the enclosure. The sterile cover for the stool and the two side sheets (optional as an added precaution) may be used to encompass the side of the operating table and the instrument table. The light is adjusted so that illumination is optimal. Range of motion of the hip may be measured for recording in the operative notes.

The electric cautery and cutting apparatus and suction tubing are now clipped to the drapes. The stool height is adjusted and its top covered with sterile pillowcases or sheets. The surgical team is now positioned for surgery (Fig. 12-1), and the entire team exchanges its outer gloves for new ones.

---

*When hexachlorophene (pHisoHex) is used for the washup, it is best left on the hands and wiped off with sterile towels.

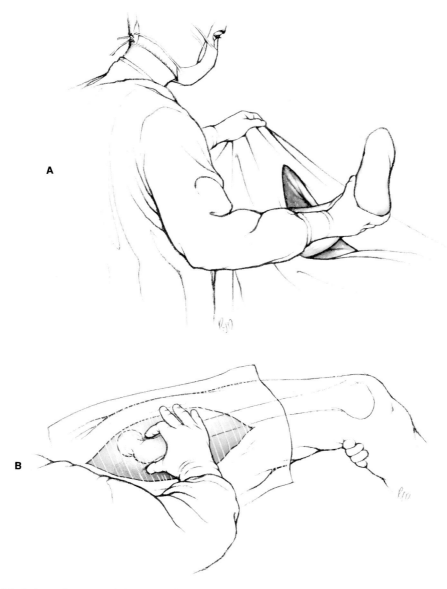

A

B

Fig. 12-8. A, Large fenestrated sheet completes draping. This drape stretches toward head of table. Fenestration is anchored to remainder of drapes with fourth towel clip to eliminate slack in aperture. **B,** Opening is scissored in stockinette centered over greater trochanter. Adhesive plastic drape (Steri-drape) is then applied to skin.

343

PHASE II: SURGICAL EXPOSURE OF HIP
Skin incision

Prior to skin incision, several requirements must be met.

1. Adequate space is provided proximal to the level of the greater trochanter.

2. The anterosuperior spine is accessible from both sides for palpation during the procedure.

3. The position of the patient is optimal on the table, since during preparation the patient is invariably moved. This is corrected now by having the second assistant place his hand onto the opposite ilium and push the patient toward the surgeon, so that, ideally, the greater trochanter is flush with the edge of the table.

4. Any pelvic obliquity resulting from fixed deformity must be noted, by palpating both anteior iliac spines through the drapes.

The skin incision is made with the hip adducted to 15 to 20 degrees and flexed only a few degrees. To determine the proper placement of the incision, an imaginary midtrochanteric horizontal line is drawn for reference, and the actual incision is made, transversing this line at the trochanteric tip, with the proximal end of the incision located 1 inch posterior to it and the distal end located 1 inch anterior to it (Fig. 12-9). The incision is approximately 6 to 8 inches long, slightly longer in an obese patient, and 1 inch proximal to the level of the anterosuperior spine at the proximal end of the incision in order to provide generous access to the acetabulum and greater trochanter.

The skin covering the trochanter must be handled carefully to avoid deviation from the center line (a particular danger in obese patients); it can either be pinched (compressed) between the index finger and the thumb or stretched over the greater trochanter. Scathing of thickened skin in individuals with loose subcutaneous tissue must be avoided.

Misplacement of the incision may occur as a result of fixed flexion deformity of the hip, improper orientation, faulty draping, excessive internal rotation, or fixed external rotation, so the surgeon must be fully cognizant of the position of the hip when the incision is made. Three major points of reference should be kept in mind: the anterosuperior spine, the greater trochanter, and the shaft of the femur. A fourth possible guideline is the configuration of the muscle planes of the thigh (the hollow area of the iliotibial tract) which can be seen by slight flexion and adduction of the hip (see Chapter 1).

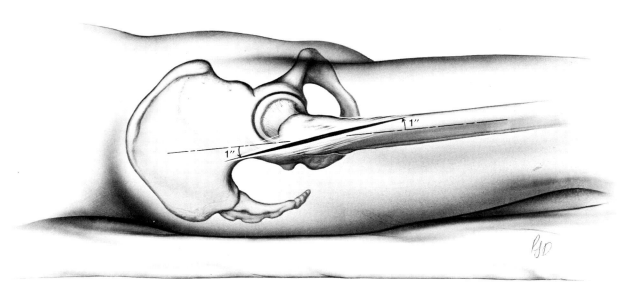

Fig. 12-9. To determine placement of incision, imaginary midtrochanteric horizontal line is considered. Actual incision is made in reference to it, traversing this line at trochanteric tip, with proximal incision end located 1 inch posterior to it and distal end located 1 inch anterior to it. Incision is approximately 6 inches long, and proximal end should reach level of anterosuperior spine to provide sufficient room above greater trochanter.

Insulation with skin towels

The skin edge is walled off with two Turkish towels, each secured by nine Moynihan clamps (complete hemostasis is attained prior to their application). The anterior skin edge towel is applied first: after centering it over the wound, the distal and proximal towel clips are applied so as to stretch the towel throughout its full length (Fig. 12-10). The remainder of the towel is secured by seven more clamps equally spaced along the edge of the wound, after which the second towel is applied to the posterior skin edge in the same manner. Four regular towel clips, two applied to either end of the incision, secure the towels together and complete the procedure. Forceful compression of the skin edge by the clamps results in skin necrosis and should be avoided. The towels should not be clipped to the drapes, nor should they be pulled by the second assistant, since they are adequately held in place by the chain and weight of the initial incision retractor.

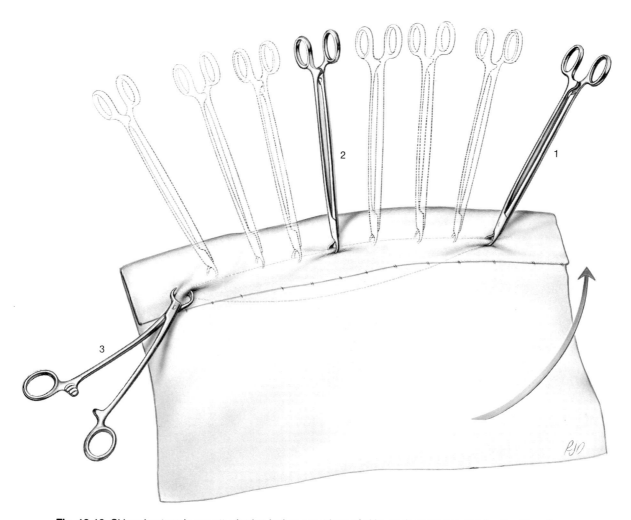

Fig. 12-10. Skin edge towels are attached to isolate cut edges of skin, each towel secured by nine Moynihan clamps. Skin protection by adhesive plastic sheet is not considered adequate by itself. Possibility of contamination from cut edges of skin exists. Anterior skin edge towel is applied first. By centering it over wound edge, distal, middle, and proximal towel clips are applied in such a way as to stretch towel throughout its full length, using three clips. Remainder of skin edge is then clipped onto towels by six more clamps equally spaced along edge of wound. Forceful compression of skin edge in clamps results in skin necrosis and should be avoided.

Incision of fat

The subcutaneous tissue is generally partially incised with the original skin incision prior to application of the towels; approximately 1 cm. of fat should have been cut with the skin knife. (A change of outer gloves by the surgeon at this point may be a good practice.) In a thin person, the incision should not be made boldly, thereby opening the fascia inadvertently; undercutting of the skin should also be avoided. Ideally, the incision of the skin, fat, and fascia is done in the same plane. Any deviation from the line of the incision should be adjusted, keeping the trochanter as a point of reference, continually palpating it as the incision is being made through the fat, and adjusting it before opening the fascia. Incision of the fat should be completed without changing the position of the limb, except in an obese patient, where it is helpful to elevate the buttock by increasing hip adduction, thereby keeping the subcutaneous tissue from falling across the wound and interfering with exposure (a common problem with obesity). The first assistant can improve exposure by retracting the anterior flap of skin and subcutaneous tissue.

Veins and small arteries often cover the outer surface of the deep fascia and should be cauterized prior to incising the innermost layer of fat covering the fascia. Temptation to undermine the fat and detach it from the fascia must be avoided; this is done *only* if the incision has deviated from its original direction. Finally, the fat incision must utilize the full length of the skin incision to maximize exposure.

Incision of fascia

The fascia is incised with the hip flexed to 20 degrees; the placement of the line of incision remains along the line of the skin incision. (The nature of the fibers constituting the fascia of the thigh at the level of the greater trochanter is discussed in Chapter 1.) The fascia should be opened sharply, avoiding bold cutting into the underlying vastus lateralis distally and the gluteus maximus proximally. From the trochanter to a point 7.5 cm. (3 inches) proximally the fascia must be carefully incised and the underlying fibers of the gluteus maximus gently separated with one finger in the line of the incision (Fig. 12-11). This is an important technical detail, for frequently the beginner attempts to split the gluteus maximus fibers without opening this fascia or tries to cut the fascia and muscle bundles as a single layer. Finding this impossible, he then usually cuts the muscle fibers deeply, not recognizing that the gluteal fascia is thin (unlike the iliotibial tract), and resistance is due to oblique fibers. But if the fascial incision is made in the lateral midline, neither the gluteus maximus insertion nor the tensor fascia femoris is cut, and gentle splitting prevents excessive bleeding and devitalization of tissue. Distal to the vastus lateralis ridge, the fascia may be split without a knife because of the parallel orientation of its fibers, but extensive distal splitting beyond the distal end of the incision makes repair difficult and may cause a dissecting hematoma over the lateral aspect of the thigh.

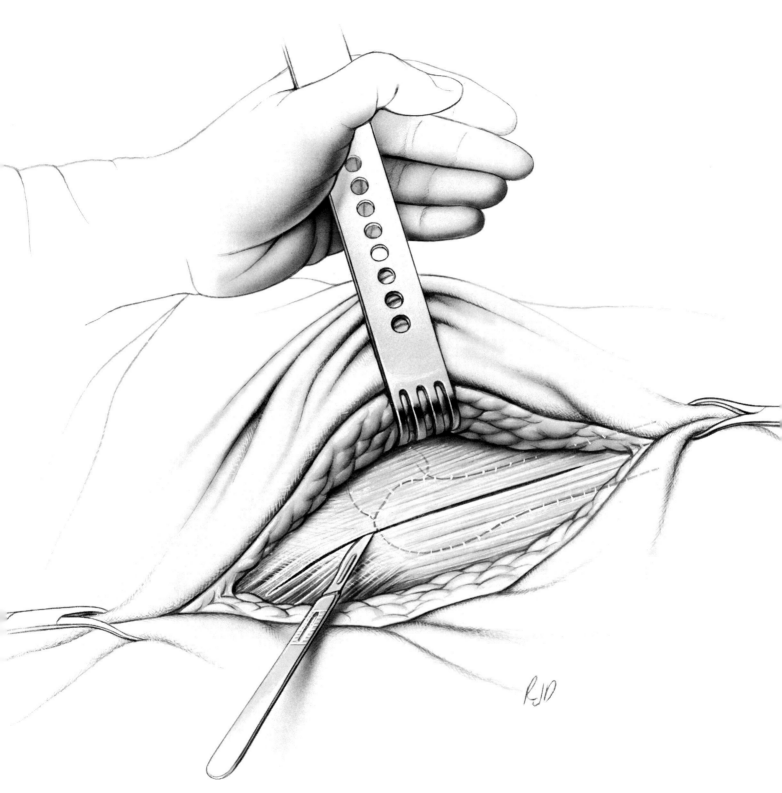

Fig. 12-11. Incision must be centered over greater trochanter. Fascia should be opened sharply with knife avoiding deep cutting into underlying vastus lateralis distally and gluteus maximus proximally. Incision is extended from tip of trochanter proximally to area of approximately 3 inches. NOTE: initial wound retractor used by first assistant holds fat to expose fascia.

Mobilization of fascia and initial incision retractor

Maximum mobilization of the fascia is necessary prior to application of the initial incision retractor. If the incision has been made excessively anterior, the iliotibial tract obstructs access to the back of the joint (this can be rectified by T-ing the fascia posteriorly); an excessively posterior placement (near the shaft of the femur) does not allow application of the retractor because of an insufficient posterior fascial edge for anchorage (Fig. 12-12).

Additional mobilization of the fascial edge may be obtained by running one's thumb beneath the edge anteriorly and posteriorly, thereby breaking up adhesions and intermuscular septae between the tensor fascia femoris and gluteus medius (Fig. 12-12)—anteriorly by placing the hip in maximum external rotation and approximately 30 degrees flexion, posteriorly by placing the hip in maximum internal rotation and 30 degrees flexion, so the posterior aspect of the trochanter can be reached for detachment of the areolar connective tissue from the fascia at the level of the gluteus maximus tendon, the gluteus medius bursa, and the trochanteric bursa.

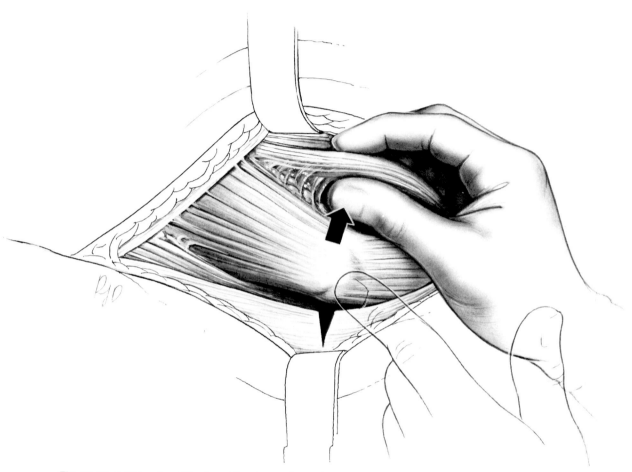

Fig. 12-12. Additional mobilization of fascia may be achieved by placing thumb onto edge of fascia anteriorly and mobilizing it from adhesions and intramuscular septa between tensor fascia femoris and gluteus medius. In this drawing tensor fascia femoris is held between thumb and index finger (for demonstration). Arrow indicates direction of thumb opening space that leads to precapsular fat and capsule. Phantom finger points to vastus ridge. Tensor fascia femoris is T'ed but not held by retractor (for demonstration). (See text.)

Since the initial incision retractor can facilitate exposure throughout the operation, it must be carefully placed. When applied properly at the trochanter level, the wound will be diamond-shaped with equal exposure proximally and distally to the trochanter. Ideally, approximately 2½ to 3 inches of abductor muscle with its tendinous insertion and about 2 to 3 inches of vastus lateralis musculature should appear in the wound (Fig. 12-13).

In an obese person the retractor may be difficult to apply. The lower jaw is applied first (detached from the frame) distal to the T incision if the tensor fascia femoris is T'd (Fig. 12-13); then the frame is inserted in situ onto the lower jaw, with the limb abducted to relax the fascia and facilitate placement. The chain and hook carrying the weight are then attached to the upper jaw to provide a somewhat horizontal plane for the retractor. The higher the level of the chain and hook, the more horizontal the position of this retractor.

Arthrotomy of hip

The anteromedial border of the gluteus medius and minimus and posterolateral border of the tensor muscle are effective landmarks for this procedure. By pressing one's thumb against the anterior border of the gluteus medius and minimus and applying a medium-sized retractor while externally rotating the hip maximally, the interval between the tensor fascia femoris and the abductors can conveniently be entered. Adipose tissue will be found in this interval. It is essential that the hip be flexed no more than 30 degrees, maximally externally rotated and slightly abducted. Precapsular fat may be removed after incising a membranous layer stretching across the space between the two muscles. At times a swab aided with the index finger readily removes the fat from this space, but complete removal is not necessary. By placing a deep retractor medially to retract the tensor fascia femoris and iliopsoas and a shallow retractor to retract the abductors laterally and cephalad, the first assistant renders the capsule available to the surgeon. To maintain this exposure, the first assistant holds both the deep and shallow retractors (since the second assistant cannot see the direction of retraction from the opposite side of the table). The retractors may be readjusted as necessary for continued maximum exposure (Fig. 12-13). The ascending branches of the lateral circumflex, the transverse circumflex, and superior gluteal vessels contributing to the anterior capsule are cauterized prior to transection; the capsule is opened in the midanterior line of the neck, the location of which is determined by palpating its inferior and superior borders. A slightly inferior position of the capsulotomy facilitates the insertion of the cholecystectomy clamp.

The tip of the greater trochanter can be used as an additional point of reference for the arthrotomy. It must be complete and synovial fluid must be observed. Capsular bleeders must be controlled prior to attempting insertion of the cholecystectomy clamp; it is futile to attempt to pass this clamp prior to actually seeing the synovial lining of the joint, and the clamp should not be passed without certainty that it is intracapsular. The superior edge of the capsular incision may be picked up with a forceps to facilitate insertion. A cruciate incision in the capsule is unnecessary if the opening along the axis of the neck is adequate.

Detachment of greater trochanter

Detachment of the greater trochanter includes: (1) the completion of the anterior capsulotomy, (2) the insertion of the cholecystectomy clamp, (3) the retrieval of the Gigli saw, and (4) the detachment of the trochanter.

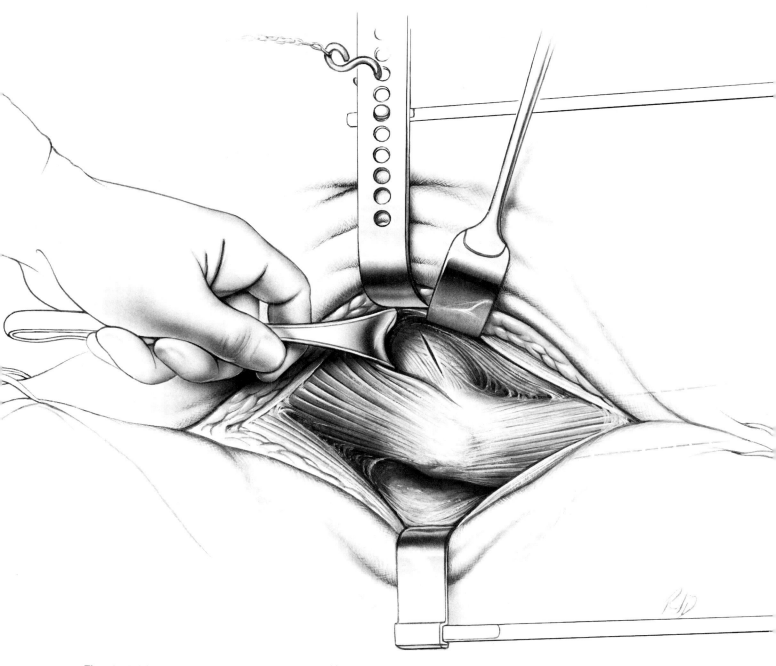

Fig. 12-13. Initial incision retractor holds cut edges of fascia lata apart. Initial incision retractor must be placed carefully to open wound in "diamond shape" with equal exposure proximal and distal to trochanter. Ideally, approximately 2½ to 3 inches of abductor muscle with its tendinous insertion and about 2 to 3 inches of vastus lateralis muscle should appear in wound centered by greater trochanter. Chain and hook carrying weight is applied to perforation of upper jaw of initial incision retractor to provide somewhat horizontal plane for this retractor. Small retractor, that is, Richardson's, pulls back anterior edge of gluteus medius and minimus, and deep retractor draws tensor and psoas muscle medially, exposing front surface of capsule of hip joint. Incision into capsule is made carefully parallel to neck of femur but somewhat distal in regard to width of neck. Synovial cavity of joint is now exposed.

353

The anterior capsulotomy must be complete and the intracapsular space well exposed, otherwise the cholecystectomy clamp and the Gigli saw may be passed external to the capsule and the greater trochanter removed without the strap of the capsule. It must be done as medially as possible, with the synovial cavity in direct view. The anterior capsulotomy may be done with an electric knife, but care must be taken so that the heat does not damage the femoral nerve or the nerve to the tensor muscle.

Difficulty in inserting the clamp may be due to:

1. Insufficient opening in the capsule
2. Extremely distal or proximal placement of the capsular incision
3. Severe hip deformity and intra-articular adhesions (slight flexion facilitating entry to the joint)
4. Misdirection of the clamp tip

Passage and retrieval of Gigli saw

This is accomplished in eight stages (Fig. 12-14):

1. The superior edge of the capsular incision is lifted with a thumb forceps and the tip of the cholecystectomy clamp is inserted into the joint cavity.

2. The tip of the clamp is passed superiorly over the neck with the concave side of the clamp facing the superior neck of the femur.

3. With the tip completely in contact with the neck (without digging into the bone of the trochanter), the handle is brought toward the patient's head, directing the tip toward the posterior aspect of the neck.

4. The tip is then forced through the posterior capsule. With the index finger of the opposite hand, the surgeon feels the tip of the clamp protruding at the back of the trochanter.

5. The jaws should protrude completely (but no more than ½ inch), to allow adequate grasping of the eye of the Gigli saw.

6. Just prior to the retrieval of the saw, the tip of the clamp is turned outward, facing the surgeon.

7. The saw is "fed" into the jaws, which firmly grasp the Gigli saw.

8. The saw is retrieved by withdrawing the clamp (in the direction of the curved tip of the clamp).

Difficulties in passing clamp

The limb must be in neutral rotation with only slight flexion and abduction while passing the clamp. The handle of the clamp is directed toward the patient's head and is not turned toward the surgeon until its tip has penetrated the posterior capsule.

Excessive extension, external rotation, or adduction of the hip tightens the capsule and anterior ligaments, thereby interfering with passage of the clamp; slight flexion and abduction relaxes the anterosuperior capsule and ligaments, thereby facilitating passage of the clamp.

If the hip is fixed in external rotation, the second assistant should be instructed to attempt to rotate the hip internally so that the surgeon can palpate the posterior ridge of the trochanter. This is necessary to ensure that the Gigli saw is medial to the trochanteric crest.

When the posterior capsule is excessively thickened or if ectopic bone is present, the clamp may be gently tapped to push it through the posterior capsule. If difficulty is encountered in passing the clamp, it is withdrawn and an osteotome is used instead for osteotomy of the greater trochanter (Fig. 12-16).

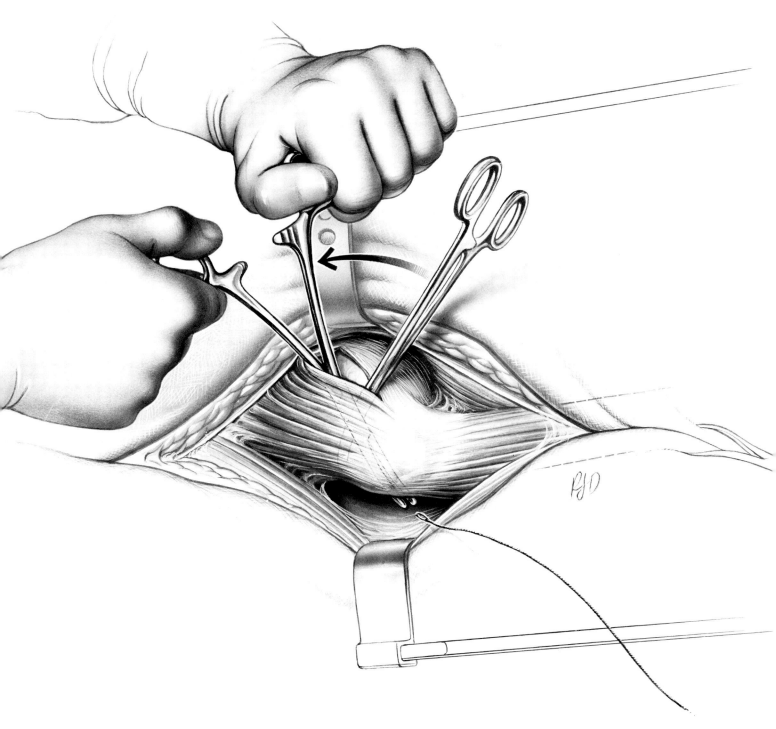

Fig. 12-14. Cholecystectomy forceps is inserted into synovial cavity of joint to pass above neck of femur and to reach posterior part of joint behind neck to retrieve Gigli saw. Tip of cholecystectomy clamp is forced through and out of posterior capsule of joint. End of Gigli saw wire is then caught in jaws of cholecystectomy forceps and pulled back through synovial cavity of joint. NOTE: first assistant has turned handles of cholecystectomy clamp to face surgeon. Jaws must be spread apart by first assistant using both hands.

Detachment of trochanter

The direction of the saw determines the size of the fragment removed from the greater trochanter, that is, the more proximal or lateral the saw emerges from the crest of the trochanter, the smaller the fragment; the more distal the saw emerges, the larger the fragment will be (Fig. 12-15, *A*). It is essential to make the osteotomy at the correct site; the optimal exit site is *just proximal* to the vastus lateralis ridge, and detachment of the vastus lateralis and periosteum from the ridge and aponeurosis of the abductor tendon prior to the actual sawing will help ensure the desired site of exit (Fig. 12-15).

After the surgeon has passed the Gigli saw, he must ascertain that:

1. The limb is in the neutral position without external/internal rotation or adduction/abduction.

2. The saw is in the correct position with respect to the greater trochanter and the femoral neck.

3. The sciatic nerve remains medial to the saw, which is verified by palpating the point of emergence of the saw (Fig. 12-15).

4. Neither the subcutaneous fat nor the anterior border of the gluteus medius are in the path of the saw. The fat is retracted as needed using a Watson-Jones gouge.

After the passage of the Gigli saw and verification of its position, it is often tempting to quickly move ahead with the removal of the trochanter without reassessing the points just outlined, but this should not be done.

Prior to cutting the trochanter, the femur must be stripped subperiosteally in order to properly reveal the vastus ridge. With a 1-inch osteotome or sharp dissecting blade, the origin of the vastus lateralis at (and slightly distal to) the ridge is cut and elevated distally until 2½ cm. of femur is visible. Likewise ½ to 1 cm. of the greater trochanter proximal to the ridge is exposed by elevating the distal fibers of the gluteus medius (Fig. 12-15, *A*). An electric knife may also be used to detach the muscle and periosteum from the bone, or a sharp chisel may facilitate this process.

The saw must be directed first toward the patient's foot, so that it will engage against the inner aspect of the base of the digital fossa. The hands and both arms must be kept well apart while holding the saw, and the osteotomy performed with smooth reciprocal motion. The first stroke must be gentle and at an acute angle to the shaft of the femur (almost parallel to the femur and thigh) so that the saw is engaged at the base of the neck onto the trochanter. After the osteotomy has been started, the saw is directed toward the exit point just above the vastus lateralis ridge (Fig. 12-15). The saw must emerge *precisely* at a point *just above* the ridge. The ridge remains on the shaft for the subsequent reattachment of the trochanter. If the saw is caught in the bone and unable to pass, it may be the result of: (1) entering the bone at an acute angle, usually resulting from not keeping the hands sufficiently apart while sawing, or (2) excessive and hasty pull, engaging the saw deep into the bone before actual cutting. A pause is essential after every few strokes to determine the direction of the osteotomy and to be sure that no skin or subcutaneous tissue are in the path of the saw. The greater trochanter is detached by five to ten gentle and controlled reciprocating strokes. Prior to completion of cutting (emergence of the saw), the surgeon must detach the remaining vastus lateralis muscle from the ridge circumferentially; failure to do this will cause this muscle to be torn off the ridge and the shaft of the femur as the saw disengages from the bone. After sawing, sudden disengagement may allow the saw to touch unsterile areas, but the assistant must not place an instrument or his hand on the trochanter to avoid this accidental contamination, since this would prevent the surgeon from assessing the exact point of the sawband's exit.

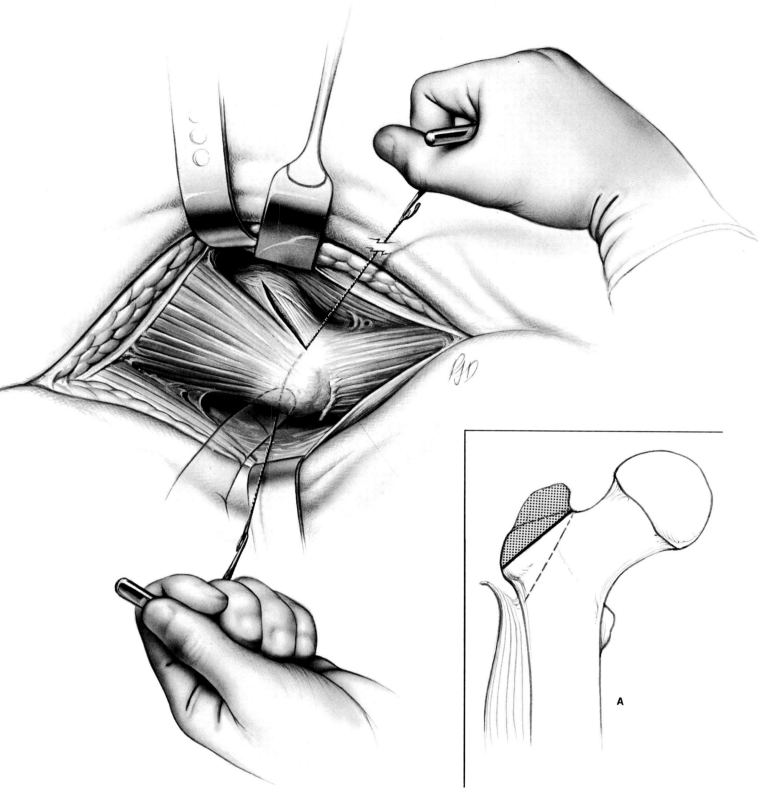

Fig. 12-15. Once Gigli saw is passed, it is laid aside for moment and surgeon palpates emergence of saw at posterior aspect of greater trochanter and ascertains its relation to crest of trochanter. It is also assured that sciatic nerve does not lie between saw and bone (phantom finger). Incision is now made onto periosteum over lateral surface of greater trochanter to detach approximately 1 cm. of vastus lateralis from ridge and 0.5 to 1 cm. of periosteum over lateral surface of greater trochanter proximal to ridge. This will expose vastus ridge and determine point of exit of saw. Direction of Gigli saw is first toward patient's foot and is then changed to cut laterally so that it emerges just proximal to vastus lateralis ridge. *Inset A,* Optimal section of trochanter to be removed. Saw must emerge just above vastus lateralis ridge. Solid line illustrates optimal site, and interrupted lines show incorrect sites of removal.

357

A common error is changing direction too early, resulting in the removal of only a small portion of the tip of the trochanter. When dealing with a severely osteoporotic trochanter, the operator may find the cutting uncontrolled if the same forces are used as in normal bone; less traction on the saw with slow emergence is important in this case (Fig. 12-15). An ascending branch of the anterior circumflex artery requires control prior to or just after detachment of the trochanter.

Trochanteric detachment failure

Optimal size and shape of the trochanter are essential to the success of subsequent reattachment, which is governed in part by the direction of the saw and its relation to the vastus lateralis ridge. Fragmentation of an osteoporotic trochanter can occur if the cholecystectomy clamp is carelessly twisted during its insertion into the digital notch. Extracapsular detachment of the trochanter divides the capsule and allows excess laxity of the abductor system.

Alternate method of detachment

If the surgeon finds it difficult to remove the trochanter with the Gigli saw, or as a result of previous surgery or certain anatomical variations the passage of the clamp is not possible, he may then osteotomize it with an osteotome or an electric power saw (Fig. 12-16).

Arthrotomy is performed as described previously. The position of the limb must be in a neutral or slight internal rotation at the time of osteotomy. The cholecystectomy clamp is inserted intracapsularly into the area of the digital fossa. This point of reference is maintained by an assistant who holds the clamp in position. After detachment of the fibers of the vastus lateralis from the ridge distally and the fibers of the anterior gluteus proximally, a 50-mm. (2-inch) wide, sharp osteotome is engaged onto the bone just proximal to the vastus ridge. Care must be taken to determine the optimal size of the trochanter to be removed. The osteotomy is completed by directing the osteotome toward the cholecystectomy clamp (Fig. 12-16).

After the trochanter is osteotomized, the capsular attachment to the base of the neck is divided, leaving it attached only to the greater trochanter. The use of a narrow osteotome will fragment the trochanter, since the planes of osteotomy may not be identical during its repeated insertion. Damage to the sciatic nerve must also be avoided; placing a flat retractor against the fatty bed of the sciatic nerve protects it from damage. (The Watson-Jones bone gouge is a useful instrument for this purpose.)

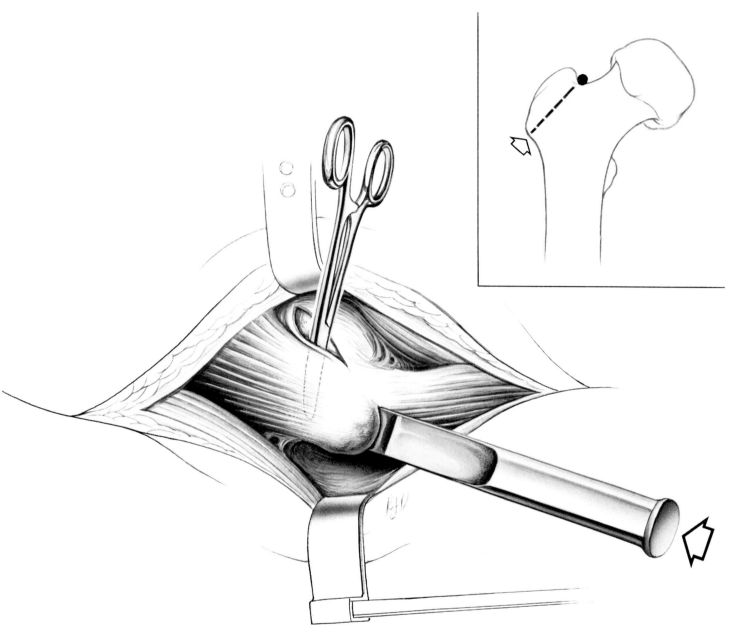

Fig. 12-16. When surgeon encounters difficulty in removing trochanter with Gigli saw, broad, thin osteotome may be used. Cholecystectomy forceps is forced through capsule into joint to point direction of osteotome, which is at junction of inner aspect of greater trochanter and neck of femur. This point of reference is maintained by first assistant as target for osteotome to reach. Inset illustrates starting point (arrow) and target for osteotome.

Completion of capsulotomy prior to dislocation

Prior to any attempt at dislocation, three steps must be taken.

Retraction of trochanter. The first assistant pulls the greater trochanter cephalad using a "Morris" or a "Hibbs" retractor. If the trochanter is severely externally rotated and requires release, it should be done at this stage (Fig. 12-17, *A*). The detached trochanter is retracted by a sharp hook to put the external rotators under tension. The external rotators stretch between the posterior part of the greater trochanter and the posterior part of the hip joint. The tip of the cholecystectomy forceps is passed from behind forward around the external rotators. The cholecystectomy forceps are chosen because of an acute curvature. They are used at this stage like a hook. A scalpel is then used to divide the rotators. This step is rarely indicated in rheumatoid hips and should be performed judiciously in osteoarthritis with fixed external rotation deformity.

It is to be noted that only the external rotator tendons are divided. The superior and anterosuperior parts of the capsule of the hip joint are left intact. This part of the capsule connects the detached trochanter to the superior lip of the acetabulum. This is a very important structure (lateral and superior capsule) connection between the detached trochanter and the acetabulum. It prevents dislocation of the joint when it is correctly tensioned during reattachment of the trochanter.

Control of posterior capsular vessels. The hip is flexed, adducted, and internally rotated to expose the posterior capsule to view (Fig. 12-17, *B*). Retinacular bleeders commonly found there must be controlled at this stage. With the hip in this position, the sciatic nerve is protected in its bed of fatty tissue by a Watson-Jones retractor held by the first assistant (Fig. 12-17, *B*). The posterior capsule is palpated against the head of the femur deep in the wound to determine where the capsular incision will be made.

Fig. 12-17. A, External rotators are divided when trochanter is severely externally rotated. Cholecystectomy forceps has been passed behind external rotators (piriformis) and scalpel is in position to divide it. **B,** Prior to attempt for dislocation, posterior capsulotomy must be completed. Posterior capsulotomy is done over flexed and internally rotated head of femur at about 6-o'clock position from surgeon's position. While capsulotomy is performed, sciatic nerve is protected by Watson-Jones gouge to visualize posterior rim of acetabulum.

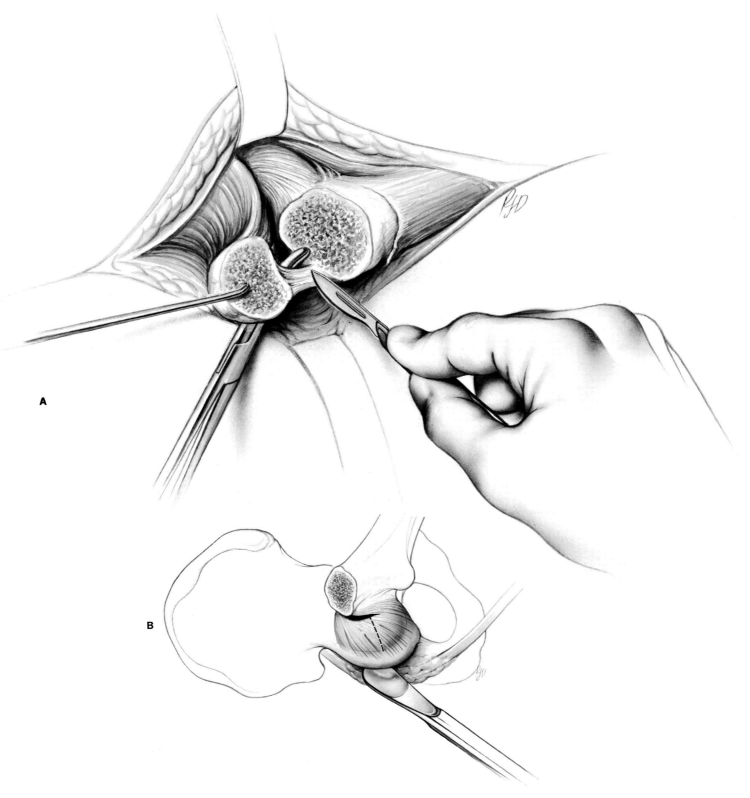

A

B

Fig. 12-17. For legend see opposite page.

Completion of capsular release. The posterior capsulotomy is then performed over the posterior aspect of the neck of the femur (at about a 6 o'clock position) (Fig. 12-18, *A*). Further diathermy of the brisk bleeders may be necessary at this stage prior to any change of position of the limb. If contracted external rotated capsules attached to the greater trochanter require release, they are sharply divided at this point close to the trochanter. While the capsulotomy is performed, the sciatic nerve is protected by the Watson-Jones gouge to visualize the posterior rim of the acetabulum.

Dislocating the hip

The second assistant adducts the limb *without* external rotation to bring the head out of the socket (Fig. 12-18, *B*). No external rotation force must be applied before the head is out of the acetabulum as it may cause a spiral fracture of the femur. Resistance may occur due to:

1. The vacuum created as the head is moved from the depth of the socket
2. Persistent posterosuperior or anterior capsular attachments
3. A peripheral osteophyte or an excessively deep acetabulum, that is, protrusio acetabuli
4. A coxa magna senilis larger than the opening of the acetabulum restricted by capsule and labrum
5. Residual ligamentum teres
6. A hypertrophied labrum

Fig. 12-18. A, Posterior retinacular capsular bleeders are controlled with hip in flexion, internal rotation, and adduction. With hip in this position again sciatic nerve must be protected in its bed of fatty tissue, while cautery forceps is used. **B,** Dislocation is accomplished by adducting limb *without* external rotation to bring head out of socket.

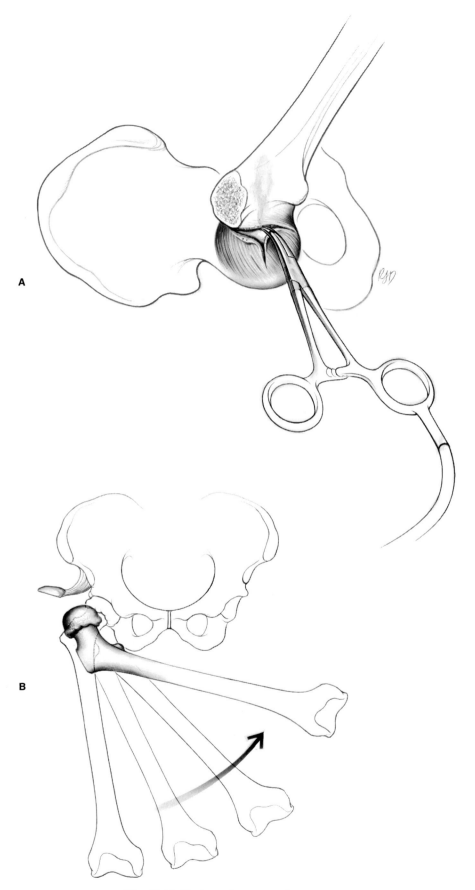

Fig. 12-18. For legend see opposite page.

363

Complete dislocation and delivery of the head into the wound may be facilitated by:

1. Placing the Watson-Jones bone gouge between the head and the acetabulum and levering the head out as the hip is adducted (Fig. 12-19)
2. Successively flexing and extending the hip to break the vacuum
3. Further release of residual capsular and ligamentous structures
4. Removal of overhanging acetabular osteophytes if present
5. Incising the labrum along the superior acetabular rim
6. Most important of all, maximal posterior capsular release (Fig. 12-18, *A*)

An excessively flexed hip in an adducted posture is more difficult to dislocate. An experienced second assistant is valuable at this stage of the operation; however, the surgeon is fully responsible for the "act of dislocation."

In summary, dislocation is achieved by maximum adduction without external rotation or flexion. External rotation can cause a spiral fracture of the femur if the head is still in the acetabulum.

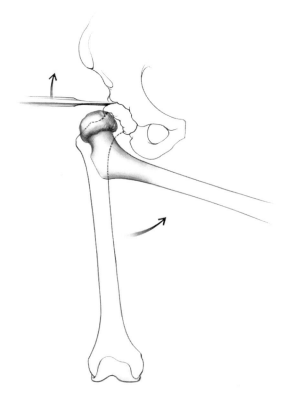

Fig. 12-19. Dislocation may be facilitated by insertion of Watson-Jones gouge between head and roof of acetabulum to pry head out of socket, while adduction force is applied to hip.

Amputation of femoral head

Before amputating the femoral head, the surgeon should divide any tight synovial or capsular bands remaining between the inferior neck and the acetabulum. Maximum adduction of the hip must be possible to allow the surgeon to pass the Gigli saw over the head and around the neck; proximal retraction of the greater trochanter is necessary to allow passage of the saw over the head.

The level of the amputation must have already been estimated by a radiographic template (see Chapter 10). The line of amputation is directed toward the proximal edge of the greater trochanteric osteotomy site (Fig. 12-20, A), and during the amputation of the head the second assistant keeps the knee flexed and the tibial shaft perpendicular (90 degrees) to the floor (Fig. 12-20). The plane of section of the neck is judged in relation to the vertical position of the tibia. It ignores any anteversion or retroversion that may be present in the femoral neck. The first assistant holds the head with a sponge to resist against the pull of the Gigli saw, thus preventing undue stripping of the capsule and detachment of the femur from the pelvic wall (especially in fragile rheumatoid patients), while the surgeon performs the amputation with a gentle reciprocating motion (Fig. 12-21).

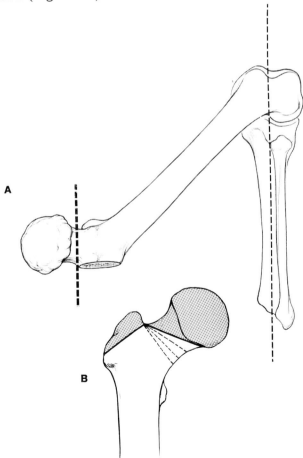

Fig. 12-20. A, Plane of section of neck is judged in relation to vertical position of tibia. This plane of section of neck ignores any anteversion or retroversion that may be present in neck of femur. **B,** Femoral head is divided by Gigli saw at "meeting point" of cut surface of greater trochanter with femoral head. In this drawing several optional lines (dashed lines) show meeting points. These optional lines indicate further shortening of neck of femur when it becomes necessary.

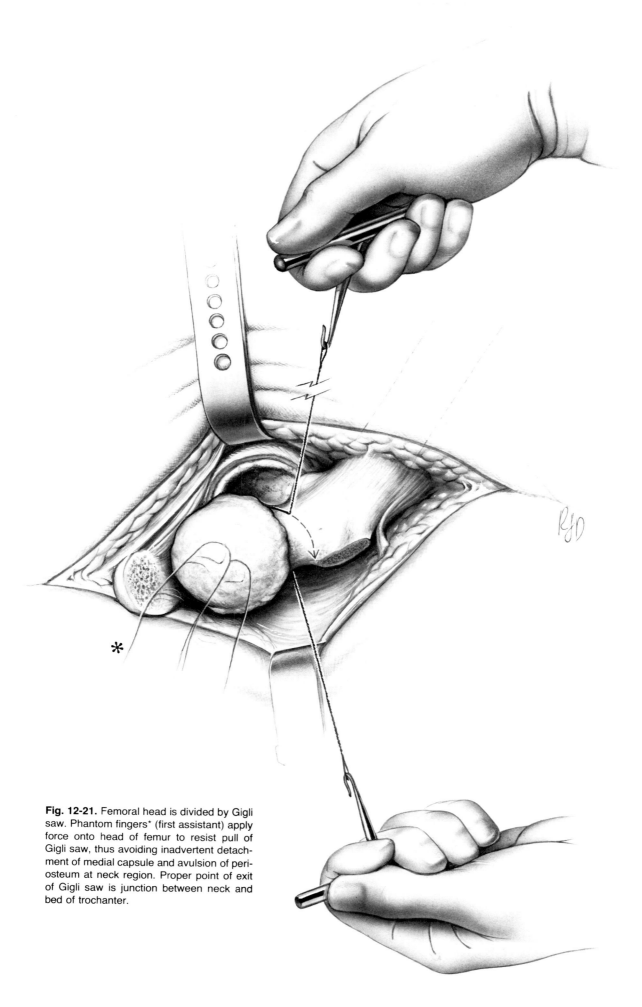

Fig. 12-21. Femoral head is divided by Gigli saw. Phantom fingers* (first assistant) apply force onto head of femur to resist pull of Gigli saw, thus avoiding inadvertent detachment of medial capsule and avulsion of periosteum at neck region. Proper point of exit of Gigli saw is junction between neck and bed of trochanter.

Common errors

1. If the plane of the amputation is not exact, the cut surface will have to be modified later with bone-cutting forceps. The common error is to leave the posterior neck longer than the anterior neck.

2. Cutting excessively proximal or distal obviously results in undesired lengthening or shortening of the limb.

3. Occasionally, for one reason or another it may be impossible to dislocate the hip, especially when the hip is ankylosed (without any motion at all) or excessive peripheral osteophytes are present. It is then necessary to amputate the head at the appropriate level in situ. In this case, use of a reciprocating power saw will prevent splitting of the neck, which can occur when using an osteotome; the head may then be subdivided with an osteotome if need be to facilitate its removal from the acetabulum (see Chapter 2, Fig. 2-4).

4. If, prior to sawing, the first assistant does not hold onto the head to resist pull by the surgeon, the result might be stripping of the capsule from the inferior neck.

5. If the first assistant is not instructed to hold onto the head, the head may "fly out" of the wound upon completion of the amputation, strike a contaminated area, and fall back onto the sterile field.

PHASE III: PREPARATION OF ACETABULUM AND CEMENTING OF ACETABULAR COMPONENT
Maximizing exposure

Since the acetabular depth and coverage for the cup are judged by observing the acetabular rim, complete exposure is necessary. Resection of the cartilaginous labrum is optional for the expert but essential for the beginner. The hip is maximally adducted across the table, and the self-retaining retractors are placed so as to give an adequate view of the acetabular cavity; sometimes additional soft tissue release is necessary for their proper application. Further division of the short external rotators and the capsule may be done to improve retraction of the greater trochanter, and the division of the remaining soft tissues will help cause the release of the proximal femur. If the capsule is constrictive and does not allow access to the acetabulum, additional resection or incision of the capsule is judiciously performed to improve the exposure.

The insertion sites of the jaws of the "east-west" and "north-south" retractors must be carefully selected (Fig. 12-22). The "east-west" retractor is used to hold the trochanter cephalad and the femur caudad. The so-called north-south retractor is used to hold the psoas muscle upward and the posterior capsule downward to expose the periphery of the acetabulum. The proximal jaw of the east-west retractor is engaged into the strap of the superior capsule proximal to the trochanter. Careless placement of the proximal jaw into an osteoporotic trochanter may fracture this bone. The distal jaw is then placed across the intramedullary canal of the osteotomized femoral neck. The posterior jaw of the north-south retractor is engaged into the posterior capsule (taking care to avoid the sciatic nerve) and the anterior jaw into the anterior capsule (under the psoas and tensor muscles). These retractors: (1) must provide maximum

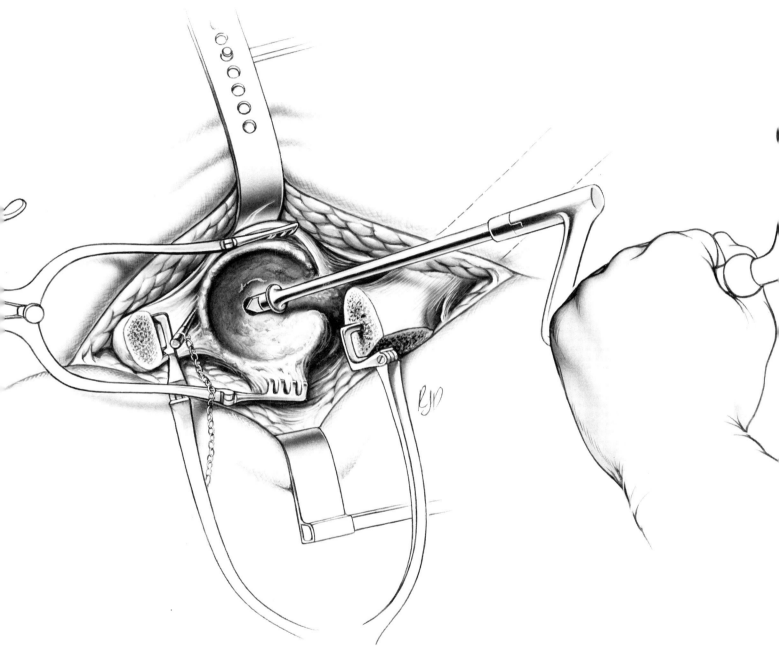

Fig. 12-22. "East-west" and "north-south" retractors are in place. Nail retractor with safety chain and detachable handle is used to complete exposure of superior rim of acetabulum. Nail retractor holds capsule in headward direction to make sure that bony margin of acetabulum is clearly visible throughout subsequent steps of operation. This visualization is most important to make surgeon sure that hip socket will be completely contained inside superior lip of acetabulum when cemented in position.

exposure of the acetabulum; (2) must not be engaged into the periphery of the bony acetabulum or the labrum; (3) must be carefully placed to avoid injury to the sciatic nerve; and (4) may be replaced by a Hohmann-type retractor engaged onto the anterior rim of the acetabulum when full exposure of the anterior wall of the acetabulum is not feasible with a north-south retractor (Fig. 12-23, *A*).

One or two "pin retractors" may be driven into the ilium just superior to the acetabular rim and external to the labrum (but intracapsularly) to allow visibility of the superior bony periphery. If it is already clearly visible, their use is optional. The pins must first be directed craniad at about a 45-degree angle to the axis of the body; then as they are hammered into place, the pin handle is brought craniad to a line perpendicular to the body's axis. Ideally, when fully engaged, they also hold the greater trochanter cephalad (Figs. 12-22 and 12-23, *A*), exposing the superior acetabular rim.

The capsule is not removed, since it may bleed excessively and since it serves: (1) as a site for application of the retractors and (2) as a protective barrier for neurovascular structures. It may be excessively thickened, however, preventing retraction with pins, in which case a posteroinferior capsular incision is necessary for relaxation prior to the insertion of pin retractors. Complete excision of the labrum is then performed (Fig. 12-23, *B*) and bleeders are controlled.

A defective anterior acetabulum (congenital dysplasia) requires additional visual exposure of the anterior acetabular wall at times, which can be attained by readjusting the north-south retractor or inserting a Hohmann retractor over the anterior acetabular rim (Fig. 12-23, *A*).

If exposure is not satisfactory at this point, the following solutions must be considered:

1. Complete detachment of contracted external rotators from the posterior aspect of the femur, to allow further mobilization of the femur
2. Tenotomy of the external rotators (piriformis), if contracted, to further mobilize the greater trochanter
3. Adequate flexion and adduction of the extremity
4. Repositioning of the limb (by even a few degrees), as directed by the surgeon, to facilitate exposure

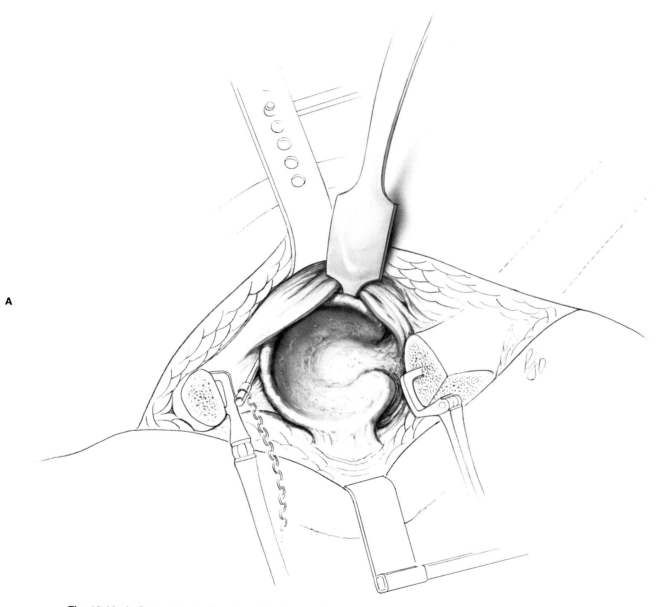

A

Fig. 12-23. A, Same visualization of acetabulum as shown in Fig. 12-22. North-south retractor has been replaced by Hohmann retractor to visualize anterior lip of acetabulum. Similar retractor may be placed additionally inferior to acetabulum at level of intercotyloid notch if necessary.

Continued.

371

Visibility of cotyloid notch and acetabular fossa (pulvinar). Complete exposure of the floor of the acetabulum is essential in order to determine the deepest possible depth for socket placement (Fig. 12-23, *B*). In arthritic hips the inferior portion of the acetabulum is filled with fibrofatty tissue (haversian fat pad and remnant of the ligamentum teres and its synovial recess) that obstructs the visibility of the nonarticulating portion of the acetabulum. In a hypertrophic osteoarthritic acetabulum, the fossa may be completely filled with bone extending from the articular portion. These osteophytes must be removed by curettage prior to reaming the acetabulum. Transverse ligament spanning the intercotyloid notch should be incised (not excised, which often causes bleeding) in order to allow full visibility of the acetabular floor. Troublesome bleeders from the obturator system require careful control at this point. The "pulvinar" nonarticulating segment of the acetabulum represents the outer margin of the "teardrop" on x-ray film and is the deepest level allowed in the preparation of the socket (Figs. 1-3 and 1-4).

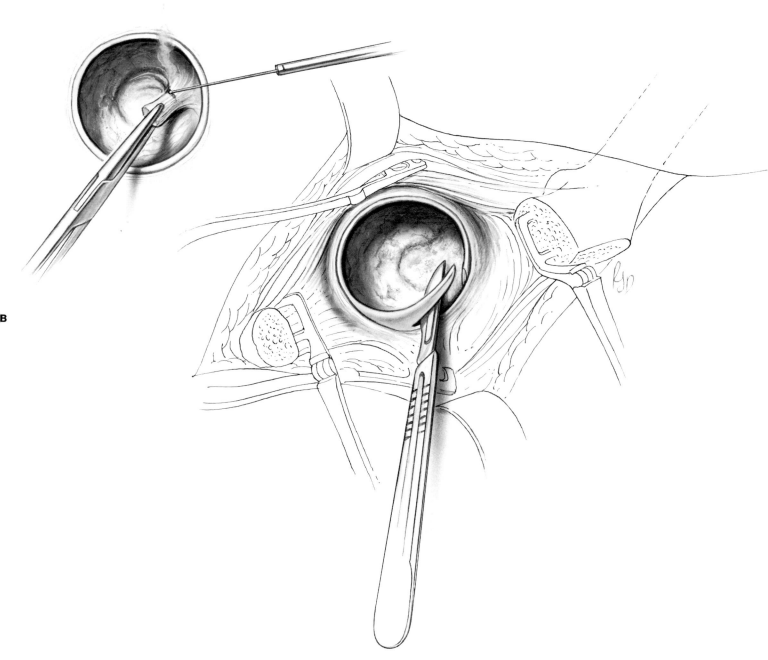

Fig. 12-23, cont'd. B, Complete excision of labrum (intracapsularly) is necessary to expose bony rim. Inset shows use of electric knife in excising ligamentum teres and fibrofatty tissue of this region to allow visualization of floor of acetabulum.

Preparing socket

Drilling pilot hole. Preparation is most effective at the site of the greatest bony mass, where a cavity can be created with minimum bone removal. The bony acetabulum must contain the prosthetic cup with maximum possible coverage. Marking the floor of the acetabulum determines the site of preparation. The transaxis of the pelvis is regarded as an important point of reference in the preparation of the acetabulum. Supine position of the patient provides an important opportunity to evaluate the orientation of the acetabulum. Depending on the pathology, that is, the size of the acetabulum and the degree of proximal migration or shortening of the neck, two types of preparation may be considered: (1) craniad deepening, at a 30- to 45-degree angle to the axis of the body and (2) transverse deepening, at a 90-degree angle to the axis of the body. The mode of preparation is determined prior to surgery (see Chapter 10, "The Use of Radiographic Templates"). Regardless of the direction of the socket preparation, the final angle of orientation of the cup is 45 degrees from the vertical axis of the body; therefore the angle of preparation is not necessarily the same as the final angle of orientation of the cup in the acetabulum. The goal is to create a cavity that will accommodate the cup in the region of the true acetabulum (Fig. 12-24). Distorted anatomy and variations in pelvis size make standard preparation impossible. For example, if the acetabulum has migrated cephalad with resultant shortening of the extremity, the goal is to lower the level of the socket while providing maximal bony coverage (Fig. 13-35) (see Chapter 13). If the acetabulum is concentrically thin medially, that area may have to be accepted as the site of preparation without further attempts to deepen the socket; in any event, the radiographic template assists in determining the proper level for the socket (see Chapter 10). (See also Figs. 10-20 and 13-14.)

Since the center pilot hole will constantly guide the deepening and expanding reamers, it is essential that it is correctly placed. Incorrect placement may result in: (1) unnecessary or excessive removal of bone; (2) the inability to remove cartilage from the acetabulum; or (3) the need for revision of the hole, which may be difficult. The transpelvic line, as indicated by the anterosuperior spine and pointed out to the surgeon by the first assistant, is a constant point of reference for preparation of the acetabulum (Fig. 12-24) (see Chapter 1).

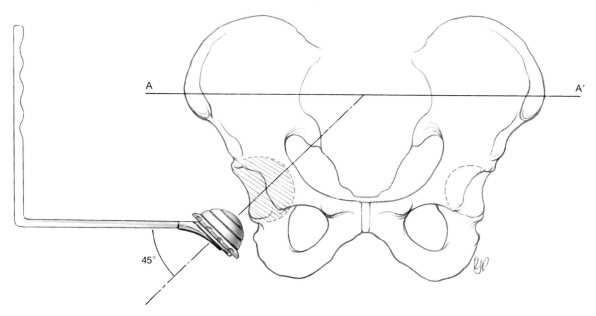

Fig. 12-24. Socket preparation is done in reference to transaxis of pelvis (line *A* to *A'*). Socket holder with plastic hip socket clipped to it is oriented in relation to transaxis line of pelvis.

Drilling pilot hole at 30- to 45-degree angle (high position). The acetabular floor must be marked for placement of the pilot hole. When the acetabulum is small or the head has migrated concentrically medialward at a 30- to 45-degree angle, the centering drill carrying the "centering ring" is placed at the depth of the acetabulum at a 30- to 45-degree angle to the transaxis of the pelvis (Fig. 12-25), which is about the same angle as the neck-shaft angle when the hip is in a 0-degree abduction/adduction position. The handle of the drill is slightly elevated (5 to 10 degrees) in order to compensate for the tilt of the patient on the operating table toward the second assistant. Following removal of the "centering ring," the marking must be checked to ascertain that it is clearly visible and appropriately placed prior to the actual drilling; if not, a second marking may be called for. The floor of the acetabulum is then perforated at the same angle using the half-inch drill. Drilling the pilot hole is a singularly important step since misplacement will direct the reamers improperly and damage the walls of the acetabulum. The direction of the drill in relation to the transaxis line of the pelvis must be constantly observed; minor deviation is permissible but must be deliberate and intentional.

Drilling pilot hole at 90-degree angle (low position). This method is typically used for dysplastic acetabuli or acetabuli that have migrated proximally—in both situations the desire is to lower the socket to the "true" level. It is also necessarily used in cases of a wandering acetabulum with proximal migration of the head; upper pole osteoarthritis and proximal migration in a large, bony man (broken Shenton's line on radiograph); or a large, inferior osteophyte formation and a short limb (usually accompanied by fixed adduction deformity with occasional dysplasia). Usually the centering device is placed against the floor of the acetabulum with the drill perpendicular to the axis of the body. Again, the handle is elevated (as much as 5 to 10 degrees) to compensate for the tilt of the pelvis toward the second assistant. Inadvertent placement of the marking device excessively cephalad will lead to the removal of important superior acetabular bone; excessive caudal placement of the marker will lead to difficulty in removing the cartilage from the roof of the acetabulum and unnecessary lengthening of the limb. Schematic drawings (Fig. 12-25) illustrate the effects of change in direction of the centering tool on the final shape and direction of the prepared acetabulum.

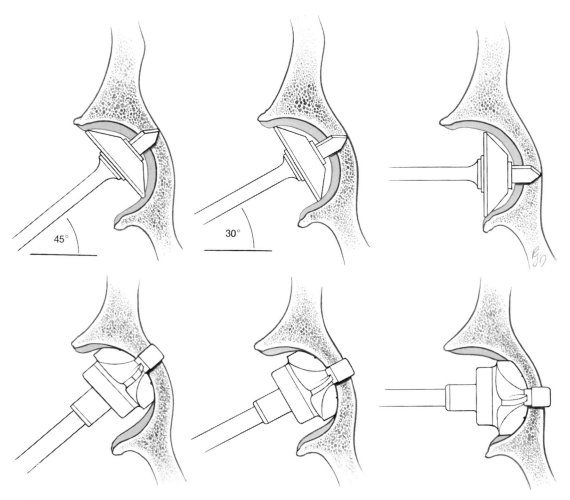

Fig. 12-25. Top shows centering drill with centering ring to find center of acetabulum where maximum deepening will be accomplished. NOTE: orientation of drill at 45 degrees, 30 degrees, and 0 degrees in relation to transaxis of pelvis. NOTE: with marking of pelvis in 45 degrees, preparation will be accomplished "high" in acetabulum with 30 degrees "intermediate" and parallel to transaxis "low." Note also, deepening and expanding will eventuate where pilot hole drill is made. It is, therefore, essential to decide mode of preparation of acetabulum, thus placing pilot hole accordingly at desired level of acetabulum (see text).

377

Deepening and expanding. The orientation of the deepening and expanding reamers will be dictated by the centering drill hole (Fig. 12-25). Four or five turns of the deepening reamer are usually sufficient to clean the innermost cartilage, and no deepening should be done beyond the level of acetabular fossa. To avoid excessive deepening it is best to remove the reamer frequently and inspect the "pulvinar." The acetabulum is then partially expanded, using the expanding reamer (Fig. 12-26). When the bony acetabular stock is good, the expanding reamer may be introduced for maximum expansion up to 50 mm., which will accommodate a 44-mm. diameter cup. If the acetabulum is small, however, only a partial expansion of the acetabulum and the use of a small cup (that is, 40 mm. outside diameter) are indicated. Note that the expanding reamer will damage the rim of the acetabulum if it is not fully inserted. Deepening and expanding must be done alternately until preparation is complete, so that the thickness of the floor and consequently the pilot hole remain adequate to support the spigots of the instrument and thereby guide its direction. Periodic inspection of the acetabulum and removal of bone dust allow the surgeon to be sure of optimal preparation of the socket. Eccentrically opened blades on the expanding reamer can damage the walls of the acetabulum, and special care must be taken to avoid overreaming of the anterior wall, which is usually defective. If the acetabulum is larger than a fully expanded reamer, it is possible to deviate the expanding reamer a few degrees from its usual orientation in order to reach the acetabular walls. For example, cartilage remaining on the posterior wall may be reamed out by dropping the handle of the expanding reamer a few degrees toward the floor.

The thickness of the medial wall may be checked by the examiner's finger or by placing an instrument in the pilot hole (Fig. 12-26). When the acetabulum is large and excess cartilage remains even after reaming, preparation may be completed by using curets and conventional Smith-Petersen acetabular gouges.

The blades of the deepening reamers must be cleaned periodically with either a clamp or a swab. Care must be taken not to dull the sharp edges of the blades. If one of the blades of the deepening reamer remains open, it will prevent the device from turning, so the reamer must be removed from the depth of the acetabulum, its blades completely opened and then all closed together. At times, the blades or the fixing screw may fall off in the wound if the nurses have not checked the instrument carefully; the surgeon must therefore check the expanding reamer prior to insertion to make sure the blades and fixing screw are tight and that the blades are sharp. A blunt instrument will be difficult to control and excessive pressure on it can damage the acetabulum.*

---

*Centering drill and deepening and expanding reamers may be powered by air or an electric motor. The use of power-driven instruments must be considered when the surgeon is well experienced with hand-operated tools.

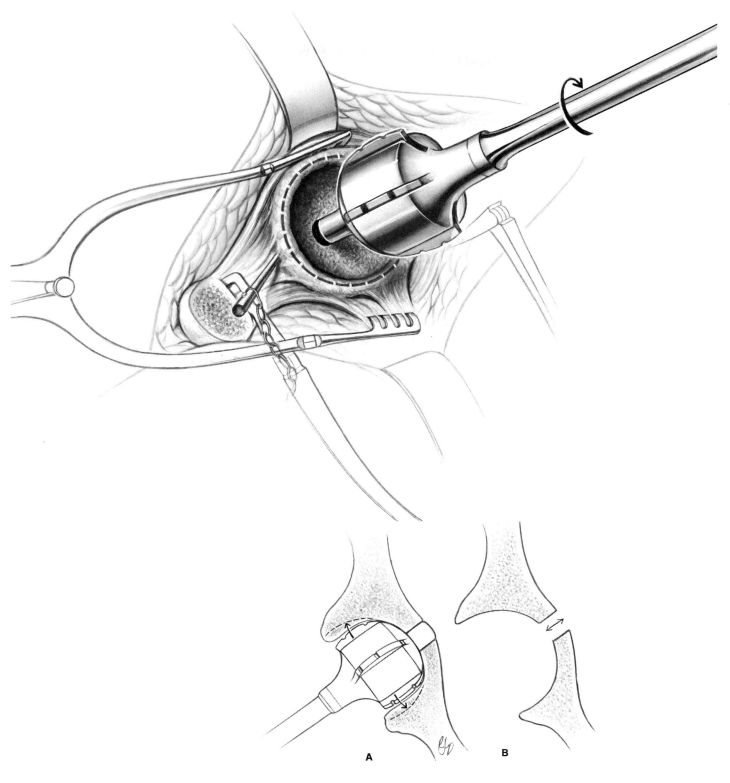

Fig. 12-26. Expanding reamer in place following use of deepening reamer. *Inset A* shows amount of bone shaving by expanding reamer. *Inset B,* Thickness of floor may be judged by thickness of pilot hole made at floor of acetabulum in addition to observing level of pulvinar. NOTE: usually pelvis is rolled away about 10 degrees so that handle of brace has to be elevated about 10 degrees above horizontal line. This simply means to elevate brace to compensate for elevation of pelvis from table on surgeon's side.

Test trial and rehearsal of cup. The acetabulum must now be completely cleansed of bone chips with a Volkmann's spoon and swabs. The small and large "cup trials" are used to determine the size of the cup to be used. The cup trial must fit into the acetabulum with good bony coverage and without impingement against the rim. The prepared socket must be larger than the outer diameter of the cup to allow a free rehearsal of the cup and a thick layer of cement about the acetabulum for fixation. The prosthetic socket, clipped to the socket guide, is then tried to make sure it fits well in the acetabulum in its proper orientation (Fig. 12-27). Correct placement of the cup on the inserter is mandatory. If the acetabular cup impinges against the rim, the anterior rim of the cup may be cut away with a knife. One must also make sure that the insertion of the socket is not impeded by the retractors or interpositioned capsules or other soft tissue. Rehearsal must demonstrate ease of insertion, good bony coverage of the socket when held in its proper position, and maximum coverage of the cup, which, ideally, is seated deep in the acetabulum and covered anteriorly and superiorly, enabling the surgeon to see the bone edge around the cup when it is fully seated. A tight fit may be rectified by using a smaller cup or by further expanding the acetabulum; if this is the case, a smaller cup is preferred in most instances so that bony stock is conserved. Occasionally (but rarely) an extra large cup (50 mm. outside diameter) may be required when the acetabulum is extremely large after preparation.

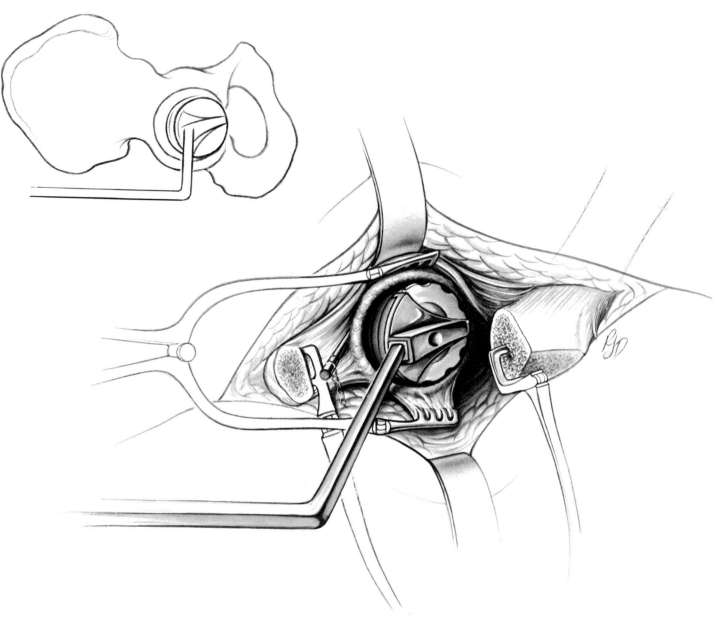

Fig. 12-27. Acetabular plastic cup is tested for orientation and coverage by bony acetabulum. Actual prosthesis clipped to holder is illustrated instead of cup size gauges to show orientation for final position. NOTE: crescent of space present between superior portion of cup and roof of acetabulum. Plastic cup has clearance within cavity created. Inset shows plastic hip socket is held by holder with which it will be oriented in relation to pelvis. It will be seen that plastic socket is oriented at 45 degrees both to longitudinal and to transaxis of socket holder. Satisfactory test is when superior bony lip of acetabulum (seen by presenting gap) is lateral to edge of socket and socket is contained within acetabulum at its final position (that is, 45 degrees to axis of pelvis).

Final preparation and anchor holes. While the scrub nurse mixes the cement, the surgeon with the short half-inch drill makes two anchoring holes in the direction of the ilium and ischium. In large, bony individuals a third hole may be drilled toward the pubis (Fig. 12-28, *A*). The bone and debris in these anchor holes must be curetted out using a Volkmann's spoon (Fig. 12-28, *B*). The cement restrictor is placed over the centering pilot hole to prevent cement from flowing into the pelvis. A small amount of cement may be used to keep it in place (Fig. 12-28, *C*). A large gauze sponge is then packed into the acetabulum, with pressure being applied on it by the first assistant using a Kocher clamp (Fig. 12-28, *D*). Meanwhile, the surgeon changes his gloves, inspects the cup on the holder and cleans the cup (if the actual cup was used for testing). He also organizes the necessary instruments for inserting the cement and cup. The following are "lined up" on the actual operating table: (1) cup on the inserter, (2) pusher, (3) small Volkmann's spoon, and (4) hammer.

The cement restrictor may be inserted immediately before the final packing of the acetabulum.

The following details must be observed.

1. If any impingement prevents the cup from entering the socket, it either must be removed or the socket edge cut away (particularly on the anterior lip). As an alternative, a smaller socket may be used.

2. In order to prevent unnecessary damage to the bone, the anchor holes need not be drilled deeper than 1 cm.

3. The pubic hole should not be routinely drilled unless the acetabulum is large and good bony stock is present in that area. In severely osteoporotic bone, a pubic anchor hole is especially unnecessary since curettage alone provides maximum surface for anchoring the cement.

4. Severe bleeding into the acetabulum from cancellous bone must be controlled by repeated tight packing with sponges to ensure a dry bed for the cement.

5. The position of the socket holder, the socket, and the edge of the acetabulum must be considered when determining the optimal position of the socket prior to its fixation by cement.

6. It is of paramount importance that time be allowed for drying and cleaning the socket before inserting the cement. Mixing the cement too soon places the surgeon in a hurried and uncontrolled situation, thus compromising the preparation.

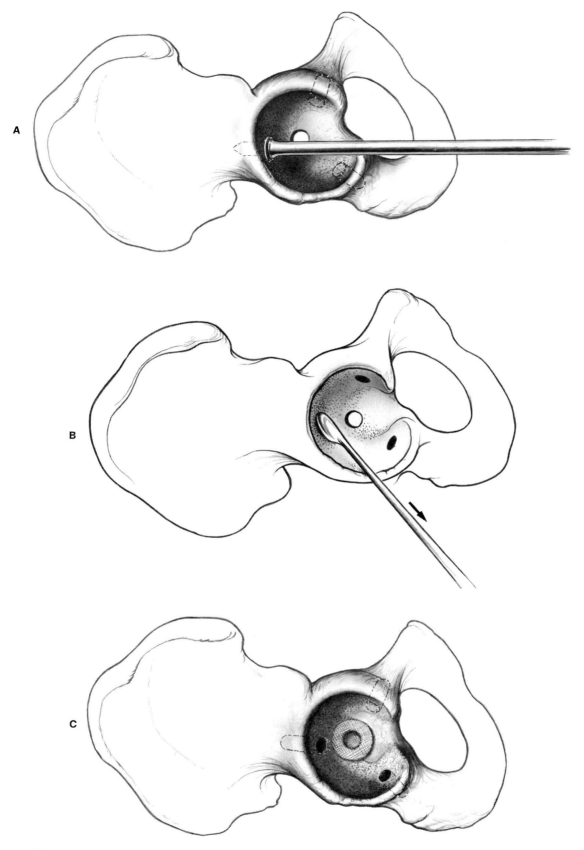

Fig. 12-28. A, Two ½-inch anchor holes for cement, one in direction of ilium and one in direction of ischium usually suffice. Anchor hole toward pubis is only used in large, bony individuals. Use of sharp, long-handled curet or bone scraper improves final preparation of acetabulum. All cartilage must be removed. **B,** Use of Volkmann's spoon. **C,** Cement restrictor used in area of pilot hole. NOTE: position of three anchor holes in pelvis. **D,** Multiple small drill holes made into subchondral bone when bone of floor of acetabulum is sclerotic and nonporous to maximize fixation. **E,** Large gauze sponge is packed into acetabulum with pressure applied by first assistant to keep acetabulum dry.

Continued.

7. As stated before, all cartilage must be removed; if the preparation of the socket cannot be completed in some areas by using the expanding reamers alone, especially in a large acetabulum, it is recommended that an acetabular gouge, that is, Smith-Petersen reverse gouge, be used for further eburnation of the bone. A sharp curet, that is, a small long-handled Volkmann's spoon, may also be used, but the use of a bone scraper is invaluable for this purpose. When subchondral bone is sclerotic, multiple ¼-inch diameter drill holes may be made to maximize the fixation (Fig. 12-28, *E*).

8. Prior to insertion of the cup, the surgeon must make sure the socket is correctly fixed (clipped) to the "holder," * noting the position of the radiographic marker and the posterior extended wall of the cup (see Fig. 3-24). Flexion of the hip about 10 to 15 degrees from the rest position by the second assistant will facilitate maximum exposure of the acetabulum prior to insertion of the cement. With experience, cement may be mixed earlier in order for it to be ready when the preparation is complete.

9. The surgeon must make sure that the self-retaining retractors and the pin retractors do not impinge against the handle of the cup holder when it is brought to its final position.

10. Readjustment of the retractors, if necessary, must be made prior to the insertion of the cement.

11. A careful final inspection of the acetabulum and removal of all bone debris is essential prior to the insertion of cement. The use of irrigation with isotonic solution is useful in removal of bone dust, finding unremoved soft tissue, and cleansing the acetabulum.

---

*This instrument is also identified as the "inserter."

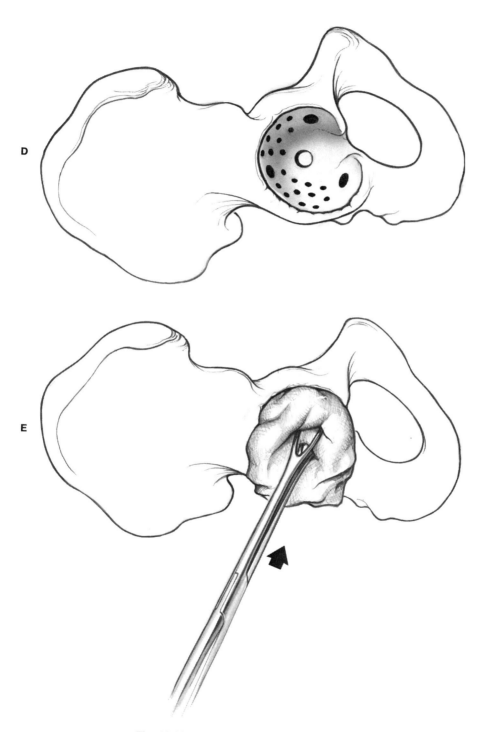

Fig. 12-28, cont'd. For legend see p. 383.

385

Cementing of acetabular component

Insertion of cement and cup. While the scrub nurse mixes the cement, the first assistant identifies the anterosuperior iliac spines in order to demonstrate the transverse axis of the pelvis.

While the assistant maintains firm pressure on the acetabular sponge (Fig. 12-28, *D*) for hemostasis (similar to packing of the dental canal by the dentist prior to insertion of a filling), the scrub nurse removes all the prepolymerized cement from the bowl and hands it in the spoon to the surgeon. (For details on preparation and mixing, see Chapter 4.) At 66° F. or 19° C., CMW cement will take 3 to 3½ minutes to set from the time it is mixed; Simplex P radiopaque cement takes 8 to 9 minutes at 66° F. after the addition of the liquid monomer to the polymer powder.* The optimal time for delivering the cement into the acetabulum is when the surgeon notes the skinning effect (evaporation of the monomer) and feels the material beginning to stiffen. Massaging or folding is avoided since it may result in lamellation of the cement or the admixture of blood. When it is fairly stiff, the assistant removes the sponge from the acetabulum and the cement is introduced immediately as a short, cylinder-shaped bolus (Fig. 12-29).

If the cement restrictor was not previously placed over the pilot hole, it should be inserted immediately before the cement. The cement should fill the entire acetabulum. With finger pressure, it is pushed against the floor and wiped off against the superior acetabular edge. Generally, in a large acetabulum no cement need be removed, and rarely, in an extremely large cavity, two batches of cement are required. If two packs of cement are necessary, both powder packages are emptied into the bowl, and both monomer vials are then simultaneously added. (See Chapter 4.)

---

*The reader is referred to discussion of "working time" of acrylic cement in Chapter 4.

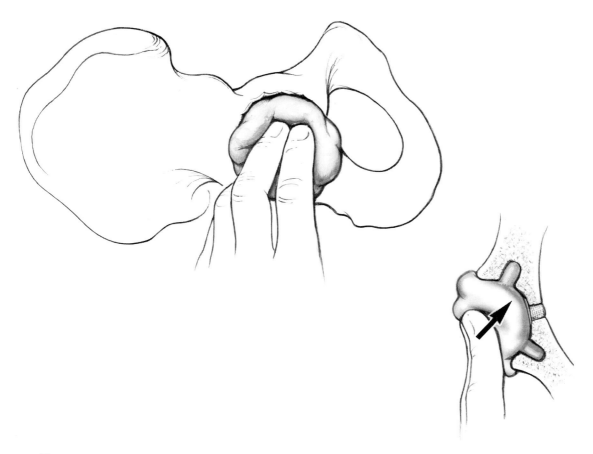

Fig. 12-29. Bolus of cement is inserted using two or three fingertips to push cement toward depth of acetabulum. Cement is pressurized especially in areas of anchor holes.

Positioning of cup and coining of cement. Once again the correct placement of the cup on the holder is verified. Insertion of the cup may be divided into six steps (Figs. 12-30 and 12-31). The *first* step (Fig. 12-31, *A*) is the insertion of the socket into the depth of the acetabulum: while pressing on the socket holder, the socket is pushed into the inferior aspect of the acetabulum (the guide handle is maximally tilted toward the patient's foot). The socket holder is oscillated back and forth a few degrees to sink the cup in deeply. The handle is not yet brought up to the final position.

In the *second* step (Fig. 12-31, *B*) the "socket pusher" is positioned into a depression in the socket holder; the handle of the holder is then gradually brought up without oscillation toward the patient's head. This causes the space between the superior aspect of the cup and the acetabulum to become filled with cement as it extrudes over the top edge of the cup. This must be pushed back into the space with the tip of a finger or the tip of a Kocher clamp to maximize filling of the superior portion of the acetabulum, although with the use of the broad rim cup* (tailored at surgery to the size of the socket) this is not necessary, since the rim of the cup will inject the cement into the acetabulum as the final position is reached.

The *third* step (Fig. 12-31, *C*) involves bringing the handle of the cup holder up to the final desired position, that is, the handle lined up with the transverse axis of the pelvis. In this way the cup assumes a 45-degree orientation to the axis of the body. No more than 5 degrees of anteversion should be allowed. Once the socket and holder are in the optimal position, the assembly is held steady—under no circumstances should the holder be readjusted, that is, by moving the socket back to a more horizontal position.

At the *fourth* step, the holder is held immobile by the first assistant, while the surgeon maintains steady pressure with the "pusher" via the depressed area of the cup holder while maintaining the 45-degree orientation with minimum anteversion. This is the *final* position of fixation, from which no further changes are made. Excess cement is removed from the anterior and posterior portions of the socket by a small Volkmann's spoon, being careful that the cement is not pulled away from underneath the cup and that this maneuver does not change the orientation of the socket. The first assistant often attempts to help remove cement, and his movement causes changes in the socket's position so he must resist this impulse and be assigned only one job, namely, holding the socket holder until it is removed by the surgeon. Excessive pressure on the pusher must be avoided, since this will cause too much cement to be squeezed out of the acetabular cavity. If this occurs (most often in a large acetabulum), the cup will reach the full depth without cement between it and the contact point of the acetabulum (Fig. 3-32).

In the *fifth* step the degree of polymerization is tested by the surgeon, using the leftover sample. When the cement is in the rubbery stage, one or two light taps of the hammer against the pusher will "coin" the socket into the cement and the cement into the bony trabeculae of the acetabulum. "Coining" must not be left to the final stage of stiffening of the cement, since it may not inject the stiff cement into the bone and might even be harmful and cause loosening of the cup.

In the *sixth* step (Fig. 12-31, *D*) the socket holder is disengaged from the cup by pressing its release mechanism. The tip of the pusher is now placed concentrically within the depth of the cup and pressure is maintained at a 45-degree angle. For the first time, the surgeon observes the true orientation of the cup. While the cement is

---

*A new cup design by Charnley.

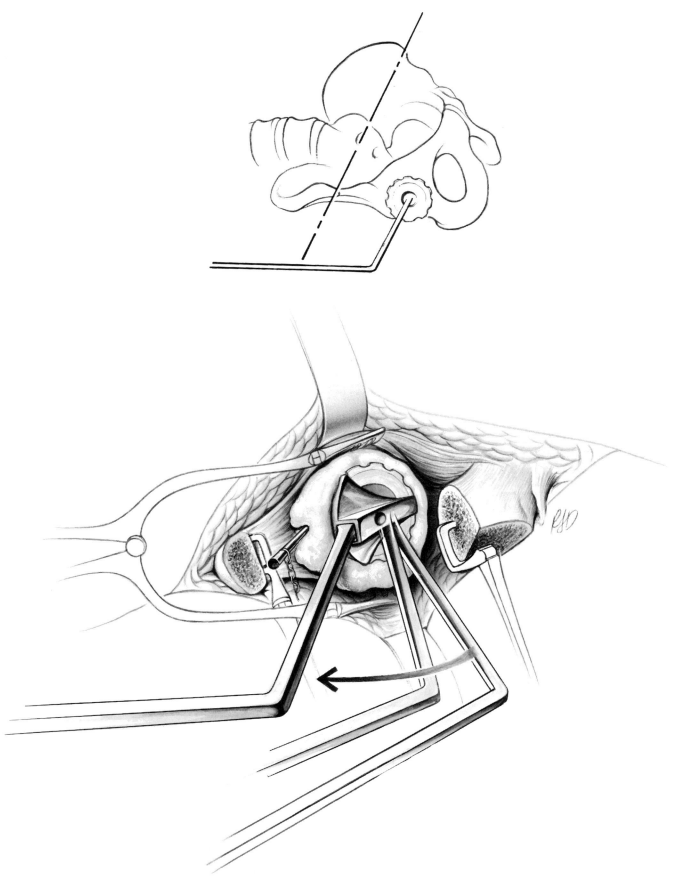

Fig. 12-30. Plastic socket fixed on socket holder is pressed into cement with face of socket directed toward patient's feet. (Transverse bar of holder is near stump of neck of femur.) When socket has reached full depth of acetabulum, surgeon presses cement with his finger into gap between socket and superior lip of acetabulum. Socket holder is maintained in position by pusher that allows socket to remain steady at depth of acetabulum. (Pusher has been removed here.) Final position of socket is obtained by moving socket holder to its final transverse position (inset).

still soft, it is "stuffed" and "buttered" into the periphery of the cup between the cup and the bone and any excess is removed with a curet. The area is thoroughly irrigated and the retractors are removed.

Art of cementing and some details

1. A steady pair of hands is mandatory. Clumsy disengagement of the socket holder from the face of the cup causes cement to pull away from the bone, creating an imperfect fit. Likewise, if the first assistant moves the holder excessively, spaces are created between the cement and bone.

2. Early excessive pressure on the cup squeezes cement from the interface, causing direct contact between bone and cup and resulting in defective fixation (Figs. 3-33 and 3-34).

3. Early removal of cement from the periphery of the acetabulum with a curet may pull cement away from the interface, which must be avoided.

4. Excessive proximal positioning of the socket holder (toward the patient's head) and later correction creates a space between the weight-bearing portion of the acetabulum and the socket.

5. An unchecked flow of cement into the anterior soft tissues is a potential hazard to the femoral nerve (see Chapter 17).

6. Poor access to the acetabulum, poor exposure, or any other factor delaying the surgeon may allow cement to harden around the holder and prevent its disengagement from the cup.

7. Unnecessary movement of the holder during disengagement leads to poor fixation, especially in a large acetabulum.

8. A steady two-handed grip by the first assistant is essential to allow the surgeon to push the cup firmly into the acetabulum as is absolute attention by the first assistant. (No talking at this stage!)

9. Excess cement must be removed prior to its polymerization and the removal of the self-retaining retractors.

10. A complete evaluation of the periphery of the cup and its relation to the acetabulum must be performed before removal of the self-retaining retractors. The amount of coverage of the cup by bone should be noted and later recorded in the operative record.

11. Complete hemostasis is attained, and irrigation with antibiotic solution to remove devitalized tissue and loose cement particles is done prior to the removal of the retractors.

12. A search for significant marginal osteophytes must be made and excision performed prior to the removal of the self-retaining retractors.

13. The jaws of the retractors must not come in contact with the cement, since this can make their removal difficult.

14. Polymerized cement on the periphery of the acetabulum (cementophytes) must be removed by a half-inch osteotome, using sharp hammer blows.

15. The capsular pin retractor(s) is removed at this point, using the cup pusher to stabilize the pelvis during extraction.

16. Removal of the self-retaining retractors completes this phase.

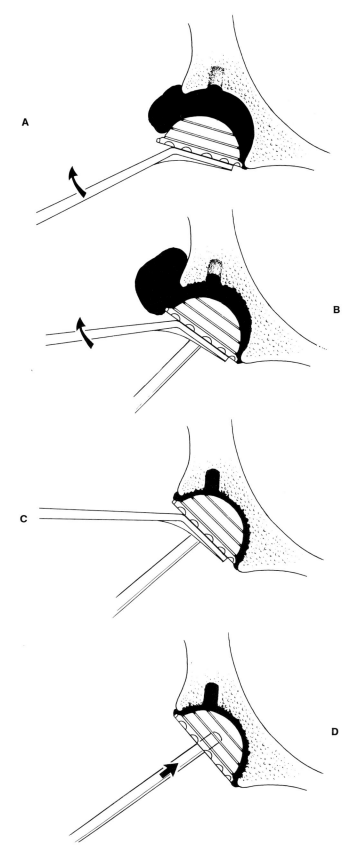

Fig. 12-31. A, Socket clipped to socket holder is pushed into depth of acetabulum pressing onto cement. Socket holder is maintained maximally toward patient's foot. **B,** "Socket pusher" is positioned into depression in socket holder to keep socket at depth of acetabulum while handle is brought up toward patient's head. NOTE: excess cement being squeezed out of depth of acetabulum toward superior lip. **C,** Handle is brought to final orientation (transverse arm parallel to transaxis of pelvis) and excess cement removed. "Coining" of cement may be done at this stage. **D,** Socket holder is removed and pusher is placed into depth of socket, and pressure is maintained until cement fully polymerizes.

PHASE IV: PREPARATION OF FEMUR
Delivery of stump of upper femur

With the self-retaining retractors removed, the stump of the proximal femur is now delivered out of the wound for preparation; excessive force is to be avoided. Delivery is best accomplished by maximal adduction of the hip without flexion by the second assistant, who supports the knee flexed at 90 degrees and places the femur across the opposite side of the table and the opposite thigh. Any medial and posterior soft tissue attachments that remain may be released if necessary at this stage. The second assistant demonstrates the knee axis and the axis of the femur to the surgeon, who can now fully assess the direction of the femur in reference to the transcondylar line and the lesser trochanter.

Further delivery from the wound can be achieved by using a posteriorly placed Watson-Jones gouge, to lever the proximal end of the femur (Fig. 12-32). The position of the instrument is maintained by the first assistant (Fig. 12-32, *inset*), while the leg position is maintained by the second assistant. The Watson-Jones bone gouge further mobilizes the iliotibial tract medially and posteriorly in relation to the femur to assist in bringing the femur out of and away from the depth of the wound. Occasionally detachment of the iliopsoas and the remainder of the contracted medial and posterior capsule may be needed, as in muscular and heavy men or obese patients, or in difficult situations where persistent adduction and flexion deformity exist. Unless complete mobilization and maximal delivery of the stump are attained, preparation of the upper femur may be severely hindered, thus complications such as misorientation, poor sense of direction, or perforation of the shaft may result (see Chapters 14 and 17). This delivery is also essential for a *valgus* preparation and a *valgus* orientation of the prosthesis.* During this stage of the operation, the greater trochanter is turned into the acetabulum by folding the tendon of the gluteus medius and minimus. Alternatively, the trochanter is pulled proximally by the first assistant—using a Hibbs or similar retractor—carefully to avoid fracture and fragmentation.

---

*The term *"valgus"* as used in this section implies and stresses avoidance of a *varus* positioning. An exaggerated valgus positioning should also be avoided.

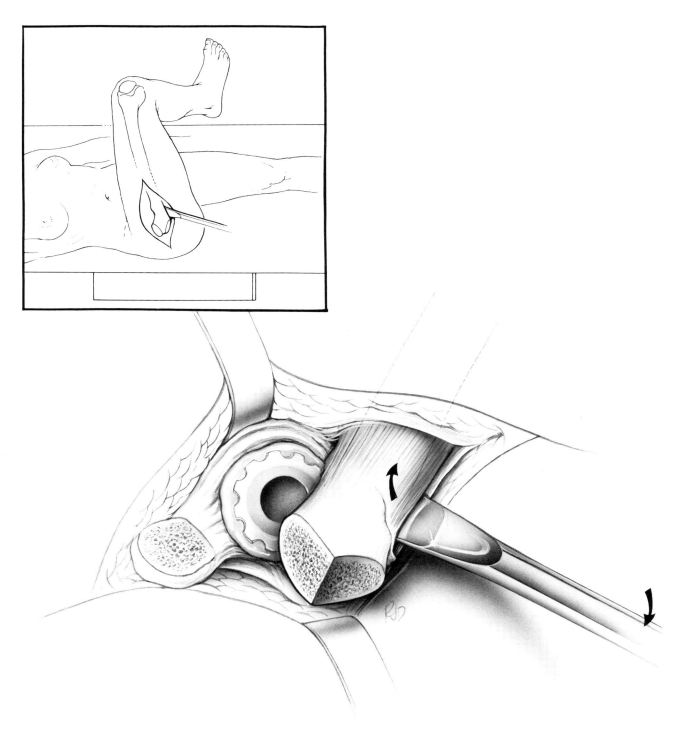

Fig. 12-32. Stump of upper femur is delivered out of wound and assisted by Watson-Jones gouge and maximal adduction of hip. With leg crossed to opposite side of table, surgeon now has complete access to top of femur. Inset illustrates cross-table position of limb during preparation of femur.

Preparation of femur

The medullary canal is opened with a tapered pin T-handle reamer (Fig. 12-33). The starting point is the junction of the cut surfaces of the trochanter and the neck. The cortical bridge dividing the stump of the neck from the site of the osteotomized greater trochanter is removed with a rongeur, unless it was removed following the resection of the femoral head. The tapered pin T-handle reamer is aimed at the knee, thereby defining the medullary canal (Fig. 12-33, *inset*). Once the reamer is fully inserted, it is shifted toward the lateral cortex to produce a slightly valgus track. This entails encroachment on the trochanteric bed. The surgeon stabilizes the knee with one hand while guiding the reamer with the other; the second assistant holds the hip in maximum adduction and neutral rotation to aid stabilization. The assistant on the far side of the table holds the tibia vertical so that the amount of anteversion in the femoral neck can be recognized. The tapered reamer must be checked to assure that it is within the medullary canal and that valgus orientation is maintained. In this way the surgeon ascertains that the reamer is not piercing the femoral cortex. The aperture is enlarged by cutting toward the trochanteric bed as it is inserted, making an oval opening for femoral broach in the correct "version." A tapered reamer attached to a wide-throw brace may be used for this purpose instead of a T-handle tapered reamer.*

---

*A tapered pin reamer attached to a power drill may be used (when power tools are used) to enlarge the cavity of the upper femur.

Fig. 12-33. Medullary canal is opened with tapered pin T-handle reamer. Starting point of insertion of tapered reamer is at junction of cut surface of trochanter and cut surface at neck. Direction of insertion of reamer is in slight valgus (to avoid any varus position), thus encroaching into bed of trochanter. Tapered pin reamer enters at somewhat posterior level of cut surface of neck and is aimed at knee joint. *A* indicates correct and *B* "faulty" insertion. In *B,* bridge between neck of femur and greater trochanteric bed is not removed thus forcing reamer into varus position.

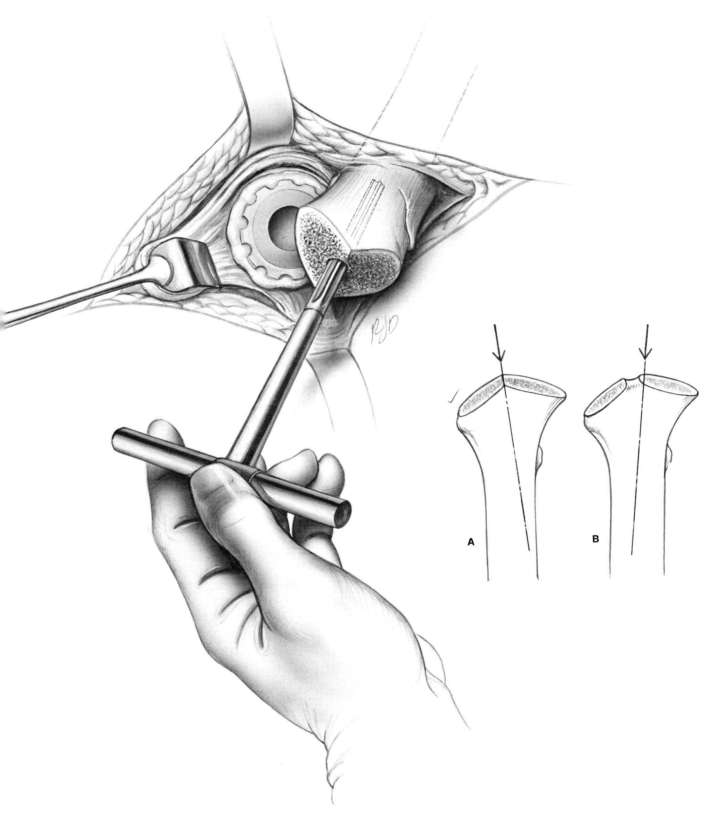

Fig. 12-33. For legend see opposite page.

Operative technique

The straight femoral broach is then hammered into the medullary canal while being held in a valgus orientation. This is best accomplished by inserting a tommy bar into the broach handle and pulling the broach toward the outer cortex (Fig. 12-34). The plane of "version" has already been determined by the tapered pin reamer. To ensure a neutral version plane, the tommy bar should be perpendicular to the floor, while the knee is in 90 degrees flexion and the tibia perpendicular to the floor. The plane of the reamer should also be parallel to the transverse intracondylar axis of the knee. In this way, there are at least four points of reference for orientation:

1. Patella and the transverse axis of the knee (transcondylar line)
2. Operating table or floor
3. Flexed knee at right angle
4. Shape of the upper femur, especially in reference to the lesser trochanter

The curved broach is hammered down the medullary canal maintaining the same orientation (Fig. 12-34). The broaches are hammered in a valgus orientation, as if cutting takes place with the convex edge of the broach (Fig. 12-34, *inset*). Should the broaches impinge against the medial calcar, they must be withdrawn and reinserted: (1) to ensure valgus positioning and (2) to prevent fracture of the calcar femorale. When the medullary canal is excessively narrow and the isthmus prevents full broaching, further widening may be accomplished by using graded reamers, such as the Küntscher reamers; broaching may then be completed. The broaches should not be driven in with excessive force, since this may shatter the upper femur. Instead, the broaches are repeatedly inserted and removed to accomplish their purpose. When the broach is jammed in the canal, it is withdrawn and the rasp action repeated using the tommy bar and oscillating motions in (external and internal) rotation, followed by reinsertion of the broach. The correct orientation of the broaches relative to the leg is constantly checked. The channel is satisfactorily prepared when the broaches can be freely inserted to their full length in optimal orientation. Ideally the channel should not be in more than 5 degrees of anteversion and should accommodate a standard (or heavy, if medullary canal is large) prosthesis. With experience the channel may be created without the use of broaches, using the tapered pin reamer and power tools.

Insertion of test prosthesis

Unless the second broach could not be inserted, a standard or heavy prosthesis is tested. If the narrow segment of the canal (usually at the isthmus) does not allow penetration of the curved broach, a straight stem may be used. The selected test prosthesis is inserted to its collar in the broached canal. The stem must fit loosely, and full insertion must be easily accomplished. If the posterior cortex of the neck is longer than the anterior, the prosthesis will be forced into anteversion; the converse is also true. Errors in orientation may also be made if the canal is excessively large, allowing unrestricted rotation of the stem in the shaft.

After insertion of the test prosthesis, reduction is attempted. This is achieved in three steps: (1) longitudinal traction, (2) flexing the hip and guiding the head into the cup, and (3) slight abduction to keep the head in. First, the greater trochanter is retracted cephalad by the first assistant. The second assistant applies longitudinal traction onto the femur; the surgeon preferentially may also apply longitudinal traction to the femur while holding the knee in a 90-degree flexed position. Keeping the knee flexed provides grasping power for traction and relaxes the flexor muscles of the hip, especially the iliotibial tract. The surgeon must make sure that: (1) the orientation of the femoral prosthesis has not changed within the canal since its insertion, which is

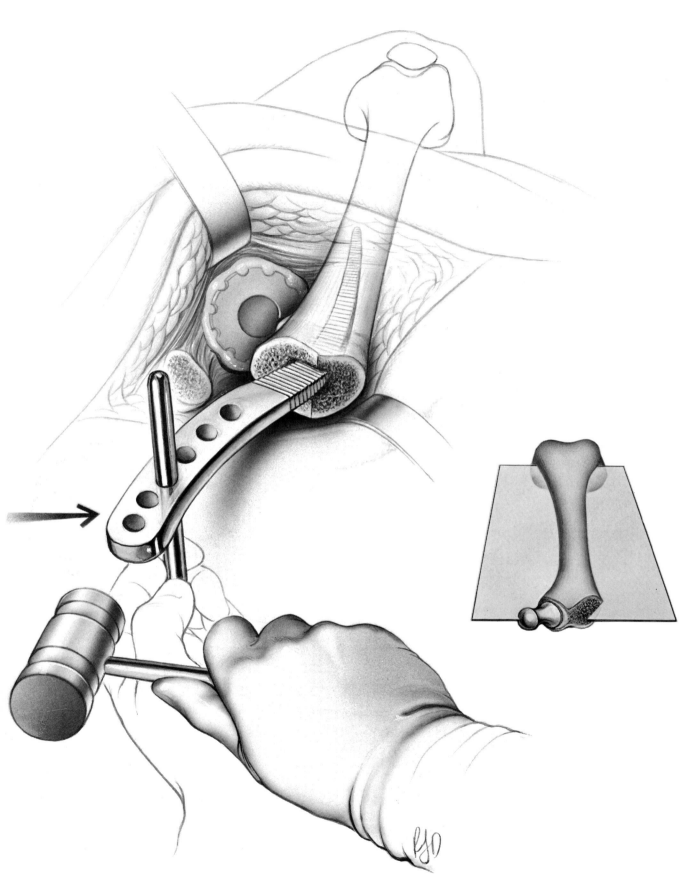

Fig. 12-34. Leg is in cross-table position with patella and flexed knee as point of reference. Transcondylar line of femur and degrees of anteversion of femoral neck (inset) determine correct plane of insertion of femoral broach. The bar inserted through broach handle is perpendicular to transcondylar line. Arrow and surgeon's left hand (phantom) thrust broach into valgus orientation as it is being driven into medullary canal. This ensures that femoral prosthesis will not lie in varus position.

accomplished by holding the femoral prosthesis in position with the middle and index fingers (this is especially important if there is an excessively large medullary canal); (2) the greater trochanter is held adequately cephalad by the first assistant (no retractors are used since they may interfere with the reduction); and (3) the hip is flexed no less than 45 degrees. No internal or external rotation is required. In addition to placing longitudinal traction on the limb, the surgeon must determine the location of the socket, and while holding the prosthesis within the femur, direct the head into the socket.

Reduction may be difficult or impossible if: (1) the patient has not been adequately anesthetized and there is insufficient muscle relaxation, (2) the femoral neck is excessively long, (3) the socket has been inserted in a low position, or (4) the soft tissues are excessively tight. If present, these impediments must be corrected, and the soft tissue then examined closely to ascertain the cause of the difficulty in reduction. Adequate muscle relaxation must be attained and soft tissue contractions should be divided, if present, prior to the decision to shorten the femur. If shortening is indicated, it must be done in stages so that excess shortening is avoided.

Testing for motion and stability

Following reduction of the prosthesis into the socket, the hip is tested in flexion, abduction, and adduction, as well as rotation. There is to be no danger of damage to the plastic socket by the test prosthesis. The anterosuperior iliac spines are demonstrated by the first assistant to define the position of the hip. If full abduction is not achieved, an adductor tenotomy should be performed (see Chapter 14, "Technique for Adductor Tenotomy"). Next, while placing strong longitudinal traction on the limb (with the knee slightly flexed), the surgeon inserts his index finger between the prosthetic components to determine the amount of separation attained (no more than 5 mm. of separation should be possible). The coverage of the head and its relation to the cup is then evaluated with the hip in neutral position. Finally, one must determine how much adduction produces dislocation—this is the real test of instability and is done with the hip in extension, including testing for "impingement" of the inferior and medial neck against the acetabular margin. By adducting the limb across the table, subluxation and dislocation are observed. A well-fitted prosthesis should not begin dislocating before 30 degrees of adduction (minimal flexion is required to allow adduction of the leg across the opposite thigh). If this occurs with less adduction, one must check for impingement of the medial femoral neck against the acetabular rim, vertical placement of the cup, laxity of the joint, or excessive valgus placement of the prosthesis. A satisfactory position of the components includes a cup oriented at 45 degrees to the axis of the body without anteversion or retroversion of either component (Figs. 12-35 and 12-36). When the head is not completely covered by the cup while the leg is in neutral position, it must be assumed that one or both of the components is malpositioned (Fig. 12-37) (see Chapter 17 and Fig. 17-2).

In summation, when the joint is reduced, several things should be noted.

1. The amount of traction required to locate the head into the socket (reduction) should be determined.

2. Flexion to 90 degrees, abduction to 30 degrees, and adduction to 30 degrees without dislocation should be present.

3. Separation of the two components by no more than 5 mm. when traction is applied (barely the tip of the index finger interposed between the two components) should not occur.

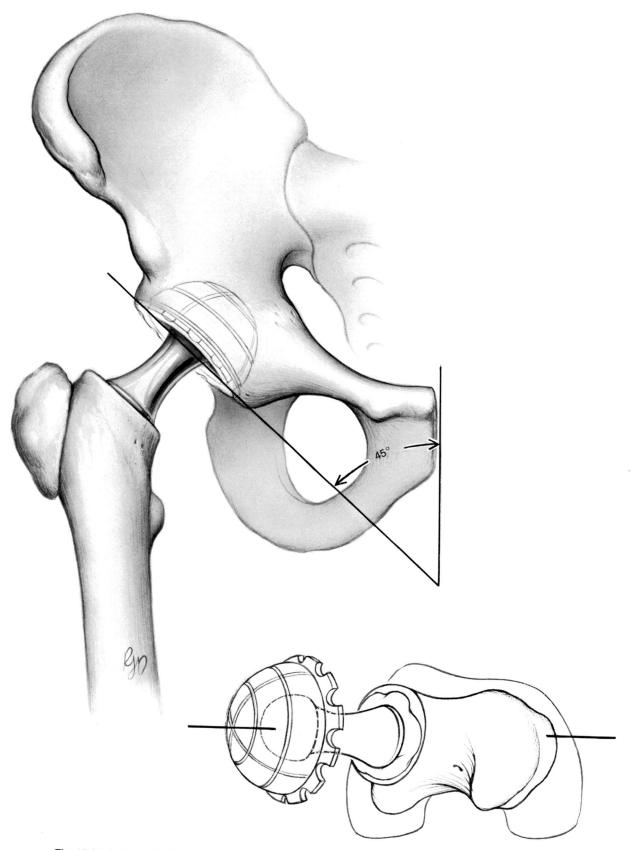

Fig. 12-35. In test reduction, both components must be in "neutroversion." Axis of cup to transaxis of pelvis or longitudinal axis of body is 45 degrees.

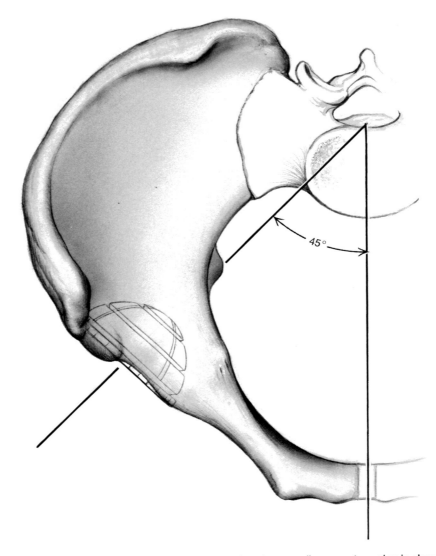

Fig. 12-36. In transpelvic view (inlet) orientation of socket revealing no anteversion is shown.

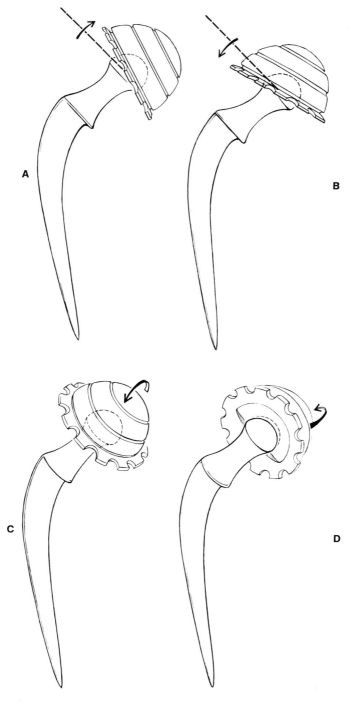

Fig. 12-37. If femoral component is inserted in proper orientation (no anteversion or retroversion), but orientation of acetabulum reveals segment of head uncovered, following defective orientation of acetabular component may be anticipated: **A,** cup is in excessive vertical orientation; **B,** cup is in excessive horizontal orientation; **C,** cup is in excess retroversion; and **D,** cup is in excess anteversion.

401

4. Full coverage of the prosthetic head by the cup when the hip is in neutral rotation should be noted.

5. Full extension capability is seen by observing the hip fully extended without any residual fixed flexion deformity.

6. A satisfactory "effective neck length" produced by the prosthesis should render equal leg length. When the limb is placed on the operating table parallel to the opposite side, both malleoli lying at the same level denote equal leg length (the malleoli can be palpated through the drapes). Ideally, dislocation will not occur with maximum internal-external rotation nor with adduction alone despite the detached greater trochanter; it will be possible, however, to dislocate the hip with maximal adduction and some traction.

As stated before, reduction as just outlined may not be possible if there is excessive neck length, unreleased contracted capsule, severe contraction of the iliopsoas tendon, or inadequate muscle relaxation. On the other hand, the reduction may be

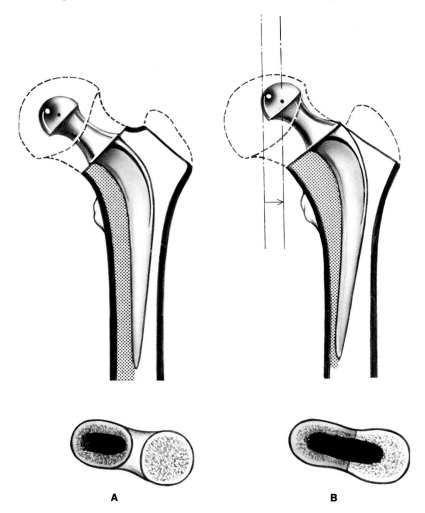

A **B**

Fig. 12-38. During preparation of canal or rehearsal, femoral axis guide and broach must be pointing slightly medial to patella in order to avoid any varus position of stem. **A,** When bridge of bone between neck and trochanteric bed is not removed, it is not possible to place stem into any degree of valgus. In **A,** canal is large and central placement was achieved. **B,** Creating good space between concave side of prosthesis and calcar by placing stem in valgus following removal of bridge between neck and trochanter. (Modified after Charnley.)

unstable if there is (1) excessive shortening of the neck, (2) a high positioning of the socket, (3) medial and anterior osteophytes or "cementophytes" about the acetabulum, (4) projecting osteophytes on the upper femur, (5) lack of clearance owing to an excessively deepened acetabulum, (6) previous surgery with subsequent loss of tissue elasticity, (7) sinking of the femoral prosthesis into the medullary canal, (8) rotation of the stem within the canal, and (9) malorientation of either component.

An unstable reduction resulting from a short neck may be rectified by placing the prosthesis in a more valgus position or by using a long-neck prosthesis. When recognized, faulty orientation of the socket or the femoral prosthesis must be corrected at once (for further details see Chapter 17). Further stability can be achieved by a firm reattachment of the greater trochanter and, in some instances, by applying a hip spica cast after surgery (see Chapter 17).

After testing for *motion* and *stability*, the hip is dislocated, the test prosthesis removed, and the stump of the femur once again delivered out of the wound. A Watson-Jones retractor may facilitate delivery. The loose cancellous bone and fatty marrow within the intramedullary canal especially in the region of the calcar femorale must be removed using a small Volkmann's spoon. Vigorous curettage is unnecessary. Curettage of the calcar area produces a space between the concavity of the stem and bone, thereby ensuring a thick layer of cement at this load-bearing portion of the femur (Figs. 12-38 and 12-39). Strong suction applied within the medullary canal also removes blood and fatty marrow. Finally, the medullary canal is packed tightly with a sponge, which further assists in the removal of debris and provides hemostasis.

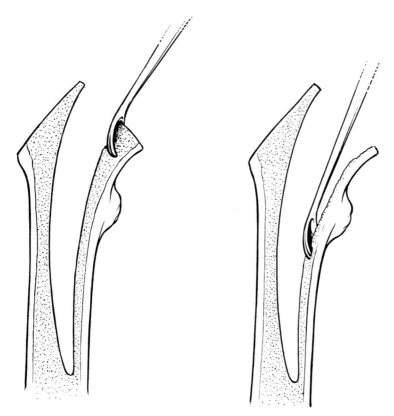

Fig. 12-39. Gentle curettage of calcar region produces space between concavity of stem and bone, ensuring thick layer of cement at this load-bearing region of femur. Additionally, strong bone of calcar will support cement.

403

PHASE V: CEMENTING OF FEMORAL COMPONENT
Insertion of wires

Different wiring techniques have been described: a single transverse loop; double vertical, single transverse; combinations of wire and screws; a bolt and screw; and other methods, all designed to improve trochanteric fixation. At the present stage of development, we feel that the surgeon must adopt and master a technique that will minimize technical complications. I have used a modification of the old "Wrightington technique" exclusively in my practice: a double vertical, single transverse loop, with great emphasis on interlocking of the trochanter to prevent forward and backward movement after fixation. Therefore the method of fixation by a double vertical, single transverse loop will be described here. Other modifications of this technique are justified when clinical results of other methods become available. (See Chapter 17 for trochanteric complications.)

The wires for reattachment of the trochanter are placed prior to the insertion of cement. In this technique, 16-gauge stainless steel wire is used. The transverse wire is 18 inches long and the vertical wire is the same length but doubled on itself. Each wire end has an identifying color-coded (silver and grey) clamp placed on it.

Transverse wires. The transverse wire is passed around the upper femur just proximal to the lesser trochanter. A curved wire passer is used. It is first passed directly on the bone around the posterior and medial surfaces of the femur, then it is brought onto the anterior and lateral aspect. After the wire has been passed posteriorly, the passer is reinserted over the anterior and medial surfaces of the femur, to pass the wire anteriorly and out laterally (Fig. 12-40). The leg must be positioned in the following way: the hip is held in adduction and internally rotated, with some flexion; the passer and wire are passed over the posterior surface, and externally rotated when they are applied to the anterior surface. Carelessness might allow the wire passer to penetrate the soft tissues, with potential risk to the sciatic nerve or femoral neurovascular structures. One must remain close to the bone at all times to prevent trapping soft tissue between wire and bone. A reciprocal, sawlike action (similar to the motion of the Gigli saw) is necessary following passage of the wire to ensure its close application to the femur. Ignoring this detail will result in either a "loose loop" of transverse wire or soft tissue entrapment between the wire and femur. The appropriate color-coded clamps are then applied to the wire ends.

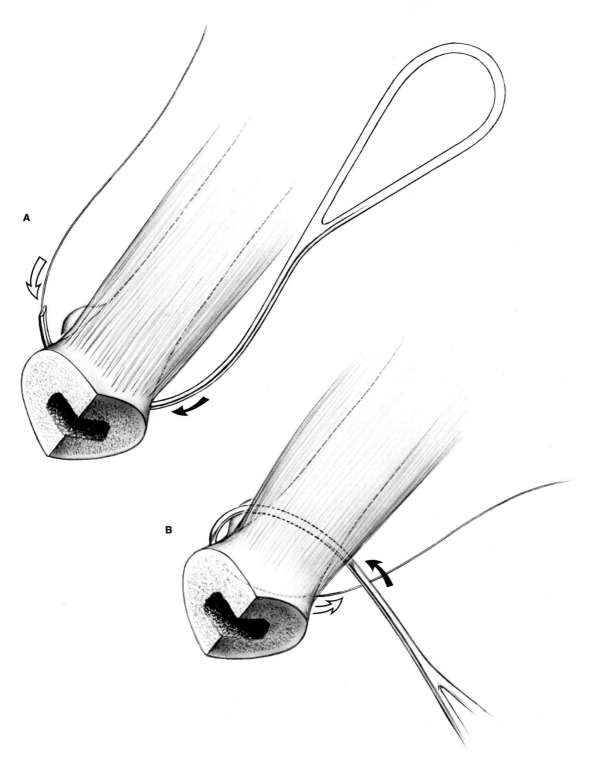

Fig. 12-40. To pass horizontal wire, wire passer is used. Wire passer is first inserted under muscle fibers of vastus lateralis and inserted as close to posterior aspect of femur as possible and revealed medially just above lesser trochanter. **A,** Wire is about to be drawn from medial to lateral side of femur. **B,** Wire passer is again inserted but this time in front of femur to recover second end of loop of wire.

Doubled vertical wire. To pass the doubled vertical wire, the hip is placed in 30 to 40 degrees flexion and 10 to 15 degrees internal rotation and adduction. The origin of the vastus lateralis is detached and the muscle belly is elevated distally with an osteotome, exposing the lateral femoral cortex for approximately 1½ inches distal to the vastus ridge (Fig. 12-41). At a midlateral position on the femur 2.5 cm. distal to the ridge, a drill hole is made through the cortex (using a 7/64-inch drill point) (Fig. 12-41, *A*). The slightly bent wire ends are then inserted and brought out of the stump of the neck, leaving a 3 to 5 mm. loop at the drill hole site. The wires are then pulled through the trochanteric bed and bent over the lateral femoral cortical margin (Fig. 12-41, *B* and *C*). Attention to the following details is essential.

1. Drilling starts perpendicular to the shaft; the drill point is then pulled out and redirected toward the opening of the medullary canal.

2. The wire loop must be of optimal size. A small loop can be inadvertently pulled through the hole into the medullary canal; the large loop may interfere with the application of the trochanter against the lateral femoral cortex.

3. If the cut ends of the wire are not even, passage may be difficult.

4. The wires are drawn through the trochanteric bed, held apart under tension, and bent sharply over the margin of the lateral femoral cortex, then they are placed along the posterior wall in the medullary canal.

5. The wire ends are placed well within the jaws of the wire holders to prevent their puncturing the gloves of the members of the operating team.

Test and rehearsal

A deliberately slow and staged rehearsal (without cement) enables the surgeon to determine the correct orientation of the femoral prosthesis within the medullary canal and to ascertain that the prosthesis can be easily inserted with the wires in place. The aim is to be able to secure the prosthesis in valgus* and neutral rotation.

After the general position of the wires is assessed, the limb is once again placed in the "cross-table position," ready to receive the prosthesis. The longitudinal axis of the femur, position of the knee and patella, perpendicular orientation of the tibia to the floor, and the relationship of the stump of the neck to the lesser trochanter are noted by the surgeon. The direction and the amount of valgus orientation are estimated, and the prosthesis is inserted into the femoral canal, rehearsing the action that will take place at insertion (following cement insertion). The position of the handle of the femoral prosthesis holder is observed. Note the longitudinal axis of the shaft of the femur and the rotational orientation of the prosthesis within the medullary canal. (Is the canal excessively large, or does the prosthesis fit snugly?) Observe the space between the medial calcar and the inferior border of the prosthesis, which has to be filled with cement (wedge-shaped). It also must be ascertained that the vertical intramedullary wires are pulled tightly against the inner wall of the lateral femoral cortex so that they do not interfere with the insertion of the prosthesis. Gentle curettage of the calcar femorale to remove marrow tissue and soft cancellous bone may be repeated at this point if necessary. Following this, the medullary canal is repacked with a dry sponge, ensuring a dry bed for the cement. Neither the prosthesis nor the packing should displace the wires. Insertion of the prosthesis in the correct orientation must be accomplished with ease prior to cementing, and a tight fit should be avoided. It must be noted

---

*The term "valgus" denotes avoidance of any "varus" positioning. Ideally, at the final step, the stem should be centered in the canal without any varus or valgus orientation.

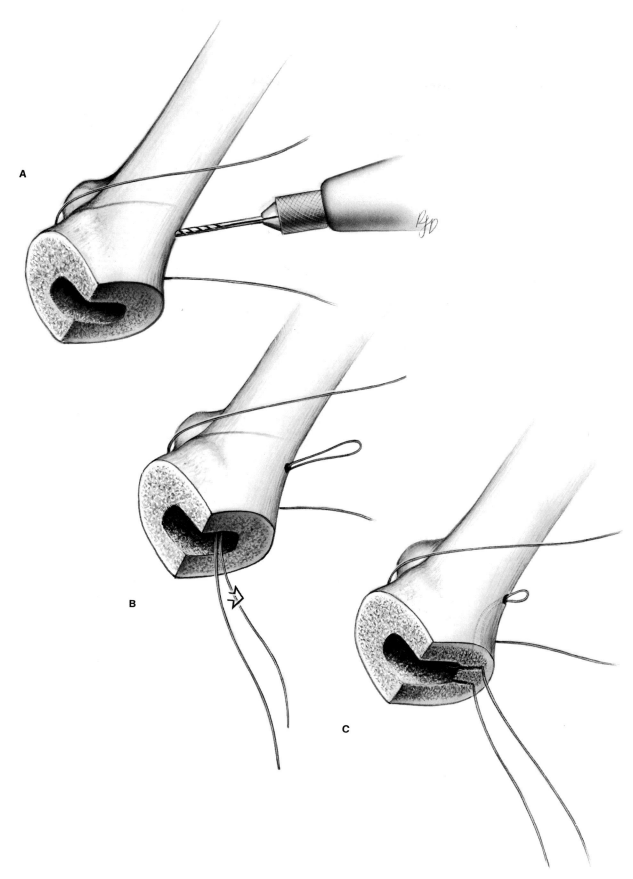

Fig. 12-41. Vertical wire doubled is passed through hole made in lateral aspect of femur. **A,** Lateral surface of shaft of femur is presented to surgeon and drill hole is made for vertical wire. Hole is at midlateral position on femur 2.5 cm. distal to vastus lateralis ridge. **B,** Vertical wire is passed through hole on lateral side of shaft of femur and emerges through opening of end of neck and finally, **C,** positioned close to outer cortex by bringing it through cancellous bone of trochanter.

that the vertical wires obviously occupy space within the medullary canal, thus broaching must take their presence into account (slightly oversize broaching).

Prior to the actual insertion of the cement, the following are to be noted:

1. Whether the prosthesis is held firmly in the holder with its stem parallel to the handle (The surgeon must check to verify that the prosthesis placed in the holder is the same as that chosen after the trial insertion, for example regular stem or straight stem.)

2. The orientation of the prosthesis in reference to the holder, the longitudinal axis of the femur, and the perpendicular line of the tibia to the floor

3. The neck of the femur's complete freedom from spicules that may puncture the surgeon's gloves during the packing of the femoral canal with cement

4. That the collar of the prosthesis is flush with the neck when fully inserted (The neck may be trimmed anteriorly or posteriorly as needed using bone-cutting forceps.)

5. Whether the prosthesis head is protected from damage when the holder is applied to it (The plastic cover is not removed until after cementing.)

6. That valgus orientation can be maintained and that the space between the medial curvature of the prosthesis and the calcar can be filled with cement

The second assistant is now instructed to hold the leg steady in the desired position (cross-table position).

Insertion

The cement is now mixed, and the surgeon puts on a third pair of gloves. It is essential that the instruments for this phase of the procedure (that is, the prosthesis itself in the holder, the long-handled curet, hammer, and prosthetic pusher) have been previously arranged on the table. The scrub nurse begins mixing the cement while the surgeon once again checks the position of the extremity (for details see Chapter 4). The second assistant is instructed to maintain the cross-table position, and the cut surface of the neck is rechecked for bone spicules. Final repacking of the canal is done by the first assistant using a fresh sponge, taking care not to interfere with the wires. If further curettage of the calcar and neck is necessary, it is done at this point. The surgeon must make sure, with several rehearsals, that the femoral stem passes smoothly and fully down the canal in the proper orientation. The novice is advised to make this determination prior to mixing the cement. If this precaution is not taken, malorientation or partial insertion may result. The greater trochanter must be retracted proximally during the insertion of the cement. Alternatively, it may be placed between the medial femoral shaft and the acetabulum. Every effort must be made to provide adequate access to the proximal end of the femur so that both thumbs can forcefully drive the cement down the canal. This is best accomplished by having the second assistant hold the leg in maximal adduction.

The surgeon receives the cement in its prepolymerized form, shaped like a sausage and ready for stuffing down the femoral canal (Fig. 12-42). At room temperature (66° F. or 19° C.), working time for CMW cement is 3 to 4 minutes; for Simplex P radiopaque, 5 to 6 minutes (see Chapter 4). A two-thumbed pressure insertion technique is preferable when possible (Fig. 12-42). Portions are advanced into the canal, with 1- or 2-second pauses between each inserting motion. With each stroke, part of the cement is advanced down the canal, and the pause aids its progress. Complete obstruction of the opening of the upper femur by the thumbs maximizes pressure behind the column of cement. Admixture of blood with cement should be avoided. A total of 10 to 15 strokes usually enables the entire batch to be inserted. All of the cement is used

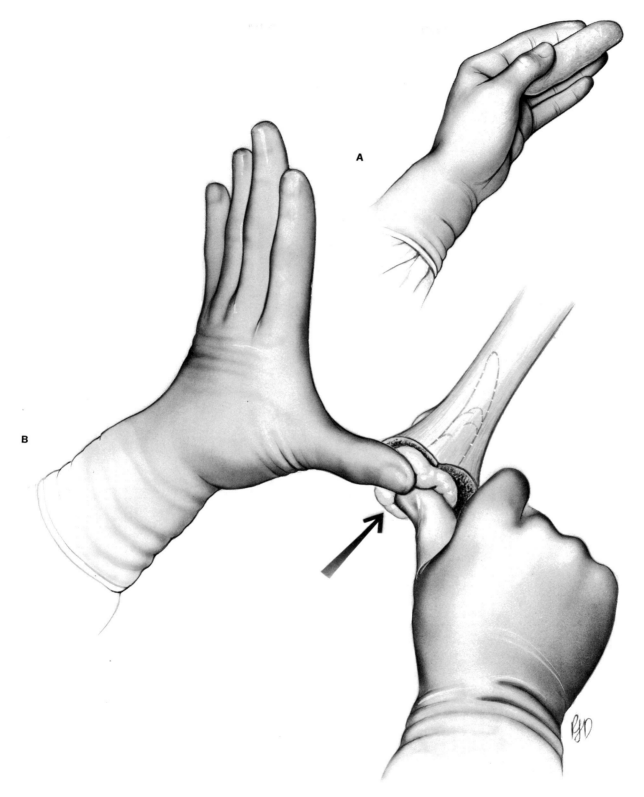

Fig. 12-42. A, Cement is shaped like sausage and ready to be inserted. **B,** "Double-thumb" technique used for insertion of cement.

in the presence of a wide medullary canal; most of it is used in most cases; about one half to two thirds of the total may suffice in a narrow canal. Cement should not be allowed to extravasate into the soft tissues, especially posteriorly. The surgeon must continually check for possible glove tears during insertion. A delicate and gentle use of fingers does not produce adequate pressure to advance the cement column inside the shaft (Fig. 12-43). The use of a catheter to vent the femur hampers peripheral injection of the cement; likewise, the use of a venting hole in the shaft is unnecessary.

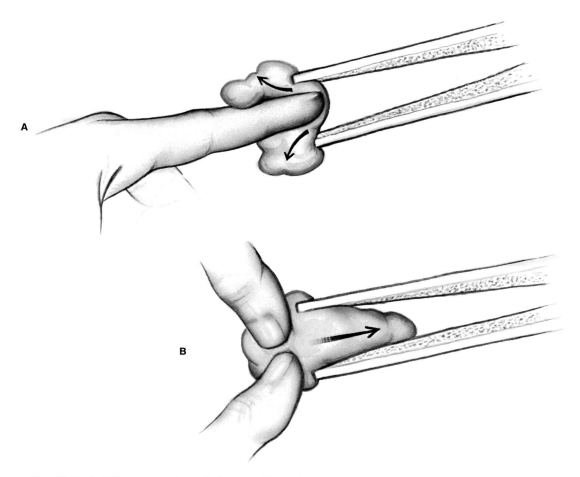

Fig. 12-43. A, Little progress is made by use of index finger singly with "delicate" and gentle handling in driving cement inside medullary canal. **B,** Effective force created by double-thumb technique in driving cement within medullary cavity.

Insertion of prosthesis

The term "neutroversion" has been applied to the positioning of the femoral component. It means that anteversion or retroversion must be avoided. However, experience suggests that in many instances, especially in patients with a narrow medullary canal, 5 degrees of anteversion, cement is better distributed in the upper femur and the possibility of contact between the metal (upper stem) and the posterior wall of the femoral canal (Fig. 12-44) is eliminated. While up to 5 degrees of anteversion may be beneficial, the prosthesis should never be orientated in retroversion because that position may prejudice the stability of the hip.

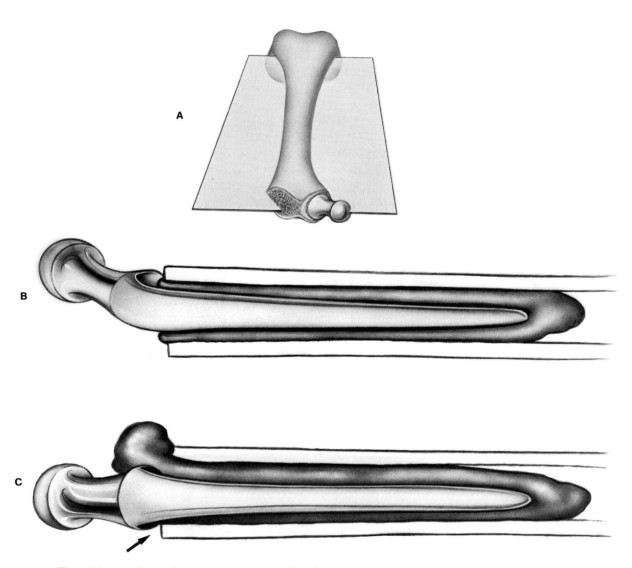

Fig. 12-44. In principle femoral component (of Charnley prosthesis) is inserted in neutroversion; however, slight anteversion (no more than 5 degrees) would allow better distribution of cement within upper end of femur. **A,** Plane of neutroversion. **B,** Five degrees anteversion. NOTE: optimal thickness of cement between prosthesis and posterior cortex. **C,** Absolute neutroversion (no anteversion or retroversion) brings stem close to posterior cortex (due to normal anteversion of femoral neck), thus eliminating thickness of cement in that region (arrow).

As in the rehearsal, the position of the knee is demonstrated by the second assistant. The tip of the stem is introduced into the prepared canal at the junction between the cut surface of the trochanter and the neck. The prosthesis (firmly held in the holder) is slowly, deliberately inserted in "neutroversion" toward the medial cortex to place it in a valgus position relative to the shaft. This valgus orientation is maximized by holding the prosthesis back against the cancellous bone area of the bed of the trochanter (Fig. 12-45). The degree of valgus is the same as that decided upon at rehearsal. An extreme degree of valgus is undesirable, especially in a very large canal. Slow and deliberate action is essential as the insertion progresses. With repeated reaming of the cement in the area between its concavity and the femoral canal, maximum cement should be present in the region of the calcar femorale. Rotation (anteversion-retroversion) or mediolateral (varus-valgus) change in direction results in a large track being made in the cement, which can lead to later loosening and should be avoided. It must also be recognized that in an extremely large medullary canal excessive valgus placement can be inadvertently produced, resulting in overlengthening of the extremity and difficulty in reducing the hip. A very large canal also may allow the prosthetic stem tip to reach the medial cortex without any cement in the region, and a prosthesis place in an excessive valgus position can also result in deficient coverage by the acetabular component. In summary, the prosthesis *must* be inserted in the rehearsed orientation.

When a heavy or extra-heavy stem prosthesis is used (Charnley's "cobra" prosthesis), the relationship of the flanges to the opening of the medullary canal is observed to ascertain that the correct degree of valgus orientation has been achieved (Fig. 12-45). The opening of the canal must be large enough to accommodate the flanges. It is important to have the opening of the femur overly reamed to allow easy penetration of the flanges; failure to do so will cause the orientation of the stem on the shaft to change as the flange contacts the opening of the upper femur.

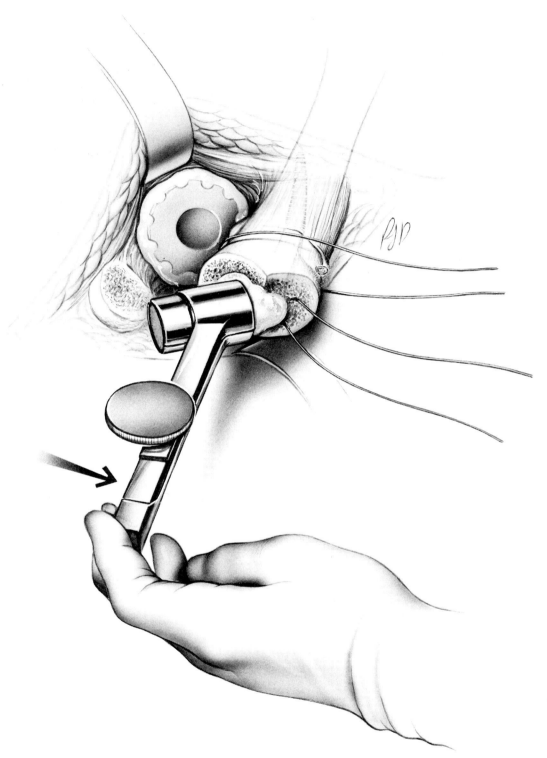

Fig. 12-45. Prosthesis is now at its full depth within medullary canal. Slight valgus position is ensured by maintaining direction of tip of stem toward medial cortex. Slight valgus position ensures that prosthesis is not in varus position and that thick layer of cement intervenes between concave surface of prosthesis and bone of calcar of femur. Holder may be detached just prior to full polymerization of cement.

415

No hammering is necessary if full insertion is easily achieved, as evidenced by the neck of the prosthesis resting flush with the entrance of the medullary canal. The holder must be carefully removed without changing the orientation of the prosthesis as the prosthesis is held in place with the pusher. The holder may be detached just before the final stage of hardening (to facilitate the removal of cement); the valgus position must remain unchanged until full polymerization. Excess cement is removed with a curet, again taking care not to move the prosthesis (Fig. 12-46). It is essential to observe the following.

1. During the final stages of polymerization, the first and second assistants must remain immobile, since any motion of the limb may change the orientation of the prosthesis within the medullary canal. Maximum adduction of the leg in the cross-leg position must be retained also.
2. Avoid scratching the femoral head if it is unprotected by a plastic cover.
3. Avoid changes of orientation during the removal of the holder.
4. Cement should be tested for hardness locally, at the neck level, prior to attempting reduction of the prosthesis.
5. The prosthesis must not be pushed into a varus position during the polymerization phase.
6. Excess force on the "pusher" is unnecessary, even harmful, since it may change the "version" of the prosthesis.
7. The position of the vertical wires (one anterior, one posterior, or both posterior to the prosthesis) must remain undisturbed.
8. All cement must be curetted away from the trochanteric bed prior to hardening. The holder may be detached just prior to final hardening of the cement.

Reduction

Phase V is completed by reducing the femoral head into the acetabular socket. This is attempted only after achieving absolute hemostasis and removing all cement debris from the wound, particularly in the socket region.

The wound is now copiously irrigated with an antibiotic solution (see Chapter 6). Cement particles and devitalized portions of muscle (usually found in the posterior aspect of the wound) are removed. Posterior capsular bleeding should be checked and controlled prior to reattachment of the greater trochanter. The reduced joint should be inspected with the leg in neutral position.

The range of motion and stability are tested at this point, and the surgeon must ascertain that the two components are in a satisfactory relationship relative to each other. *The hip must be stable prior to reattachment of the greater trochanter.* Ideally, the orientation of the components relative to each other should be exactly the same as that noted prior to the cementing of the femoral component.

Some technical details

Since successful cementing depends on firm injection of the cement into the femoral canal, delicate handling should be avoided. Double-thumb, or single-digit, forceful but steady pressure not only results in excellent distal filling but also injection into the peripheral cancellous bone. Wide exposure, especially at the proximal end of the wound, full mobilization of the upper femur, and adequate retraction of the trochanter allow the surgeon optimal access to the medullary opening during cement insertion.

Beginners are usually concerned about the "working time" of the cement and, as a

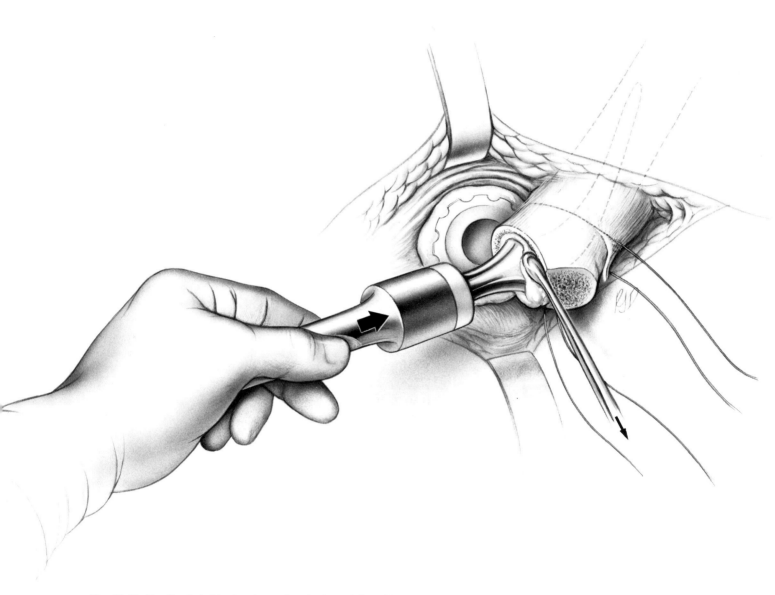

Fig. 12-46. Prosthesis holder has been detached carefully, without jarring stem. Pusher maintains position of prosthesis while excess cement is curetted away. It is essential not to move prosthesis within cement while cement is being polymerized.

result, may use it too soon following mixing. This only makes the process of insertion difficult and actually prolongs the time of insertion, since the cement adheres to the gloves. Likewise, hasty insertion with short rapid strokes does not move the cement down the canal as well and results in a greater admixture of blood (Fig. 12-43). The temptation to pick up the cement from the mixing bowl too early, while it is still at the tenacious stage, must therefore be avoided. Allowing the cement to stiffen slightly by aeration not only minimizes absorption of monomer but also makes insertion easier. The surgeon must be aware of the room temperature and observe the 10-minute check for "setting time"; the temperature of the mixing bowl and storage area should also be checked, since this has a profound influence on the setting time of the cement (see Chapter 4). The cement is ready when it no longer sticks to the gloves. A small amount of excess cement left over from the same batch is observed for stiffening while awaiting full polymerization.

Full cooperation of the assistants is essential so that the entire process can be executed in an organized fashion with minimal effort. Excessively slow insertion of the cement or the prosthesis can be disastrous, since the cement may harden inside the canal before the surgeon has fully inserted the prosthesis.

PHASE VI: REATTACHMENT OF GREATER TROCHANTER

Prior to reattaching the greater trochanter, the following steps must be completed: (1) The hip must be placed in some degree of adduction to create a space between the trochanter and the upper end of the femur. (2) The surgeon, having identified the vertical and transverse wires, assesses the location and direction of the abductor muscle fibers, the greater trochanteric axis, and their relationship to the midlateral cortex of the femur. The desired position of the greater trochanter against the femoral shaft must be determined. If there is a fixed external rotation deformity, the piriformis tendon should be divided. Release of the piriformis (short rotator) often allows the trochanter to rotate forward along its longitudinal axis (Fig. 12-47). Excess forward displacement of the trochanter should be avoided since it reduces the coaptation. (3) A sharp bone hook is applied just proximal to the greater trochanter at the insertion of the abductor tendon; this gives the surgeon control over the greater trochanter during preparation and positioning (Fig. 12-47). (4) The hip is then brought to neutral position and the site most suitable for trochanteric attachment is determined. Ideally, the center of the trochanter should lie at the level of the vastus ridge, requiring no more than 5 or 10 degrees abduction of the hip and no more than a moderate degree of tension on the abductor mechanism (Fig. 12-47). If the greater trochanter cannot be brought distally to the level of the ridge, the lateral posterior and superior capsule and/or short rotators can be detached from the greater trochanter at the site of their insertion. If this maneuver must be done, bleeders must be looked for and controlled.

418

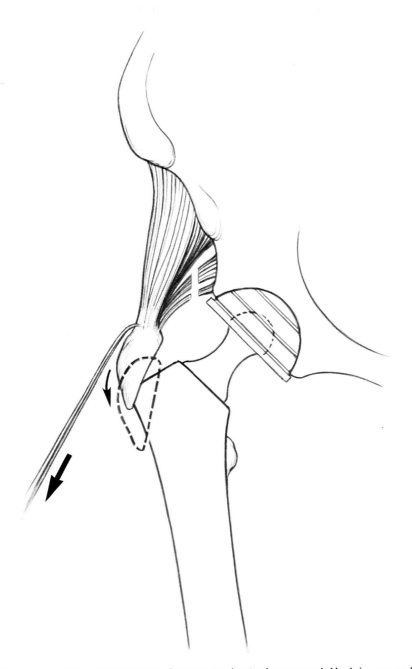

Fig. 12-47. Amount of distal displacement of greater trochanter is assessed. Hook is engaged onto outer aspect of trochanter and hip is brought to a few degrees of abduction. Release of short rotators and superior capsule may be needed if trochanter does not conveniently reach level of vastus lateralis ridge.

Passage of vertical and transverse wires

The two vertical wires (identified by dark-handled clamps) are passed through the tendon of the abductors as close as possible to the greater trochanter. This can be accomplished by using a wire passer or directly by straightening the end of the wire and pushing it through the soft tissues using the wire-holding forceps. The anterior and posterior ends of the doubled vertical wire must be kept approximately 1 cm. apart to distribute the forces over the top of the greater trochanter (Fig. 12-48). Care is taken to avoid puncturing one's gloves (by not touching the tips of the wires as they are passed through the abductor tendon). The black-handled clamps are reapplied to the ends of the vertical wires once they are recovered.

Fig. 12-48. A, Drill holes are being made to pass transverse wires. Trochanter is held in suitable position by trochanteric clamp. NOTE: position of doubled vertical wire and transverse wire. **B,** Wire passer has been pushed through abductor tendon just above trochanter keeping as close to bone as possible. Two ends of verticle (double) wire are being inserted into wire passer in order to pull them through abductor tendon above trochanter.

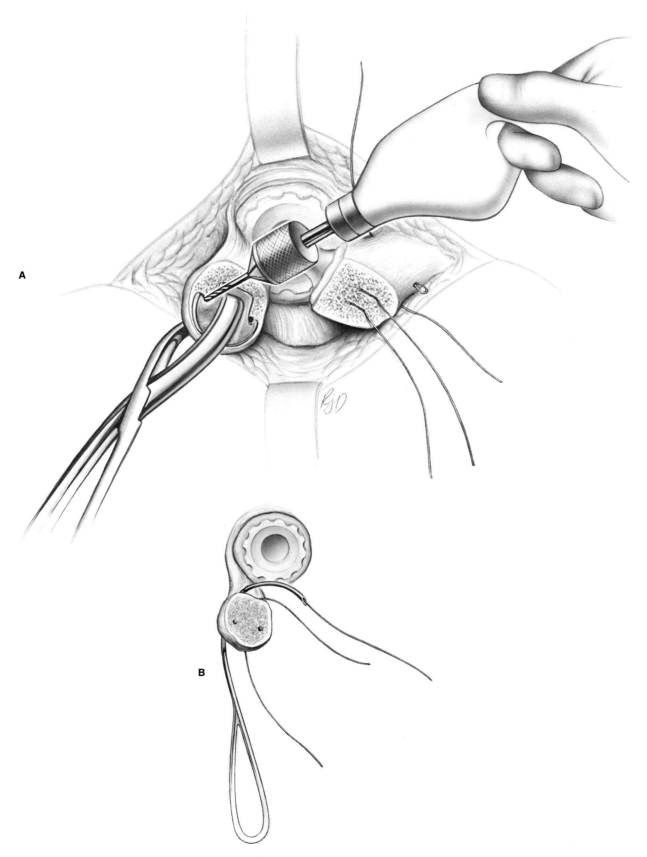

Fig. 12-48. For legend see opposite page.

The trochanteric clamp is now applied, holding the trochanter in its optimal orientation and against the vastus ridge as if it were to be fixed in position. This enables the surgeon to drill the holes through the trochanter in the proper orientation (Fig. 12-48). A line drawn between these two holes should be perpendicular to the longitudinal axis of the trochanter. The trochanteric clamp is held firmly by the first assistant while the surgeon drills two holes using a $7/64$-inch drill point. The wires are passed from within outwards, identified, and grasped by wire clamps (Fig. 12-49). In doing so, three minor details must be observed: (1) the distal inch at the ends of the wires should be straightened out to ease their passage through the drilled holes; (2) care must be taken with an osteoporotic trochanter so that it is not fragmented by the trochanteric clamp; and (3) the ends of the wires are identified and held by silver-handled clamps to prevent perforation of the gloves.

Fig. 12-49. A, General view of both wires passed and in position following disengagement of trochanteric-holding forceps. NOTE: osteotome is beveling anterior aspect of shaft of femur at area of vastus lateralis ridge. Similar beveling is done posteriorly. **B,** Pyramidal-shaped prominence created in region of vastus lateralis ridge is shown. NOTE: location of vertical wire loop in relation to prominence. **C,** Hollowing of cancellous surface of greater trochanter by ½-inch gouge is also shown.

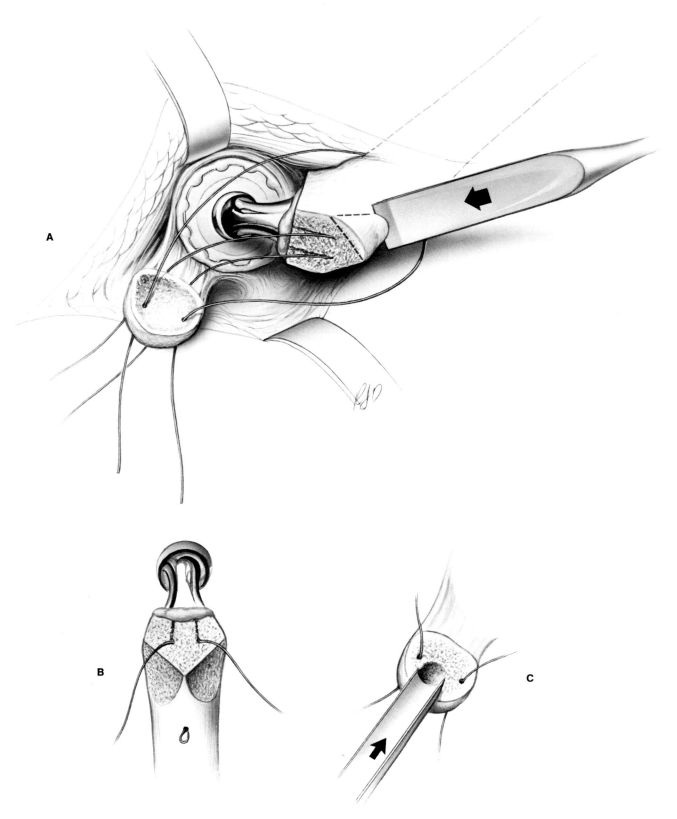

Fig. 12-49. For legend see opposite page.

423

Interlocking of trochanter

Prior to tightening the wires, the site where the greater trochanter will be interlocked is determined. The site of the eminence is determined by holding the trochanter at the desired site. The anterior and posterior aspects of the shaft of the femur are then bevelled in this area at the level of the vastus lateralis ridge, leaving a pyramid-shaped prominence (Fig. 12-49, *B*). Hollowing out of the cancellous surface of the greater trochanter is now done using a ½-inch gouge (Fig. 12-49, *A*), as care is taken not to disturb the transverse wires while the bone is being removed. The pyramid-shaped prominence created in the region of the vastus ridge is now inserted into this hollowed out area, achieving a mechanical interlocking. Full penetration of the prominence into the trochanter must be achieved before attempting to tighten the wires. This maximizes the bony contact necessary for rapid union; it also provides a bed for the trochanter away from exposed cement and prevents forward and backward motion of the trochanter, the cause of early fatigue fracture failure of the wires.

Prior to tightening the wires the surgeon must make sure that: (1) the limb is in neutral position while the trochanter is fitted onto the eminence; (2) the prominence and the hollowed trochanter fit together snugly without excessive abduction of the extremity; (3) no kinks or loose loops of wire are present, especially medial to the shaft and proximal to the trochanter; and (4) the femoral prosthesis is located within the socket, determined by placing the index finger along the neck of the prosthesis reaching the junction of the head and the socket.

Tightening of wires

Tightening of the longitudinal and transverse wires is preferably done simultaneously using two wire tighteners but may be done in sequence. After identifying the anterior and posterior transverse wire ends, a single overhanded throw is made tying them over the outer aspect of the trochanter (Fig. 12-50). The wires are gripped in the jaws of the tightener (for example, Kirschner's bow) and fully tightened. An occasional pull on the bow during the tightening will eliminate any residual laxity (looseness) in the wire, but at the same time care must be taken not to pull the femoral prosthesis out of the socket. The vertical wires are then brought through the arc of the bow and over the lateral aspect of the greater trochanter; they are pulled distally by the second assistant, while the transverse wires are tightened (Fig. 12-51). A gentle hammering of the trochanter against the shaft provides for a "snug" coaptation. A second wire tightener is now applied to vertical wires (which have been passed in the opposite direction) through the loop of the vertical wire (Fig. 12-50).

A slight loosening of the transverse loop may take place as the result of a subsequent distal shift of the trochanter, which will be rectified by further tightening of the transverse loop (via the first tightener). This alternate tightening may be repeated until a firm fixation is accomplished.

When distal movement of the trochanter has taken place (while tightening the vertical wires) and firm contact between the trochanter and the shaft is apparent, further tightening may damage (split) the trochanter; care must be taken therefore not to overtighten the wires. The end longitudinal wires are then twisted upon themselves, turned, cut short, and buried in the soft tissues. If the trochanter has been ideally reattached by the method described, it should be in the desired position relative to the shaft (centered over the ridge) and exhibit no forward or backward motion in relation to the shaft of the femur when tested at surgery.

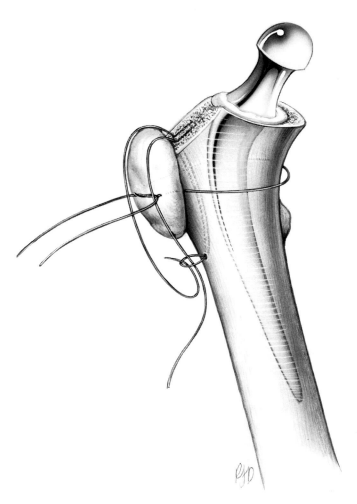

Fig. 12-50. General view of wires just prior to tightening. Trochanter is in position and held by traction on double wire. Ends of transverse wire have been passed through trochanter and tied. Vertical wire ends are passed over trochanter and in and out of loop of same wire.

425

Common sources of failure. An excessively small trochanter makes interlocking difficult or impossible. On the other hand, an excessively large trochanter containing the ridge renders the creation of the prominence impossible. The wires may be damaged by the clamps and weakened by careless handling. If the wires are passed through the substance of the abductor tendon carelessly, damage to the abductor muscle or puncturing of the surgeon's gloves may occur.

The transverse wires may be ripped out of the trochanteric drill holes and through the substance of the trochanter if they are carelessly pulled while bringing the trochanter down upon the shaft. If the limb is not continuously held in neutral rotation during the tightening of the wires, the trochanter may be fixed excessively anteriorly or posteriorly. If the longitudinal wires are placed too far posterior or too far anterior to the longitudinal axis of the trochanter, the trochanter may rotate when the wires are tightened. The transverse wire must not be tightened over the greater trochanter prior to pulling the loop snugly against the medial side of the femur shaft. Excessive tightening of the longitudinal wires may fracture the trochanter, especially if the bone is osteoporotic. The trochanter may escape between the longitudinal wires (due to the pull of the abductors) if the wires are placed too far apart. Tying the wrong wire ends (for example, one end of the transverse to the vertical) leads to failure of trochanteric fixation.

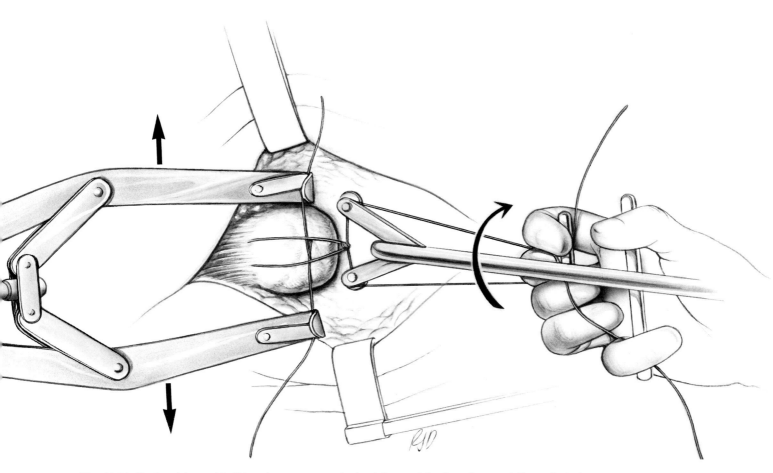

Fig. 12-51. Having tightened half-knot in transverse wire by tightener (Kirschner bow, to left), vertical wire passed through loop is being tightened by second wire tightener. Distal movement of trochanter as result of tightening of vertical wire now may loosen transverse wire, which is corrected by further tightening. This alternate tightening of wires allows perfect adjustment of wires. Final maneuver includes twisting of both vertical and transverse wire ends. (Wire tightener was designed by author and is supplied by Codman & Shurtleff, Inc.)

Repair of vastus lateralis cuff

After the wires have been tightened, it is essential to bring the detached proximal end of the musculotendinous vastus lateralis "cuff" over the wires and suture it to the abductor tendon and aponeurosis. Nonabsorbable suture material is used. After this is done, the wires are no longer visible (Fig. 12-52). This can successfully be achieved if the cuff has been well developed at the time of its detachment from the shaft. A good closure of wires will prevent development of bursitis around the exposed wires.

Insertion of Hemovac drains

Two medium-sized Hemovac drains are placed along the space between the vastus lateralis and the deep fascia. The two ends are brought out through the skin away from the incision; one drain is placed next to the arthroplasty anteriorly, the other is placed posteriorly. Both are then connected to the suction tubing temporarily to avoid clotting during the completion of wound closure. To avoid communication between the deep and superficial layers of the wound, the drains must not be brought through the opening in the tensor fascia femoris.

The initial incision retractor is now removed and wound closure begins.

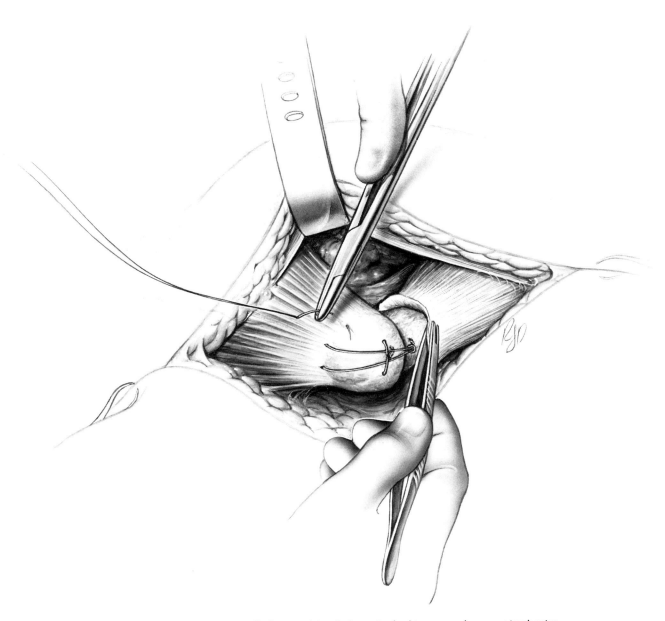

Fig. 12-52. Musculotendinous cuff of vastus lateralis is reattached to cover wires over trochanter.

429

Alternative methods of trochanteric fixation

It should be emphasized that no wire technique is 100% successful by itself if the patient resumes early postoperative activities without a walking support. Furthermore, it should be realized that interpositioning of soft tissue and muscle at the trochanteric fixation site impedes early healing, thus loss of fixation following the rupture of the wires.[3] To enhance the trochanteric fixation, Charnley has recently introduced a cruciform method (three-strand wire technique) (Fig. 12-53, *A* to *C*) in order to prevent forward and backward motion of the trochanter. In this technique, the trochanter is fixed in six directions, and the wire encompasses the trochanter as if held by a basket of wires (Fig. 12-53, *C*). The pulley arrangement by the two transverse wires doubles the tension in a transverse plane, while the double longitudinal wires hold the trochanter in place along its longitudinal axis. The trochanter is removed at the level of the ridge (not above the ridge as described in the previous technique in this chapter), and only a minimum distal transfer of the trochanter (projection) is allowed so that the trochanter will be fixed to its removal site (bed) (Fig. 12-53, *A*). The double vertical wire is tightened first, followed by the tightening of the cruciform system (Fig. 12-53, *C*).

An additional supplemental fixation of the trochanter can also be achieved by the use of a staple clamp, which is introduced to maximize the fixation of the greater trochanter.[3] The staple clamp is an optional supplement to any wire technique the surgeon may chose. When properly applied, this apparatus will prevent forward and backward motion of the trochanter during flexion and extension of the hip, which is detrimental in trochanteric fixation methods (Fig. 12-53, *B* to *D*). The staple clamp in Fig. 12-53 is demonstrated in conjunction with a cruciform method of fixation of the trochanter. It should be noted that prior to reattachment of the greater trochanter, a groove is created to accommodate the screw portion of the staple clamp. The wires are tightened prior to tightening the staple clamp. The excess length of the screw is cut off by a double-action wire cutter following the completion of the fixation. As indicated previously, the staple clamp may also be used in a standard double-wire method or with a double vertical wire.[1,3]

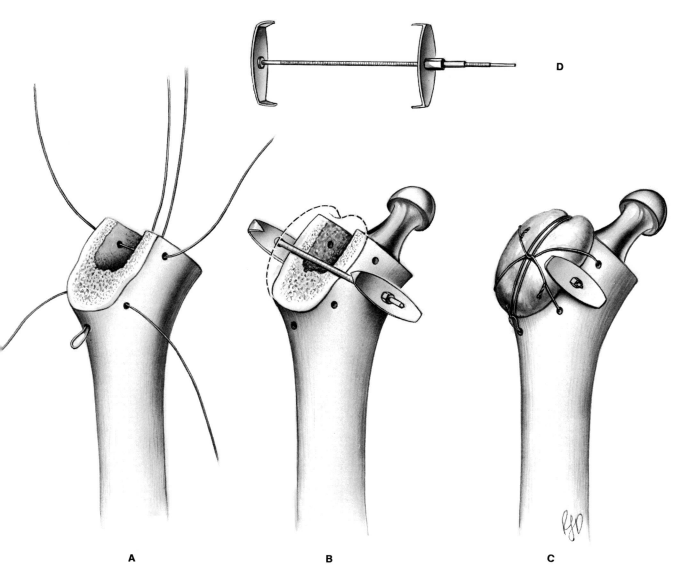

Fig. 12-53. A, Site of insertion of two transverse wires and one vertical double wire. Medial transverse wire passes through canal, but lateral transverse wire remains within lateral wall of femur. NOTE: both transverse wires are parallel and vertical wire is passed through hole in medullary canal of femur. **B,** Site of application of staple clamp and orientation of greater trochanter in relationship to staple. **C,** Configuration of wires at completion of tightening. NOTE: cruciform arrangement of wires and final position of staple. (Posterior staple clamp is not seen in this figure.) **D,** Staple clamp designed by Charnley.

431

PHASE VII: WOUND CLOSURE AND APPLICATION OF DRESSING

Wound closure consists of closure of the fascia, fat, and skin.

Closure of fascia

Preferably, nonabsorbable sutures such as No. 1 cotton monofilament or No. 1 Teftek are used to achieve a perfect watertight closure of the fascia. The tensor fascia femoris, which separates the superficial layers of the wound from the deep layers, and the artificial joint must be respected. The first assistant retracts the proximal corner of the wound; the hip is placed in some flexion to provide maximum visibility of the proximal fascia. Fascia closure begins proximally and proceeds distally. Special care must be taken to avoid inadvertent inclusion of the drains in the closure. A watertight repair of the fascia is essential and is achieved by placing the sutures at a modest distance from the fascial edge, thereby causing the edges to overlap when the sutures are tied. Having the hip in abduction at the time of closure enhances the stability of the hip and relaxes the fascia, easing closure.

Fat closure

Utilization of the pull-out retention sutures that have become popular is an excellent method of wound closure in total hip replacement. The importance of good closure of the fat cannot be overemphasized; this is crucial in the prevention of hematoma formation and infection. Using No. 1 nylon, the full thickness of the skin and fat are brought together with five stitches, passing the needle on either side from within the wound outward. The large curved needle is introduced at the deepest level of the fat and brought out through the skin 1 inch lateral to the skin edge (Fig. 12-54). The depth and level of the sutures must be the same on both sides so that no dead space is left behind. In a thin person the sutures must be brought out closer to the edge of the skin, that is, ½ to ¾ inch away from the edge so that the wound will not be excessively everted. A second pair of Hemovac drains is placed deep in the subcutaneous tissue to prevent hematoma formation in both very obese and extremely thin individuals (Fig. 12-54).

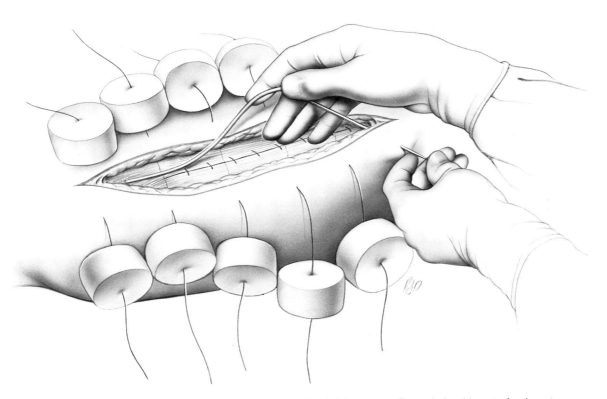

Fig. 12-54. Fascia lata is closed with interrupted nonabsorbable sutures. Deep drains (deep to fascia not seen in this figure) are inserted. Second set of drains (if used) is placed superficial to fascia. Pull-out fat sutures are U-shaped and can be seen at depth of wound.

433

Skin closure

Prior to tightening the retention sutures, the skin is meticulously closed with a running 3-0 Dermalon mattress stitch. The retention sutures are then tightened. At the completion of the skin closure the retention sutures are passed through the center foam pads and suture buttons. The buttons are fixed to the nylon traversing the wound and held in place using a "button crusher" (Fig. 12-55, *A*). The foam pads should be compressed only to half of their thickness to allow adjustment of the wound postoperatively without skin necrosis. A Hibbs strip soaked in povidone-iodine (Betadine) solution is applied over the suture line. Finally, the entire wound area is covered by a compression dressing with the drainage tubes exiting from the distal end (Fig. 12-55, *B*). The drainage tubes are not sutured in place but are secured along with the rest of the dressing with adhesive tape so that they can subsequently be removed without disturbing the dressing. The method for removal of retention sutures is illustrated (Fig. 12-56).

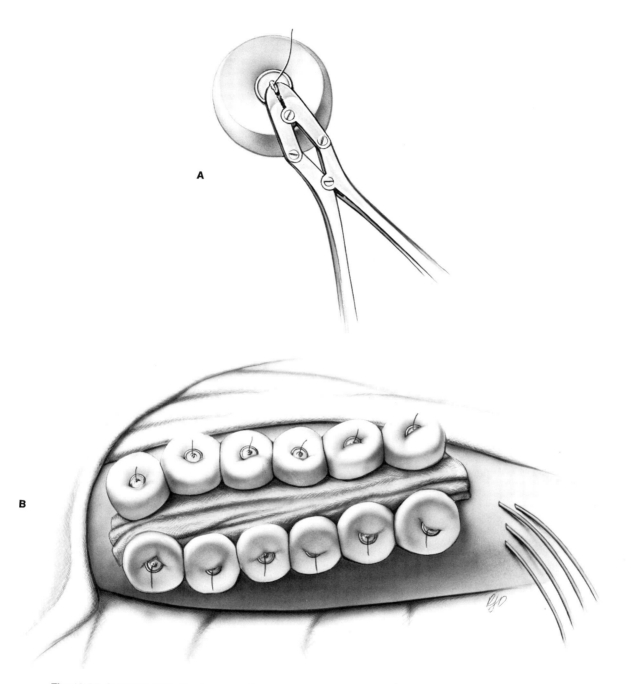

Fig. 12-55. A, Aluminum button is crushed to secure suture over foam pads used in retention sutures. **B,** Final dressing held in position by pressure pads. Position of drains in lower end of wound is shown. NOTE: only half of thickness of pressure pads has been compressed to allow swelling of wound without undue pressure necrosis on skin.

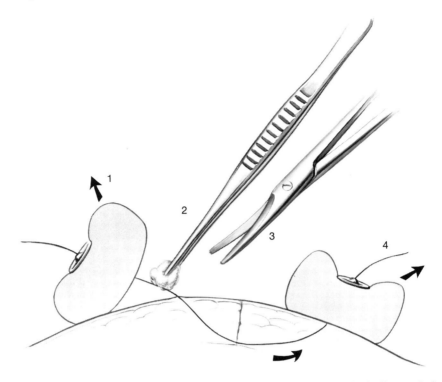

Fig. 12-56. Pressure pads and skin sutures are removed 13 to 14 days postoperatively. Removal of retention sutures by *(1)* pulling on one end of suture, *(2)* iodine swab to clean emerged suture from skin, *(3)* suture is cut, and *(4)* opposite end of suture is removed.

Application of antiembolic stockings and abduction splint

While the patient is still under anesthesia, elastic bandages (that is, Ace bandages or antiembolic stockings) and an abduction splint are applied. Transfer from the operating room table to the bed is supervised by the surgeon and first assistant, with special care being taken to avoid dislocating the hip while the patient is still under the muscle relaxing effect of anesthesia.

■　■　■

All details are considered essential. This chapter is not summarized.

REFERENCES

1. Charnley, J.: Personal communications.
2. Charnley, J.: Operative technique of low friction arthroplasty of the hip joint, Internal Publication No. 6, 2nd revision, Centre for Hip Surgery, Wrightington Hospital, England, February, 1971.
3. Charnley, J.: Total hip replacement, low friction technique, Slide-Tape Presentation by Professor Sir John Charnley, C.B.E., F.R.S., F.R.C.S., Courtesy of Chas. F. Thackray, Ltd., 1977.
4. Müller, M. E.: Total hip prosthesis, Clin. Orthop. **72:**46-68, 1970.

CHAPTER 13

Variations in technique and specific considerations

'Surgical technology' should not be allowed to triumph over 'clinical judgement.'

ROBERT B. SALTER

In Chapter 12 the technical details of a standard (routine) total hip arthroplasty were discussed; this chapter deals with their *clinical application* and with surgical techniques that deviate from those used in a standard operation and are necessitated by specific anatomical and pathological conditions. These specific conditions include congenital dysplasia and dislocation of the hip, Paget's disease, rheumatoid arthritis, juvenile rheumatoid arthritis, ankylosing spondylitis, protrusio acetabuli, bone tumors, and productive osteoarthritis.

CONGENITAL DYSPLASIA AND DISLOCATION OF THE HIP

Because of the great percentage of predictable successful results, total hip replacement has been extended to the treatment of secondary osteoarthritis resulting from congenital dysplasia and dislocation of the hip.

Unfortunately, arthrodesis, osteotomy, and cup arthroplasty are not suitable alternatives to total hip replacement for these conditions: arthrodesis in women is undesirable, and a varus or displaced osteotomy may aggravate an already significantly shortened extremity; mold arthroplasty results are not satisfactory because of the lack of a bony stock in the acetabulum and excessive anteversion of the femoral neck. In the past, such operations yielded poor results, but early results of total hip replacement for congenital subluxation have been extremely encouraging. However, patient selection must be done with special care because of the age factor and the possibility of a persistent defective abductor mechanism and a permanent limp, which may follow despite surgery. The mechanical behavior and "life of fixation" of the prosthesis, es-

pecially if it is subjected to vigorous physical activities, remain unknown.

Undoubtedly, early recognition of congenital dysplasia and dislocation and efforts toward restoration of the normal anatomy in the early months of life are ideal. Unfortunately, since unrecognized early childhood dysplasia may remain a common cause of degenerative osteoarthritis of the hip (despite the advent of total hip arthroplasty), orthopaedic surgeons must continue to strive for early recognition and successful treatment.

Prior to the evolution of total hip arthroplasty, many surgeons expressed the opinion that no operation could be successful in certain cases of complete hip dislocation. It was feared that with an unsuccessful attempt at a reconstructive procedure, patients who originally had no pain might become symptomatic; therefore many patients with a completely dislocated hip were not treated, despite an unacceptable gait remaining throughout their lives. It is now apparent that a long-standing dislocated hip is a major disability and will ultimately cause pain.[8,14,20]

With the advent of total hip replacement, it is now possible to rectify failed operations, that is, Colonna arthroplasty or Chiari osteotomy,[6] when an acetabulum has been created by one of those operations. Therefore, even if surgery in childhood fails to achieve a "perfect result," the attempt to reduce a dislocated hip should be made, even when a complete dislocation is present. In older children 6 to 8 years of age when bilateral hip dislocation is present, a compromised result with a stiff hip owing to late treatment (as with capsular arthroplasty and the like) is far easier to manage later in life than a completely dislocated hip. Reconstructive efforts by replacement in

437

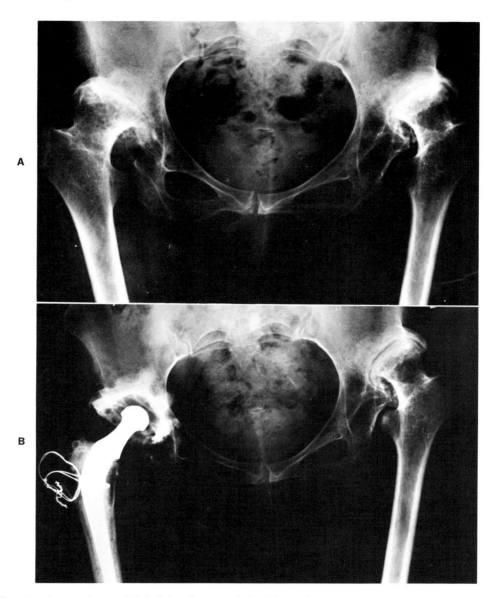

Fig. 13-1. Intermediate and high dislocations usually lend themselves well to hip replacement. True acetabulum is usually well formed and floor of acetabulum is thickened; it is technically feasible to deepen acetabulum at site of triradiate cartilage. **A,** Preoperative bilateral hip dislocation: right, intermediate, and left, high dislocation. **B,** Postoperative replacement by low-friction arthroplasty of left hip. NOTE: preparation of socket at original site of acetabulum. Good coverage could be obtained by modest deepening of existing bone at site of original acetabulum. Left hip was ankylosed, free of pain, but in adducted position. Patient became fully active following replacement and no further surgical intervention of left hip was necessary. Preoperative grading B-right, 2,3,4; left, 5,3,1. Postoperative grading right, 6,5,6; left, 6,5,1.

untreated dislocations are technically difficult and, at times, impossible.

Symptomatic adolescent hip dysplasia generally should be treated conservatively or by improving the mechanics of the hip with a femoral or pelvic osteotomy or shelf procedure (Fig. 8-11).

A general philosophy for surgical indications has been advanced in Chapter 8. In adults with good function, radiological evidence of dysplasia, even with minor to moderate osteoarthritis, does not necessarily indicate surgery; such patients should certainly be encouraged to delay surgery

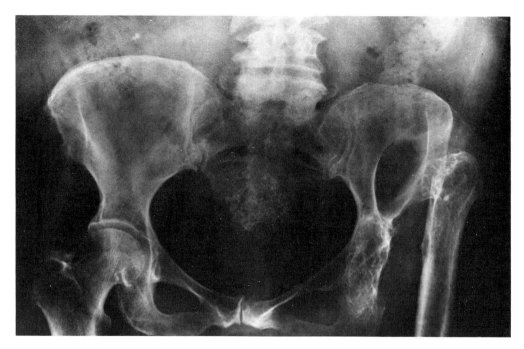

Fig. 13-2. Preoperative radiograph of 73-year-old woman with unilateral completely unreduced dislocated hip. Attempt at reconstruction of this hip was made; however, site of acetabulum was found to be completely unsuitable for smallest available acetabulum. Consideration of bone graft was given but surgery was terminated without replacement in view of narrow anteroposterior diameter of pelvis at site of original acetabulum. Width of narrow "band" of bone at site of triradiate cartilage measured 15 mm. In fact, medial lateral thickness of bone was considerably greater than anteroposterior diameter.

until their disability becomes intolerable. This applies specifically to young patients who wish to be rid of their limp and become more active, the main concern here is cosmesis and not disability.

There is no disagreement among surgeons that indications for total hip arthroplasty for congenital subluxation and dysplastic hips with degenerative osteoarthritis are the same as those outlined for osteoarthritis without dysplasia.

Generally, intermediate and high dislocations lend themselves well to hip replacement.[7,16] The true acetabulum is usually well formed, and, technically, replacement is no different than that for osteoarthrosis (Fig. 13-1), providing that surgical and technical details are carefully considered. Reconstruction, however, may be formidable or impossible on a completely unreduced dislocated hip with no evidence of any development of the acetabulum (Fig. 13-2). Even where a new acetabulum can be created and a total prosthesis inserted, it is doubtful whether the extremely atrophic and perhaps shortened abductor muscles would allow a satisfactory gait following recovery. Fortunately, contact between the upper end of the femur and the pelvis in completely dislocated hips has usually been minimal throughout life, and there is no true "constrainment osteoarthritis," so that these patients generally have a pain-free hip. However, back pain, shortening of the extremity, and a gross limp are the main complaints.

When hips have been bilaterally dislocated throughout life and no false acetabuli have been formed, leg length is equal and back pain is usually negligible, with fewer adaptive changes in the spine and knees. Generally, these patients should be discouraged from having surgery because of the obvious technical problems and the fact that they may undergo a dangerous operation without improvement of the basic problem, that is, the limp, which is generally related to the underdeveloped adductor muscles (Fig. 8-10).

Unreduced congenital dislocations

There are those who feel that a completely dislocated hip (unreduced) is a distinct contraindication for total hip replacement surgery.[5,10,16]

439

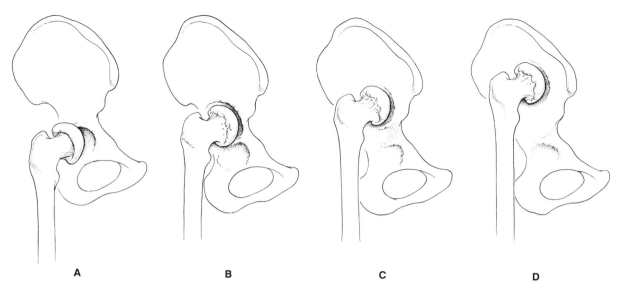

Fig. 13-3. Four stages of hip dislocation from dysplasia to complete dislocation. **A,** Acetabulum is slightly elongated and appears dysplastic, accommodating flattened mushroom-shaped femoral head. **B** and **C,** Intermediate and high dislocation. True acetabulum is poorly developed, but floor is thick and easily identifiable following removal of fibrofatty tissue from original site of true acetabulum. Lower border of false acetabulum identifies roof of original acetabulum. **D,** Old, unreduced dislocation (similar to Fig. 13-2). Head actually has never been in contact with ilium. There is no pseudoacetabulum, and original site of acetabulum can hardly be recognized. It only represents a narrow "isthmus" at site of triradiate cartilage.

This view is expressed because of the technical hazards involved in this type of reconstructive surgery, and because in most instances the prime motive is not relief of pain but elimination of an unsightly gait and fatigue, usually resulting from the underdeveloped and disadvantageous adductor mechanism.

Our own policy in the past has been not to attempt reconstruction of unreduced dislocations of the hip.[10] It is felt, generally, that this type of high dislocation is too extreme for reconstruction, inviting more hazardous complications than the degree of disability warrants. In a few instances where reconstruction was attempted, the results have been less than satisfactory (Fig. 8-15).

Reconstructive surgery in congenital dysplasia and dislocated hips is generally more difficult than a standard operation and requires experience and special attention to specific technical details.[4,16] Surgeons are well advised to postpone this type of reconstructive operation until they are totally familiar with its technical details.[8,12-14,20]

Specific considerations

In congenital dysplasia and dislocation there are many considerations, such as: anatomical

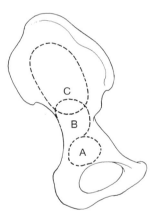

Fig. 13-4. Represents site of acetabulum accommodating femoral head in various situations. *A,* Original site of acetabulum in normal and dysplastic hip. *B,* Site of intermediate and high dislocations. *C,* Site of high untreated and unreduced "ancient" dislocations.

pathology, exposure and handling of soft tissue, preparation and conservation of the acetabulum, bone graft to provide coverage, femoral dysplasia, shortening of the femur versus length, and aftercare.

Anatomical pathology. The anatomy of congenital subluxation must be considered sepa-

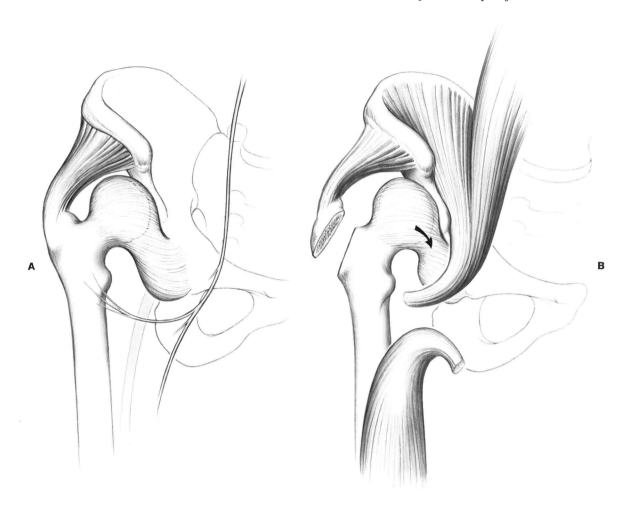

Fig. 13-5. A, Shortened soft tissue including all muscle groups and neurovascular structures must be considered in congenitally dislocated hip. Location of femoral and sciatic nerves are shown. In lowering head of femur to original site of acetabulum, contracted soft tissue must be released, while respecting neurovascular structure. **B,** Abductor muscles are detached via greater trochanter. Hourglass capsule is shown accommodating femoral head. Arrow indicates direction of capsule communicating with site of original acetabulum (see text).

rately from dislocation. In congenital subluxation the head still articulates with a shallow acetabulum, which is partially developed at the original site. However, the acetabulum is elongated and slopes proximally, with a flattened (mushroom-shaped) femoral head (Fig. 13-3, *A*). The distortion of the femoral head generally accompanies a thickened capsule that supports it only partially and a greater trochanter that is located posteriorly with an excessively anteverted femoral neck (Fig. 13-4, *A*). Fixed contractures are present in the medial aspect of the hip joint between the proximal end of the femur (to the lesser trochanter) and the pelvic wall (contracted capsule). Soft tissue contractures such as short-

ening of the adductors and the iliopsoas are common (Fig. 13-5).

In congenital dislocation the head has escaped from the scarcely developed original socket and is now located at the site of the false acetabulum against the thin wing of the ilium. (Figs. 13-3, *B* to *D*, and 13-4, *B* and *C*). The innominate bone is poorly developed. The true acetabulum is also poorly developed and usually is not easily identifiable since it is filled with fibrofatty tissue. The site of the true acetabulum (a rudimentary rough surface) can be seen only after complete excision of the capsular and fibrous tissue in this region. The femur is placed posteriorly in relation to the site of the false acetabulum (Fig.

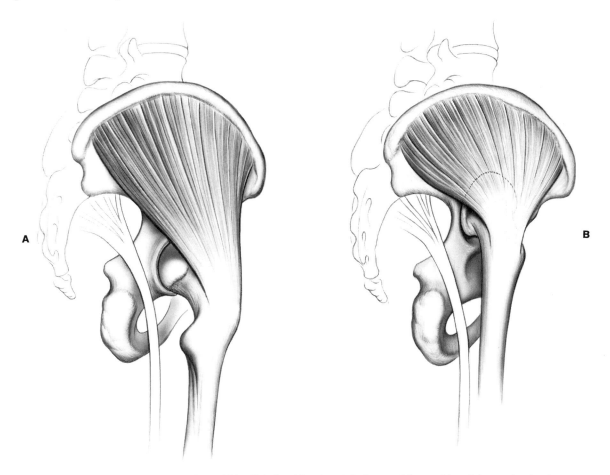

Fig. 13-6. A, Posterolateral view of hip. Relationship of acetabulum and femoral head, lesser trochanter, ischium, and sciatic nerve is shown. **B,** Same view of congenitally dislocated hip, emphasizing relationship of femoral head with ilium, shortened abductor muscles, and somewhat posteriorly located femoral shaft in relation to wing of ilium. NOTE: proximity of sciatic nerve and its potential danger of being stretched or damaged during elongation of limb.

13-6). The false acetabulum is markedly displastic or underdeveloped if the head has never been in contact with the wing of the ilium (Fig. 13-2). The site of the original (true) acetabulum is markedly narrowed in its anteroposterior diameter (oval shaped). It is notably lacking an anterior wall but is usually thickened in depth (at the level of the site of the teardrop on radiographs) medially (Fig. 13-7).

The femoral head is small and the femoral neck shows a severe degree of anteversion (sometimes as much as 80 or 90 degrees). The greater trochanter is located markedly posterior, with a marked forward twist of the femoral neck. The narrowing of the femoral canal with its thick and strong cortex is striking (Fig. 13-8).

Fixed adduction and flexion deformity is a common finding. With the fascia enveloping the hip joint and thigh, the iliopsoas, rectus femoris, and adductors are contracted. Any attempts to gain length by lowering the level of the socket to its original site must be accompanied by a complete release of these structures. It must, however, be noted that unlike a normally developed anatomy, the neurovascular structures are not developed, and any attempt to lengthen the extremity may jeopardize their integrity and function (Figs. 13-5 and 13-6).

Dense fibrous tissue found at the level of the original acetabulum site and extending between the medial aspect of the femoral neck and the wall of the pelvis requires sharp incision or exci-

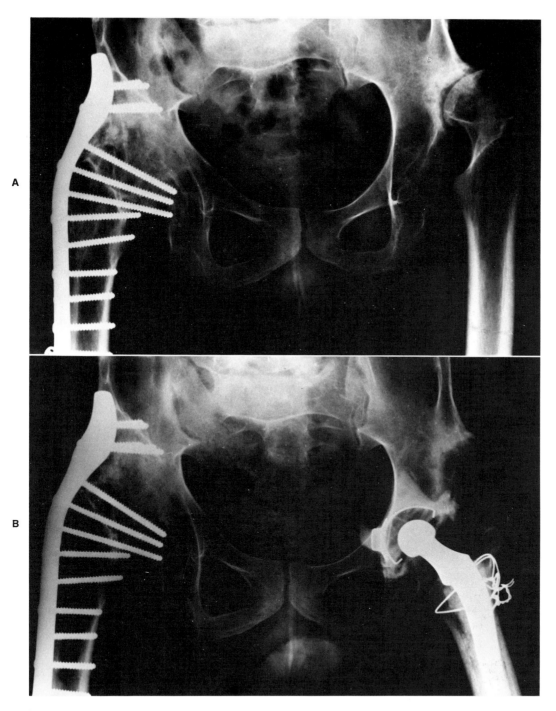

Fig. 13-7. A, This 42-year-old man with history of bilateral congenital dislocation had severe back pain as well as left knee instability as result of hip fusion performed. **B,** Low-friction arthroplasty was performed. Adequate acetabular cup could be created at original site of triradiate cartilage, without need for bone graft. NOTE: small acetabular cup (40 mm. outside diameter) could be accommodated. Preoperative grading B-left, 2,3,1; postoperatively, 5,4,6.

443

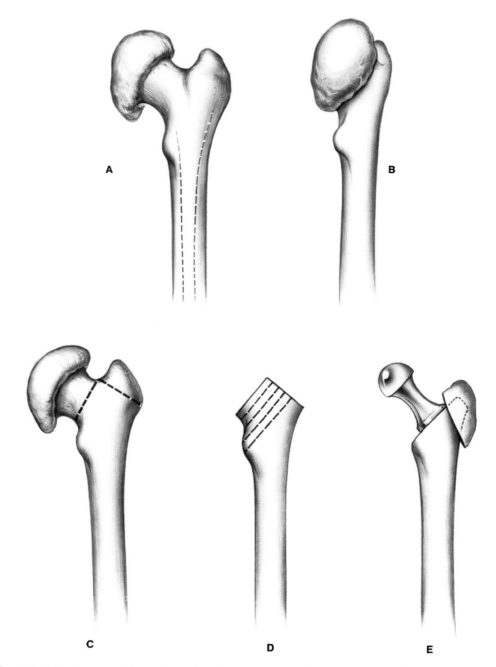

Fig. 13-8. A and **B,** Illustrate front view and profile of upper femur in severe dysplasia. Femoral cortex is usually thick and strong but extremely narrow within medullary canal. Head is mushroomed-shaped and neck is markedly anteverted. **C** to **E,** Illustrate site of osteotomy of greater trochanter and neck with sequential shortening as needed to accommodate prosthesis, while leaving spike on lateral cortex for interlocking of greater trochanter (see text).

sion to allow mobilization of the upper femur. Preoperative skeletal traction is of no value and does not help in lowering the femur.

As stated previously, the abductors are underdeveloped and shortened. The greater trochanter often is small and located posteriorly; its removal must be inclusive, which is best accomplished with a broad osteotome. The poorly developed femoral head is supported by the superior capsule, thickened within the substance of the abductors and the iliopsoas muscles (Fig. 13-5). In an untreated congenital dislocation, the head may be at the level of the iliac crest, especially in unreduced, untreated bilateral conditions (Fig. 13-2).

Exposure and handling of soft tissue. The incision is similar to that of a standard operation, but it must be at least 2 to 3 inches longer than in conventional operations. Exposure must be maximized and no effort should be made to attempt replacement prior to a complete exposure. A wide exposure of the original site of the acetabulum is essential.

To obtain a wide exposure the gluteus maximus muscle fibers may be split approximately beyond and proximal to the level of the skin incision. This can be done blindly by digital separation of bundles of this muscle. The sciatic nerve must be located and palpated, and its location in relationship to the acetabulum kept in mind. To allow better access to the back of the hip joint (unlike conventional operations), a large sandbag (placed under the flank and in the sacroiliac region) may be useful. This sandbag may be removed when orienting the acetabular components. However, if the exposure is satisfactory, the surgeon must keep in mind the degree of the patient's tilt to the opposite side if the sandbag is not removed.

Removal of the greater trochanter must be done with extra care in that a large-sized trochanter is being removed. The trochanter should include the vastus lateralis ridge and a small portion of the upper shaft. Because of the posterior placement of the trochanter on the shaft in congenital dysplasia of the hip, the hip must be internally rotated and held in that position at the time of the osteotomy of the greater trochanter. Conventional removal of the greater trochanter with a cholecystectomy clamp is not indicated, as it may lead to removal of a very small trochanter. Instead, the cholecystectomy clamp is inserted and used as a target at the junction of the

neck and the greater trochanter, and a broad osteotome is used to reach this target to be sure that the large-sized fragment removed includes the entire abductor mechanism (Fig. 12-16).

External rotators are detached from the upper femur, and the piriformis is detached from its insertion into the digital fossa of the greater trochanter.

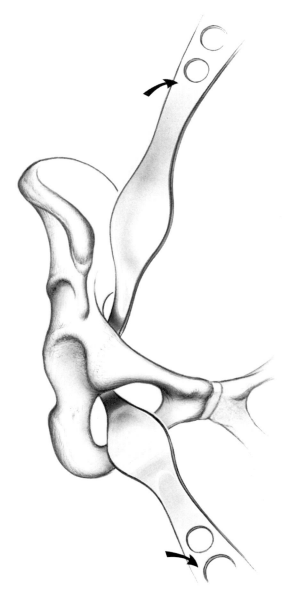

Fig. 13-9. To maximize acetabular exposure, Hohmann retractor is placed anteriorly engaging it onto inner wall of pelvis at junction of ilium and pubic ramus, and second similar retractor is placed below intercotyloid notch. Second retractor is extremely useful in order to define lowest possible location for preparation of acetabulum. Arrows indicate direction of pull on retractors.

445

A complete excision of the capsule is necessary. This is done best by incising the capsule on the head of the femur then, following dislocation, the insertion of the capsule on the neck is removed. By holding onto the capsule with a Kocher clamp, the remainder is excised, working from the femoral head toward the periphery of the acetabulum. Often, dense capsule and scar are present and require sharp dissection and careful protection of the neurovascular structure of the hip joint. To improve exposure it is often necessary to release the iliopsoas tendon from the lesser trochanter, to remove the origin of the rectus femoris, and occasionally section the iliotibial tract of the tensor fascia femoris.

To achieve abduction it is often necessary to do a percutaneous adductor tenotomy at this stage of the operation (see Fig. 14-3).

To maximize the exposure of the acetabular site a Hohmann retractor must be placed anteriorly, engaging it onto the inner wall of the pelvis at the junction of the ilium and pubis ramus. It must be placed deeply to prevent accidental fracture of the anterior wall of the acetabulum.

A second smooth-tipped Bennett retractor or a second Hohmann retractor is placed inside the obturator foramen just beneath the intercotyloid notch of the acetabulum. This retractor will maximize the exposure of the inferior boundary of the acetabulum (Fig. 13-9) and best locates the site of the original acetabulum.

The problems of excessive shortening and underdeveloped abductor muscle may be overcome by dissecting along the anterior and posterior border of the abductors and mobilizing this muscle using an osteotome in the region of the super

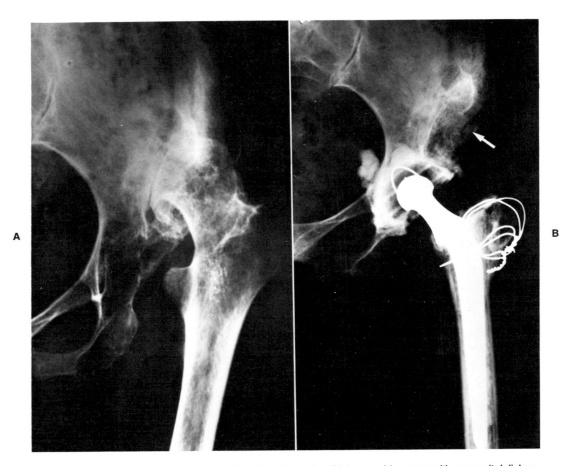

Fig. 13-10. Preoperative, **A,** and postoperative, **B,** radiographs of 64-year-old woman with congenital dislocation of hip and secondary osteoarthritis. NOTE: lowered site of acetabulum, roof of new acetabulum, and floor of false acetabulum. Abductor shortening was severe and only position of abduction could facilitate reattachment. Patient was placed in hip spica cast in abduction for 4 weeks, which subsequently was followed by exercises to mobilize and stretch abductors. Arrow, **B,** indicates site of false acetabulum. (See text).

446

acetabular area. Z-plasty of abductor muscle is not satisfactory and should be avoided. At the end of the operation, the abductor muscle may be too short to be conveniently reattached to the femur, therefore the femur must be brought to the greater trochanter by maximal abduction of the hip (Fig. 13-10).

Preparation and conservation of the acetabulum. In congenital subluxation, the volume of the acetabulum is usually small, with reduced dimensions at the site of prosthetic implantation. It is therefore imperative to preserve as much bone as possible, especially in younger patients where future revision surgery might become necessary. The smallest possible cavity should be created where maximum bone exists, that is,

at the original site of the acetabulum. It is of paramount importance to carefully define the site of the original acetabulum and dissect the capsule and soft tissue at its periphery in order to maintain exposure and to evaluate the amount of existing bone (Fig. 13-11). Despite scrupulous preparation of the acetabulum, at times its superior portion may not be adequate to accommodate a small socket. Thus a peripheral margin of the acetabulum may be exposed and augmented by bone graft for improved coverage and with the hope of creating a bone stalk for future revision surgery (Fig. 13-12).

Generally, the posterior wall of the acetabulum is thicker than the anterior wall; in deepening the socket, the reamers should be directed

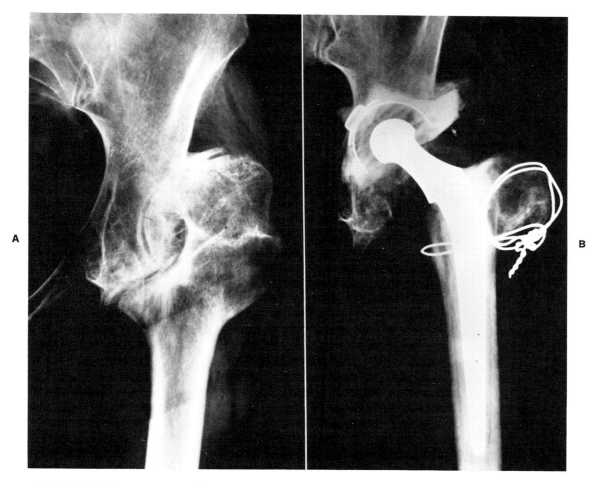

Fig. 13-11. A, Preoperative and, **B,** postoperative radiographs of unilateral congenital dislocation in 44-year-old female. NOTE: postoperatively remarkably good acetabular coverage could be provided for cup without bone graft only by deepening socket at original site of acetabulum. Also note that marked shortening of femur was necessary (down to lesser trochanter) in order to reduce hip. This postoperative radiograph was taken 8 years following surgery. Preoperative grading A-3,3,1; postoperative grading of the left hip, A-6,6,6.

447

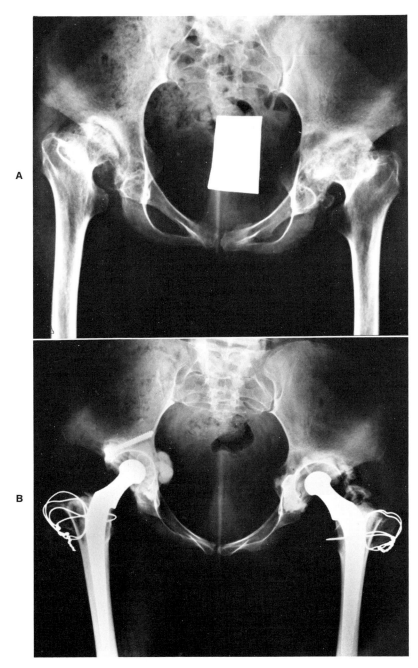

Fig. 13-12. A, Preoperative radiograph of 19-year-old female with multiple epiphyseal dysplasia and severe hip disability (C-2,2,2, right and 2,2,2, left). Extent of dysplasia was not fully appreciated until time of surgery. At surgery left hip and right hip were both defective not only anteriorly but posteriorly as well. Superior wall was defective and in continuation of wing of ilium. **B,** On right side by maximum deepening small socket could be used but approximately 15% of superior weight-bearing portion of acetabular cup was uncovered. Two screws were used to augment fixation. Left hip was similarly defective but bone chips were obtained from head and shavings were packed around acetabulum both superiorly and posteriorly. NOTE: bone formation 1 year following surgery on left may have resulted from fragments of bone graft. Postoperative grading, B-right, 6,6,6; and B-left, 6,6,6.

448

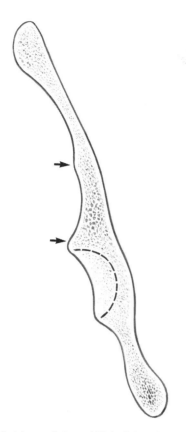

Fig. 13-13. In intermediate and high dislocation, ridge (lower arrow) separates true acetabulum from false acetabulum. Space between two arrow sites indicates false acetabulum. In lowering socket to original site, special care must be rendered to preserve ridge between two acetabulae (see text).

more toward the posterior wall than the anterior segment; that is, the handles of the reamers should be inclined 20 to 30 degrees in reference to the operating table.

The first step in the preparation of the acetabulum involves identification of the original site of the acetabulum, which is often filled with fibro-fatty tissue. This is best done by palpation and by placing two pointed retractors (such as a Hohmann) to maximize the exposure: one anteriorly, within the inner wall of the pelvis, and one into the intercotyloid notch. Excision of all soft tissue, including fibro-fatty elements, at the level of the original acetabulum, is essential. This step is tedious and time-consuming but must be performed thoroughly to expose the true acetabular site. The soft tissue at the inferior margin of the true acetabulum is sharply excised to provide exposure and to facilitate insertion of a Hohmann retractor into the inferior border of the true ace-

tabulum (the superior margin of the obturator foramen). Generally, a bony ridge separates the false acetabulum from the original site of the acetabulum (Figs. 13-7, 13-10, and 13-13).

With standard instrumentation, at times, the centering device may not reach the depth of the acetabulum to mark the center. In this case the centering drill may then be introduced (without the centering disc), estimating the drill site by direct vision ("eyeballing"). Because of the minuteness of the acetabulum site, the direction of the deepening reamer must be carefully observed as any deviation from the center of the "bony mass" in the region of the true acetabulum may remove one or more of the acetabular walls. The periphery and depth must be frequently checked. Care must be taken not to interfere with the "ridge" between the true and false acetabuli, which forms the roof for the newly prepared acetabulum (Fig. 13-13).

It is essential to proceed slowly in preparing these small acetabuli and to examine the walls of the socket as preparation progresses to avoid the danger of removing one or more walls because of defective bone. Generally, the deepening reamer should suffice. The expanding reamers should never enlarge the socket to 50 mm. After the deepening reamer, a sharp, long-handled curet can enlarge the acetabulum wherever necessary.

Without exception, a false acetabulum on the lateral wall of the ilium in "intermediate" and "high" dislocations is not suitable for prosthetic fixation. The bone at that level is not sufficiently thick to withstand any deepening to support the prosthesis. (See Figs. 1-4 and 1-7.) As already indicated, the newly prepared acetabulum must accommodate a small cup (that is, 40 mm. or less outer diameter). When bone is markedly dysplastic, an even smaller diameter socket should be used. The Charnley (22 mm. diameter) head is quite suitable; it provides the maximum thickness of plastic with the smallest outer diameter.* The thickness of the acetabular floor can be judged by radiographs. At surgery, however, the medial wall of the pelvis can be palpated with the index finger inside and the thumb outside, in order to assess the area of greatest thickness. As an alternative method fol-

---

* A 40-mm. outer diameter Charnley low-friction arthroplasty cup is often used, but the extra small and the offset bore cup are particularly prescribed for severely dysplastic acetabuli.

lowing exposure of the acetabular site, the centering drill hole allows insertion of a finger to estimate thickness. The pulp of the index finger palpates the inferior margin of the pilot hole. When extreme dysplasia is evident, standard gouges and chisels should be used in preference to standard reamers in order to avoid damage by reamers.

During preparation of the socket, it is most important to preserve the roof, medial wall, and anterior and posterior lips of the acetabulum. The deepening should never violate the "inner table" of the pelvis. A ½-inch anchor hole can usually be made in the direction of the ilium, but because of the defective bony structure of the floor, additional anchoring preparation must be limited to several small anchor holes. A sharp long-handled curet or a bone scraper is the best instrument for removing the remainder of the cartilage from the acetabulum.

Occasionally, a slightly higher level than the true site of the acetabulum may be preferable, particularly when the acetabulum has been expanded proximally by disease or previous surgery, such as when a shelf Chiari osteotomy cup or endoprosthesis has created a "high socket" with good bony coverage (Figs. 13-14 to 13-16).

The concern in these situations is a thin floor at the site of the true acetabulum with a well-formed cavity at a more proximal level. The decision regarding the site may be determined finally by observing the thickness of the pelvis through the pilot hole (in the floor of the acetabulum) or by digital palpation from within the pelvis.)

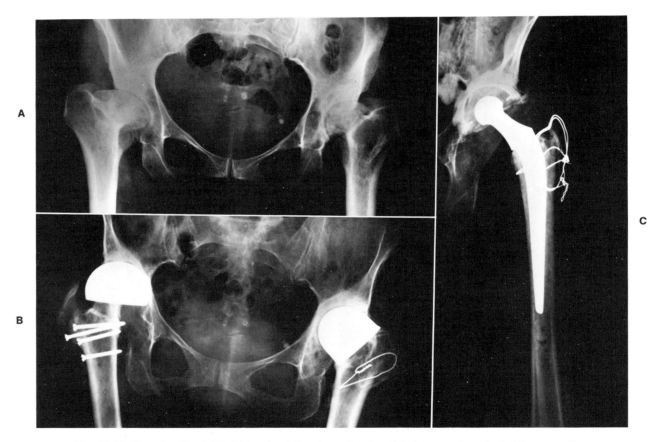

Fig. 13-14. Occasionally slightly higher level than true site of acetabulum may be selected for cementing socket. This is especially true if previous operations such as cup arthroplasty or shelf procedure have created good bony stock at slightly higher level. **A,** Preoperative radiograph of 52-year-old woman with bilateral degenerative osteoarthritis of hip secondary to congenital dysplasia. Patient had multiple surgical procedures as child and in adolescence. **B,** Following bilateral mold arthroplasty, note proximal migration of both hips as result of previous surgery and bone absorption. **C,** Hip following low-friction arthroplasty. Selected site of socket was high because of marked opening of acetabulum in craniad direction.

450

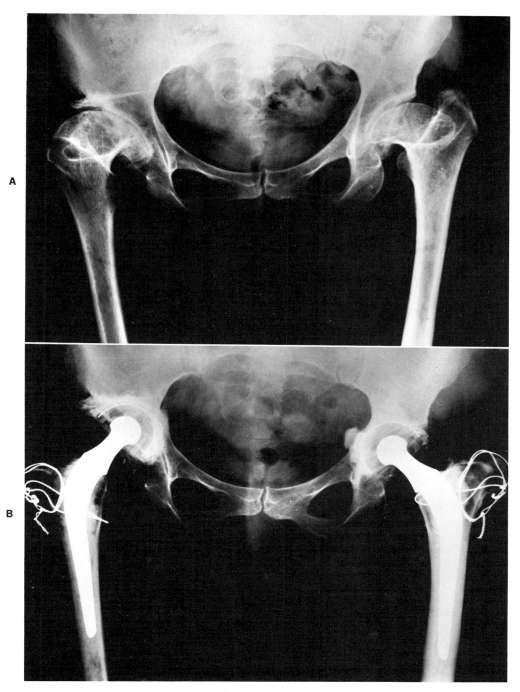

Fig. 13-15. A, Preoperative radiograph of 58-year-old female with bilateral congenital dislocated hips and multiple surgical procedures in past. NOTE: left hip had been treated by shelf procedure that had provided support for femoral head. **B,** Eight years following bilateral low-friction arthroplasties. NOTE: slightly higher selected socket site on left than right was to take advantage of good support by previous shelf surgery.

451

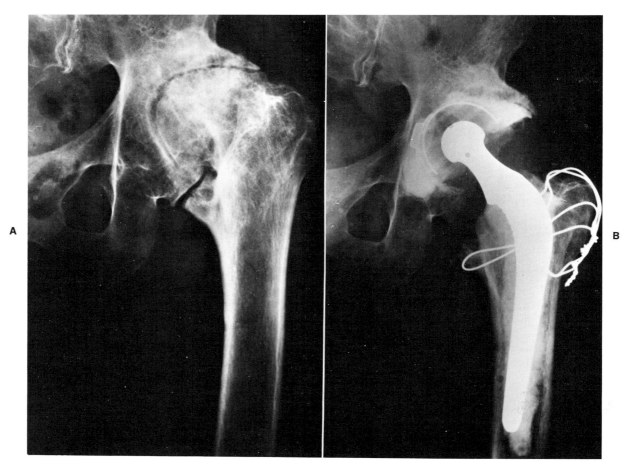

Fig. 13-16. Congenital dislocation of hip, **A,** treated by Colonna and shelf procedure in 38-year-old male has created high position for socket. **B,** Similar to postoperative case Fig. 13-15. Shelf is utilized to support socket. Socket is lowered to provide length and wedge of cement is interposed between roof of acetabulum and cup (see Fig. 13-35).

Bone graft to provide coverage. Only after the acetabulum is fully prepared and the superior and posterosuperior walls are assessable can a decision regarding bone graft necessity be made. If the walls of the acetabulum remain deficient, as when, in testing, the ability to provide support for the smallest acetabular cup (special CDH cup with 34 mm. outside diameter) is not present, then a bone graft must be considered. It is possible to insert two or three screws into the superior acetabular area and leave the ends projected to be incorporated in the cement, which can then provide coverage for the cup (Fig. 13-12). Although it might appear satisfactory on radiographs and at surgery, this system may not be as satisfactory as having the entire prosthetic component and cement covered by bone. Therefore, preferentially, bone grafting must be done

in cases where the coverage of the acetabular cup is deficient. There are at least three ways in which a bone graft may be used to improve the coverage of the prosthetic component when the acetabular bone is deficient:

1. Packing autogenous bone chips around the uncovered segment of the cemented cup (Fig. 13-12)
2. Autogenous bone-block grafting, secured with screws (Fig. 13-17)
3. Autogenous bone grafting using the femoral head[12,13] and bolts for fixation (Fig. 13-18)

Of these three methods, bone chips reinforcing the uncovered cup is the easiest and carries the least morbidity; local bone from the femoral head or "bone paste" from shavings of the acetabulum is available for packing around the

452

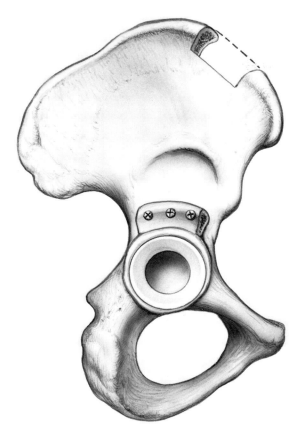

Fig. 13-17. Autogenous bone graft may be obtained from crest of ilium and screwed onto acetabulum to provide support for socket. NOTE: bone graft is screwed onto site of false acetabulum just above ridge. False acetabulum is shown just above bone graft. Smallest size prosthesis is used to contain socket and conserve bone.

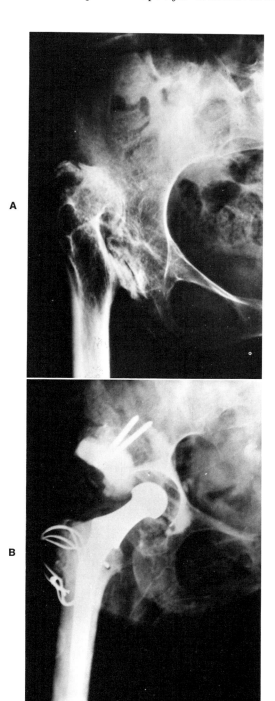

Fig. 13-18. Preoperative, **A,** and postoperative, **B,** radiographs of 51-year-old woman with congenitally dislocated hip treated by low-friction arthroplasty and bone graft procedure. **B,** Immediate postoperative film taken through plaster hip spica cast, showing position of bone graft using two screws. Hip was in abduction in order to approximate greater trochanter because of short abductors.

cup. This method is particularly useful when more than 80% of the total weight-bearing portion of the acetabular cup is covered. Therefore chips are used to augment the coverage and to produce additional bone stock for the pelvis against the possibility of arthroplasty revision at a later date.

However, where the coverage of the acetabular cup is defective and more than 20% of the weight-bearing portion of the acetabulum is not covered (by the superior and posterior wall of the acetabulum) a bone graft fixation is advisable. The insertion of a bone block includes:

1. A satisfactory and generous bone block must be obtained from the ipsilateral or contralateral pelvis, including the crest of the ilium and both tables (Figs. 13-17 and 13-18).

2. A bed at an appropriate site on the wing of

453

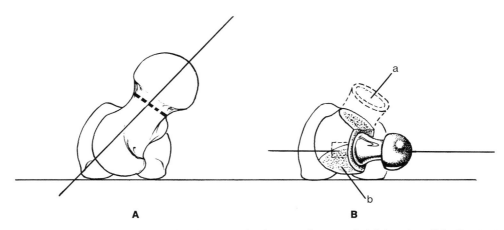

Fig. 13-19. A and **B,** At times, femoral neck anteversion is severe in congenital dislocation of hip. Greater trochanter is located posteriorly in addition to narrowing of femoral shaft. *a,* Indicates amputated site of neck; *b,* indicates site of removal of greater trochanter. Attempt is made to keep femoral component in neutroversion plane; nevertheless, slightly anteverted position of stem may be selected to allow insertion. This compromise is exception to rule, which may be carefully considered in severe narrowing and anteverted femurs.

the ilium must be carefully prepared to receive the graft. This includes a sharp dissection and reflecting the gluteal origin. An area at least 20 mm. wide must be thoroughly cleaned of the soft tissue and roughened to receive the graft. This area usually is best determined following a complete visual examination of the rim of the acetabulum.

3. The site of the graft must be carefully determined by testing a variety of positions to observe the improved contact and fit of the graft.

4. The block(s) of bone must be transfixed with two or three screws (the length of the screws must be measured by a depth gauge and the holes drilled and tapped using A-O cancellous screws).

5. Care is taken not to split the carefully prepared double-thickness graft obtained from the ilium and to be sure that after fixation cement will not extrude between the bone graft and the ilium.

Femoral dysplasia. Anatomical changes of the femur include: (1) excess narrowing of the medullary canal, (2) excess anteversion of the femoral neck, and (3) posterior location of the greater trochanter.

Excessive narrowing of the medullary canal is a most serious problem and requires reaming for the insertion of the stem. We find a graded, straight Küntscher reamer (up to 12 mm. in diameter) useful and safe; however, most femurs are less than 12 mm. wide (as measured by preoperative radiographs), and reamers must be used with extreme care to prevent perforation of the shaft. Direct access to the upper femur is necessary, with entry to the shaft from the posterior aspect of the cut surface of the stump (because of excessive anteversion) following resection of the femoral head. At times the opening of the neck leading to the medullary canal may have to be ignored entirely and a new perforation made on the top of the femur in the direction of the knee joint. It is important to enter the shaft as far posteriorly as possible to avoid penetration (Fig. 13-19). It is essential to have the femur maximally adducted, using the knee joint and patella as a point of reference when directing the reamers (see Chapter 12). Whenever possible, it is better to ream the medullary canal to accommodate a straight, narrow stem or a CDH stem rather than to use an excessively thin prosthesis (custom-made). (See Chapters 3 and 17.)

In extremely narrow canals with anterior bowing of the femur, it is difficult to insert the broaches in a neutral plane; because of excess anteversion, usually it is only possible to insert the stem in an anteverted position. For this reason, it may be necessary to compromise and accept 10 to 15 degrees of anteversion in order to allow insertion of the stem (anteverted channel) (Fig. 13-8, *A* and *B*). However, this must be done with caution since the hip may become unstable, thus inviting anterior dislocation following surgery.

Although the heaviest straight stem prosthesis is ideal, a straight, narrow stem is usually all that can be accommodated in this case. An "extra–short neck prosthesis" (¾ neck length) may obviate the need for unnecessary shortening of the femur by removing bone. A progressive and successive shortening of the femur may be necessary to allow reduction following cementing of the socket. This process creates the additional problem of the prosthesis reaching the narrow segment of the femur—the isthmus, thus difficulty in expanding the femur in this narrow segment. A rechannelization drill-guide system may be used (see Chapter 14) with a straight but narrow stem and a short-neck prosthesis.

Shortening of femur versus length. Following the cementing of the socket, the neck is invariably too long to allow reduction. Prior to deciding to shorten the femur, one must make sure that all of the soft connecting tissue (capsule, fibrous scars, and so on) has been severed and the upper femur is completely detached from the pelvic wall (Fig. 13-8) and mobilized. If reduction is not possible despite soft tissue release, the femur must then be shortened. Five to six centimeters of lengthening will usually result because of the lowering of the acetabulum site. Forceful traction to obtain maximum length may be unsafe. It is important to preserve the lateral cortex as much as possible during this procedure so that the trochanter can be reattached with a good bony contact. The femur is shortened in successive stages, removing no more than 2 to 3 mm. of bone at a time until successful reduction is accomplished. It should be possible to abduct the limb to allow the greater trochanter and abductor muscles to reach the outer upper end of the shaft. Usually a relatively large trochanter can be easily fitted onto a "spike" created at the proximal lateral cortex (Fig. 13-8). Following release, however, the trochanter must be under minimum tension to allow subsequent fixation. When the socket has been lowered from its original site, it is often necessary to mobilize the detached greater trochanter by bringing it downward against the shaft of the femur. This requires division of most of its capsular attachment, external rotators, and often blunt elevation of the musculotendinous portion of the abductors from the wall of the pelvis (Fig. 13-18); despite this, some abduction may be required at the time of fixation of the greater trochanter, even cast immobilization, to avoid detachment (Fig. 13-5).

Aftercare. Following a reconstructive procedure for congenital dysplasia and dislocation of the hip, most patients may manifest a weak gluteus medius gait (positive Trendelenburg sign). They should be told prior to surgery that the purpose of the operation is properly to relieve pain, and an existing limp following surgery may denote a weak musculature about the hip resulting from a congenital condition. They should be encouraged to use a cane postoperatively if they demonstrate a positive Trendelenburg sign and a weak gluteus medius gait.

Another deviation from routine for the postoperative course is the use of a balanced suspension apparatus for approximately 6 weeks following surgery or, alternatively, a unilateral short-hip spica cast worn for the same period of time. This is used because of tenuous fixation of the greater trochanter as a result of shortening of this muscle and additional bone graft procedure accompanied by total hip arthroplasty. If a bone graft is used, an additional period of protective weight bearing may be indicated, which may range from 3 to 6 months, allowing incorporation of the bone graft. The resumption of weight bearing may be gradual, that is, the first 3 months with partial weight bearing, starting "toe-touch," and subsequently, increased to full weight bearing within 6 months. If abductors are extremely short at surgery even with advancement of the glutei and the attachment was only feasible by maximum abduction of the hip, a hip spica cast must be applied in that position for 4 to 6 weeks and subsequently removed and followed by a regimented exercise program.

While physiotherapy and an extensive exercise program will not be prescribed for patients with degenerative osteoarthritis undergoing a routine total hip replacement, in contrast, abductor strengthening exercises with the use of a powdered board and progressive resistive exercises of this type would be indicated in cases of congenital dysplasia and dislocated hips with a weak adductor mechanism (see Chapter 11). It is most essential that these patients keep their weight at an optimal level, since weight reduction by even a few pounds may alleviate considerable demand on the poorly developed abductor mechanism.

PAGET'S DISEASE

Experience with total hip replacement in Paget's disease has proved to be highly successful in relieving pain, although occasional unexplained pain has been reported following total hip arthroplasty in Paget's disease.[19]

Personal experiences and several studies[15,18] now indicate that surgical results can be as good as in the so-called idiopathic osteoarthritis of the hip joint. Because of the gradual process of "bone deformity" and rapid "turnover" of the bone in this disease, it remains to be seen whether the good early results can be maintained as well as those with normal bone. Undoubtedly, cement fixation has greatly contributed to the success of total hip arthroplasty in this condition in lieu of seeking a better mechanical fastening method. It is a known fact that most conventional operations, that is, osteotomy, mold arthroplasty, and so on, were notably difficult and unsuccessful in the past. Our experiences with Paget's disease indicate that the so-called pagetic pain originating from the bone of the pelvis or femur is usually the result of the arthritic process within the joint itself, even though the radiological changes of the femur or pelvis may be impressive so as to suggest severe osteoporosis and sclerosis.[9]

Fractures of the neck of the femur are notoriously known for their slow rate of healing and also for the poor result of those treated by hemiarthroplasty.[2,11] Similarly, if a prosthetic replacement has been used without cement, the failure of resorption and acetabular changes have been observed commonly in this condition. We feel, therefore, that a total hip replacement may be preferentially indicated in Paget's disease complicated by fracture of the neck of the femur. The possibility of gradual morphological changes in pagetic bone of the pelvis and femoral neck, although a possibility, has not yet been seen. Of 16 patients with Paget's disease I treated by hip replacement, two have demonstrated a nonprogressive line of demarcation at the acetabular site between the cement and bone. The follow-up range was between 6 months and 6 years.

Excessive osteophyte formation contributes to the deep seating of the femoral head, prohibiting clearance between the greater trochanter and the pelvis and sometimes resulting in extreme stiffness and causing difficulty in dislocating the hip.

The femur and acetabulum may both exhibit marked density or osteoporosis, which in either case may cause technical difficulty in preparing the acetabulum or the femur. Often cystic changes (osteoporosis circumscripta) may be present in the upper femur or in the acetabulum, especially within the region of the hip joint. Pathological fractures on the tension side of the femur are rather frequent, thus radiographs of the entire shaft of the femur are essential. We have not experienced excessive bleeding from pagetic bone. The blood loss at hip replacement has been comparable to that in osteoarthritic replacement.[10] (See Figs. 8-30, 8-31, 10-2, and 17-8.)

Specifics of technique

The technical difficulties and problems encountered are not related to Paget's disease itself but to the accompanying anatomical changes of the hip. The problems include the following.

High incidence of protrusio acetabuli. Difficulty in dislocating the hip at surgery is caused by protrusio acetabuli. The greater trochanter should be osteotomized as in other cases involving protrusion of the acetabulum. The bone of the trochanter may be excessively osteoporotic, requiring special handling during detachment and subsequent reattachment. A good reattachment of the trochanter is essential to avoid nonunion and other complications. Prior to dislocation, osteophytes around the acetabulum may be excised to facilitate dislocation. In preparing the acetabulum, special attention is required to prevent damage to the thin floors, which could result in loosening and intrapelvic protrusion of the components. No pilot hole is necessary for reaming, and in most instances only expansion of the periphery of the acetabulum is necessary, as the acetabulum is already sufficiently deep (Fig. 13-25). Curettage of the floor with a curet or bone scraper will maximize the bony contact. Large cystic changes (osteoporosis circumscripta) of Paget in the region of the pelvis near the acetabulum may be left alone if they are not communicating with the acetabulum; on the other hand, smaller cysts may be curetted and packed with cement. All fibrous tissue within the acetabulum must be cleaned, while conserving the good and strong bone within the periphery and the floor of the acetabulum.

Difficulty in preparation of the femur. Due to excess bone formation in the medullary canal, difficulty may be encountered in preparing the femur (Fig. 17-11). The use of a special drilling jig or power reamers may be necessary. Reamers must be directed carefully within the medullary canal to avoid perforation of the shaft through the weakened area of the bone (unrecognizable on x-ray film) while working in the area of dense bone within the medullary canal. Unrecognized radiolucencies within the shaft of the upper femur may lead to fractures during or after operation (Fig. 10-2). The deformity of the upper femur must be recognized, and an enlarged medullary canal requiring extra care in reference to packing of the cement or the use of a thick-stem prosthesis must be noted. Often two doses of cement may be required to fill up the medullary canal within the region of the prosthesis (Fig. 8-31).

Excessive bleeding from pagetic bone. Excessive bleeding (similar to that encountered at long bone fractures) has not been observed, as stated before. Occasional arterial bleeding during broaching of the medullary canal may be controlled by packing the femoral canal; total blood loss has been consistently comparable to other total hip replacement cases.

Excessive heterotopic ossification. Although our experience with Paget's disease is admittedly limited, we have not found excessive heterotopic ossification to be a problem.

RHEUMATOID ARTHRITIS AND OTHER INFLAMMATORY TYPES

A combined group of patients will be considered in this category, including those with classic rheumatoid arthritis, chronic juvenile polyarthritis or Still's disease, ankylosing spondylitis, psoriatic arthritis, Reiter's disease, and other collagen disorders. Of these conditions, total hip replacement is most commonly performed for rheumatoid arthritis, juvenile rheumatoid arthritis, and ankylosing spondylitis. There are several problems common to these patients: previous steroid treatment with chronic dermatitis, vasculitis, susceptibility to bruising, and fragility with advanced degrees of osteoporosis, thus making these patients prone to fractures during surgery.

The type of anesthesia administered is of special consideration, since stiffness of the neck and the temporomandibular joint may make intubation difficult. On the other hand, spinal anesthesia may be difficult because of the high incidence of spinal deformities and arthritis of the spine with accompanying interspinal ligament ossification. At times, tracheotomy may be needed and should be planned prior to surgery if

difficulty in intubation is anticipated. Intubation while the patient is awake is often a good solution (see Chapters 5, 9, and 11 for further details). The use of fiberoptic light facilitates this procedure in most cases.

The position of the arms and shoulders during surgery must be carefully considered because of the common involvement of the upper extremities. A careful evaluation of other joints is also necessary prior to surgery, especially when planning bilateral hip replacement, as well as a thorough assessment regarding the involvement and anticipated treatment of other joints. Details of the surgical correction of other joints in relation to hip surgery must be considered; for example, in doing major lower extremity surgery, hip surgery must precede surgery of the knees (see Chapter 8).

Specific postoperative exercises and a program designed to meet the unique needs of the patient with multiple joint disability must be planned. For example, a general muscle-strengthening regime longer than that for routine hip replacement must be carried out in most cases. Special crutches or walker modifications may be needed. Preferably, the second hip is operated on during the same hospitalization to facilitate postoperative ambulation (see Chapter 11).

As one may expect, a higher rate of postoperative complications may be anticipated if the details of surgery and postoperative management are not carefully planned and executed.[1,21] Myositis ossificans is one specific complication related to the hip joint, which has been reported to be higher in ankylosing spondylitis than in osteoarthritis. From the technical standpoint, operations with these complications are more difficult because of the severe deformity in the majority of the cases and the severe osteoporosis that accompanies stiffness of the hip, thus rendering the hip prone to fractures of the femoral neck or shaft during dislocation or preparation. Pathological anatomical complications such as complete ankylosis of the hip in ankylosing spondylitis and protrusio acetabuli in rheumatoid arthritis require special attention. In juvenile rheumatoid arthritis, a special prosthesis of small dimensions is required, sometimes necessitating modification of the available prosthesis to accommodate a bone that is typically extremely underdeveloped in these individuals. They also require special care, owing to the fragility of their skin, which may be seriously damaged by manipulation of the limb during surgery, and strict aseptic technique, as these cases are often prone to a higher rate of infection (see Chapters 6 and 17).

Most of these patients have suffered from chronic disability for many years, and their general condition is usually poor, with considerable muscle waste. Most have received corticosteroids and cytotoxic agents, and at times the physical and psychological stress of coping with the disease may have altered the patient's mood and ability to cooperate in the rehabilitation program postoperatively. These factors are best assessed and managed when a combined team of rheumatologists and orthopaedic surgeons participate in the patient's care. Often it is important to time the surgery based on psychosocial factors in combination with physical function, for example, in a young patient who is undergoing academic training or a young housewife whose family life is in great distress owing to her wheelchair confinement. Every effort must be made to plan for surgery prior to the patient's becoming chairbound.

Specifics of technique

Technical considerations in rheumatoid arthritis include careful handling of the greater trochanter to avoid fragmentation owing to severe osteoporosis; preservation of an acetabular floor, defective as the result of protrusion; and careful handling of the femoral shaft to avoid fracture, especially during dislocation and preparation of the femur.

To avoid damage to the greater trochanter, it is advisable to remove a slightly larger than usual size trochanter, and avoid placing retractors directly on the bone of the greater trochanter. The short rotators, usually removed in hips with osteoarthrosis, need not be removed in rheumatoid arthritis. We regard the osteotomy of the greater trochanter as an essential feature in the management of rheumatoid arthritis, although greater trochanteric fixation and union may be more difficult to achieve than in osteoarthrosis. The soft tissue generally causes more bleeding, and patience and care are necessary to avoid damage to the soft tissue. In preparing the acetabulum, in both "concentric" and "destructive" types (see Chapter 10), curettage of the floor without the use of deepening or expanding reamers may be

sufficient to remove the soft tissue and fibrocartilage. When the floor is thin or any degree of protrusion is present, the centering drill must not be used and the floor of the acetabulum should not be violated. The main anchoring holes should be drilled in the ilium and ischium, and, if necessary, several small drill holes at the periphery of the acetabulum may add surface contact for the cement. When a portion of the floor is membranous and devoid of any cortical bone whatsoever, the use of a wire mesh with or without a bone graft may be advisable. The bone graft may be obtained from the femoral head or from the wing of the ilium. Maximum contact between the cement and bone can be achieved by careful curettage and scraping of the bone where needed. The use of standard instruments, that is, deepening and expanding reamers, may be dangerous and may remove bone unnecessarily from the periphery or especially from the depth of the acetabulum. If protrusion is severe, two doses of cement may be required (see section on "Protrusio Acetabuli").

Preparation of the femur must also be done with care to avoid damage to extremely osteoporotic bone. Special care at the time of dislocation is essential to avoid a spiral fracture of the femoral shaft. It is best to insert a Watson-Jones gouge between the femoral head and the acetabulum and lever the head out of the socket rather than use conventional methods of dislocation by manipulating the limb (Figs. 12-18 and 12-19). External rotation at the time of dislocation must be avoided. The medullary canal of the femur is usually large, and fatty marrow may be easily curetted out. This curettage must be done to the level of hard bone, producing a large cavity requiring a greater amount of cement (similar to the acetabular component); if required, two doses of cement may be used (Fig. 13-20). The orientation of the femoral component in a very large (wide) medullary canal must be observed to avoid excessive varus or valgus orientation. Likewise, during polymerization of the cement in these types of medullary canals, the prosthesis must be held firmly without any movement, while the cement is polymerizing. Gentle handling of the limb during preparation and fixation of the femoral component is essential. Damage to the knee and especially the skin of the lower extremity is a common complication in these patients during the procedure.

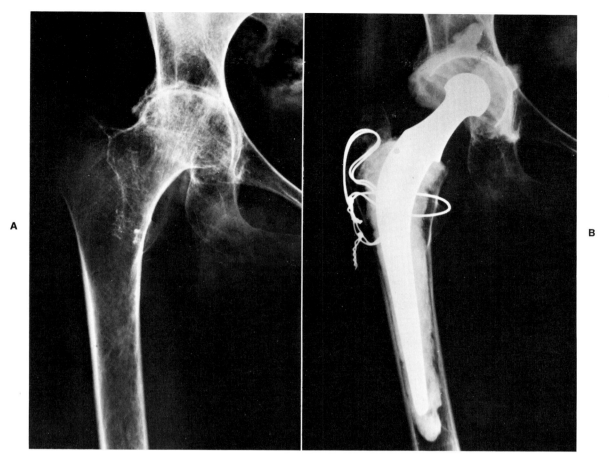

Fig. 13-20. A and **B,** Preoperative and postoperative low-friction arthroplasty, respectively, in 44-year-old female with advanced rheumatoid disease. NOTE: osteoporosis as evidenced by lack of bone trabeculi. Large medullary canal required two packs of cement. Preoperative grading of hip, C-left, 3,2,1; postoperative, C-6,4,6.

JUVENILE RHEUMATOID ARTHRITIS

In juvenile rheumatoid arthritis patients, the hips are small, and a "childlike" anatomy is present (Fig. 13-21). Additionally, bone is often osteoporotic, requiring particularly careful handling. Hip stiffness is often another complicating factor that may lead to catastrophies such as fracture of the femur or damage to the soft tissue when attempting to dislocate the hip. The soft tissue is extremely underdeveloped, thus preservation of the musculature of the hip is essential. The bones of the acetabulum and femur are severely dysplastic. Removal of the greater trochanter facilitates exposure and, especially, preparation of the femur.

Specifics of technique

Acetabular preparation should be done with curets and gouges if the conventional instruments (reamers) cannot be inserted. Reamers are used with care; expanding reamers are rarely used. The goal is to insert a small acetabular cup similar to a CDH cup. As in congenital dysplasia of the hip, damage to the floor of the acetabulum should be avoided. This can be achieved only by using a small socket in these cases, which often can be accommodated without the need for bone grafting (Fig. 13-22). To expose the upper end of the femur or the acetabulum to view, adductor tenotomy or iliopsoas tenotomy may be performed.

459

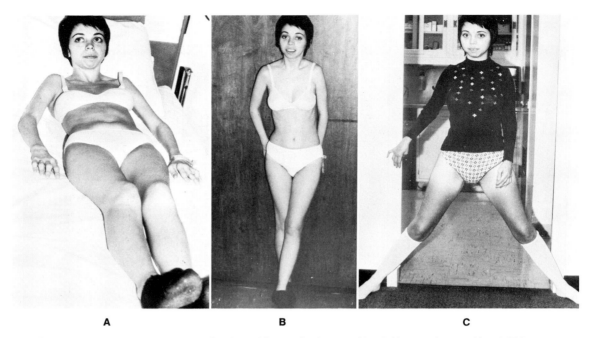

Fig. 13-21. A, "Childlike" anatomy of patient with juvenile rheumatoid arthritis must be considered. This 21-year-old female with juvenile rheumatoid arthritis was only able to get about with aid of two crutches. Bimalleolar separation was 2 inches because of severe adduction deformity bilaterally. In standing, preferred position was standing on one leg with further adduction of opposite leg, **B.** Following bilateral low-friction arthroplasty, range of motion was full bilaterally; patient's ability to abduct is demonstrated in **C.**

The most difficult aspect of the technique in these dysplastic hips is reaming the femoral canal. The cortex is thin and does not allow expansion in most instances. A narrow or especially "narrowed-down stem" is required. A careful preoperative x-ray measurement of the medullary canal is necessary to determine if modification of the existing prosthesis is necessary. Reaming with graded Küntscher reamers is useful in preparing these medullary canals (Fig. 13-23). (Also see Fig. 17-12.)

ANKYLOSING SPONDYLITIS

The problems of technique in ankylosing spondylitis include:

1. The presence of a severe deformity of the hip, for example, flexion, abduction or adduction
2. Severe stiffness, for example, often complete ankylosis
3. Severe osteoporosis
4. Young patients with a considerable demand in performance (when other joints are spared)
5. Anesthesia—specifically related to ankylosis of the temporomandibular joint as well as the cervical spine in addition to restricted chest expansion

Specifics of technique

To achieve exposure in these patients, removal of the greater trochanter is essential. The neck must be osteotomized in situ using a reciprocating or an oscillating saw as opposed to an osteotome, which may fracture the posterior or inferior neck.

Following the division of the neck, the hip must be adducted, and a complete soft tissue mobilization of the upper femur is necessary in order to view the site of the ankylosed head and the acetabulum. Exposure of the site of the acetabulum is essential to avoid the tendency to prepare the socket too high, leading to shortening or instability of the hip. (See Fig. 14-34.) If the hip is fixed in adduction, an adductor tenotomy may be necessary. The muscles about the hip are usually remarkably good and appear healthy.[3,10] The trochanter with the abductor mechanism must be mobilized to reach the lateral shaft for a good fixation. Soft tissue release must be done,

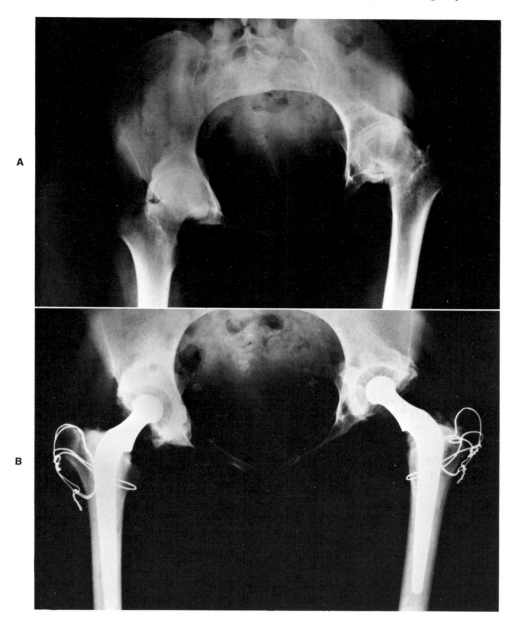

Fig. 13-22. Preoperative and postoperative radiographs of patient shown in Fig. 13-21. Rimless, 40 mm. outside diameter acetabular cups and extra-narrow straight stems were used. **A,** Ankylosis of both hips; preoperative grade was C-right, 5,2,1; left, 5,2,1. **B,** Postoperative grade 7 years following surgery: right, 6,6,6; left, 6,6,6. This patient has no other restricting factor.

accordingly, in order to overcome preexisting deformities (see Fig. 14-2). Severe preexisting flexion deformity, for example, at times requires shortening of the femur in order to achieve full extension. Obviously, this must be done only after verification of the status of the soft tissue causing flexion contractures. In other words, the release of soft tissue must precede the shortening of the femur. The acetabulum is prepared using conventional acetabular gouges to remove the femoral head piecemeal. When a cavity is created, then deepening and expanding reamers may be used in the conventional manner. Judicious use of the expanding reamers is of paramount importance in order to avoid damage to the pelvis (Fig. 13-24).

461

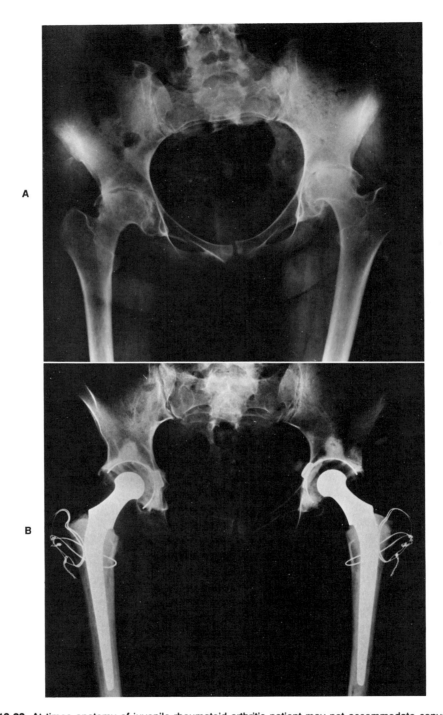

Fig. 13-23. At times anatomy of juvenile rheumatoid arthritis patient may not accommodate conventionally available prostheses, and special provisions must be made for these individuals. **A,** Preoperative radiograph of 23-year-old female with bilateral involvement of hips and severe disability, C-right, 2,2,1 and left, 2,2,1. **B,** Following bilateral low-friction arthroplasty within 2 weeks apart, hip grades at 4 years following surgery, right, 6,4,6, and left, 6,4,6. NOTE: straight narrow stem could not be accommodated in either hip. On both sides prosthesis was used in which stem was especially thinned down to accommodate narrow canal. Graded Küntscher reamers were used up to only 9 mm. prior to insertion of stem.

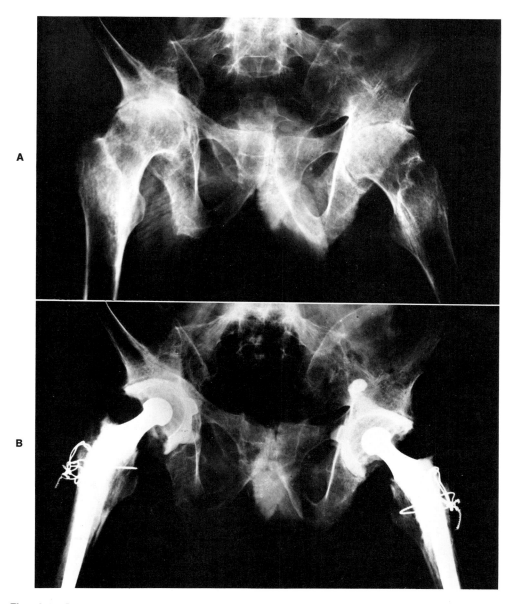

Fig. 13-24. Despite radiographic joint space in both hips in ankylosing spondylitis, dislocation may be impossible and retrograde removal of femoral heads may be necessary. **A,** Preoperative radiograph of 32-year-old banker with ankylosing spondylitis, preoperative grade C-right, 4,2,1 and left, 4,2,1; postoperative results C-right, 6,5,6; left, 6,5,6. **B,** Postoperative radiograph shown here is at 6 years following surgery. Patient was able to resume work full time following surgery. NOTE: socket demarcation of nonprogressive nature on right side and to lesser extent on left.

PROTRUSIO ACETABULI

The indications for surgery, the radiological morphology, and the etiology of protrusion of the acetabulum are discussed in Chapters 8 and 10. Technical details related to the handling of protrusion are further discussed in the section on rheumatoid arthritis.

Specifics of technique

Regardless of the etiology, there are several technical aspects of protrusion of the acetabulum that must be considered: (1) removal of the trochanter, (2) dislocation, (3) visual exposure of the acetabulum, (4) preservation and preparation of the acetabular floor, (5) fixation of the

463

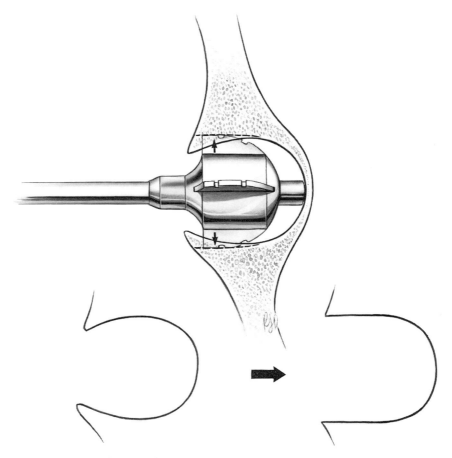

Fig. 13-25. Periphery of protusio acetabuli may be expanded by inserting expanding reamer into socket without drilling centering pilot hole, which should be avoided in these cases. Sharp curet used following expanding reamer is all that is needed to remove fibrocartilage from periphery and depth of this type of acetabuli.

acetabular component, (6) leg length discrepancy, and (7) the occasional need for bone grafts.

In removing the greater trochanter, a broad osteotome may be used in preference to a Gigli saw (see Fig. 12-15). Because the greater trochanter has shifted medially, its medial border is often in contact with the superior and lateral aspect of the acetabulum, thus difficulty is encountered in passing the cholecystectomy clamp to retrieve the Gigli saw. The abductor mechanism must be mobilized and retracted cephalad in order to see the periphery of the superior acetabulum. Dislocation may be difficult as the result of medial migration of the head, but usually adduction of the hip produces the head out of the socket after a complete conventional capsulotomy (see Chapter 12 and Figs. 12-18 and 12-19). Marginal osteophytes, which do not allow the

head to escape from the depth of the acetabulum, can be removed with an osteotome to facilitate head dislocation. No external rotation must be attempted prior to disengagement of the head from the socket.

Exposure of the acetabulum is facilitated by removal of any marginal osteophytes, which also permits the reamers and the cup to enter the acetabulum. As the acetabulum is often "barrel-shaped" with a narrow entrance and a large diameter at its depth, we have found it convenient to expand its periphery with the expanding reamer without drilling the centering pilot hole. This maneuver conveniently opens up the entry to the acetabulum for further preparation as needed (Fig. 13-25). A sharp curet or bone scraper is useful to remove the fibrocartilage from the periphery. The goal is to maximize fixation in the periphery of the acetabulum and con-

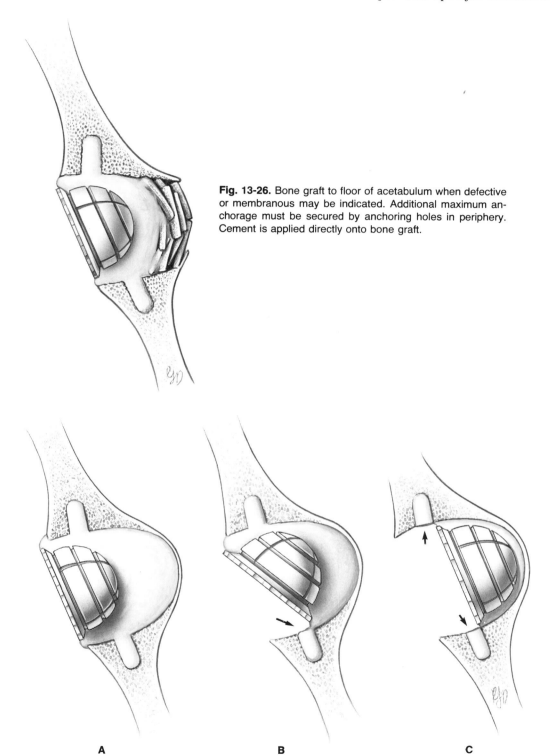

Fig. 13-26. Bone graft to floor of acetabulum when defective or membranous may be indicated. Additional maximum anchorage must be secured by anchoring holes in periphery. Cement is applied directly onto bone graft.

A   B   C

Fig. 13-27. A, For maximal fixation of acetabulum with cement, maximize anchoring holes in periphery and avoid deep penetration of socket into cement mass. **B,** Extra care is necessary to avoid problem shown here. Cup is pushed in somewhat horizontal plane (20 to 30 degrees to transaxis of pelvis), thus causing ischium anchor hole to become superficial in relation to edge of cup. **C,** Note discontinuity of cement between anchor holes; cement medial to cup is eliminated when cup is placed too deep.

465

serve the bone of the floor when the acetabulum is thin or defective. Removal of bone from the floor of the acetabulum and the use of conventional centering pilot holes must be avoided. The use of wire mesh is discouraged if the floor is intact and a good cortical thickness is present in the protruded segment of the acetabulum. A bone graft to the floor of the acetabulum (defective and membranous floors) may be indicated (Fig. 13-26) (see "Rheumatoid Arthritis" and Chapter 14). For maximal fixation of the acetabulum with cement, one must: (1) maximize anchoring holes in the periphery and avoid medial placement of the anchor holes; (2) avoid deep penetration of the socket into the cement mass (Fig. 13-27, *A*); and (3) use a stiffer cement than usual to avoid its early escape (squeeze) from the depth of the acetabulum. Often, the tendency is to push the socket too far medially too soon (Fig. 13-27, *C*). If the acetabular cup is set deeply in the protrusion, the continuity of the cement on the deep side of the acetabular component with the recessed holes made in the ilium, ischium, and pubis may be lost. This is especially true when the acetabular component is oriented in a somewhat horizontal plane, that is, 20 or 30 degrees in relation to the transaxis of the pelvis. It is important to take extra care in placing the anchor holes and in placing the acetabular component in relation to these holes to prevent the holes from becoming superficial in relation to the margin of the cup once it is set (Fig. 13-27, *B*).

One of the problems of medial migration or protrusion is often a weak and thin medial cortex, which is also brittle and hard.[17] This sclerotic bone sometimes does not allow good penetration of the methyl methacrylate, and therefore there is an increased risk of loosening of the acetabular component. Care must be taken to roughen the surface of hard cortical bone without fracturing the thin and brittle floor. Scoring of the bone is easily done with a small, sharp curet, or multiple small drill holes may enhance cement fixation. Fracture of the thin plate of the dense bone at the floor must be avoided. A proximally migrated protrusion (Fig. 13-28, *A*) is a serious problem, since the bone stock is inadequate inferiorly for lowering the socket, and at the time of insertion of the acetabular component the cup may assume a position higher than the level of the true acetabulum. This not only invites instability and possible dislocation, but it

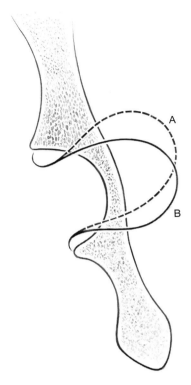

Fig. 13-28. Two modes of proximal, **A**, and transverse, **B**, appearance of protrusio acetabuli are shown. Proximally migrated protrusion is serious problem since bone stock is inadequate inferiorly for lowering of socket at time of insertion. It is advisable to protect floor of acetabulum in both cases and maximize fixation via periphery.

also shortens the extremity (Fig. 14-11). Additionally, if the prosthesis migrates too far proximally, it is possible that the continuity between the cement in the recess hole of the ischium and pubis and the cement in the region of the ilium will be lost. In this situation it is best to use two doses of cement, to pack the superior portion of the acetabulum well, and to make efforts to keep the level of the socket as low as possible (Fig. 14-11). It is occasionally advisable to use a wire mesh reinforcement, which may also assist in creating a floor. A special protrusion cup has been helpful in keeping the socket superficial in a severely damaged and deep acetabulum, resulting from previous surgery (see Chapter 14). The clearance between the upper end of the femur and the rim of the acetabulum must be assured, otherwise the periphery of the acetabulum will act as a fulcrum, causing dislocation. This is especially true if the acetabular cup is placed too deep within the dome of the protruded floor. A bone graft to a defective and membra-

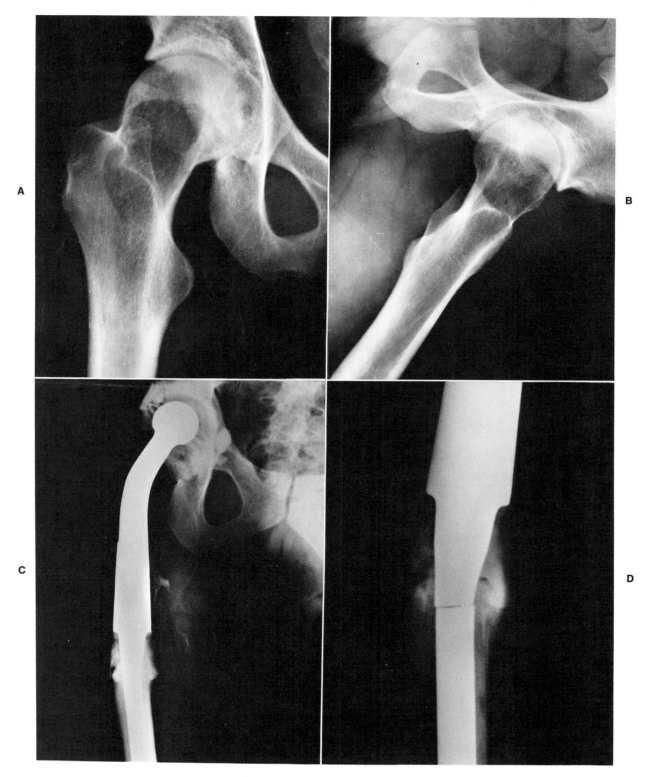

Fig. 13-29. A and **B,** Preoperative radiographs of right hip of 26-year-old man with giant cell tumor of upper femur with breakage through posterior cortex into soft tissue. **C,** One year following surgery by segmental resection of upper femur owing to invasiveness of tumor and its invasion of acetabular region. **D,** Fracture of stem at junction of "resection segment" and remainder of shaft. *Continued.*

467

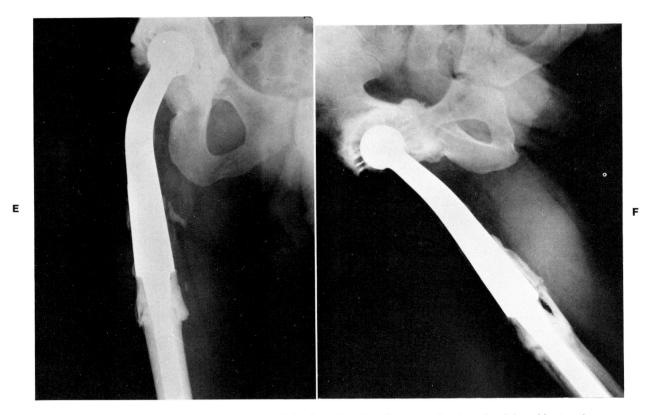

E   F

Fig. 13-29, cont'd. E and **F,** Three months following reinsertion of new prosthesis and revision of fractured stem. NOTE: dimensions of stem inserted within medullary canal were largest possible. Patient's age and vigor undoubtedly have contributed in addition to mechanical situation leading to breakage of first stem.

nous floor is indicated. The bone graft may be obtained from the ipsilateral ilium or the femoral head removed at surgery may be used.

Leg length discrepancy often accompanying protrusio acetabuli may be improved by using a long-neck prosthesis, providing reduction is feasible after insertion of the femoral prosthesis and abductors can conveniently reach the site of reattachment to the shaft.

BONE TUMORS

Certain primary and metastatic lesions about the pelvis and upper femur may be treated by total hip replacement (see Chapter 8). The location of the tumor, the extensiveness of the destructive lesion involving the hip joint, the extent of the soft tissue involvement about the hip, the nature of the tumor, its invasiveness, and the modes of treatment available must all be appraised prior to reaching a decision regarding replacement. Naturally, the most important consideration is the proper oncological treatment of the lesion. With careful selection of patients for this procedure, certain low-grade sarcomas such as chondrosarcoma, fibrosarcoma, and periosteal osteogenic sarcoma may lend themselves favorably to local en bloc resection. A giant cell tumor with low-grade malignancy may also be treated by this method (Fig. 13-29) as well as a reticulum cell sarcoma, solitary myeloma, and pigmented villonodular synovitis. There is less concern if the proposed segmental resection is palliative than when it is definitive. In the former category, the patient is usually older or the life expectancy is short; on the other hand, when the tumor is benign, the patient is young, and a permanent cure is expected, the concern is the demand of the young person on the use of the artificial hip joint (Fig. 13-29).

Primary tumors about the hip that may indicate total hip replacement include lesions that are in the upper end of the femur and have infiltrated the region of the pelvis. Tumors of the upper femur are either in the head and neck, the trochanteric region, or the subtrochanteric areas. Tumors located in the head and the neck or within the intertrochanteric line may lend themselves to conventional total hip replacement, and the basic technique involved is no different from conventional operations. This type of replacement most often may be done in cases of pathological fracture of the neck of the femur; that is, metastatic lesions, where considerable osteoporosis is present in the acetabulum, and simple prosthetic replacement and cement fixation are feared because of the possibility of proximal migration of the replaced femoral prosthesis into the acetabulum.

The most challenging area of replacement is the location of the tumor in the subtrochanteric region below the level of the lesser trochanter, when the tumor has invaded local soft tissue including the adductors, flexors, occasionally the extensors, and the greater trochanter. In this situation replacement by a special "segmental-type" prosthesis will be necessary. The abductor mechanism may have to be partly removed and stability for the joint provided by adequate "spacing" with careful selection of the length of the segment between the upper end of the femur and the pelvis. In addition to the problem of instability as the result of resected soft tissue, fixation of the prosthesis to the remainder of the bone below the level of the isthmus and the stability of the prosthesis itself are problems to be considered.

Specifics of technique

The following must be given consideration:
1. Adequate exposure and soft tissue resection
2. Respect for the principles of tumor surgery
3. Level of resection of the femur
4. Accurate measurement of the resected segment and spacing by a "segmental prosthesis"
5. Transfer of the abductors to the tensor fascia femoris
6. Postoperative care

Exposure is required not only for total hip replacement but for a successful tumor surgery. A "goblet" or T-shaped incision may be used in order to provide access to the front and back of the joint and the soft tissue for en bloc resection. The proximal limb of the incision is directed and spanned between the anterosuperior iliac spine to the ischium; the distal limb of the T-shaped

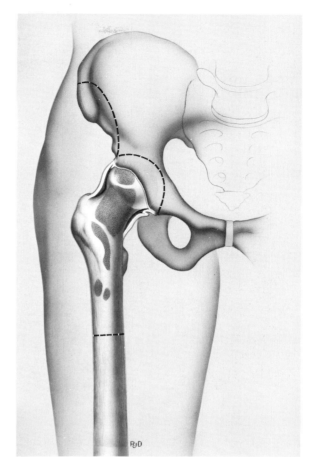

Fig. 13-30. Pathology of upper femur, showing extent of tumor invasion. Dotted lines illustrate segments of bone to be resected in conjunction with replacement. Same hip as shown in Fig. 13-29.

incision bisects the proximal limb at the midportion and extends for 2 to 3 inches distal to the level of the lesion. Following resection of the soft tissue by dissecting around the lesion on the femur, the hip joint is then dislocated and the proximal end of the femur is removed as distally as needed. The level of resection of the femur is determined by radiological assessment of the tumor invasion of the bone, which is confirmed at surgery by histological examination of the tissue to assure the proper level of the resection (Fig. 13-30).

For the measurement of the segment to be replaced, an "adjustable" prosthesis such as one designed by Charnley (with perforations on the outer aspect) may be used. Alternatively, preoperative x-ray examination may determine the

469

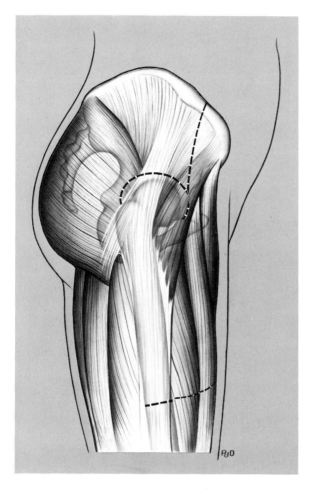

Fig. 13-31. Soft tissue resected segment with bony tumor shown in Figs. 13-29 and 13-30.

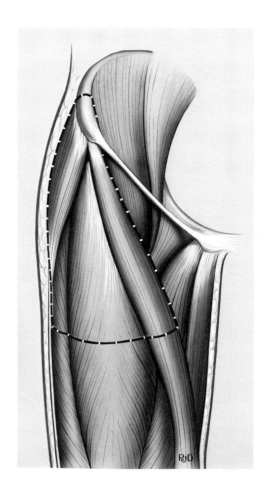

Fig. 13-32. Anterior aspect of hip. Dotted line illustrates extent of soft tissue accompanying resected bone based on invasion of tumor anteriorly.

length of the segment to be replaced and the segmental prosthesis selected accordingly. It should be recognized that a large margin of normal tissue must be removed en bloc with the tumor and often includes the adductor muscles, the vastus lateralis, psoas, short external rotators, glutei, and a portion of the gluteus medius and maximus (Figs. 13-31 and 13-32). Removed muscles and complete capsulectomy both contribute to the instability of these joints; it is therefore of paramount importance that the "spacing" and the length of the segment be determined carefully at surgery in order to prevent postoperative dislocation (Fig. 13-33).

Restoration of abduction power is principally through the tensor fascia femoris and by reattachment of the remainder of the abductor muscle onto the iliotibial tract and a tight imbricated

closure of the enveloping fascia of the thigh (Fig. 13-33). Insertion of more than two drainage system Hemovacs may be needed in different layers of the wound. A good hemostasis is necessary. The fascia must be closed with the hip in maximum abduction, producing a tight fascia when the hip is adducted postoperatively. This augments the stability of the joint.

Postoperative care

Characteristically, two types of problems are inherent in this type of replacement: (1) immediate dislocation postoperatively because of musculature removed from the upper end of the femur and (2) loosening and fracture of the stem of the prosthesis in young and active individuals whose medullary canal does not allow insertion of a large-sized prosthesis at the distal end of the

470

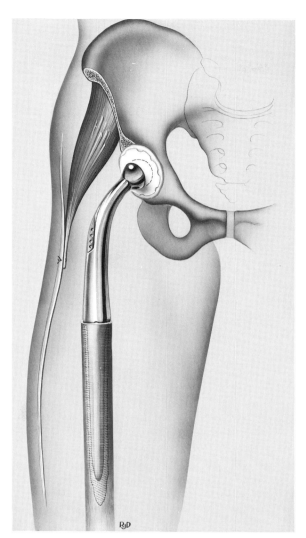

Fig. 13-33. Implanted segmental prosthesis following resection of upper femur, acetabulum, and portion of ilium as well as muscle groups as shown in Figs. 13-31 and 13-32. NOTE: remainder of gluteus medius and minimus is sutured to tensor fascia femoris to provide stability for hip joint.

femur. These young and vigorous patients subject the prosthesis to enormous wear and tear (Fig. 13-29). It is important that during the first 6 weeks postoperatively the hips are protected by either a hip spica cast or a balanced suspension apparatus to keep the hip in an abduction position. Further rehabilitation is cautiously undertaken. Following this, ongoing use of a cane (for life) may be a sensible approach in view of the difficulties in obtaining a good fixation of the stem and the dimensions of the prosthesis.

PRODUCTIVE OSTEOARTHRITIS IN MALES

This group typically includes large, bony men, with productive osteoarthritis as manifested by x-ray examination, who generally show coxa magna senilis at surgery. Their weight is usually over 170 lb., and at surgery they demonstrate a very large acetabulum corresponding to the large size of the femoral head. Radiologically, often an upper pole type III osteoarthrosis with a broken Shenton's line (see Chapter 10) is demonstrated. In addition to marked external rotation deformity, they exhibit one or more inches of shortening, and often some degree of adduction deformity of the hip is present. It is of incidental interest that these patients usually form heterotopic bone postoperatively (see Chapter 16). Because there are several unique features of surgical management by total hip arthroplasty in this group, some technical details should be considered.

Specifics of technique

1. Removal of the greater trochanter
2. Acetabular exposure
3. Lowering of the socket level
4. Stabilization of the hip and equalization of the leg length
5. Avoidance of impingement
6. Augmentation and protection of the trochanteric fixation

Because of marked external rotation deformity, the greater trochanter has reached the posterior wall of the acetabulum and its removal may be difficult, requiring the use of an osteotome (see Chapter 12). Removal of the greater trochanter is essential in these cases because of the large volume of the total abductor muscle mass, which would otherwise be damaged and difficult to retract without osteotomy of the trochanter.

To expose the acetabulum it is best to use pin retractors to be able to see the superior lip and the roof of the acetabulum to prepare the socket and provide complete coverage for the socket.

Capsular excision should be restricted, especially from the superior portion of the joint medial to the abductor muscles. The inferior capsule may have to be resected in order to allow exposure of the inferior portion of the acetabulum. Large marginal inferoposterior and anterior osteophytes are common. They may be extensive, reaching the area of the acetabular fossa, covering the "pulvinar."

The site of preparation of the socket is best de-

471

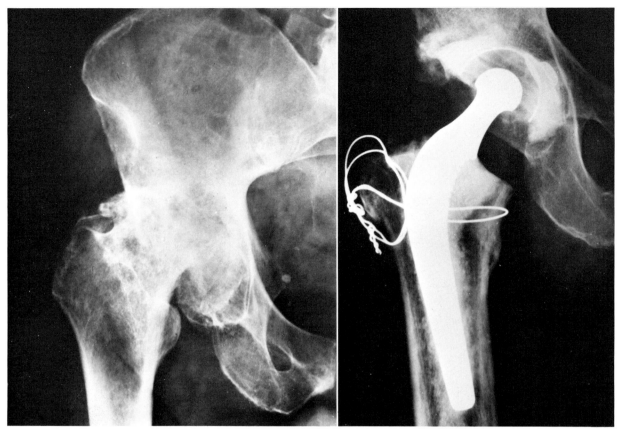

Fig. 13-34. Productive osteoarthritis in male with large skeleton requires special preparation of socket and femur. **A,** Preoperative x-ray film of degenerative osteoarthritis in 64-year-old man weighing 180 pounds. NOTE: large medullary canal and marginal osteophyte formation as well as external rotation deformity of hip. **B,** Postoperative x-ray film illustrating satisfactory replacement by lowering socket level with wedge segment of cement in outer margin between cup and acetabulum. NOTE: removal of inferior marginal osteophyte as well as valgus orientation of stem within shaft. Valgus is somewhat exaggerated, but note size of medullary canal in proportion to extra-large stem of Charnley low-friction arthroplasty used in this case (see text).

termined by radiographic template preoperatively (see Chapter 10). If one places the "pilot hole," using a centering device, transversely (parallel to the transaxis of the pelvis), this automatically lowers the socket, and reamers will subsequently prepare the acetabulum in a horizontal manner (Fig. 12-25). In doing so, the expanding reamer may not reach the roof of the acetabulum, and cartilage and subchondral bone have to be curetted out of this area as an independent process (Fig. 13-34). A standard-sized cup may be used if the preparation is correctly accomplished, so there is no need for expanding the entire acetabulum. By using a standard size acetabular socket, the bone of the pelvis is conserved. Following cement fixation of the cup,

efforts are made for complete clearance between the marginal osteophytes of the acetabulum and the upper neck of the femur, accomplished by removing the osteophytes with a Watson-Jones gouge and an osteotome. Fig. 13-35 illustrates the lowered position of the socket within the site of the acetabulum. A segment of the cup is covered by the cavity created in the floor of the bony acetabulum and a segment by the roof of the old acetabulum. The bone supporting the wedge segment of cement is specially prepared, using a scraper to remove cartilage and multiple drill holes to enhance the fixation.

Preparation of the femur in these patients requires special attention because of the large medullary canal, which at times may be two to

472

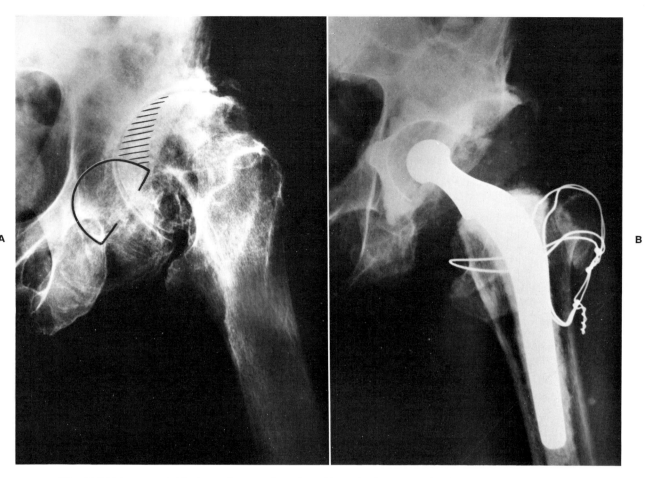

Fig. 13-35. Two essential features of surgery in patient with productive osteoarthrosis and large bony skeleton are demonstrated in this case. **A,** Site of preparation of acetabulum and its relationship to teardrop and obturator foramen. NOTE: large marginal osteophyte present in this individual. Marked external rotation of femur and lateral subluxation in addition to proximal migration of head should be observed. **B,** Replacement following lowering of socket. NOTE: lateral portion of acetabulum is supported by cement, which in turn is supported by outer segment of old acetabulum (shaded area in **A**).

three times the normal size. This may place the orientation of the stem in jeopardy, and careless cementing may result in an excessive valgus or varus orientation of the stem in the canal. At the test rehearsal, the femoral prosthesis is held within the medullary canal manually, while observing its relationship to the neck at the time of reduction. Excessive valgus orientation of the femoral stem inside the shaft may create instability (a portion of the femoral head remains uncovered by the acetabular cup); on the other hand, an excessive varus orientation may result in shortening of the distance between the femoral head and the cup, leading also to instability of the joint. Selection of a prosthesis with a large offset (distance between the femoral head and

the axis of the shaft) is preferred in these cases so that the head will reach the depth of the socket without being levered out by the margin of the acetabulum (see Chapters 3 and 17).

The greater trochanter requires careful handling. It is important to mobilize the trochanter and achieve maximum bone contact between the trochanter and the outer side of the femur. Use of supplemental screws or trochanteric staples is advisable in heavy muscular men with large bones. Excessive early postoperative flexion or positional external rotation must be avoided.

■ ■ ■

All details are considered essential. This chapter is not summarized.

473

REFERENCES

1. Arden, G. P., and Ansell, B. M.: Total hip replacement in inflammatory arthritis. In Jayson, M., editor: Total hip replacement, Philadelphia, 1971, J. B. Lippincott Co., pp. 86-102.
2. Barry, H. C.: Fractures of the femur in Paget's disease of bone in Australia, J. Bone Joint Surg. **49A:**1359-1370, 1957.
3. Bisla, R. S., Ranawat, C. S., and Inglis, A. E.: Total hip replacement in patients with ankylosing spondylitis with involvement of the hip, J. Bone Joint Surg. **58A**(2):233-238, March, 1976.
4. Charnley, J., and Cupic, Z.: The nine and ten year results of the low friction arthroplasty of the hip, Clin. Ortho. **95:**9-25, 1973.
5. Charnley, J., and Feagin, J. A.: Low friction arthroplasty in congenital subluxation of the hip, Clin. Ortho. **91:**98-113, 1973.
6. Chiari, K.: Medial displacement osteotomy of the pelvis, Clin. Orthop. **98:**55-71, 1974.
7. Coventry, M. B.: Total hip arthroplasty in the adult with complete congenital dislocation. In The Hip Society: The hip, proceedings of the fourth open scientific meeting of The Hip Society, 1976, St. Louis, 1976, The C. V. Mosby Co., pp. 77-87.
8. Dunn, H. K., and Hess, W. E.: Total hip reconstruction in chronically dislocated hips, J. Bone Joint Surg. **58A:**838-845, 1976.
9. Eftekhar, N. S., and Roy, D.: Diphosphenates in treatment of Paget's disease (unpublished data).
10. Eftekhar, N. S., and Stinchfield, F. E.: Experience with low friction arthroplasty, a statistical review of early results and complications, Clin. Orthop. **95:**60-68, 1973.
11. Grundy, M.: Fractures of the femur in Paget's disease of bone. Their etiology and treatment, J. Bone Joint Surg. **52B:**252-263, 1970.
12. Harris, W. H.: Total hip replacement for congenital dysplasia of hip; technique. In The Hip Society: The hip, proceedings of the second open scientific meeting of The Hip Society, 1974, St. Louis, 1974, The C. V. Mosby Co., pp. 251-265.
13. Harris, W. H., and Crothers, O. D.: Autogenous bone grafting using the femoral head to correct severe acetabular deficiency for total hip replacement. In The Hip Society: The hip, proceedings of the fourth open scientific meeting of The Hip Society, 1976, St. Louis, 1976, The C. V. Mosby Co., pp. 161-185.
14. Hass, J.: Congenital dislocation of the hip, Springfield, Ill., 1951, Charles C Thomas, Publisher.
15. Jackson, C. T.: The results of low friction arthroplasty of the hip performed in Paget's disease, Internal Publication No. 47, Centre for Hip Surgery, Wrightington Hospital, England, January, 1974.
16. Lazansky, M. G.: Low friction arthroplasty for the sequelae of congenital and developmental disease. In American Academy of Orthopaedic Surgeons: Instructional course lectures, vol. 23, St. Louis, 1974, The C. V. Mosby Co., pp. 194-200.
17. Salvati, E. A., Bullough, P., and Wilson, P. D.: Intrapelvic protrusion of the acetabular component following total hip replacement, Clin. Orthop. **III:** 212-227, 1975.
18. Stauffer, R. N., and Sim, F. H.: The total hip arthroplasty in Paget's disease of the hip, J. Bone Joint Surg. **58A**(4):476-478, June, 1975.
19. Stinchfield, F. E.: Discussion, Ann. Surg. **174:** 662, 1971.
20. Tronzo, R. G., and Okin, E. M.: Anatomic restoration of congenital hip dysplasia in adulthood by total hip replacement, Clin. Orthop. **106:**94-98, 1975.
21. Welch, R. B., and Charnley, J.: Low friction arthroplasty of the hip in rheumatoid arthritis and ankylosing spondylitis, Clin. Orthop. **72:**22-32, 1970.

CHAPTER 14

Revision arthroplasty for failed previous surgery

There is no situation so complicated which cannot be made more complicated.
ALEXANDER GARCIA

This chapter deals with hips that have undergone previous surgery and, because of unsuccessful results, need further reconstruction. These failures may be due to immediate complications of previous surgeries, such as failed fracture fixation, or they may be due to pain resulting from failure of previous operations. Revision arthroplasty for the following operations will be discussed in detail: failed endoprosthesis, failed cup arthroplasty, failed osteotomy and fracture fixation, failed arthrodesis, failed pseudarthrosis, and failed total hip replacement.

Several problems specific to this group of patients and common in all types of revision for failed surgery deserve comment.

Social and psychological aspects

Failure of one or more previous operations makes these patients generally fearful and undermines their confidence in further surgery since the proposed surgery is usually of greater magnitude, and, in view of previous disappointments, they are very doubtful regarding future recovery. This is especially true in those patients whose operations were complicated by thromboembolic disease, since such a complication may be life-threatening should it occur again. Multiple hospitalizations, which often exhaust finances, further complicate the problem. Finally, total hip replacement becomes especially difficult technically after previous operations and makes the patient prone to a higher incidence of complications and infection. In some there is a feeling of guilt (in which case they are sympathetic with their surgeons), while in some there is a deep-seated hostility that may not even be apparent at first but reveals itself as further treatment is carried out.

Technical problems

Revision surgery is especially prone to technical pitfalls related to distorted anatomy, scars, ectopic bone, and joint stiffness.[8,9,12,13] Osteoporosis from disuse increases the potential risk of fracturing the femur during surgery. Damage to the shaft of the femur and acetabulum is a potential risk because of these combined anatomical problems (see Chapters 16 and 17). These patients also are more prone to postoperative instability and dislocations (see Chapter 17). Unless the preoperative state of the hip is carefully evaluated, there will be a higher rate of infection than with a primary intervention; there is also a considerably higher percentage of positive cultures obtained in revision cases than "virgin" hips (see Chapter 16). Trochanteric nonunions and other technical complications are also more common (by far) in these cases than primary operations.

Careful preparation is essential.[1,3,9,19] This includes having a radiographic machine or image intensification available in the operating room in anticipation of any complication, such as fracture, and also provision for adequate blood transfusion. The preoperative evaluation of radiographs is of paramount importance (especially in the case of displaced osteotomy) to verify the amount of angulation and displacement in two planes. Every effort must be made to rule out the possibility of preexisting infection.

The precise and "generous incision" length is of primary importance in revision operations. Because of one or more previous incision scars, the surgeon may have difficulty in choosing an optimum incision site and obtaining adequate exposure. In our experience, previous scars are best ignored and the new incision placed at the most favorable site. We have not encountered healing problems as the result of crossing the old scars about the hip, regardless of their direction or shape and design (Fig. 14-1). The surgeon must take care to remove previously inserted internal fixation devices or prostheses without damaging the shaft of the femur or the acetabulum. Mobilization of the upper femur and complete division of the structures in the medial aspect of the upper femur to the level below the lesser trochanter is essential in most instances; not only must the posterior, medial, and inferior capsule and capsular adhesions be severed, but the iliopsoas and the hip adductors must also be released if necessary. The hip is mobilized to the extent that the ipsilateral heel may easily reach the opposite shoulder by maximum flexion, adduction, and external rotation; to obtain this exposure it is important to find and detach all contracted structures at their points of attachment to the upper femur (Fig. 14-2). Adductor tenotomy is performed during or at the end of the procedure as illustrated in Fig. 14-3.

The lateral approach with removal of the greater trochanter is indispensable to aid the visual accessibility of the anatomy without damage to the osseous structures in these cases.[6,7,15] The need for trochanteric osteotomy is agreed upon even by those surgeons who do not routinely remove the trochanter. A slightly larger portion of the greater trochanter than in standard operations must be removed (Fig. 14-4) and then carefully reattached as distally as possible to enhance the stability of the hip joint, since these hips are generally more prone to dislocation (Fig. 14-5). Further immobilization

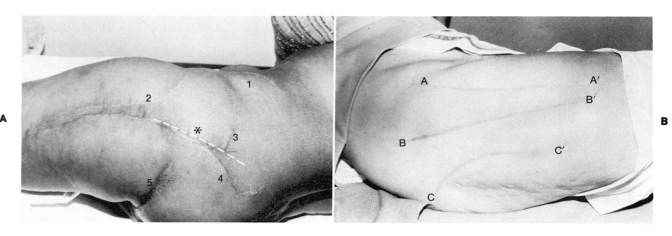

Fig. 14-1. A, Multiple scars of previous operations about left hip of 38-year-old female, whose last two operations included insertion and revision of total hip arthroplasty. Scars have been numbered to indicate each operation. NOTE: in all operations wound healed without skin necrosis. * Indicates proper site of incision used to revise fourth operation. **B,** Common revision operations for revision of failed endoprosthesis following failed fracture fixation. Usually incision for insertion of prosthesis is posterior, C to C′, and insertion of nail anterolateral, A to A′. Most suitable line of incision for transtrochanteric approach is one shown here, B to B′. Anterior and posterior incisions should be disregarded and appropriate line of incision, B to B′, made to provide maximum exposure. Middle line, B to B′, was used for total hip arthroplasty.

Fig. 14-2. Mobilization of upper femur following dislocation and removal of head. Hip is mobilized to extent that ipsilateral heel may easily reach opposite shoulder (inset) by maximum flexion, adduction, and external rotation. To obtain this exposure it is important to find and detach all contracted structures at their attachment to upper femur as shown here (dotted line). Inset illustrates position of limb at completion of release and delivery of stump of femur out of wound.

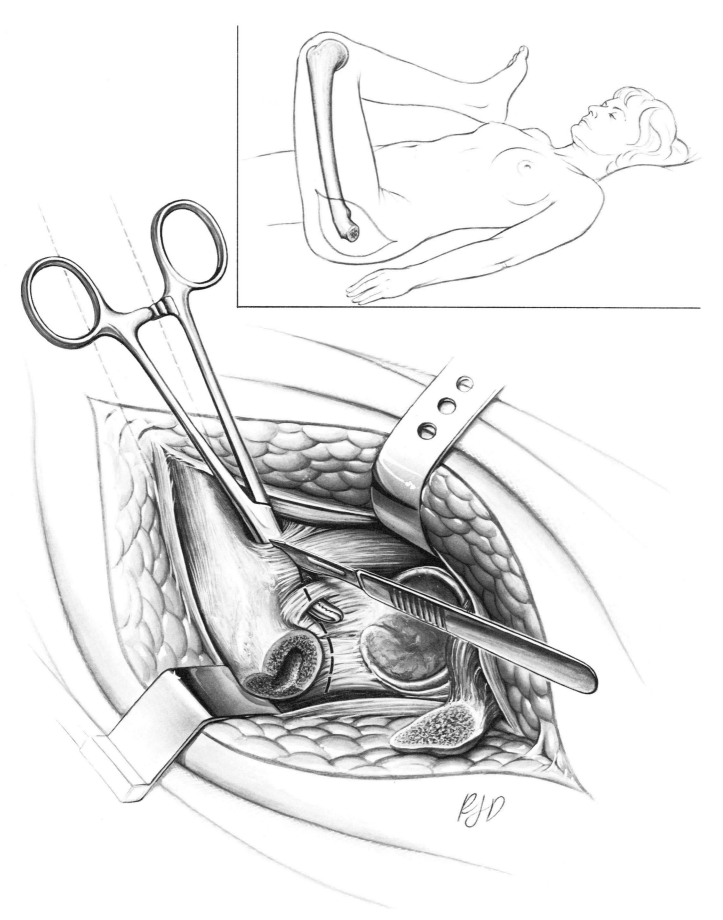

Fig. 14-2. For legend see opposite page.

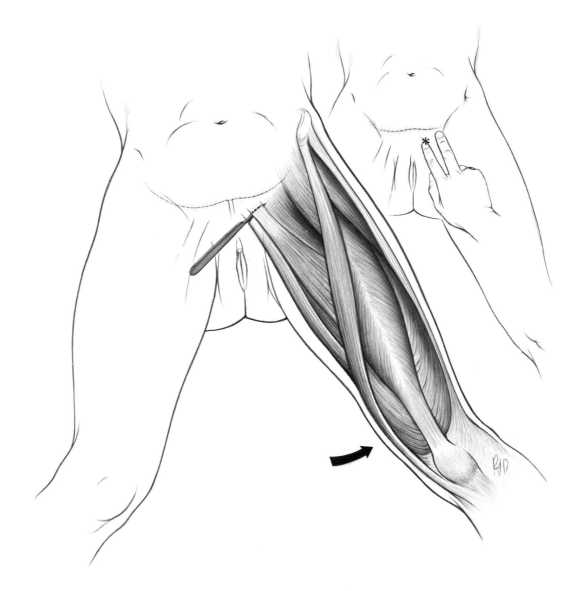

Fig. 14-3. Position of hip at time of adductor tenotomy. NOTE: adductor longus and major portion of adductor brevis can be made prominent by maximal abduction of hip. Tenotomy is done as close to bone as possible using tenotome knife percutaneously. Inset shows surgeon's index and middle fingers pressing skin to make tendon become prominent. * Indicates pubic tubercle.

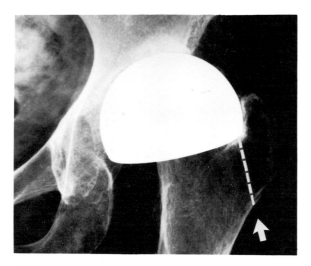

Fig. 14-4. In revision surgery larger than conventional size greater trochanteric segment must be removed. Vastus lateralis ridge is important landmark, but osteotomy site must be distal to ridge. Trochanteric osteotomy must be performed with osteotome as indicated in Fig. 12-16. Arrow points to proper site of osteotomy.

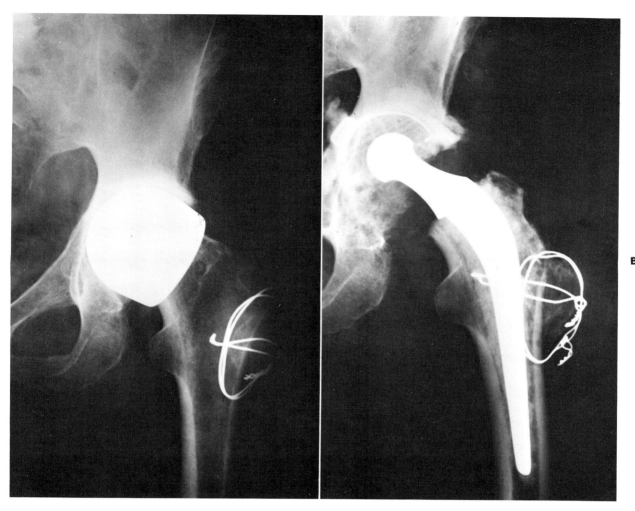

Fig. 14-5. In revision surgery abductor mechanism may have been elongated or scarified. **A,** Marked distal transplantation of greater trochanter following cup arthroplasty. Reattachment of greater trochanter must be attempted as distally as possible to enhance stability of hip joint since these hips are generally more prone to dislocation than in primary operations. **B,** Further distal transplantation of trochanter was necessary to achieve stability at surgery in this case (7½ year postoperative radiograph).

by a balanced suspension apparatus or by a hip spica cast may be necessary when marked instability is present at surgery (Chapter 17).

Preparation of the acetabulum and the femur deserves extra time and effort: The bone of the acetabulum is often sclerotic following the removal of the implant, so it needs careful scraping and eburnation. The medullary canal of the femur likewise is not usually a suitable site for fixation if it has been violated by previous surgery. In revision of failed total hip replacement, testing for loosening of the components is done by direct pressure onto the prosthetic device and observing the blood or froth expressed at the interface between cement and bone. A complete visualization is essential. The entire periphery of the bony acetabulum must be exposed using a blunt instrument; the cup is tilted in several directions while observing the interface. A similar testing is done to identify the femoral loosening, which is usually less difficult to detect (Fig. 14-6). Minor loosening should not be ignored. The acetabular cup must be revised in "questionable situations."

One prosthesis that is especially suited for most types of revision has a straight stem, which can be inserted even when the neck of the femur is absent. In revision cases, the neck of the

479

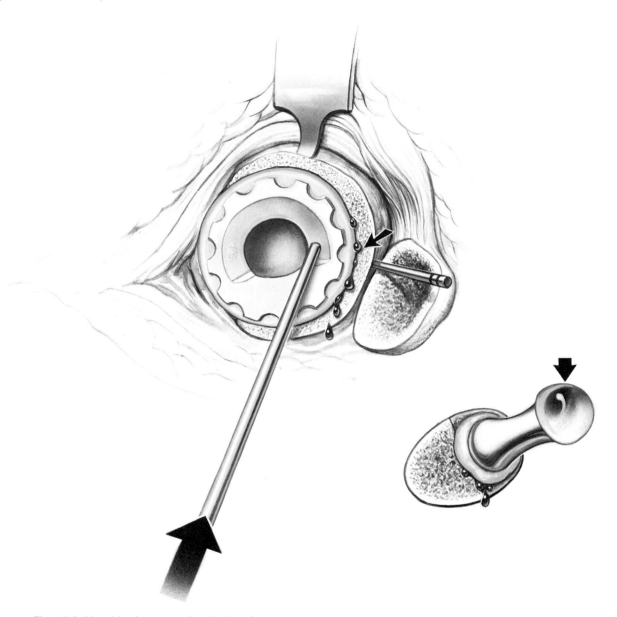

Fig. 14-6. Note blood expressed at the interface between cement and bone in testing prosthetic cup and femoral prosthesis. Full exposure of cement-bone interface is essential.

femur is often short or absent, that is, absorbed or removed at previous surgery, and the shaft begins at or just above the level of the lesser trochanter. A spiral fracture of the femoral shaft is a common complication in revision surgery; it is usually due to a hasty removal of the previous prosthesis without adequate mobilization of the upper femur (Fig. 17-5). This can easily be prevented if the upper end of the femur is complete-

ly avulsed from the wall of the pelvis to allow the surgeon to directly appreciate the axis of the femur while removing the intramedullary stem of the previous prosthesis. Since it is advantageous to preserve length in the limb where excessive shortening is a result of previous operations, the natural course of action would be to use a prosthesis with a long neck. However, equalization by this extreme method should be avoided, as one then loses the opportunity of advancing the greater trochanter to ensure good lateral fixation of the trochanter to the femoral shaft. In other words, a slight shortening in favor of better advancement of the adductor mechanism and proper attachment of the trochanter is acceptable. Every effort must be made to remove all of the cement interposed between the site of the removed trochanter (trochanteric bed) and the trochanter itself to facilitate a better union (see Chapter 17); if a satisfactory trochanteric reattachment has been unsuccessful by conventional means, we strongly advise extending postoperative immobilization with an abduction splint for 2 to 3 weeks and protective crutch walking for the first 6 to 12 weeks postoperatively. Alternatively, a unilateral hip spica cast may be applied.

In the following sections, the specifics of the clinical and technical problems related to the revision of different operations will be discussed.

REVISION OF FAILED ENDOPROSTHESIS

With the exception of revision of a failed total hip replacement, revision of a failed endoprosthesis is the most difficult conversion operation. Problems that arise include difficulty in dislocating the prosthesis as a result of its protrusion into the pelvis and/or ectopic bone formation. Fibrous or bony growth in the fenestration presents an added disadvantage of the Moore self-locking prosthesis during extraction. Because of the growth of abnormal bone and fibrous tissue in the medullary canal and the formation of the cul-de-sac at the tip of the femoral prosthesis, cement fixation may be jeopardized. Above all, diagnosing a low-grade infection in a failed endoprosthesis is sometimes impossible (see Chapter 16). Removal of the cement from the shaft in cemented endoprostheses requires deliberate effort to avoid damage to the shaft.

To counter these problems, one must pay strict attention to the technical details, which include: (1) removal of all scar tissue and ectopic bone for good visual exposure, (2) mobilization of the upper femur, and (3) careful dislocation (without forceful external rotation) to avoid fractures. The fenestration bone of the Moore self-locking prosthesis must be removed; curettage of the fibrous canal must be complete, and special attention to the preparation of the socket is mandatory, as medial or proximal migration

wears the medial wall of the acetabulum quite thin. Lengthening the extremity with a longer neck prosthesis is only indicated when instability is noted at reduction. Overenthusiasm for gain in length may place the fixation and union of the trochanter in jeopardy. Because of the problem of instability coupled with a distal attachment of the trochanter, a longer period of immobilization may be indicated.

Technical modifications in the revision of a failed endoprosthesis include:
1. Removal of the trochanter and exposure of the hip
2. Extraction of the prosthesis
3. Preparation of the acetabulum
4. Preparation of the femur

Removal of trochanter and exposure of hip

Because the prosthesis is usually sunk into the shaft of the femur, the greater trochanter appears larger with its tip close to the acetabular roof; the proper size to be removed must be assessed by the study of the radiographs (Fig. 14-7). During exploration of the hip the fascia must be fully mobilized. Because most prostheses have been inserted through a posterior approach, the interval between the tensor fascia femoris and the abductors is readily identifiable, but thick scar tissue should be entered by a sharp incision with a scalpel or an electric cutting knife down to the neck of the prosthesis. The cholecystectomy clamp is placed at the junction between the prosthetic neck and the medial aspect of the greater trochanter as a "target" to identify the junction of the trochanter and the top of the prosthesis. With the lower extremity in 20 to 30 degrees internal rotation and slight adduction, the trochanter is osteotomized at the level of the vastus lateralis ridge with a broad osteotome (5 cm. wide), which will prevent fracture (Figs. 12-23 and 14-7). To prevent fragmentation also, the osteotomy must be completed before attempting to retract the trochanter cephalad. Maximizing exposure by removal of the posterior scar tissue and mobilizing the femur by removing all scar tissue and the pseudocapsule from its periphery allows visual exposure of the head of the prosthesis to take place. Here, if ectopic bone has bridged between the femoral neck, trochanter, and acetabulum, it must be removed (Fig. 16-23). Dislocation of the prosthesis is accomplished without any external rotation. With maximum adduction, a Watson-

Fig. 14-7. Failed Moore self-locking prosthesis in 80-year-old man (otherwise in good health) requiring revision. **A,** Note marked proximal displacement of greater trochanter and distal migration of prosthesis to level of below lesser trochanter. Larger than conventional sized trochanter should be removed, but proper site of osteotomy must be determined by review of radiographs. **B,** Note use of long-neck prosthesis and interlocking of greater trochanter to lateral aspect of femur. Large-sized fragment of greater trochanter is necessary for good subsequent reattachment. Bed from which trochanter is removed also allows removal of bone from fenestration.

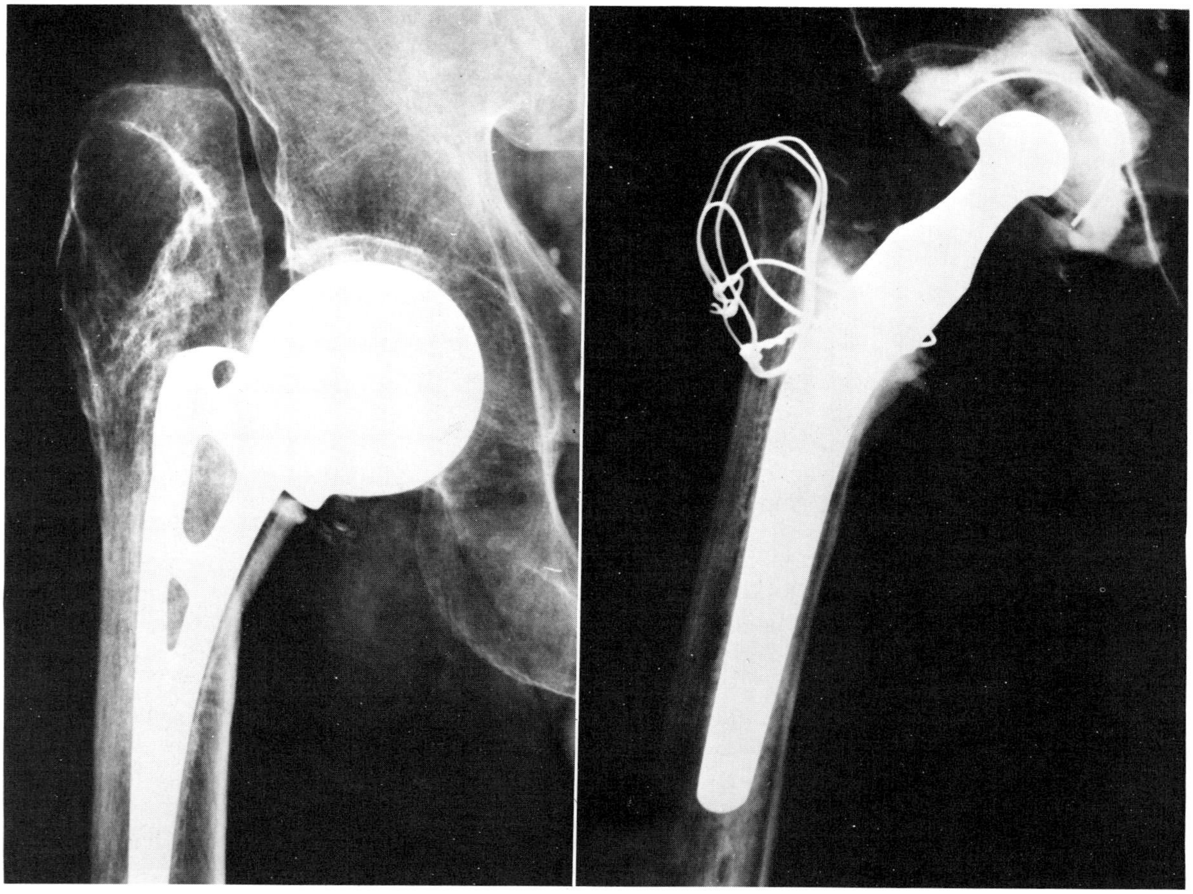

Jones skid is inserted between the head of the prosthesis and the acetabulum, and the head is levered out of the socket (Fig. 12-19). It is essential to avoid external rotation at the time of dislocation to prevent a fracture of the femur (see Chapter 17).

Extraction of prosthesis

Mobilization of the upper femur is a fundamental step prior to removal of the prosthesis and may include iliopsoas tenotomy and release of the short rotator to deliver the upper end of the femur into the wound. The bone and fibrous tissue from the fenestrations are removed through the bed of the greater trochanter with a reciprocating thin-bladed automatic saw (Fig. 14-8). The hip is then flexed to 60 to 70 degrees with some external rotation delivering the prosthesis and upper femur out of the depth of the wound. A blunt engineering "cold chisel" is placed at the inferior aspect of the neck of the prosthesis, which is then driven out of the channel by steady and strong hammer blows, while ascertaining that the position of the limb does not vary. The cold chisel must be placed under the collar of the prosthesis at the margin between the collar and the neck. Because of the telescoping effect of the "trapped stem" during extraction, a standard Austin Moore extractor or a blunt hook should be engaged on the prosthe-

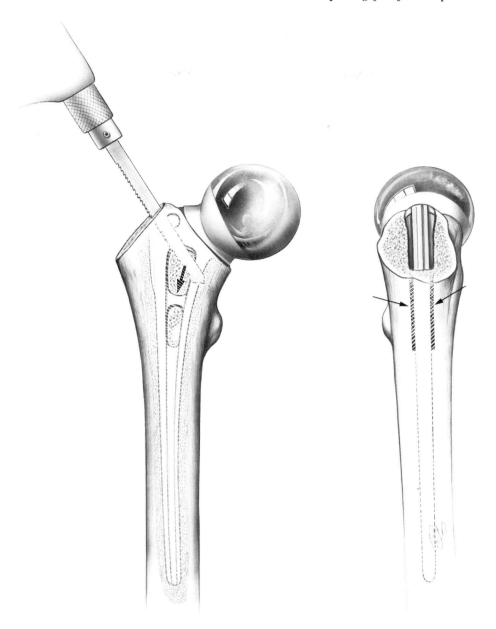

Fig. 14-8. Bone of fenestration of Moore self-locking prosthesis is best removed by reciprocating thin-bladed saw. Saw blade is inserted through bed of trochanter (arrow) both in front and in back of prosthesis and parellel to it (arrows). Attempt to remove bone of fenestration with conventional osteotome renders hazard of fracture of femur.

sis and then pulled by the assistant in the direction parallel to the shaft of the femur to facilitate its extraction (Fig. 14-9). Prior to attempting removal, the entire junction of the neck and the prosthetic collar must be inspected for soft tissue or ectopic bone holding the prosthesis to the shaft. If heavy hammer blows did not dislodge

the prosthesis, the soft tissue or bone of the fenestration must be reevaluated and removed; repeated heavy hammer blows may fracture the posterior wall of the upper femur, with or without a spiral fracture extending into its upper third. A standard inertia, mechanical hammer extractor is not sufficient to remove a fenestrated

483

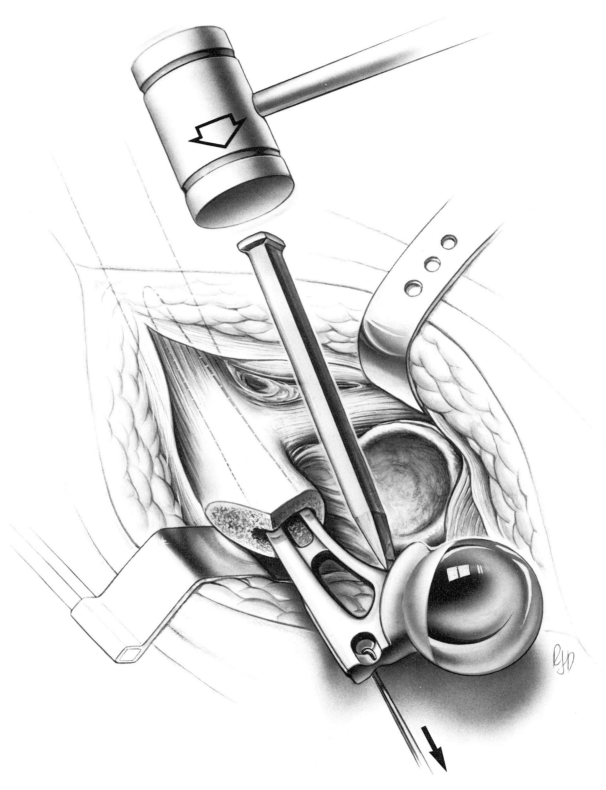

Fig. 14-9. In removing Moore self-locking prosthesis, hook assists prosthesis to maintain direction of extraction parallel to shaft of femur, while engineering cold chisel is applied to neck of prosthesis.

stem of the prosthesis; the use of a standard or even flexible, thin osteotome to remove the fenestrated bone may fracture the upper femur. The fibrous tissue filling the fenestration is troublesome at times, as when an osteotome or saw fails to remove it. However, steady traction coupled with heavy hammer blows to the collar (via the cold chisel) will eventually remove the prosthesis—provided that the bony segment is cut off from the fenestration.

Preparation of acetabulum

The lining of the acetabulum is a fibrous layer that should be curetted out to observe the state of the acetabular floor. If there is a sclerotic, but brittle, cortical layer of bone present immediately under the fibrous layers, it provides unsuitable ground for fixation of the cement. On the other hand, complete removal of this sclerotic bone may lead to fracture of the floor (which is often thin and brittle). Cavitation in the superior acetabulum with proximal migration of the socket is common, resulting in shortening of the extremity. An "eggshell" thin and often defective acetabulum may fracture while conventional deepening reamers are being used. If medial migration and protrusion of the head into the acetabulum are present, no centering drill hole should be used; the floor should be gently curetted of all soft tissue without disturbing the hard but thin cortical bone in the floor of the acetabulum. Reinforcement of the floor by bone graft may be advisable (Fig. 14-10). It is essential to preserve the "eggshell"

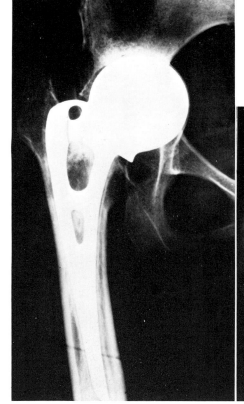

A

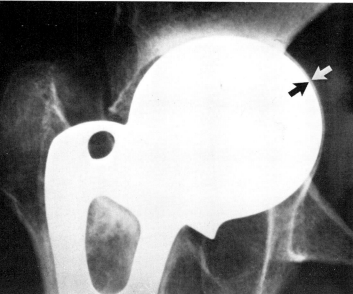

B

Continued.

Fig. 14-10. With severe protrusion of prosthesis, floor must be protected by gentle curettage of soft tissue without disturbing hard but thin cortical bone in floor of acetabulum. **A,** Ten years following Moore self-locking prosthesis inserted in 32-year-old female for revision of failed Judet prosthesis, which had been inserted at age 12 for slipped capital femoral epiphysis. NOTE: marked medial migration of prosthesis resulting in protrusion. **B,** Close-up of socket revealing very thin "eggshell-like" cortical bone. **C,** Seven years following low-friction arthroplasty, which was supplemented by primary bone graft procedure utilizing struts of iliac bone. Cement was inserted in conjunction with graft, and patient was protected 6 months postoperatively by walking aids and progressed to full weight bearing on gradual basis. **D,** At 7 years following surgery patient has grading of A-6,6,6 and is fully active and gainfully employed. NOTE: arrows indicate graft reinforcing floor of acetabulum, which still can be identified from floor of acetabulum by thin radiolucent line. Graft remains in continuity with ilium, ischium, and pubis.

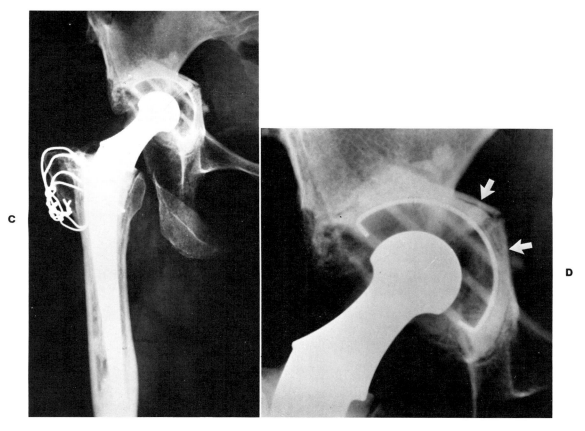

Fig. 14-10, cont'd. For legend see p. 485.

support of the floor. If a defect is found at surgery, it may be reinforced by supportive metallic mesh (Fig. 14-11). It must be recognized that metallic mesh does not provide an improved fixation element to the bone, but it simply:

1. Increases the strength of methyl methacrylates where they are thinly applied
2. Maintains continuity for the layer of cement
3. Prevents extrusion of cement into the pelvis, partially at the thin segments especially in the floor, thus building up pressure behind the cement mass at insertion

It is best therefore to sandwich the mesh in the cement by applying half of the cement dose before the insertion of the mesh, then the remainder of the cement and finally the cup. It should be noted that as the cup is being introduced, the mesh may move out of the acetabulum, which may result in "layering" of the cement and partial extrusion of the mesh; this must be avoided by actually anchoring the mesh

to the periphery of the acetabulum (see Chapter 13).

Proximal migration is a more difficult problem because at the time of the cementing of the socket, the proximal defect must be filled while the socket is kept at the lowest possible level (for the best fixation and lengthening of the limb). A special protrusion cup (designed by the author) is helpful,* and extra support may be obtained from the periphery of the acetabulum. It is particularly helpful when the bone of the pelvis is abnormal (such as in Gaucher's disease) and the use of bone graft may be of questionable value. The use of such cups would allow a better pressure injection of cement and provide extra support from the periphery of the acetabulum in addition to safeguarding the socket should medial migration occur (Figs. 14-11 to 14-13). (See

---

*Protrusion cup and extra large cups designed by author are manufactured by Cintor Division of Codman & Shurtleff, Inc. in the United States.

486

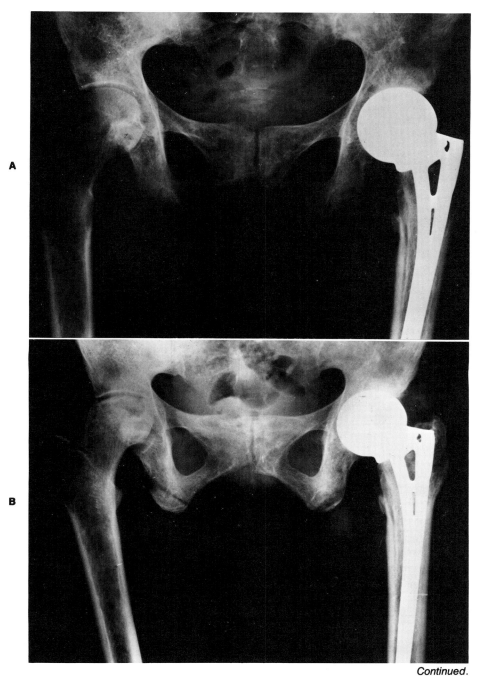

Continued.

Fig. 14-11. A, Bilateral hip disease secondary to avascular necrosis owing to Gaucher's disease in 34-year-old female was treated by left Moore self-locking prosthesis. **B,** One year following insertion of prosthesis because of collapse of femoral head and pain, similar operation was performed on right side, **C. D,** Two years following insertion of right hip femoral prosthesis, medial migration of both prostheses was so severe that patient lost complete range of motion in both hips and became chairbound. Arrows indicate medial migration of femoral prosthesis, but unlike hip shown in Fig. 14-10 there is no evidence of cortical bone at floor of acetabulum. **E,** Three years following bilateral low-friction arthroplasties. NOTE: use of large amount of cement and wire mesh in addition to use of "protrusion cup" in this situation. **F,** and **G,** Lateral view of hip showing inlet view of pelvis demonstrating lack of bone at site of floor of acetabulum (arrow). See also Fig. 14-12 for illustration of technique used in this case.

487

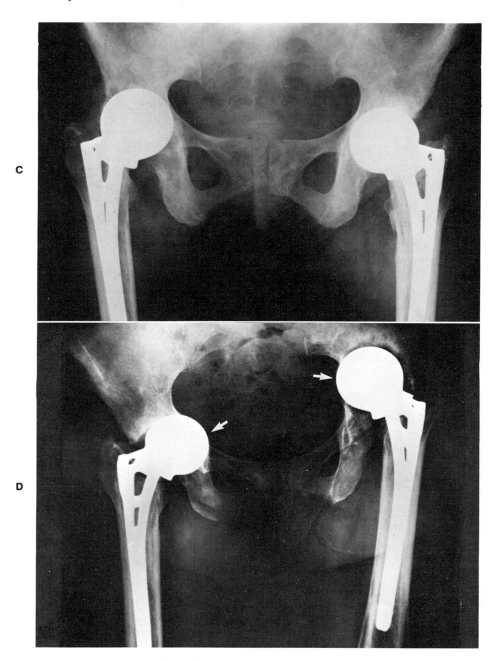

Fig. 14-11, cont'd. For legend see p. 487.

Chapter 13, "Technique for Protrusio Acetabuli.") It is necessary at times to use an extra large cup in order to reduce the amount of cement in extreme conditions of proximal and medial migration (Fig. 14-13). In the case of protrusion, the aim should be to maximize peripheral fixation of the acetabular component (Fig. 13-27). If the acetabulum is excessively large, two packs of cement may be used. It is essential that the cup be inserted slowly and not too deeply into the protruded acetabulum. Excessive penetration of the cup into the cement bypasses the peripheral anchor holes made for extra fixation, eliminating the advantages of the anchor holes made in the ilium, pubic, and ischial bones (Fig. 13-27), in addition to loss of clearance between

488

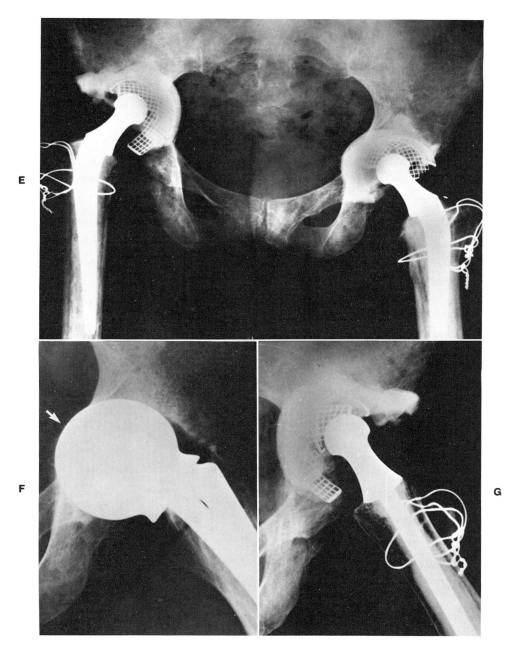

Fig. 14-11, cont'd. For legend see p. 487.

the upper femur and the acetabulum, predisposing the hip to instability.

The thin layer of bone formed in the acetabular floor against the femoral head may be sclerotic and hard; this nonporous segment of the acetabulum must not be removed. It can be improved for fixation by being roughened by a gouge or a sharp curet. A bone scraper is a useful tool for this purpose. At times, multiple drilling by a ¼-inch drill may be the best solution. Roughening of the surface should be done after anchor holes are made in the ilium and ischium. One must pay special attention to avoid excessive deepening, since in most instances there is already some degree of medial migration of the prosthesis. A sharp curet is useful in producing

489

irregularities for "keying" of the cement. Multiple small holes, that is, ⁷/₆₄-inch drill holes (Fig. 12-28), may be used to increase the surface contact. After fixation, the socket must be tested to see that it has been firmly fixed. If the socket has been inserted too deeply and large marginal protrusion (especially medial and inferior) has been created, this marginal extension of bone must be removed to provide clearance (see Chapter 17).

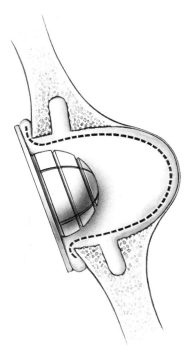

Fig. 14-12. Special protrusion cup is used in conjunction with large amount of cement, which is well anchored peripherally and augmented in strength medially by wire mesh. Wire mesh (optional) is shown in dotted lines. NOTE: rim of cup is anchored outside as safeguard to prevent medial migration should loosening occur (see Chapter 13).

Preparation of femur

The specific problems of the femur include: (1) shortening, (2) fibrous sleeve, (3) cul-de-sac, (4) abnormal orientation of the old track, and (5) presence of cement in the shaft. Because of the gradual sinking of the prosthesis, the femoral neck is often absent and the femur is shortened to the level of the lesser trochanter. Following removal of the stem, a protective fibrous sleeve remains in the shaft and must be removed. A long Kocher clamp may remove this fibrous tissue in its entirety with a direct pull and twist on the sleeve. On the other hand, long-handled curets (Volkmann's spoon) are best for curetting out the soft connective tissue from the femoral shaft. It is essential to remove all soft tissue and the thin cortical bone that have formed (the innermost layer of bone next to the prosthesis), and to curet the femur completely (especially on the concave side of the prosthesis) in preparation for the new prosthesis. Generally, tapered reamers inserted in a valgus position are most useful. The new direction must disregard the path of the original stem since most prostheses have drifted into a varus position (Fig. 14-14); the new path must take a slight valgus orientation. An optimal "version" must be observed. The previous prosthesis has usually been inserted in too much anteversion or (most often) retroversion to be acceptable for the channel of the new stem (Fig. 14-15).

The stems of most noncemented prostheses, for example, Moore self-locking prosthesis, are usually longer than those of total hip replacement, that is, Charnley's low-friction arthroplasty stem; however, in preparing the shaft, the new channel must extend beyond the site of the old stem tip. A cul-de-sac of sclerotic bone

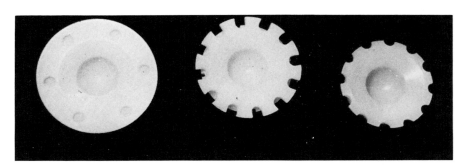

Fig. 14-13. Acetabular protrusion cup with broad rim as used in Figs. 14-11 and 14-12. On right, standard Charnley low-friction arthroplasty acetabular cup (44 mm.). In middle is similar prosthesis but with outer diameter of 57 mm. "Protrusion cup" with outer diameter of rim of 65 mm. is on left.

formed at the tip of the femoral prosthesis must be removed so that the methyl methacrylate cement can enter this zone. Failure to do this, with air or fluid trapped in this area, leads to inadequate cement fixation (Fig. 14-16). The cul-de-sac may be entered by a straight taper pin reamer (Fig. 14-17). In the case of a previously cemented prosthesis, the cul-de-sac may be left undisturbed if the length of the channel accommodates the new prosthesis; a venting hole through the vastus lateralis region into the shaft of the femur allows the cement to flow to the tip

level (Fig. 16-22). When a long neck prosthesis is to be used for stability, the abductors must oppose the shaft without undue tension for a satisfactory fixation. The abductors must be attached against the shaft as distally as possible to produce stability and ensure union. Compromised circulation of bone as the result of previous intervention may lead to nonunion of the trochanter if extreme care is not taken to achieve good bony contact between the trochanter and the shaft (see Chapter 17).

For revision of cemented endoprostheses the

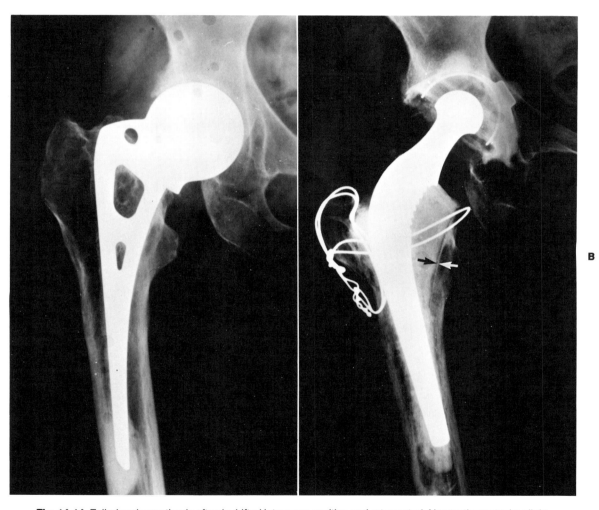

Fig. 14-14. Failed endoprosthesis often is drifted into varus position and retroverted. New path must take slight valgus orientation and neutroversion. **A,** Failed Moore self-locking prosthesis in 52-year-old woman who was treated for fractured neck of femur 3 years prior. Preoperative grading was A-2,3,5. **B,** Postoperative x-ray film of same woman 3 years following replacement. NOTE: good acetabular fixation and trochanteric reattachment. Valgus positioning was somewhat overdone; nevertheless, excellent support on medial side of prosthesis by cement is produced. Arrows indicate hard cortical bone often present at region of calcar, which must be curetted and drilled into (via medullary canal) at time of preparation. NOTE: old channel of previous prosthesis has been disregarded.

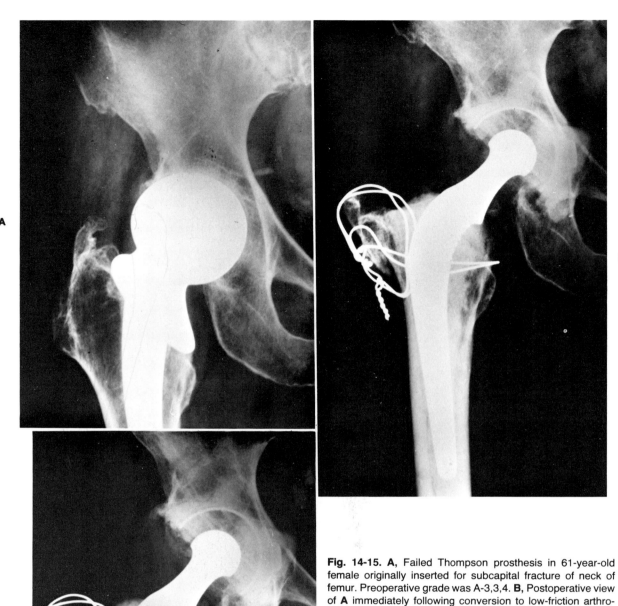

Fig. 14-15. A, Failed Thompson prosthesis in 61-year-old female originally inserted for subcapital fracture of neck of femur. Preoperative grade was A-3,3,4. **B,** Postoperative view of **A** immediately following conversion to low-friction arthroplasty. At surgery it was noted that prosthesis had been inserted 30 degrees anteverted and bone absorption was noted to level of lesser trochanter. **C,** Four years following insertion of low-friction arthroplasty, postoperative grade was A-6,6,6. NOTE: because of valgus orientation of stem in medullary canal and lowering of socket, effective neck length has restored stability for hip in addition to equalization of leg length without use of long-neck prosthesis (see text).

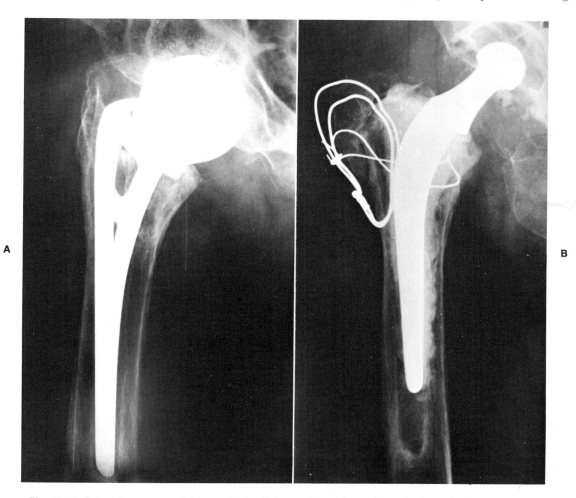

Fig. 14-16. Failure to remove cul-de-sac of sclerotic bone at tip of femoral prosthesis can lead to inadequate cement fixation. **A,** Loose Moore self-locking prosthesis in 61-year-old woman requiring revision. **B,** Immediate postoperative x-ray film of **A,** indicating inadequate cement at distal portion of stem especially on lateral side. Cul-de-sac had not been opened at surgery.

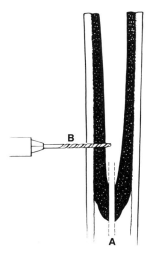

Fig. 14-17. Two alternative methods of venting cul-de-sac. **A,** Drilling of shaft is done through hole on lateral aspect with small drill, that is, $^7/_{64}$-inch through vastus lateralis muscle without exposing shaft. **B,** Use of long ¼-inch drill via intramedullary canal of femur (see Fig. 16-22).

493

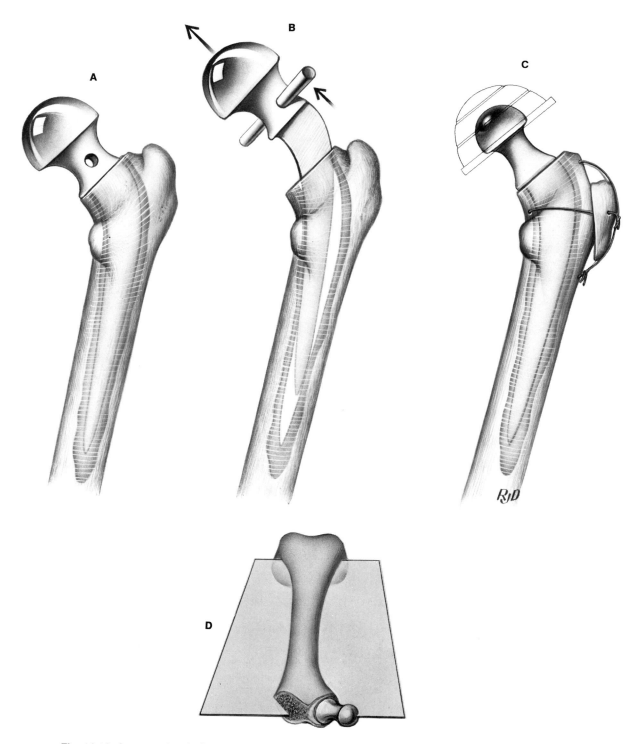

Fig. 14-18. Concept of replacing cemented endoprosthesis is illustrated. **A,** Cemented endoprosthesis stem is identical to Charnley's stem but 10% proportionally larger. **B,** Endoprosthesis being removed. **C,** Standard low-friction arthroplasty inserted adding only minimum amount of cement. **D,** Neutral plane (neutroversion) to be used for both replacements (see text).

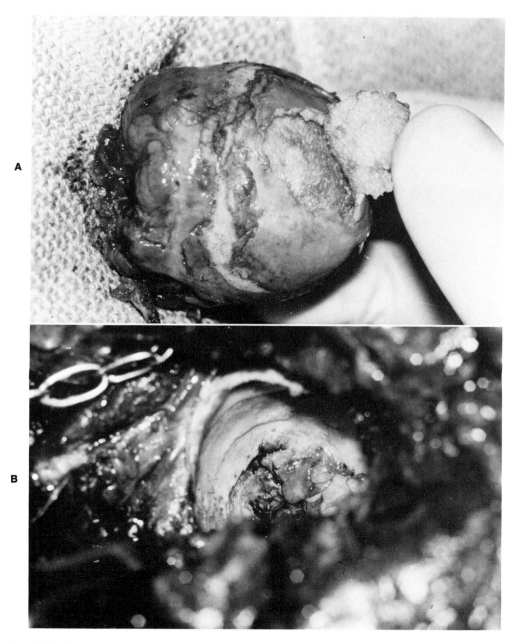

Fig. 14-19. Femoral head, **A,** and acetabulum, **B,** respectively, as observed at surgery in 51-year-old man undergoing hip arthroplasty for avascular necrosis. Because of relatively minor changes of acetabulum and in view of patient's young age, hemiarthroplasty was performed utilizing cemented endoprosthesis (see also Fig. 14-20).

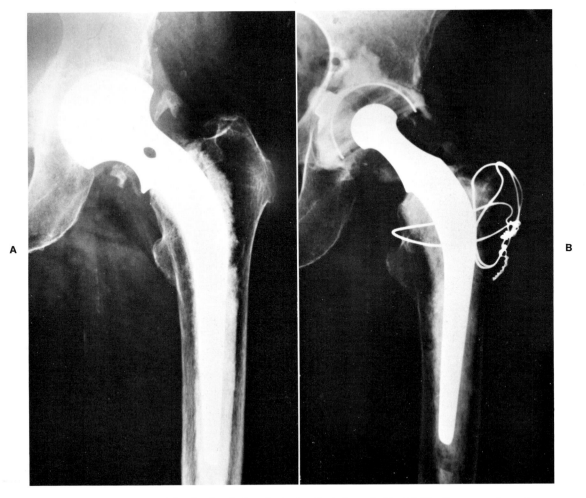

Fig. 14-20. A, Three years following hemiarthroplasty of patient shown in Fig. 14-19 with progressive pain as result of acetabular changes. **B,** One year following total hip arthroplasty replacing cemented endoprosthesis by low-friction arthroplasty.

reader is referred to the section on revision of total hip replacement. Revision of previously cemented endoprostheses may be facilitated if the original design of the stem is similar to that of the stem of total hip prosthesis. Such a prosthesis developed at New York Orthopedic Hospital by the author has been in use since 1969.* At revision, following removal, only a small amount of cement need be used, utilizing the old channel (see Chapter 4) (Fig. 14-18), which is only 10% proportionally larger than the standard stem of a Charnley prosthesis. Figs. 14-19 and 14-20 illustrate a case where such a prosthesis was used and subsequently converted to a low-friction arthroplasty.

---

*Manufactured by Howmedica, Inc., Rutherford, N.J.

496

REVISION OF FAILED CUP ARTHROPLASTY

With the exception of those patients with ectopic bone formation and marked stiffness, conversion of a failed cup arthroplasty to a total hip replacement has proven to be relatively easy. If the greater trochanter has been transferred during previous surgery, care must be taken to avoid its fragmentation when the wires are being removed. Because most cup arthroplasties have been performed through the Smith-Petersen approach, there may be considerable scarring in the interval between the abductor mechanism (glutei) and the tensor fascia femoris, which must be incised for exposure. Extreme stiffness may make femoral neck osteotomy necessary to facilitate removal of the cup from the acetabu-

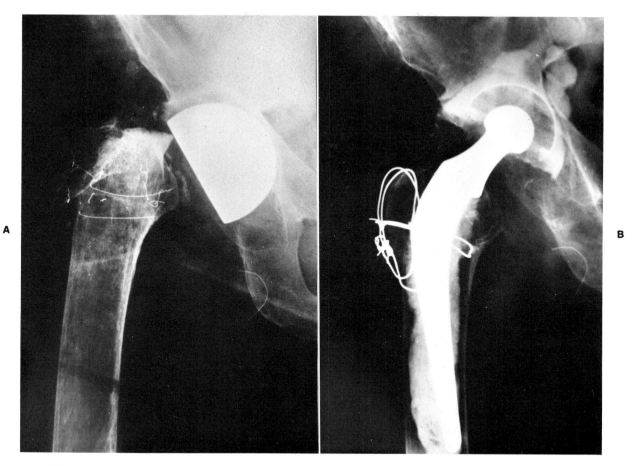

Fig. 14-21. A, Four years following cup arthroplasty in 52-year-old female. Operation had been performed for degenerative osteoarthritis. Fracture of neck of femur had occurred 3 months prior to radiographs shown here. **B,** Postoperative radiograph following revision by low-friction arthroplasty. NOTE: marked osteoporosis resulting from non-weight bearing.

lum. The head and the cup are then removed in a retrograde manner following mobilization of the upper femur. If a large cup was used originally, necessitating deepening of the acetabulum, or if medial migration has occurred, the huge cavity and the thin medial wall of the pelvis will require an extra-large acetabular cup and/or two packs of cement. The details cited in revision of failed femoral prosthesis must be observed. The sclerotic and reactive bone found in a failed cup arthroplasty is similar to that present in a failed femoral head prosthesis, which must be roughened for good fixation (Fig. 14-21). Because of continuous bone absorption of the head of the femur under the cup, shortening of the extremity is often present, but here again, the level of neck resection and leg length is gauged by the abductor length and the mobility of the greater trochanter as well as the stability of the hip. Because a number of cup arthroplasties have originally been performed for degenerative osteoarthritis secondary to congenital dysplasia, the bony structure of the acetabulum and upper femur may be underdeveloped, in addition to the presence of osteoporosis as the result of disuse. It may be well to ignore the original site of the acetabulum and accept the existing high position for the new joint. Special attention must be directed toward preparation of the underdeveloped shaft. A small or extra-small cup and stem may be required (see Chapter 13 and Figs. 13-18 and 13-22).

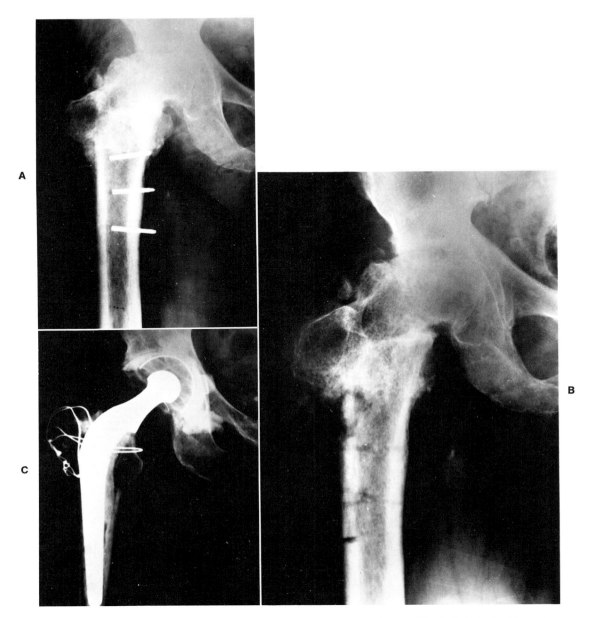

Fig. 14-22. Occasionally, removal of previously inserted screws may be so difficult that shaft of femur is excessively traumatized and operation may have to be terminated prior to replacement. **A,** Patient was referred for removal of screws and insertion of total hip prosthesis. **B,** Immediately after surgery, during which extensive damage to shaft "lateral cortex" was introduced. Operation took 60 minutes to perform. **C,** Patient was readmitted subsequently 4 months later and total hip arthroplasty was performed.

REVISION OF FAILED OSTEOTOMY AND FRACTURE FIXATION

Failed osteotomies and fracture fixations are combined here because both share the following common problems: (1) difficulty in removal of internal fixation devices and (2) displacement of the upper femur, rendering preparation of the femoral canal difficult.

Removal of nails, plates, and screws

Extraction of the screws may be difficult, adding an hour or more to the surgical procedure. The surgeon must be equipped with an appropriate type of screwdriver tip and nail extractor. Occasionally, removal may be so difficult that the shaft of the femur is excessively traumatized and the operation may have to be termi-

498

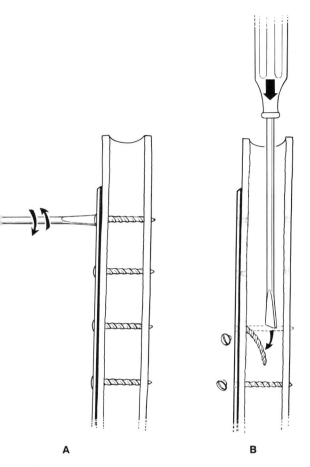

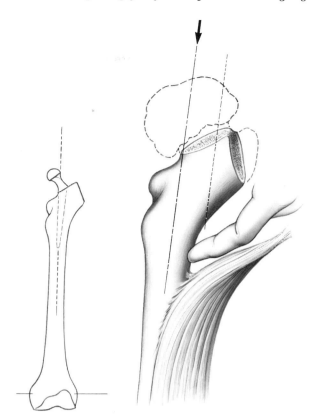

A   **B**

Fig. 14-23. A, Slight turn (⅛ or ¼ turn) in direction of tightening may loosen screw prior to reversing direction for removal. **B,** When screw heads are broken and screws are left within shaft, blunt instrument such as screwdriver may be inserted into shaft to clear way for insertion of stem. If fragments of chromium and cobalt screws cannot be removed, they may be left in place.

Fig. 14-24. Arrow indicates selection of site of entry to femur (long dashed lines) and compares it with erroneous entry (short dashed lines) of medullary canal if osteotomy site is not observed. Straight, narrow stem is ideal in this situation.

nated prior to replacement (Fig. 14-22). Fracture of the femur may occur during dislocation in a femur weakened from screw extraction. At times, the screw head may break off, and the screw shaft creates a problem with the insertion of the prosthetic stem. Rather than damaging the shaft of the femur by trephine holes through the shaft of each screw, it is possible to break the screws without attempting to completely remove all broken pieces. It is quite possible to break screws inside the medullary canal with a long metallic device such as a screwdriver or "punch." Leaving the Vitallium screws behind might be theoretically objectionable when using a stainless steel prosthesis, but in practice this has not created a problem, perhaps

because the fragments of chromium and cobalt screws (Vitallium) are insulated from the steel stem by cement inside the shaft of the femur (Fig. 14-23). To remove a very tight screw, the screwdriver must fit exactly to the screw head before attempting removal. A slight turn (eight- or quarter-turn) clockwise (direction of tightening) may loosen the screw prior to reversing the direction for removal (counterclockwise) (Fig. 14-23). Following removal, plates and screw sites must be carefully observed for purulent material. These sites must be cultured and a Gram's stain obtained for possible bacteria. Occasionally, following removal of the side-plate, the extraction of a nail or screw from the neck is not possible without damage to the trochanteric area. In this situation, it is best to remove the head of the femur at an appropriate level and then tap the nail out of the neck and trochanteric

499

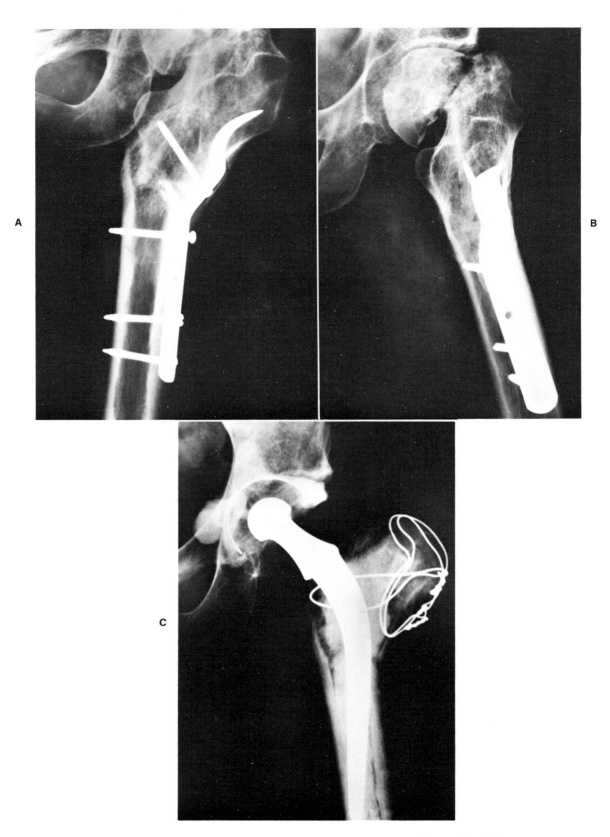

Fig. 14-25. A and **B,** Anteroposterior and lateral view of left hip in 48-year-old housewife. Valgus osteotomy had been performed 4 years previously following failed union of fractured neck of femur. NOTE: amount of displacement in both planes. **C,** Postoperative radiographs 3½ years following replacement. NOTE: straight, narrow stem is accomodated within shaft of femur. (See also Fig. 14-24.)

region. As a rule, it is best to dislocate the hip joint prior to removal of the internal fixation device, which may weaken the bone at removal.

Displacement of upper femur

It is of paramount importance to obtain a good lateral view radiograph in addition to the routine anteroposterior view of the pelvis and the hip (two perpendicular planes) (Fig. 17-5) in order to evaluate the exact amount of displacement of the femoral fragments. It is also essential to have a straight, narrow-stem prosthesis available. With a markedly displaced osteotomy, it is essential to find the actual medullary canal at a straight line from the top of the shaft down to the direction of the patella; this can be facilitated by using a straight tapered pin reamer, which may be introduced from the outside of the opening of the upper femur when a grossly displaced osteotomy had been performed (Figs. 14-

24 and 14-25). Additionally, we have found it helpful to expose the lateral cortex (by splitting the vastus lateralis for a distance of 1 to 2 inches from the lateral aspect of the shaft of the femur) and directly observe the direction of the femur below the site of osteotomy. With severe displacement in two planes, it is advisable to use the guide and drill to open the medullary canal. It is most essential to completely mobilize the upper femur before attempting its preparation so that direct access to the top of the femur is possible (Fig. 14-2). The second assistant must stabilize the knee and demonstrate the patella for reference during drilling of the upper femur. As stated, direct palpation of the upper femur (through the split vastus) is an important additional guide in assessing the accurate direction of the tapered pin reamer or drill. A radiograph or image intensifier will guarantee proper orientation. In a markedly displaced proximal frag-

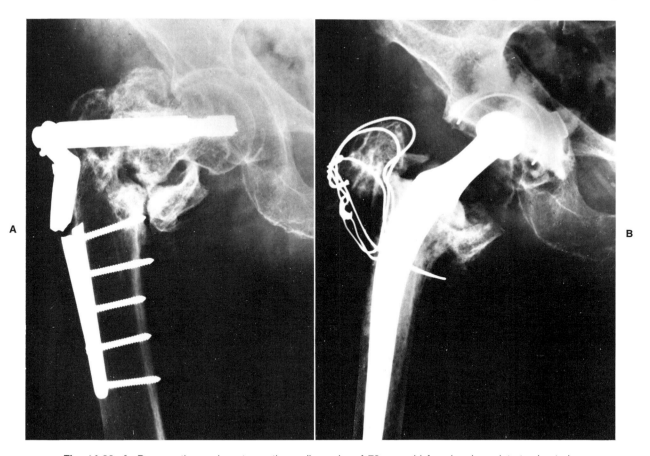

Fig. 14-26. A, Preoperative and postoperative radiographs of 73-year-old female whose intertrochanteric fracture of right femur was complicated by nonunion and breakage of internal fixation device. Entire upper femur was removed down to level of lesser trochanter and straight, narrow-stem, long-neck prosthesis was used. **B,** Radiograph at 4½ years following surgery by low-friction arthroplasty.

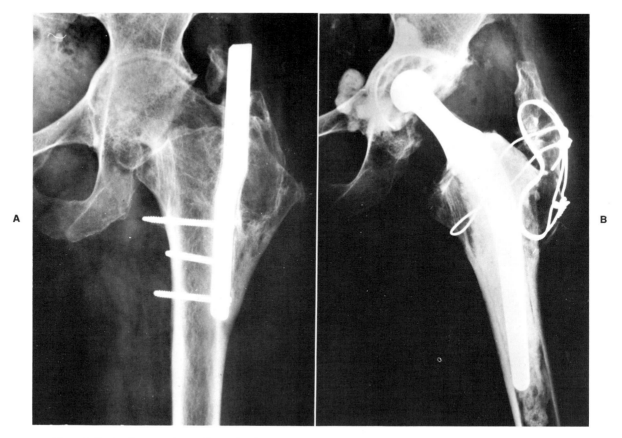

Fig. 14-27. A, Preoperative radiograph of 62-year-old male with advanced degenerative osteoarthritis of hip, for whom intertrochanteric osteotomy had been performed. Marked displaced proximal segment of upper femur (although not appreciated by preoperative radiographs) had to be removed. Hip was stabilized at surgery by use of long neck–straight stem prosthesis. **B,** Five years following low-friction arthroplasty (see text).

ment or nonunion of intertrochanteric fractures, it is possible to sacrifice the entire proximal segment down to the level of the lesser trochanter and to use a straight-stem prosthesis, although this will obviously lead to some shortening of the lower extremity, which can be partly compensated for by the use of a long-neck prosthesis (Fig. 14-26). When the proximal fragment is to be removed in this manner, the greater trochanter may have to be osteotomized below the vastus ridge, thus leaving a generous fragment for subsequent fixation. The problem of instability created following removal of the neck must be compensated for by a long-neck, straight prosthesis (Figs. 14-26 and 14-27). (See Chapter 17.)

Other considerations

Complications of fracture fixations are now best treated by total hip replacement (Figs. 14-

28 and 14-29). There is usually no problem with nonunion of the neck of the femur proximal to the intertrochanteric line.

Following removal of the greater trochanter, the pseudoarthrosis site is explored and the head of the femur is removed in a retrograde manner. From this point the operation is carried out in a routine manner. However, when nonunion occurs intertrochanterically with an extension to the subtrochanteric level, sufficient bone stock may not be available for the insertion of the stem of the prosthesis. In the case of nonunion of the neck of the femur, extensive scarification of soft tissue and hyperemia often exist at the site of nonunion, and surgery is considerably more difficult than in a straightforward operation. Bone is often more osteoporotic than normal, and trauma to the upper femur is a likely possibility.

Avascular necrosis, a common complication of

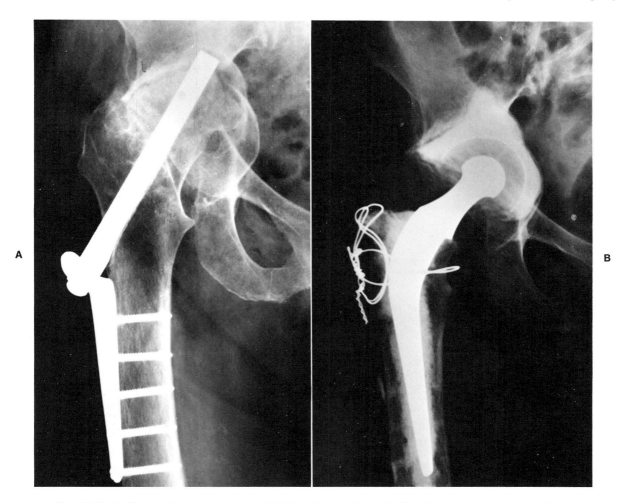

Fig. 14-28. A, Preoperative radiograph of right hip following 3-year fixation of intracapsular fracture of hip in 68-year-old female who also developed protrusio acetabuli following fracture fixation. **B,** Four years following low-friction arthroplasty.

fracture fixation, can be conveniently handled by total hip replacement. The results of this type of revision surgery are the most gratifying and technically there usually are no extra risks or complications that exist. One of the difficulties often encountered with avascular necrosis is the small size of the acetabulum, since in most cases, the size of the bony acetabulum is unchanged and the acetabular cartilage is only fibrillated. The size of the head is usually small, and typical reactive changes similar to those of osteoarthrosis are not present. Attempts should not be made to expand the acetabulum to a standard size, but a small acetabular cup should be used for these individuals, who are usually younger, thus preserving bone stock for future

revision should it become necessary (Fig. 14-30). As indicated elsewhere (see Chapter 8), one should resist the temptation to replace only the necrotic femoral head when there is any evidence of fibrillation of the cartilage present in the acetabulum (Figs. 14-19 and 14-20). Fractures of the pelvis involving the acetabulum must be carefully evaluated for the presence or absence of bony stock as well as the orientation of the bony acetabulum, which may have been altered as the result of trauma (Fig. 14-31). With prior surgery resulting in scar formation, the operation is usually more difficult and makes the sciatic nerve more vulnerable to injury. At times, a bone graft procedure may be needed (if pelvic fracture includes a displaced

503

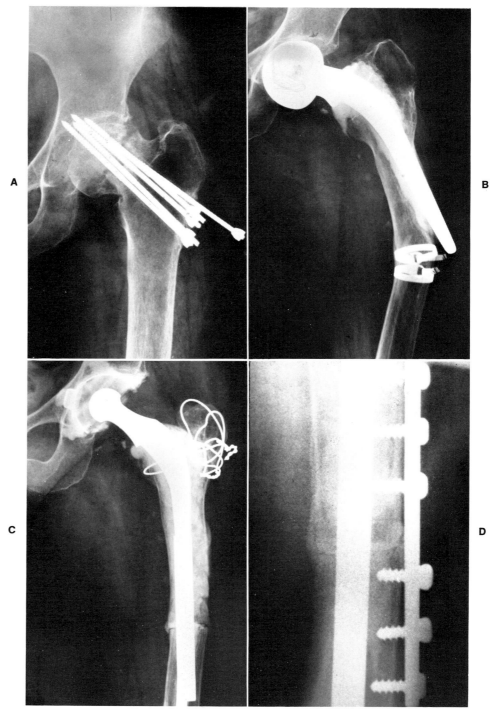

Fig. 14-29. For legend see opposite page.

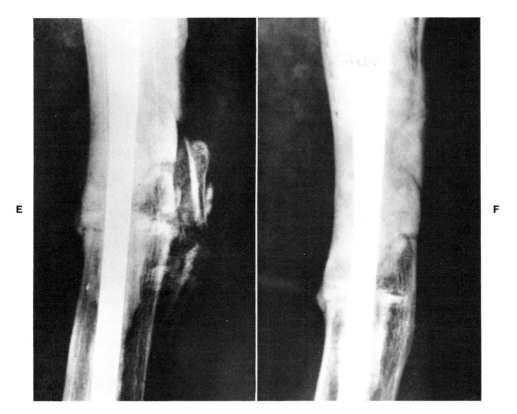

Fig. 14-29. A, Fifty-one-year-old female whose subcapital fracture of neck of femur was treated by multiple pinning. It resulted in nonunion with migration of pins both proximally and distally. **B,** Following removal of pins hemiarthroplasty had been attempted using cemented endoprosthesis resulting in intraoperative fracture of upper femur. Parham bands had been used to secure fracture, but angulation and nonunion developed at fracture site. (Operations performed in another institution.) **C,** Patient had been immobilized at this point in hip spica cast for nearly 18 months. NOTE: marked osteoporosis of femur. Low-friction arthroplasty was performed using long-stem prosthesis, which was supplemented by unicortical screw and plate fixation to augment cement fixation at fracture site. NOTE: extensive damage to lateral aspect of shaft. **D,** Lateral view of femur at site of fracture fixation and use of unicortical screws in addition to long stem of prosthesis. **E,** Six weeks following insertion of total hip prosthesis, plate was removed and area of fracture was supplemented by iliac bone graft. **F,** Complete bony union occurred at 1 year following surgery.

acetabular fragment or is defective) as an adjunct to the total prosthesis. Bone graft procedure may be done in conjunction with the total prosthesis (at the same operation) or as a staged procedure (Fig. 14-32).

REVISION OF FAILED ARTHRODESIS

A painful hip following arthrodesis (failure of fusion) or deformity of the hip following arthrodesis can be rectified by total hip replacement and may prove most gratifying.[2,4,8] (See Chapter 8.) Other indications for converting a fusion to a total hip replacement include a painful or deformed knee (contralateral and ipsilateral) or back pain as a result of a malpositioned hip fusion. Two basic principles must be recognized.

1. No hip fusion should be revised without objective clinical findings of pain in the hip as a result of pseudoarthrosis or deformity.

2. Prior infection in the ipsilateral hip for which a fusion was undertaken must not be taken lightly, regardless of the time lapsed between the fusion and the contemplated replacement (Fig. 8-17).

Regardless of the type of arthrodesis performed, two technical details must be considered: (1) the state of the trochanter and abductor mechanism and (2) the potentials of limitation of range of motion following conversion of an arthrodesed hip to a total hip replacement.

Although we are concerned with the physiological aspect of muscles (especially abductors),

Fig. 14-30. A, Femoral head collapse and avascular necrosis following fracture fixation in this 51-year-old woman required revision. **B,** Following removal of nail at surgery, replacement did not take place because of suspicious granulation-type tissue found at surgery in addition to appearance of mottling around nail track shown on radiographs. **C,** Six weeks following removal of nail. Negative cultures obtained at time of removal of nail. Low-friction arthroplasty was performed. **D,** Five years following replacement patient has excellent functional result. Hip grade A-6,6,6. Line of demarcation between cement and bone has remained unchanged since surgery.

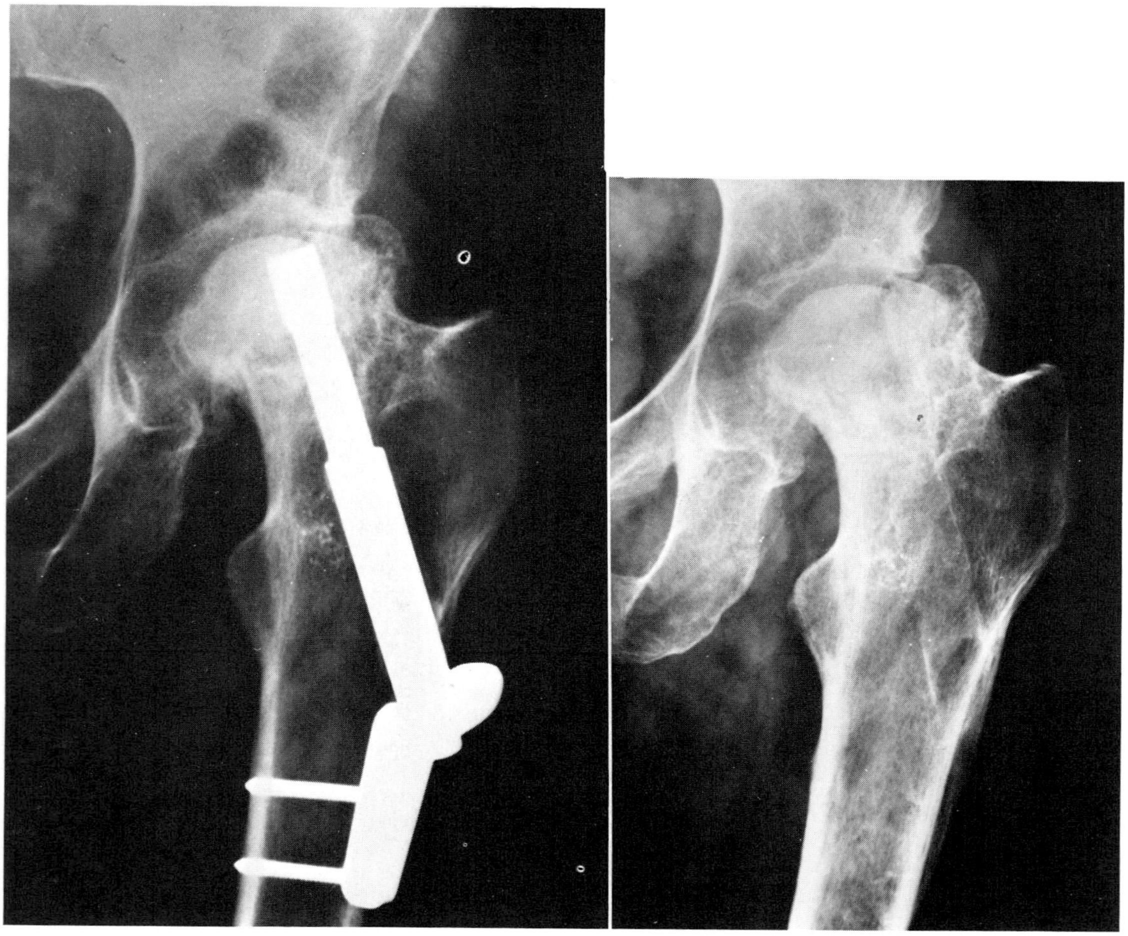

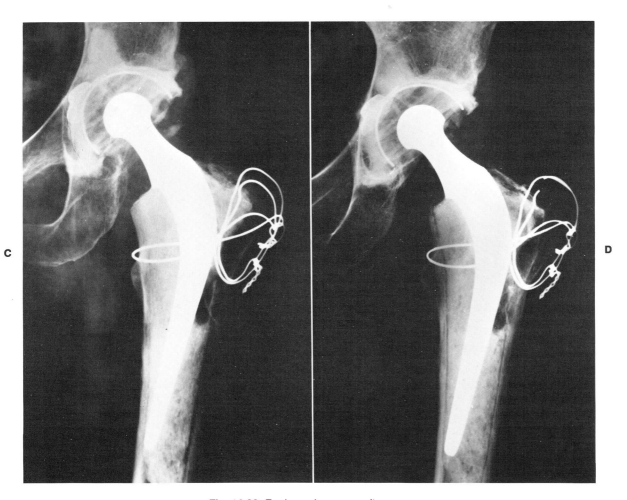

C

D

Fig. 14-30. For legend see opposite page.

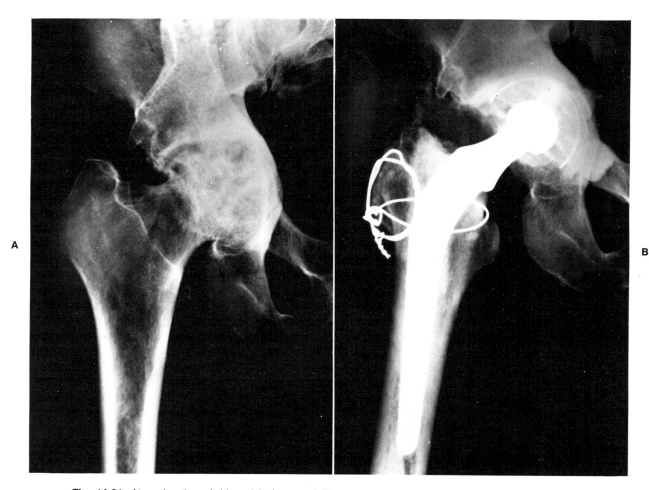

Fig. 14-31. At exploration of this pelvic fracture (with central acetabular protrusion) of 49-year-old man, marked posterior and medial displacement of posterior column of pelvis was observed. Defective area was grafted with bone obtained from femoral head to provide bony stock for posterior wall of acetabulum. Bone was packed into defect without use of internal fixation device. **B,** Two years following replacement.

a good functional result may be expected despite many years of muscular inactivity. Regardless of the state of the abductor mechanism, considerable improvement can be achieved in regard to pain and relief of back and knee "strain" following conversion of a failed fused hip to a total hip replacement.[4,8] While careful muscle strength testing and electromyography studies are of academic interest,[2] this information is less important than the overall clinical examination of patient and x-ray findings. It is not always possible to determine the degree of muscle function when the hip has been arthrodesed, either clinically or by electromyography. Furthermore, in many instances the hip muscles increase in strength following revision. The function of the

abductor muscles is ordinarily compromised but usually will suffice, providing the abductors have not been excised by the original arthrodesis and the trochanter is identifiable by radiography. A limited range of motion may be expected following conversion of a failed arthrodesis hip to a total hip replacement; nevertheless, concerning relief of pain, most patients with a successful arthroplasty are pleased with the outcome despite a weak gluteus medius gait (Figs. 14-33 and 8-29).

From the technical standpoint, a routine lateral approach and removal of the greater trochanter are essential. It is important to enter the original site of the neck of the femur and osteotomize the neck as proximally to the ace-

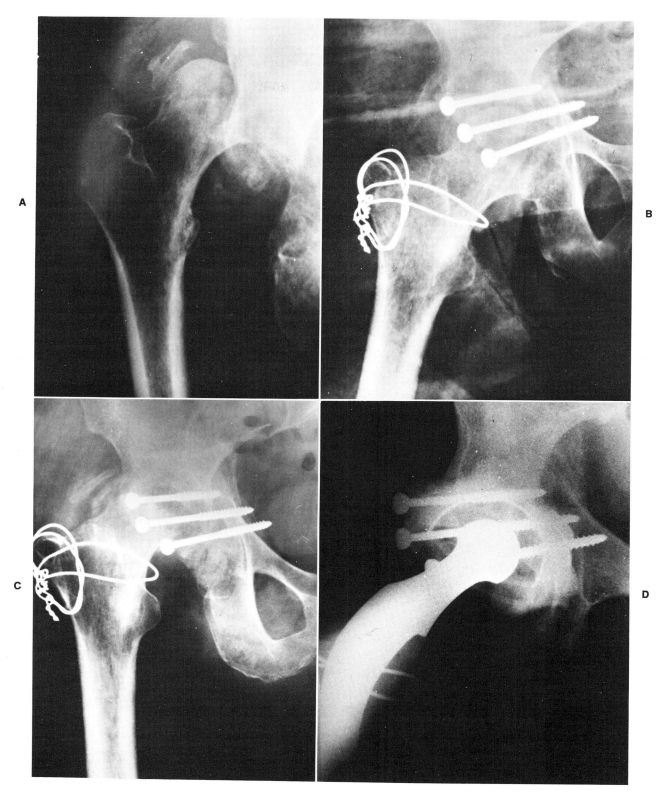

Fig. 14-32. A, Recurrent posterior dislocation of hip following two attempts of closed and one open reduction at another institution. Patient, 38-year-old housewife, also suffered head injuries as well as sciatic nerve palsy following automobile accident. **B,** Immediate and, **C,** 6 months following bone graft procedure to posterior aspect of acetabulum. **D,** Hip immediately following total hip replacement by low-friction arthroplasty.

Continued.

509

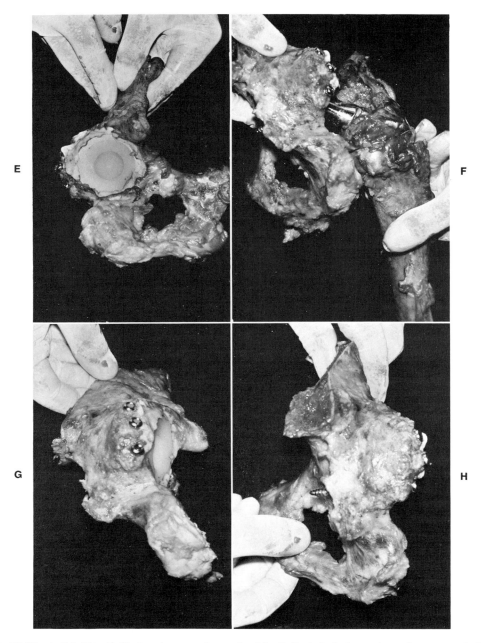

Fig. 14-32, cont'd. E to **H,** Postmortem specimen of pelvis. Patient died of massive pulmonary embolism. NOTE: excellent coverage of acetabulum by bone graft and also complete healing of bone graft to posterior wall of pelvis as indicated in **F** to **H.** No line of separation between bone graft and pelvic bones can be identified.

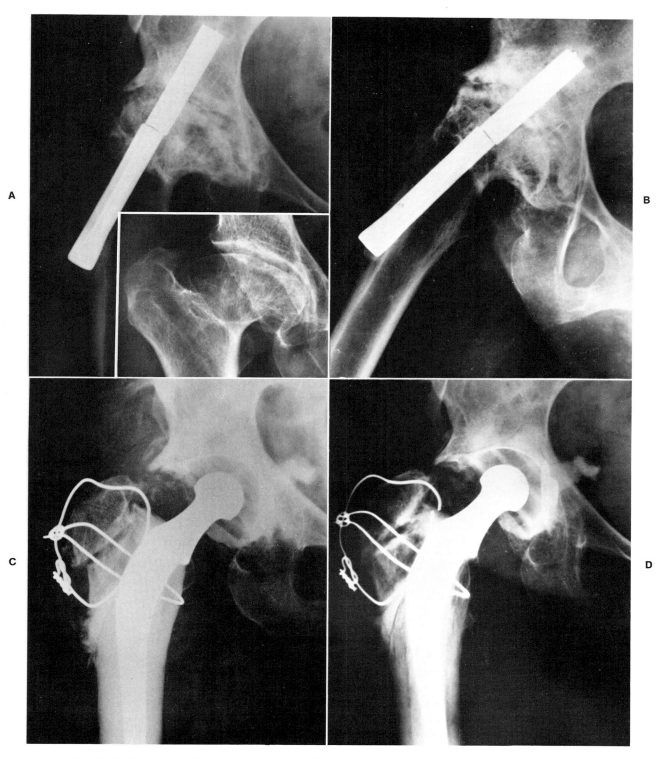

Fig. 14-33. Conversion of failed arthrodesis to total hip arthroplasty at times may be most gratifying. **A,** Degenerative osteoarthritis of hip (inset) in 64-year-old college professor whose hip was arthrodesed 6 years prior. Reattempt at fusion on two additional occasions failed to produce pain-free hip. **B,** Malposition of femur as well as fractured nail; evidence for minor motion at arthrodesis site although clinically hip was ankylosed. **C,** Immediately following low-friction arthroplasty. **D,** Eight years following low-friction arthroplasty. Although trochanteric wire is fractured (delayed), patient's grading at this time is A-6,6,6.

511

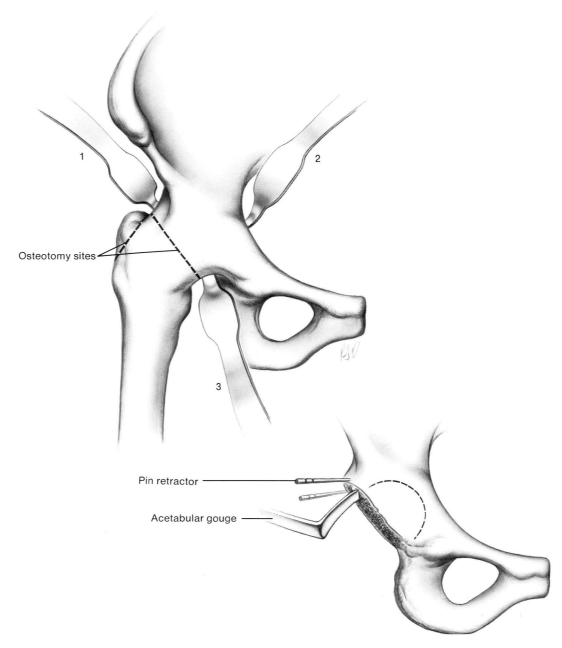

Fig. 14-34. Line of osteotomy of fusion mass and greater trochanter as well as proper site for preparation for acetabulum (curved line, bottom) are shown. NOTE: insertion of pin retractors to visualize periphery of acetabulum as well as use of acetabular gouges to create and "excavate" new acetabulum. This drawing is based on Fig. 8-29 (see text). *1, 2,* and *3* represent Hohmann retractors.

tabulum as possible in order to gain length. By exposing the original site of the acetabulum with Hohmann retractors, one can carefully examine the exact location of the site of the original acetabulum. Error in selection of the site, that is, high-level osteotomy on the pelvis,

may lead to a fractured pelvis or marked shortening of the limb. Excavation of the head of the femur follows a complete exposure of the acetabular rim with one or two pin retractors (Fig. 14-34). Depending on the surgeon's preference, a conventional gouge and curets or the standard instrumentations such as deepening and expanding reamers are used to remove the fused head from the acetabulum. It is most essential that the acetabular site be exposed fully and maintained using Hohmann retractors during removal of the head. One such retractor should be placed inferior to the acetabulum to expose the lower limits of the boundary of the acetabulum (Fig. 14-34). The depth is determined by a pilot hole in the floor or by direct palpation of the thickness of the wall via the inner side of the iliac bone. Stability for the artificial hip joint may be provided by proper selection of the acetabular site, appropriate placement of the socket, and maintenance of the soft tissue tension across the hip joint using the appropriate prosthetic neck length. The stability is then augmented by the transfer of the greater trochanter as distally as possible. It is equally essential to provide maximum clearance between the upper end of the femur and the wall of the pelvis. Because of the contracted soft tissue about the hip, it may be necessary at times to shorten the upper femur in order to accommodate the soft tissue or to use a prosthesis with a short neck. Extra care must be exercised to protect the sciatic and femoral nerves during the exploration and preparation of the acetabular site. The femoral shaft is often osteoporotic, and during mobilization of the upper femur gentle handling is necessary to prevent accidental fracture of the shaft.

In summary, we consider a total hip replacement an excellent way to salvage a "failed hip fusion" that is characterized by a painful hip after fusion or malposition, substantial low back pain, and ipsilateral knee pain requiring mobilization at the hip joint. A number of potential complications are inherent in this surgery, and a surgeon without extensive experience with surgery of the hip joint should not undertake this type of reconstructive surgery. The principal goals are to gain some motion (even if a full range is impossible), to alleviate strain from the back and ipsilateral knee, and, in the case of nonunion or malunion of hip fusion, to correct deformity and relieve pain.

REVISION OF FAILED PSEUDARTHROSIS

Pseudarthrosis following the failure of previous surgery, that is, head and neck resection in the absence of infection, may be converted to a total hip replacement when pain and instability exist. Generally, these patients show considerable shortening in that extremity and the abductor mechanism is in poor mechanical condition, as evidenced by the telescoping effect of the upper femur on examination, the inability to raise the leg straight, or to abduct against gravity. Trendelenburg's sign is often positive, and these patients often manifest fatigue, pain in the hip, and low back or ipsilateral knee pain as in the conversion of a failed arthrodesis. The history of infection as an indication for a pseudarthrosis must be verified, since an infected pseudarthrosis owing to failure of previous hip surgery may be less amenable to correction than a pseudarthrosis without infection.

The quality of the results obtained from this revision is gratifying and this operation should be attempted despite the common presence of poor abductor function.[15] It must be noted that if a classic Girdlestone pseudarthrosis has been performed, the resected superior acetabular lip may be too deficient to allow consideration of replacement. The history of previous operations must identify whether or not the acetabular wall has been removed. A laminagram of the hip may be helpful in estimating the available bone stock. One of the major concerns and technical details of this type of procedure is a complete mobilization of the upper femur from the wall of the pelvis (Fig. 14-2). This involves resection of the soft tissue scarring about the hip as well as tenotomy of adductors and the psoas tendon in order to mobilize the upper femur. The extensive soft tissue release in a severely scarred region of the proximal femur is usually accompanied by excessive blood loss. Release is necessary to provide space for the prosthesis and consequently lengthening of the extremity. Occasionally, however, it is necessary to additionally shorten the proximal end of the femur in order to provide space to insert the prosthesis. The decision regarding the amount of shortening must be made following a complete soft tissue release and the cementing of the socket. A straight-stem, short-neck prosthesis is usually ideal if a standard neck length (straight stem) appears too long in the test trial. Occasionally at surgery it is possible to gain length and enhance stability by using a long-neck prosthesis. We believe that preoperative skeletal traction in these cases is futile, especially since the scar tissue will not yield under traction; additionally, traction can be poorly tolerated by elderly patients.

513

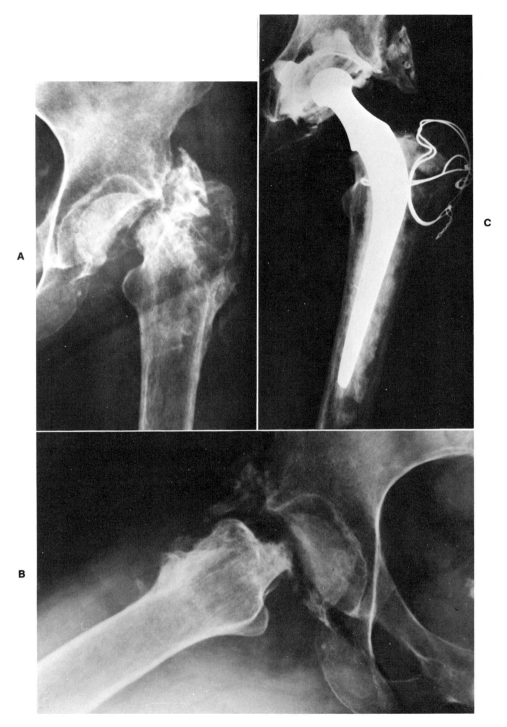

Fig. 14-35. Revision of pseudarthrosis involves extensive mobilization of upper femur in order to gain length following removal of scar tissue from pseudarthrosis site. **A** and **B,** Preoperative radiograph of ununited femoral neck fracture in 61-year-old female. NOTE: marked shortening and proximal migration of upper end of femur. **C,** Postoperative radiograph 7 years following replacement; 2½ inches of preoperative shortening were corrected using standard neck length prosthesis.

The bony acetabulum is usually extremely osteoporotic (as the result of non-weight bearing) and filled with fibrous tissue. Occasionally, the site of the acetabulum is obscured and efforts must be made to enter the original site of the acetabulum by removing all scarred tissue from this region. Fear of neurovascular compromise following elongation of the leg is unfounded because reduction of the prosthesis and excessive elongation are impossible in view of the muscle fascial length of the thigh.

A wide range of prostheses of different neck lengths and stem thicknesses should be available. A straight stem (narrow or thick) with a standard neck length (28-mm. Charnley straight-stem prosthesis) is often applicable (Fig. 14-35). The greater trochanter presents a twofold problem: (1) inadequate abductor mechanism, which is scarified and shortened, and (2) when the leg has been lengthened, inability to fasten the trochanter onto the shaft with wires at the optimal level. At times, prior to reattachment, it is necessary to mobilize the abductors in order to gain length. Short rotators must often be released in addition to psoas tenotomy and adductor release. We feel that this type of conversion is difficult and at times formidable, especially in a high-riding femur in the presence of fixed adduction and flexion deformity, and it requires a complete understanding of the surgical technique and familiarity with the procedure. The gain in neck length and resultant elongation of the extremity in a severely shortened limb are the most gratifying aspects of converting a pseudarthrosis to a total hip replacement.

REVISION OF FAILED TOTAL HIPS (IN ABSENCE OF INFECTION)

Further surgical intervention may be necessary as the result of failures of total hip arthroplasty other than those caused by infection. The most common failures may be attributed to:

1. The use of uncemented varieties of total hip prostheses
2. The loss of the mechanical fixation of cemented prosthetic components of total hip replacements
3. The mechanical failure of the stem (fractured stem)
4. Recurrent dislocation and instability
5. Traumatic conditions following total hip replacement (such as fracture of the femur or pelvis) leading to loss of fixation

Revision of a painful total hip replacement is a procedure that challenges the most skilled orthopaedic surgeon.[5] Except for failures resulting from infection, reoperation to rectify mechanical failures, such as the loss of fixation of the components, may become necessary with increasing frequency as more total hip replacements are performed, especially in younger and more active individuals. As this demand increases, so may the need for specialized centers and personnel to be trained to cope with revision surgery. A thorough understanding of the technical difficulties is mandatory prior to undertaking this procedure. Infection, the prime cause of failure of total hip replacements, must be fully recognized prior to reoperation. While this might not be possible in all cases, when infection is strongly suspected, the total hip replacement may have to be converted to a pseudarthrosis and not revised with a new prosthesis (see Chapter 16).

Diagnosis of mechanical failure

One of the most difficult aspects of revision surgery is the correct preoperative diagnosis of the cause of failure. This is essential to ensure proper management of the patient. Diagnosis of a low-grade infection is difficult, and at times impossible, as mechanical loosening can mimic infection clinically and radiologically, especially if it has been of long standing. Differential diagnosis of mechanical loosening and infection has been discussed in Chapter 16. Clinical signs of loosening are most helpful criteria for the diagnoses of cemented total hips[14,16,17,19]; a sudden onset of pain in a previously pain-free hip joint was recorded in all but one of the cemented hips in our series. In eight of the nine hips where the prosthesis had not been cemented, however, the pain was insidious and gradual. The intensity of the pain was much greater in the loosened cemented prostheses than in the uncemented one. In most cases, the onset of the pain was attributed to trauma or a vigorous physical activity such as lifting heavy objects.

Loosening of a cemented cup produced severe pain in the groin on weight bearing or on attempts at sharp internal or external rotation. With the exception of two, all patients with femoral loosening experienced instability while walking or standing, and most of the patients resorted to canes or crutches. An antalgic gait with a positive Trendelenburg's sign and the inability to raise the leg straight were predominant fea-

515

tures in 18 of 21 loosely cemented total hips, which previously were stable and pain free.[10]

It has been stated elsewhere (Chapter 16) that repeated aspiration has not been our routine practice because of the false negative and false positive interpretation of this technique. *Staphylococcus epidermidis* found in subcultures of two of the hips were felt to be due to laboratory contamination.[10] X-ray diagnosis of distal migration of the femoral components, changes of the orientation of cement in relation to the bone, appearance of a radiolucent zone between cement and bone, or interruption of the cement column suggesting loosening of the femoral component were of considerable help. Varus-valgus strain films were of no value; arthrographic studies[18] in 17 of 21 cemented total hips yielded 14 negative and 3 positive diagnoses of loosening.[10] Of eight cases in which a laminagram was done, two showed no signs of loosening in the standard x-ray films, but the laminagram revealed loosening. A laminagram (magnified or localized conedown views) proved useful in determining the level of cement interruption that is suggestive of loosening.

The surgeon must be acquainted with several aspects of total hip replacement when considering revision of failed total hip replacements, including histology, lateral exposure and removal of the component, mobilization of tissue and removal of the femoral component, and rechannelization of the femur.

Histology. The biological reaction to acrylic cement has been discussed in Chapter 3; in the histology of the interface, the bone as well as the soft tissue varies greatly from case to case depending on the duration and severity of loosening. These changes must be interpreted correctly and differentiated from infection by a pathologist familiar with tissue reactions to implanted plastics (see Chapter 3).

An opaque, whitish fibrinous film, resembling purulent material, was removed from the stems of most of the cemented prostheses. Although its gross appearance resembled "pus" and suggested infection, all cultures proved negative; microscopically this material is amorphous and is interpreted as fibrinoid necrosis. At times, severe histiocytosis or fibrosis is present in addition to fibrinoid necrosis. While the presence of fibrinoid necrosis alone may suggest infection, its presence is also common in situations without infection; it is typically found in relation to femoral prostheses without cement (Fig. 3-5).

During exploration, a metallic stain resembling particulate material of metal is found in most metal-against-metal prostheses, as well as a granulation type of tissue about the periphery of the acetabulum, which may be the result of loosening and not infection.[19,20] Definitive replacement was postponed until a later date, but no positive organism could be cultured from the specimens obtained.[10]

Lateral exposure and removal of the previous prosthesis. A lateral approach in the removal of the trochanter has proved the best method in revising these difficult cases. The existence of previous incisions about the hip does not preclude the suitability of that region for another incision, as we found no skin necrosis at such sites when the incision crossed previous scars (Fig. 14-1). In any event, the incision must be made at the most suitable site for the present surgery, that is, 1 inch posterior at its proximal end and 1 inch anterior at its distal end in relation to an imaginary midtrochanteric line (see Chapter 12). It must provide abundant room proximal to the trochanter for adequate acetabular exposure. A generous exposure is essential as minor loosening of the acetabular cup cannot be ascertained by exploration until a wide exposure of the entire periphery of the acetabulum is accomplished. This can be achieved only after the removal of the fibrous tissue from the critical zone of the cement-bone interface. The pin retractors and Hohmann retractors are used for this purpose. Minor loosening can then be detected by expressing blood from the zone between the cement and bone by firm pressure at the edge of the cup (Fig. 14-6). Minor loosening of the femoral component is readily recognized since the cement-bone junction is well exposed once the hip is dislocated. The femoral component, as the acetabulum, is subjected to a tilting force and the bone-cement interface observed for blood or froth extrusion.

Mobilization and removal of femoral component. Mobilization of the upper femur is routinely done prior to attempting removal of the femoral component. The femoral component should be removed routinely even when not loose (by a blunt chisel at the medial aspect of the neck of the prosthesis), as this facilitates the visibility of the acetabulum. No attempt should be made to remove it prior to the complete mobilization of the femur from the wall of the pelvis, as forceful external rotation at that point could cause fracture of the shaft.

516

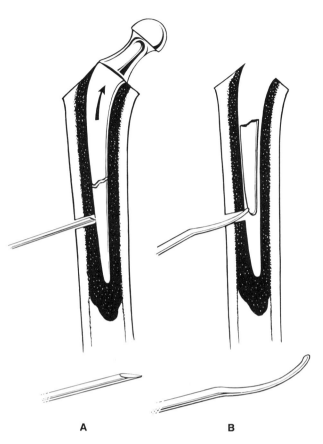

Fig. 14-36. A, Proximal fragment is extracted with ease (arrow). Fractured distal stem fragment may be removed by engaging small gouge via perforation directly onto its lateral aspect. **B,** Once distal fragment is disengaged, it is pushed into medullary canal using a curved narrow instrument such as one shown here.

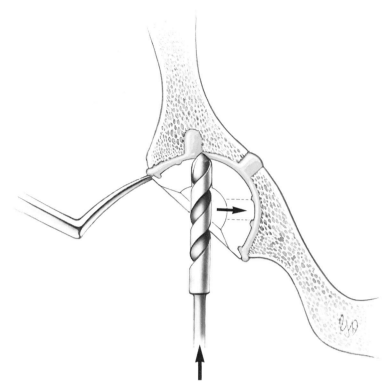

Fig. 14-37. Acetabular cup is usually removed by insertion of acetabular gouge between cement and bone. If it is desirable to remove cup without cement (to protect bony acetabulum from damage), gouge should be inserted between plastic cup and cement. Preferably plastic cup is drilled at 2 or 3 areas to ease its collapse for ease of extraction.

Removal of components. In noncemented prostheses, for example, a Ring prosthesis, the fenestration bone of the prosthesis is removed by a reciprocating saw and dislodged from the canal in the same manner as the cemented prosthesis. Removal of the trochanteric wire prior to removal of the femoral component must be executed with caution to avoid fragmentation.

If the stem of the prosthesis is fractured and this is recognized preoperatively, a small window is made in the anterolateral aspect of the shaft at 1 to 2 cm. distal to the level of the fractured stem. A narrow gouge is then engaged onto the outer aspect of the distal fragment, which is tapped out of the channel into the femoral canal (Fig. 14-36). It is essential to avoid making an excessively large window or placing it too distally, since the former predisposes the shaft to frac-

tures and the latter prevents the lengths of the gouge to reach the stem once the fractured fragment is advanced into the canal.

A special engineering tap also may be helpful in fixing it to the distal fragment through the opening of the medullary canal for extraction. This system is at its developmental stage but has a great advantage over the previous methods, since it alleviates the need for perforating the shaft. The acetabular component may be easily extracted by placing a curved Smith-Petersen gouge at the cement-bone junction (Fig. 16-17); however, if there is excessive acetabular damage, it is best to remove the cup and leave the cement undisturbed at the floor of the acetabulum. We found that reaming out the high-density polyethylene socket with a special reamer is a most suitable method. Removal of the socket may be achieved also by drilling two or three half-inch drill holes through the thickness of the plastic, thus bending the cup on itself and prying it out of its cement bed (Fig. 14-37).

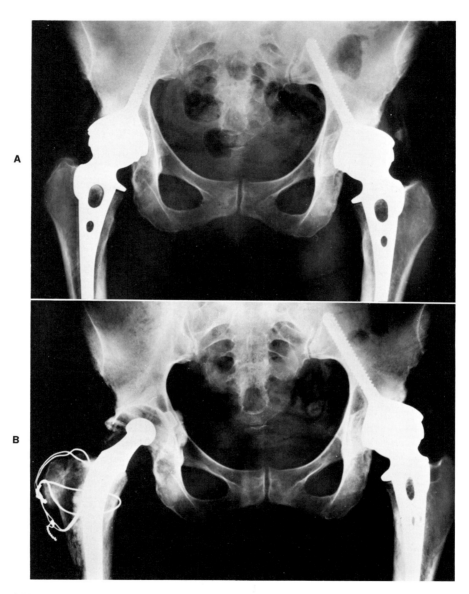

Fig. 14-38. A, Bilateral Ring total hip prostheses were inserted in 51-year-old female for degenerative osteo-arthritis. **B,** Because of pain in right hip, conversion was done 1 year following insertion of Ring prosthesis. **C,** Following total hip replacement by low-friction arthroplasty on right hip, patient became active but sustained fracture of stem of Ring prosthesis of left hip. Arrow indicates fracture site. **D,** Retained portion of Ring prosthesis (arrow) following low-friction arthroplasty. At surgery it was not possible to remove fractured stem from pelvis.

518

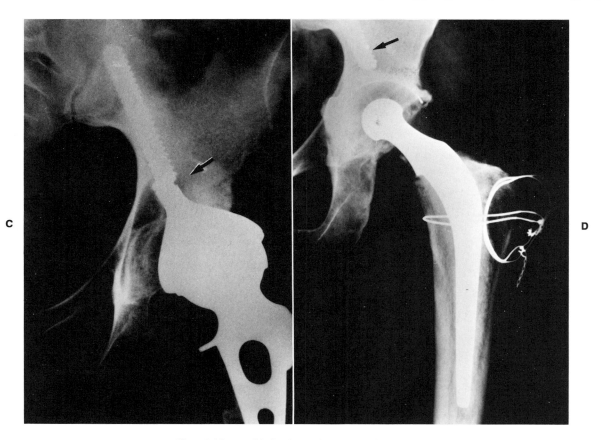

Fig. 14-38, cont'd. For legend see opposite page.

Plates, screws, cement fragments, or the broken stem of a Ring acetabular cup may be difficult to extract; these devices may remain in the pelvis, providing they do not interfere with the preparation or implantation of the new prosthesis (Figs. 14-38 and 14-39).

Rechannelization of femur. Complete removal of the cement from the femoral canal may not be necessary, as it will bond satisfactorily with the new cement (see Chapter 3) (Figs. 14-40 and 14-41); loose fragments, however, must be completely removed. It is essential in reaming out the old cement that no damage is done to the shaft, since perforation may prevent adequate fixation, weaken the femur, and create a new path for the revised prosthesis (Fig. 17-19). Rechannelization is necessary, and often minimal reaming may be sufficient to accommodate the new prosthesis (Fig. 14-42). The new channel must be in an optimal position with adequate valgus orientation for the stem. It is essential to avoid the old track (channel) when inserting the new stem (Fig. 14-43). At times, large pieces of cement fragments may be extracted through the medullary canal of the femur by a crochet-type hook or a pituitary-type forceps. A tapered corkscrew-like tap inserted into the cement channel may also assist in extracting cement fragments. Thin and narrow gouges and narrow osteotomes specially designed for the removal of cement from the shaft also may facilitate removal. High-speed drills may further facilitate removal of cement by a grinding mechanism. A fiberoptic light is a useful source of illumination of the canal during preparation. The canal must be carefully dried after irrigation, prior to the application of cement.

The rechannelization guide and drill system devised by the author[11] (Fig. 14-44) is used with the following instructions:

1. The greater trochanter and femoral components are removed as previously described; the femoral prosthesis is knocked out of its bed by an engineering cold chisel. *Text continued on p. 530.*

519

Fig. 14-39. A, Posterior fracture dislocation of pelvis following automobile accident in 53-year-old female had been treated by open reduction and screw fixation of posterior fragment. **B,** Two years following insertion of Tronzo prosthesis that has been cemented in place. NOTE: extreme damage to floor of pelvis and extent of cement into ilium toward sacroiliac joint. **C,** Following revision note superior defect was supported by wire mesh. Screw is left in place and portion of cement that could not be extracted from pelvis remains in situ. **D,** Removed prosthesis showing only portion of cement attached to base of stem could be extracted. Considerable force was necessary to extract this prosthesis from pelvis.

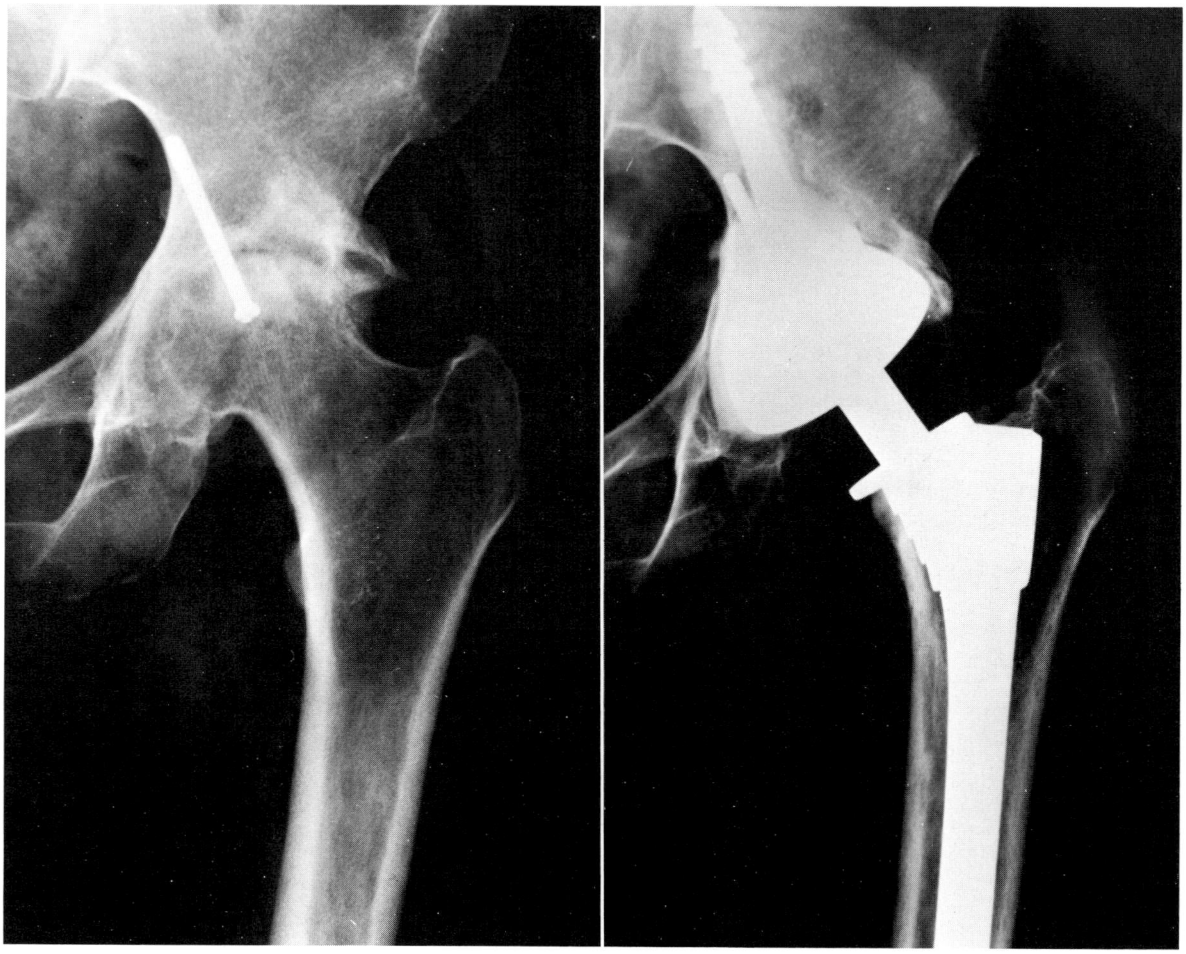

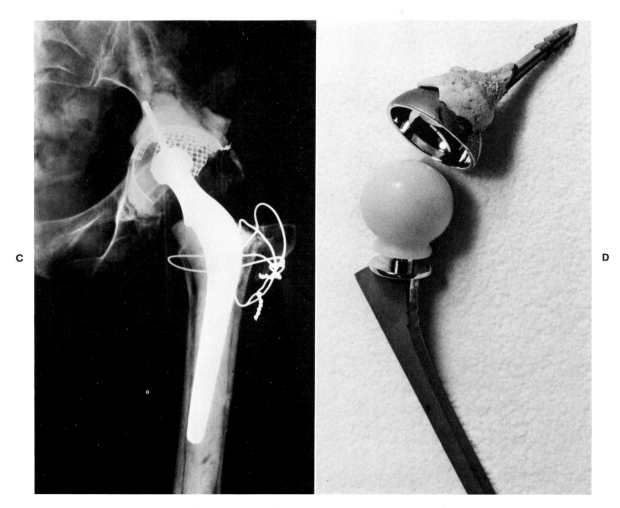

Fig. 14-39, cont'd. For legend see opposite page.

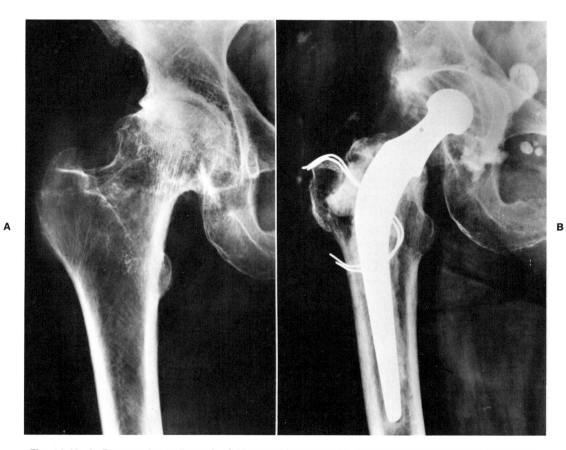

Fig. 14-40. A, Preoperative radiograph of 68-year-old woman with degenerative osteoarthritis of right hip. **B,** Postoperative radiograph following low-friction arthroplasty performed in another institution, after which partial removal of wires was done because of persistent pain in thigh and trochanteric region. NOTE: inadequate cementing of stem evidenced by sclerosis of tip of stem and inadequate cement between shaft and lateral cortex of femur at distal end. Also note radiolucent zone appearing between convex side of prosthesis and cement. **C,** "Successful arthrogram" performed without evidence of leakage of dye between femur and stem. Bottom arrow indicates needle inserted in joint and middle arrow indicates radiolucent zone between convex side of prosthesis and cement. Top arrow shows dye but without any communication between joint space and space between prosthesis and cement. **D,** Three years following revision arthroplasty by rechannelization of femur and insertion of heavy-stem prosthesis. At surgery clinical impression of femoral loosening was confirmed (see text).

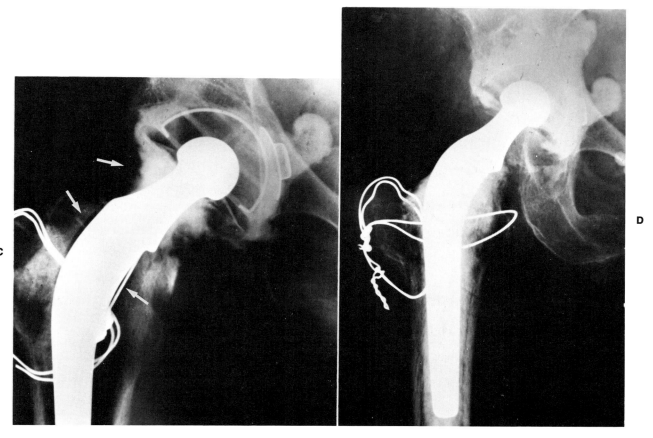

Fig. 14-40, cont'd. For legend see opposite page.

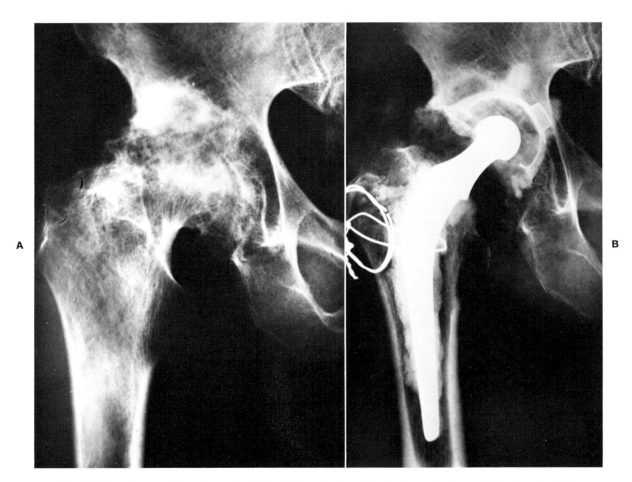

Fig. 14-41. A, Preoperative radiograph of right hip; low-friction arthroplasty was indicated. Patient's weight at surgery was 178 pounds. **B,** One year following surgery patient remained asymptomatic except for occasional painless "click" in hip in certain ranges of motion. Vertical wire is fractured. NOTE: large medullary canal of femur and inadequate cement technique. Patient's weight was 225 pounds at this point. **C,** Two and one-half years following surgery, there is evidence of subsidence of stem of prosthesis with further breakage of wires. NOTE: varus shift of prosthesis and radiolucent zone between outer aspect of stem and cement. **D,** Revision of loose stem by insertion of heavy-stem prosthesis following rechannelization of femur. NOTE: slight valgus orientation achieved to produce thick layer of cement at region of calcar and concave side of prosthesis as well as laterally between stem tip and outer shaft of femur.

C
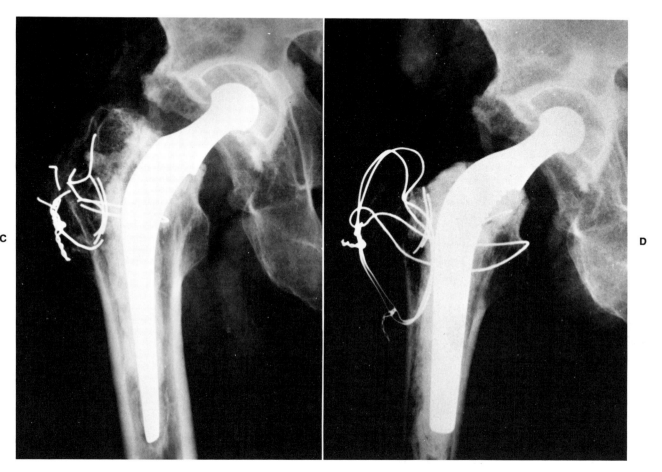
D

Fig. 14-41, cont'd. For legend see opposite page.

Fig. 14-42. A, Painful Thompson prosthesis in 52-year-old woman with history of congential dislocation of hip who had previously been treated by bone graft and shelf procedure. NOTE: prosthesis has been end bearing as evidenced by sclerosis at level of tip. **B,** Following revision by total hip replacement, perforation of shaft of femur and extrusion of stem and cement are noted. **C,** Insertion of new prosthesis was possible following rechannelization of femur without disturbing old cement. Cup was also found to be loose, thus requiring replacement. NOTE: old cement was not removed from femur for fear of damage to shaft.

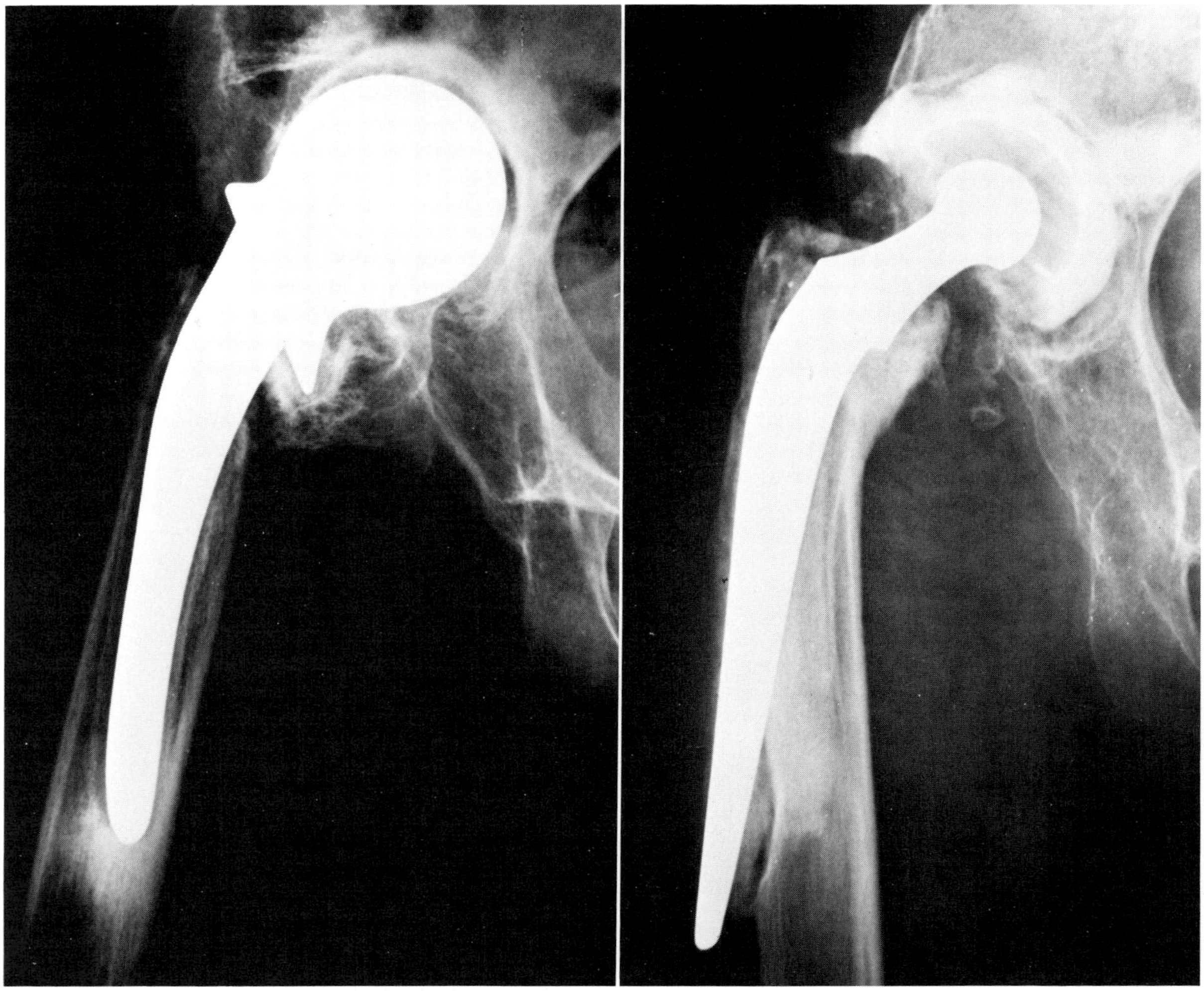

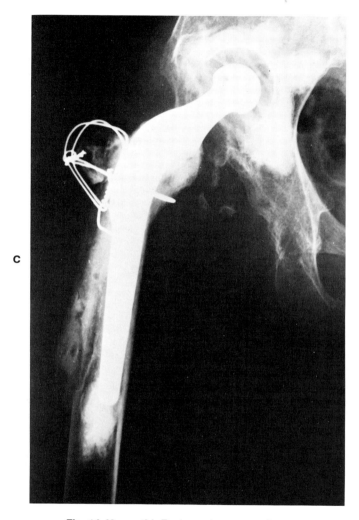

C

Fig. 14-42, cont'd. For legend see opposite page.

Fig. 14-43. Following rechannelization in optimal position, it is essential to avoid old tract (channel) at insertion of new stem. **A,** Failed McKee-Farrar total hip prosthesis inserted for complication of fracture of neck of femur in 62-year-old librarian. NOTE: prosthesis was inserted in marked varus orientation; radiolucent cement had been used. **B,** Rechannelization of femur was successfully performed, but stem of new prosthesis was inserted through old tract. Thus prosthesis is again in a varus orientation.

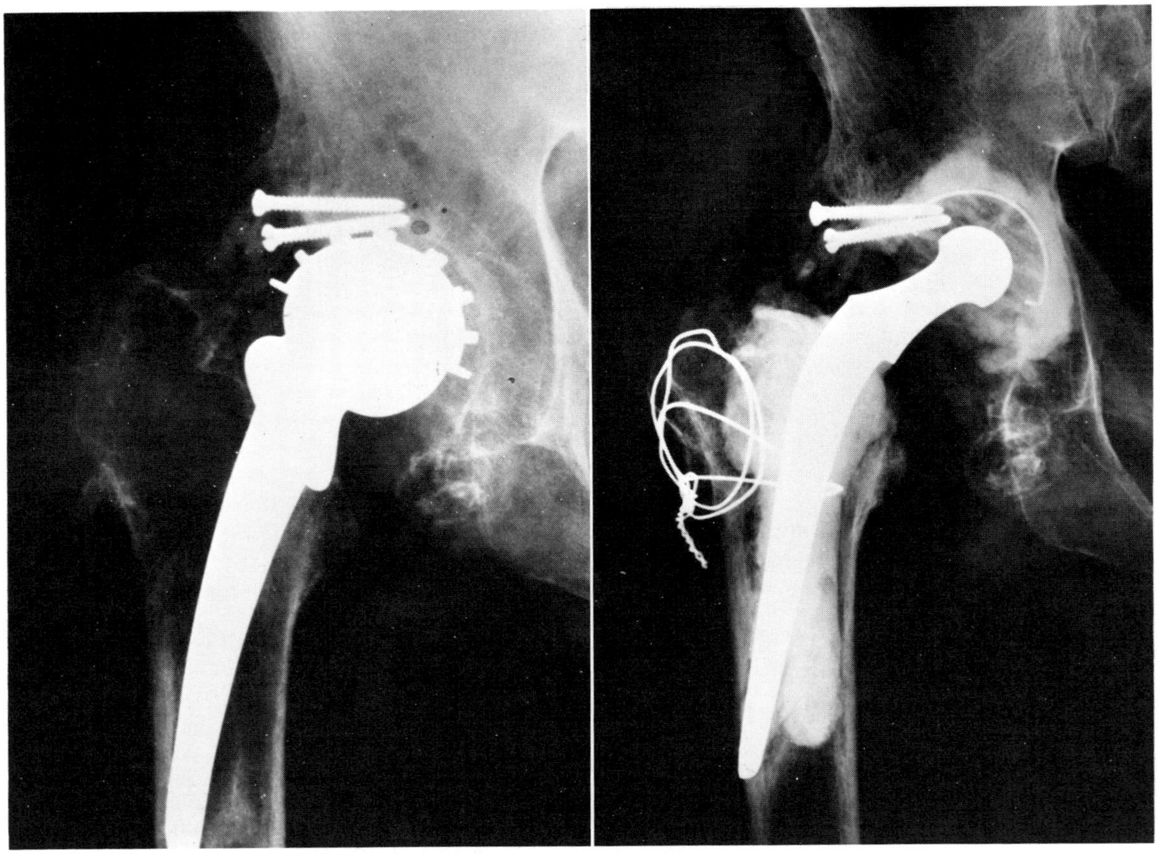

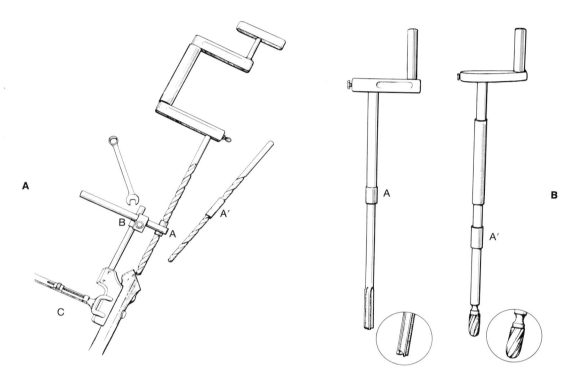

Fig. 14-44. A, Guide drill system using wide throw brace and twisted drill bits with chip clearance and terminal cutting tip. Drill guide consists of three parts: part *A* consists of bushing that is fixed to transverse bar of instrument. Each drill and expanding reamer carrying its own sleeve (*A'*) is fixed to transverse bar of guide at point *A*. Universal joint *B* allows transverse bar to move in all planes and directions. By friction lock at point *B* optimal position can be maintained for orientation of drills and reamers. Main segment of guide (side bar) is clamped by conventional Lowman clamp to lateral aspect of shaft at point *C*. Position is maintained rigidly throughout procedure of drilling and reaming. **B,** Reamers similar to drills carry their own bushings (*A* and *A'*) but are used with narrow-throw handle brace. It is essential that correct angle of reaming be selected, otherwise penetration of shaft may occur (see text). (From Eftekhar, N. S.: Clin. Orthop. **123:**29-31, 1977.) Rechannelization guide and drill system devised by author and manufactured by Codman & Shurtleff, Inc.

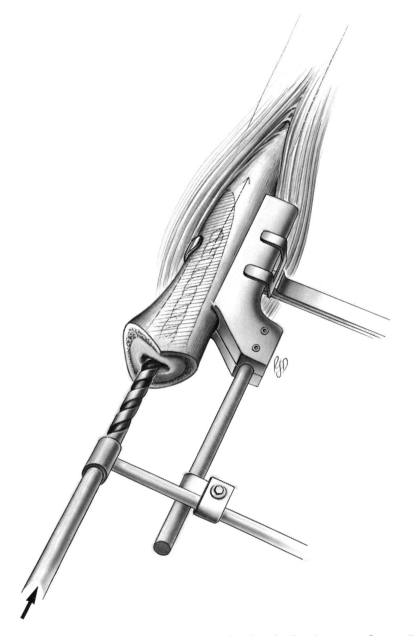

Fig. 14-45. Application of rechannelization instrument and direction of drill and reamers. Correct direction of drill and reamers may be verified by radiograph (if necessary) on operating table (see text).

2. The vastus lateralis is detached from the ridge and also split midlateral similar to the method used for nail and plate fixation of fractures.

3. The single prong of the Lowman clamp is passed posterior and medial to the side of the shaft of the femur holding the side bar of the guide against the shaft.

4. Having the universal friction bolt loosened at point "B" (Fig. 14-44), the surgeon will guide the drill toward the desirable direction for the preparation of the channel.

5. Once the desired direction is established, the correct direction of the drills and reamers is assisted and maintained by the bushing carried on each drill and reamer (Fig. 14-45).

■ ■ ■

All details are considered essential. This chapter is not summarized.

REFERENCES

1. Amstutz, H. C.: Complications of total hip replacement, Clin. Orthop. **72:**123-137, 1970.
2. Amstutz, H. C., and Sakai, D. N.: Total joint replacement for ankylosed hips, J. Bone Joint Surg. **57A**(5):619-625, 1975.
3. Andersson, G. B. J., Freeman, M. A. R., and Swanson, S. A. V.: Loosening of the cemented acetabular cup in total hip replacement, J. Bone Joint Surg. **54B:**590-99, 1972.
4. Brewster, R. C., Coventry, M. B., and Johnson, E. W.: Conversion of the arthrodesed hip to a total hip arthroplasty, J. Bone Joint Surg. **57A**(1): 27-30, 1975.
5. Charnley, J.: Editorial comment, Clin. Orthop. **72:**2, 1970.
6. Charnley, J., and Ferreira, A.: Transplantation of the greater trochanter in arthroplasty of the hip, J. Bone Joint Surg. **46B:**191-197, 1964.
7. D'Aubigne, R. M., and Postel, M.: Functional results of hip arthroplasty with acrylic prosthesis, J. Bone Joint Surg. **36A:**451-475, 1954.
8. Dupont, J. A., and Charnley, J.: Low friction arthroplasty of the hip for the failures of previous operations, J. Bone Joint Surg. **54B:**77-87, 1972.
9. Eftekhar, N. S.: Mechanical failure in low friction arthroplasty. In American Academy of Orthopaedic Surgeons: Instructional course lecture, vol. 23, St. Louis, 1974, The C. V. Mosby Co., pp. 230-242.
10. Eftekhar, N. S.: Revision of failed total hip replacement by Charnley low friction arthroplasty. In The Hip Society: The hip, proceedings of the fourth open scientific meeting of The Hip Society, 1976, St. Louis, 1976, The C. V. Mosby Co.
11. Eftekhar, N. S.: Rechannelization of cemented femur using a guide and drill system, Clin. Orthop. **123:**29-31, 1977.
12. Eftekhar, N. S., and Stinchfield, F. E.: Experience with low-friction arthroplasty. A statistical review of early results and complications, Clin. Orthop. **95:**60-68, 1973.
13. Eftekhar, N. S., Smith, D. M., Henry, J. H., and Stinchfield, F. E.: Revision arthroplasty using Charnley low friction arthroplasty technic. With reference to specifics of technic and comparison of results with primary low friction arthroplasty, Clin. Orthop. **95:**48-60, 1973.
14. Evarts, C. M., Gramer, L. J., and Bergfeld, J. A.: The Ring total hip prosthesis. Comparison of results at one and three years, J. Bone Joint Surg. **54A:**1677-1682, 1972.
15. Ferrari, A., and Charnley, J.: Conversion of hip joint pseudarthrosis to total hip replacement, Clin. Orthop. **121:**12-19, 1976.
16. Lazansky, M. G.: Complications in total hip replacement with the Charnley technic, Clin. Orthop. **72:**40-45, 1970.
17. Patterson, F. P., and Brown, C. S.: The McKee-Farrar total hip replacement. Preliminary results and complications of 368 operations performed in five general hospitals, J. Bone Joint Surg. **54A:** 257-275, 1972.
18. Salvati, E. A., Freiberger, R. H., and Wilson, P. D., Jr.: Arthrography for complications of total hip replacement. A review of thirty-one arthorgrams, J. Bone Joint Surg. **53A:**701-709, 1971.
19. Wilson, J. N., and Scales, J. T.: Loosening of total hip replacements with cement fixation. Clinical findings and laboratory studies, Clin. Orthop. **72:** 145-160, 1970.
20. Wilson, P. D., Jr., Amstutz, H. C., Czerniecki, A., Salvati, E. A., and Mendes, D. G.: Total hip replacement with fixation by acrylic cement. A preliminary study of 100 consecutive McKee-Farrar prosthetic replacements, J. Bone Joint Surg., **54A:**207-236, 1972.

PART FIVE

CLINICAL RESULTS AND COMPLICATIONS

CHAPTER 15

Clinical results

The life of the law has not been Logic: it has been experience.

JUSTICE OLIVER WENDELL HOLMES, JR.

I know of no way of judging the future, but by the past.

PATRICK HENRY

The best of prophets of the future is the past.

LORD BYRON

DEVELOPMENTAL YEARS

Undoubtedly, the objective value of any surgical procedure is judged by the clinical results obtained. For a better understanding of the evolution of successful total hip replacement, a background of statistical data concerning its development is helpful. The various clinical results reflecting a variety of the techniques and devices cited have been divided into two main groups: group 1—those with metal-to-metal bearing, with and without cement; and, group 2—those with metal-against-plastic bearings, with cement.

METAL-TO-METAL BEARING TOTAL HIP REPLACEMENT PROCEDURES
Noncemented varieties

In this category Ring and Sivash prostheses were widely used. In 1964 Peter Ring of Redhill, England, began to use an uncemented metal-to-metal total prosthesis made of cobalt-chromium alloy; he reported on the development and early results of this prosthesis in 1,000 arthritic hips,[65-70] 942 hips were evaluated, with a mortality rate of 1.1%. Deep wound infection (0.7%) and dislocation (0.3%) followed this procedure. By comparison, of the 159 hips of "earlier" design that he followed for 5 to 8 years, 45% had remained excellent and 29% good, but 14% needed reoperation because of loosening of the femoral compound. From his study Ring concluded that of 535 patients followed for 1 to 5 years, 69% showed excellent results; results were good in 21%, and revision was necessary in only 2%.

He also obtained better results with improved cortical fit by introducing a tapered screw thread on the pelvic component of the prosthesis.

The Russian-designed "Sivash" prosthesis—one unit metal-against-metal lock fit—has been used widely in the Soviet Union since 1956.[71,73,85] It was first tested for 3½ years in 38 dogs, and Wolkow,[81] in 1959, reported encouraging results in 158 patients. The prosthesis is designed to fit mechanically into the cancellous bone of the acetabulum by impaction of its sharp perforated blades into the bone's substance. No acrylic cement is used for fixation. At this time it is estimated that approximately 500 Sivash arthroplasties have been done in the United States,[81] and Russins'[71] report on 120 such cases indicates that not only does it not offer advantages over other designs, but it is especially ineffective because of the severe constrainment of metal against metal and the small bearing contact of ball and socket, which create high-rising stresses of the articular surfaces.

Breck[3,4] reported his experiences from 1969 to 1973 with the use of a Urist socket combined with a Thompson prosthesis; he concluded that there was no need for acrylic cement based on the excellent results obtained in 21 of 47 cases, good results in 18 cases, fair results in 5 cases, and poor results in only 3 cases.

Between 1961 and 1972 R. D. Smith[75,76] developed a metal-against-metal set by matching a Gaenslen cup with a Moore self-locking prosthesis. He performed the longest follow-up (11½ years) and reported that improvement occurred

535

Clinical results and complications

in all but a small number of patients. There are several other accounts (of small series) of metal-to-metal prosthesis in both the United States and Europe with limited follow-up indicating gradually increasing rates of complications and failure; among them are Wilson and Scales,[83] who performed 108 total hip arthroplasties using a Stanmore (metal-on-metal) socket with three obliquely set round pins on the convex side of a cup similar in design to Urist's. Their 1½ to 9-year follow-up showed unsatisfactory results (loosening), and most of the prostheses were replaced with high-density polyethylene sockets. They concluded that a metal-on-plastic component would be preferable to the metal-on-metal prostheses because of the higher frictional properties of the design.

An uncemented Moore femoral prosthesis against a McBride acetabular component was used by Shorbe[72] and Lunceford[50] with limited experiences and short-term follow-up results.

Debeyre and Goutallier[22] used a combination of metal-to-metal prosthesis with a Moore femoral component against a Urist cup in 63 hips. Early results were satisfactory, but later follow-up revealed a high percentage of loosening and fixation failures.

The main problem with the metal-to-metal prosthesis was the high-frictional torque and the attendant inadequacy of fixation owing to the high concentration of stress at the fixation site, making the results of this type of prosthesis universally unpredictable. (See Chapter 3.) (The author has no personal experience with prostheses of this category except for converting several failed prostheses of this type to a cemented design of total hip replacement [see Chapters 3, 4, and 14]. A true incidence of successful metal-to-metal bearings without cement over a period of 10 years remains unknown.)

Cemented varieties

The most widely used prosthesis of this type in the United States and abroad is the McKee-Farrar prosthesis; Kenneth McKee and Watson Farrar are credited with the development of this type of prosthesis at Norwich Hospital, England. McKee's work was entirely independent of Charnley's, and it featured a metal-to-metal bearing (chromium and cobalt alloy). According to McKee,[54] the first model was constructed in the 1940s but was never inserted into a patient. Between 1956 and 1960 a prototype was used in

40 cases with a success rate of 54%. In 1960, after a review of the first series, they improved their results with modifications, including the use of acrylic cement. In their second 100 cases, although there were four deaths, there was a success rate of 94%; further improved results (as high as 98%) were reported in their third 100 hips.[54] A recent study of total hip replacement in 300 consecutive operations (using the McKee-Farrar method) revealed the following complications: sepsis, 4%; dislocations, 2%; revisions, 8%; pulmonary embolism, 3%; deep vein thrombosis, 1.3%; femoral shaft perforation, 1%; fracture of the femoral shaft, 0.3%; allergy to cobalt-chromium alloy, 0.3%.[52,53,55,56] Good to excellent results from McKee-Farrar hip replacements have similarly been observed and reported by other surgeons.[7,36,41,42,48,80]

Other surgeons who experimented with metal-to-metal designs were less enthusiastic because of the problem of loosening. Patterson[64] reviewed and reported the clinical results of 368 McKee-Farrar prostheses used in five hospitals in Canada in 1972, as did Wilson and associates[84] during the same year.

METAL-TO-PLASTIC BEARINGS WITH CEMENT

To my knowledge no series of cases has been reported using a metal-to-plastic bearing without cement.

Charnley's greatest contribution to total hip arthroplasty has been the use of plastics for bearing surfaces and the fixing of components to bone with acrylic cement. In his classic descriptions of early results, he states, "On removal of the splint, after three weeks, most patients can execute a 'straight-leg raise' and have no pain or spasm on passive movement. After a week out of plaster they have recovered the preoperative range of movement."[8,17] Charnley[8] exercised caution when reporting "spectacular results," and in his first report on 97 hips he clearly defined the "experimental nature" of the operation. He stated, "though my experience of using polytetrafluorethylene for arthroplasty of the hip extends over three years, the technique in its present form has been used only since January, 1960."[8] There were no deaths except for one coronary occlusion 6 weeks after the operation, and the only serious complication was one deep venous thrombosis.

In his exhaustive efforts to identify pitfalls and

536

complications, Charnley continuously surveyed his early results. Because of pressure from colleagues to make public his technique and prosthesis, he periodically reported clinical results and complications in a series of Internal Publications at the Wrightington Hospital, but there was no publication on a worldwide basis and little data were available. Following his failure with Teflon (PTFE), he further cautioned against the massive embarkment on a new procedure (such as total hip replacement) because of its uncertain future, and restricted the procedure to those who had attended the Wrightington Hospital for firsthand observation and apprenticeship. In these early reports two outstanding features are noted: (1) advocacy of restricting this operation to the old and disabled and (2) caution against the possibility of tissue reaction and mechanical failure of the device.[11] As late as 1972, he stressed the immense responsibility of surgeons performing these operations toward their patients, that is, the potential failure and complications—not likely to be anticipated except by a casual operator practicing occasional total hip replacement.[14]

Marshall Urist[81] of the United States recognized the importance of statistical data and follow-up of patients undergoing total hip replacement—and the effect the implant material might have on the body. He devoted three issues of *Clinical Orthopaedics and Related Research* to the subject of total hip replacement and summarized the status of the art of using acrylic cement in surgery in a recent monograph.[81]

Charnley[10] abandoned Teflon in November of 1962—some 2½ years after it was first used. In January 1963, as president–guest lecturer to the American Academy of Orthopaedic Surgeons in Miami, he pointed out the mechanical and biological defects of Teflon and the suitability of high-density polyethylene (RCH 1,000) by reporting clinical data related to the latter's superiority to polyfluoroethylene (Teflon).

Like Charnley,[11] McKee[56] recognized the importance of acrylic cement in hip replacement. It may be stated that the "spectacular" results of the technique of total hip replacement prove that the defects of past methods were due to the diseased acetabulum when left in situ. Furthermore, it may be stated that the loss of movement from fibrous ankylosis and ectopic bone formation (which commonly followed replacement arthroplasty) must have been due to irritation caused by motion between the implant and living bone. By eliminating such motion, fibrous ankylosis is less likely to occur. With reports of outstanding early results, it became evident that if a total hip replacement is properly performed on a suitable candidate that the following outcomes may be expected: (1) total absence of pain, (2) consistent improvement in range of motion shortly after the operation, and (3) maintenance of range of motion.

Improved functional activity with excellent gait is another typical achievement characterizing total arthroplasty using acrylic cement. Surgeons' experiences with cemented prostheses leave little doubt that these outstanding outcomes are due to the excellent fixation of the prosthesis to the bone.

SHORT- AND LONG-TERM RESULTS OF CHARNLEY LOW-FRICTION ARTHROPLASTY

Our experiences with over 3,000 low-friction arthroplasties at the New York Orthopaedic Hospital and more than 10,000 operations performed at Wrightington Hospital in England (with supporting literature), all demonstrate that the most rewarding aspect of total hip replacement by low-friction arthroplasty are the "predictable" and "reproducible" results. While the early results of this operation are gratifying, we continually urge a conservative attitude in patient selection, always keeping in mind potential complications (serious when they do develop). Thus the careful selection of patients and strict adherence to technical details are essential factors in contributing to satisfactory results.

Charnley and his associates* have continued surveillance on the results of low-friction arthroplasty since its inception at Wrightington Hospital. He and Cupic[18] reported that 92% of 106 low-friction arthroplasty total hip replacements showed complete success, with no evidence of deterioration after 9 and 10 years. In this group the failure rate was as follows: infection, 6.6%; mechanical loosening, no more than 1.6%; dislocation, 1.6%. No case was found with enough "wear" to require replacement—75% of these cases showed an average wear of 1 mm./5 years; the remaining 25% showed wear three times greater than average. A special feature of this study concerned bone resorption in the region of

---

*See references 9, 12, 13, 15, 16, 18, 19, 25, and 82.

Table 15-1. Systemic complications of low-friction arthroplasty

Source	Institution	Date of report	Period operations performed	No. of hip operations	Follow-up period (yr.)	Gastro-intestinal complications	Renal failure	Urinary retention
Charnley[13]	Wrightington Hospital	1970	1962-63	138	6-7			(10)
Eftekhar[26]	Wrightington Hospital	1971	1962-63	138	7-8			
Charnley[16]	Wrightington Hospital	1972	1962-65	$\frac{379}{582}$	4-7			
Charnley and Cupic[18]	Wrightington Hospital	1973	1962-63	106	9-10			
Coventry et al.[21]	Mayo Clinic	1974	1969-74	$\frac{2012}{333}$	$\frac{1\text{-}2}{\text{Min.2}}$	2.4%	0.5%	22%
Lazansky[45]	Hospital for Joint Diseases	1973	1966-72	501	½-6	(1)		
Eftekhar et al.[31]	New York Orthopaedic Hospital	1976	1969-74	800	2-4	(10) 1%		(281) 35%

Table 15-2. Local complications of low-friction arthroplasty

Source	Institution	Date of report	Period operations performed	No. of hip operations	Follow-up period (yr.)	Deep vein thrombosis	Deep wound hematoma	Superficial wound infection	Deep wound infection
Charnley[13]	Wrightington Hospital	1970	1962-63	138	6-7	(4)	(5)	(7)	3
Eftekhar[26]	Wrightington Hospital	1971	1962-63	138	7-8	(4)	(5)	(7)	5
Charnley[16]	Wrightington Hospital	1972	1962-65	$\frac{379}{582}$	4-7	5.5%			3.8%
Charnley and Cupic[18]	Wrightington Hospital	1973	1962-63	106	9-10				6.6%
Coventry et al.[21]	Mayo Clinic	1974	1969-74	$\frac{2012}{333}$	$\frac{1\text{-}2}{\text{Min.2}}$	3.4%	1%	1.3%	0.6%
Lazansky[45]	Hospital Joint for Diseases	1973	1966-72	501	½-6	(7)	(18) 3.5%	1.7%	0.8%
Eftekhar et al.[31]	New York Orthopaedic Hospital	1976	1969-74	800	2-4	(54) 7%	(55) 7%	(25) 3%	(4) 0.5%

Nonfatal pulmonary embolism	Fatal pulmonary embolism	Paralytic ileus	Pulmonary complications other than pulmonary embolus	Coronary thrombosis and heart failure	Cardiac arrest at operation	CVA	Postoperative psychosis	Death related to surgery
(3)		(4)	(3)	(1)				
(3)		(4)	(3)	(1)				
3.2%	1.4%							2.1%
2.2%		(19)	1.7%	1.7%	(1)	(1)	(8)	0.4%
(6)	(2)	1		(1)				1.1%
(58)		27	(16)	(11)				(6)
7%		3%	2%	1%			3%	0.5%

Sciatic and peroneal nerve palsy	Femoral nerve palsy	Dislocation	Subluxation	Trochanteric bursitis	Trochanteric nonunion	Ectopic bone formation	Loosening socket	Loosening femoral component	Late dislocation	Unexplained pain
2		1	1	(6)			(2)			
2		1	1		3%		(2)			
		1.5%			4.2%	5%	1%		0.17%	0.17%
1.1%		1.6%								
		1.6%	1.1%		2.7%					
(12)	(5)	3%	Few					(2)	4.2%	
(6)	(1)	1%	3.2%		1.8%	8.1%	0.4%	1%		
(9)		(4)	(16)		(25)	(85)	(2)	(1)		
1%		0.5%	2%		(3%)	10%				

the calcar femorale (in a small percentage of the cases); it was postulated to have been due to tissue reaction not present in previous studies. However, there was no correlation between the amount of wear of the socket and the bony absorption at the region of the neck.[18] Although the author has used a number of different types of prostheses and surgical techniques, his main clinical experiences have been with Charnley low-friction arthroplasty.

EXPERIENCES WITH CHARNLEY LOW-FRICTION ARTHROPLASTY

In March 1971, I[26] was permitted (by Sir John Charnley) to make a separate and independent study of the long-term results of low-friction arthroplasty involving 580 patients who were operated on prior to that date at Wrightington Hospital. Of 256 operations performed between 1962 and 1963, an unselected series of 138 hips in 120 patients who qualified for long-term study (a minimum of 7 and maximum of 8 years' follow-up) were subject to this personal study. Clinical and radiological observations were made at 6 months, 5 years, 7 years, and 8 years, based on prospective evaluation records at Wrightington Hospital. In more than one third of the cases there remained a functional restricting factor (especially in polyarthritic rheumatoid patients), but the two most remarkably constant features were freedom from pain and the mobility gained after surgery. The most serious complication was deep wound infection in five hips, and its delayed appearance in one hip 4½ years following surgery. The only other failure was bilateral loosening of the socket in one patient with rheumatoid arthritis. In no case was there loosening of the femoral component, nor was there any clinical or radiological evidence of tissue reaction to cement or high-density polyethylene. The average wear rate of high-density polyethylene ranged from 0 to 1.5 mm./5 years at the 7- to 8-year follow-up. Similar studies but with a shorter term follow-up have shown a greater number of complications by several investigators—as one might expect, surgeons faced a great number of complications at first—such as nonunion, trochanteric problems, and dislocations,[21,34] but with extended experience desirable results were obtained efficiently with low-friction arthroplasty.* As Charnley's low-friction

---

*See references 20, 27, 30, 39, 43, 44, 56, 63, 78, and 79.

arthroplasty technique became more prevalent both in Europe and the United States, there appeared reports of early results of the use of this procedure as adopted by others. One can conclude from these statistics that Charnley's procedure was replicable and most effective when adopted without major modifications.

The largest series of low-friction arthroplasties with the longest follow-up was done at Wrightington Hospital and involved more than 10,000 operations using one standard technique.

An in-depth study of the problems associated with total hip replacement was initiated at The New York Orthopaedic Hospital at Columbia-Presbyterian Medical Center in New York, following the introduction of the technique of total hip replacement by low-friction arthroplasty. It was decided to adopt Charnley's low-friction arthroplasty procedure with only minor modifications. Summarization of the details of the operative technique and evaluation of the pre- and postoperative findings were initiated for the sake of future studies of the clinical results (see Chapters 9 to 11). A modified D'Aubigne and Postel method was used to evaluate the results (Table 15-4). A statistical review of early results and complications of low-friction arthroplasty was published in 1973,[29] and systemic and local complications following low-friction arthroplasty were reanalyzed and reported in 1976[29] (Figs. 15-1 to 15-3 and Table 15-3).

A special record containing preoperative history, general physical and hip examination, x-ray details and analysis, and the details of operative procedure and postoperative complications was designed (Chapters 9 to 11), and the results of 6 months to 3½ years follow-up of 700 hips were evaluated. The follow-up figures represented the entire series of 700 operations on 518 patients—320 women and 198 men; although 212 patients suffered bilateral disease, only 91 required bilateral operations. The results of the first 300 operations were evaluated in detail after a minimum of 2 years follow-up. The list of diagnostic categories and the age distribution in the major categories are represented in Fig. 15-2.

These operations constituted the first series of total hip replacements and were performed in a conventional operating room with the patient in a supine position, under general anesthesia and endotracheal intubation. The greater trochanter was routinely osteotomized and a whole blood transfusion of 1,000 to 2,000 ml. was given to most. The sterile compression dressing was not removed until 1 week after the operation; the hips were maintained in a position of abduction by a special splint; weight bearing was resumed after 6 days. (See Chapters 6 to 9 and 11.)

A modified D'Aubigne and Postel method was used to evaluate the results: subsidence of pain was dramatic and consistent in most cases and, as in previous studies, unrelated to the condition of the hip prior to surgery. Functional activities (walking and so on) were remarkably improved provided there were no other restraining factors, such as systemic disease or other joint disabilities. Only those patients with rheumatoid arthritis who had previously been quite restricted remained so after the operation. Most patients dis-

pensed with their walking aids 3 months postoperatively; in most instances there was a gradual improvement of gait over a period of 1 year or more following the operation, and the improved gait (achieved at about 6 months to 1 year after surgery) was preserved.

Improvement in passive and active range of motion was parallel to improvement in function, and most patients gained adequate range of motion to be compatible with normal functions for their age. Although gain in mobility was not as dramatic as relief from pain and functional improvement, nevertheless, most patients were able to sit comfortably (although about one fourth [26%] of them were not able to touch their toes and were rated 3 or 4 for mobility). Figs. 15-1 and 15-2 graphically illustrate these preoperative conditions and postoperative improvements. They represent unilateral and bilateral hip disorders and those with and without systemic disorders—that is, rheumatoid disease with multiple joint involvement.

Stability of the joint and ability to abduct and flex the hip against gravity were assessed by Trendelenburg's test and the straight-leg raising test; the latter is a very important achievement after total hip replacement, and all patients demonstrated good to excellent results. Only in five cases (which were considered failures) were the patients unable to perform straight-leg raising or unable to abduct against gravity (due to infection or mechanical failure).

POSTOPERATIVE COMPLICATIONS

Most of the series cited in this section have reported systemic and local complications related

Table 15-3. Diagnosis in 700 hip arthroplasties (518 patients)

Diagnosis	Number
Primary degenerative osteoarthritis	372
Failed previous operation	144
Secondary degenerative osteoarthritis	119
Congenital hip dysplasia	30
Avascular necrosis	21
Slipped femoral epiphysis	15
Protrusio acetabuli	10
Gaucher's disease	5
Paget's disease	5
Acromegaly	4
Legg-Calvé-Perthes disease	4
Miscellaneous	25
Rheumatoid arthritis	65

Table 15-4. Grading of the hip according to a modified 6-point system of D'Aubigne and Postel's classification

Grade pain	Function	Mobility (degrees)
1 Severe and spontaneous	Few yards or bedridden; two canes or crutches	0-30
2 Severe on attempting to walk, prevents all activities	Time and distance very limited with or without canes	31-60
3 Tolerable, permitting limited activities	Limited with one cane; difficult without cane; able to stand long periods	61-100
4 Only after some activity, disappears quickly with rest	Long distance with one cane; limited without a cane	101-160
5 Slight or intermittent pain on starting to walk, less with activities	No cane, but a limp	161-210
6 No pain	Normal	211-260

541

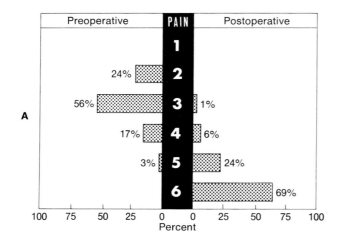

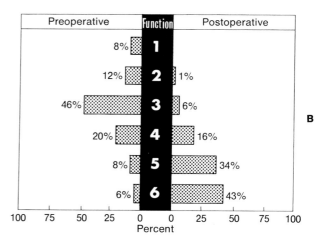

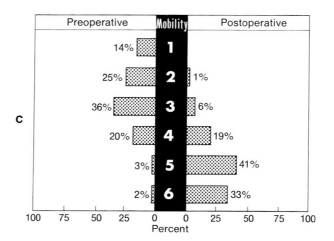

Fig. 15-1. Preoperative and postoperative grading of hip according to D'Aubigne and Postel's numerical classification. It should be noted that most dramatic improvement following low-friction arthroplasty was freedom of pain. **A,** Grading of pain. **B,** Grading of function. **C,** Grading of mobility. (From Eftekhar, N. S., et al.: Clin. Orthop. **95:**48-59, 1973.)

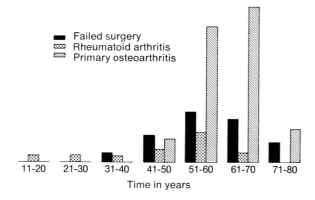

Fig. 15-2. Age distribution in 700 consecutive operations as applied to three major categories of osteoarthritis, rheumatoid arthritis, and revision of failed surgery. NOTE: relatively high proportion of rheumatoid patients in younger age groups. (From Eftekhar, N. S., et al.: Clin. Orthop. **95:**48-59, 1973.)

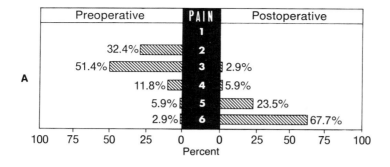

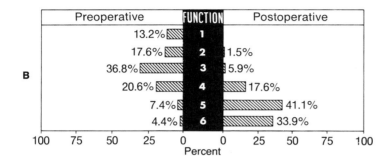

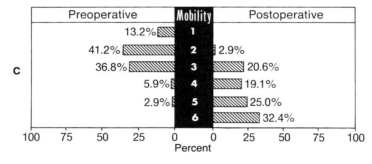

Fig. 15-3. Preoperative grading of hip and postoperative condition in revision arthroplasty cases. Grading: **A,** pain; **B,** function; and **C,** mobility. (From Eftekhar, N. S., et al.: Clin. Orthop. **95:**48-59, 1973.)

to total hip replacement; a study of 800 consecutive low-friction arthroplasties at our institution—with a maximum of 7 years follow-up—also revealed local and systemic complications, as summarized in Tables 15-1 and 15-2.[31] It can be seen from them that while the rate of infection was low (less than 1%), the incidence of thromboembolism and deep vein thrombosis was high—despite the prophylactic anticoagulation regimen. There were no deaths during or immediately following surgery, but six occurred within the next 6 weeks. Autopsy revealed that two were due to massive pulmonary embolism, one to a perforated cecum, and two had a clinical diagnosis of myocardial infarction. The incidence

of mechanical and technical failures was relatively low and comparable to results reported by others.[31] Details of the major systemic and local complications following low-friction arthroplasty as performed in different institutions are also summarized in Tables 15-1 and 15-2.

COMPARISON OF RESULTS BY DIFFERENT TECHNIQUES

Because of the introduction of several techniques of total hip replacement in the past decade, surgeons have attempted to compare the merits of one prosthesis with another. We must not ignore the fact that these studies are related to early experiences and do not necessarily reflect valid comparisons with more modern mechanical devices and methods. Furthermore, since the variables are numerous and many techniques have evolved through the years, these studies may be of limited value; on the other hand, such reviews show that in most instances the trend has been away from metal-to-metal prostheses and toward metal-to-plastic components. Bently and Duthie[2] compared 201 patients who underwent 101 McKee-Farrar and 128 Charnley total hip replacements between 1968 and 1971. The results were assessed for pain, function, and mobility. Relief of pain was demonstrated following 83% of the McKee-Farrar implants, as compared to 96% for the Charnley replacements; function was rated 4 or better in 85% of the McKee-Farrar replacements, and in 97% of the Charnley replacements; total range of movement of more than 100 degrees was reported in 88% of the McKee-Farrar prostheses and in 89% of the Charnley prostheses. Complications included three deep wound infections and three cases of loosening of the femoral component with the McKee-Farrar replacement; none were reported using the Charnley replacement. The incidence of thromboembolism was rare (about 2%), and no pulmonary emboli were observed in patients on adequate warfarin therapy. The incidence of complications in patients with rheumatoid arthritis was no higher than in the others. Bently and Duthie[2] concluded that the Charnley prosthesis was superior to the McKee-Farrar throughout the series, including bilateral cases. Morris and associates[58] and Nicholson[62] also made comparisons between the Charnley and the McKee-Farrar methods: after reviewing 1,025 hip replacements using the Charnley prosthesis in 939 hips, and the McKee-Farrar prosthesis in 86, Nicholson concluded that long-term results (revealed in follow-ups of up to 5 years) were favorable to the Charnley prosthesis.[62] A similar conclusion favoring the metal-on-plastic total hip prostheses was drawn by other surgeons—that is, Wilson and associates,[84] whose early experiences also included metal-to-metal prostheses. Other surgeons such as Leinbach and Murray favored metal-to-plastic components because loosening occurred less frequently.[48,61,83]

Freeman and associates[36] compared results between the McKee-Farrar and the Howse designs in patients with osteoarthritis and rheuma-

toid conditions, and found no statistical difference between the two.[36] In both types, the incidence of complications was greater in patients with rheumatoid conditions than with osteoarthritis.

Smith and Turner,[77] under the auspices of the Food and Drug Administration of the United States, tabulated the results of operations involving 3,482 patients and several types of total hip prostheses (with acrylic cement). They concluded that postoperative mobility was either good, very good, or excellent in 83% of the cases. Serious side effects and complications were relatively few, and only 1.6% of the cases developed infection. (No differences relating to the type of prosthesis or technique used were noted.)

Moczynski and associates[57] evaluated 150 cases where the Charnley prosthesis was used and 94 cases where the Müller prosthesis was used; they found the early results satisfactory in most of the cases. They were unable to detect any differences between the two types of prostheses.

Several efforts were made to show the advantages of performing total hip replacement without the routine trochanteric osteotomy and with the use of a large femoral head prosthesis as technique improvements.[34,51,74] However, because of the shortness of the follow-up period and the resulting lack of information regarding the long-range effects of these techniques, these reports must be considered tentative. Mallory,[51] in a comparison of two groups of patients (one with and one without trochanteric osteotomy), observed that the exposure was better (with less damage to the abductor mechanism) and the biomechanical equilibrium was restored when the total hip replacement was preceded by a trochanteric osteotomy, although both operations consistently relieved pain, eliminated limping, and improved both walking (endurance) and (active) abduction against gravity.

MODIFICATION OF CHARNLEY'S PROSTHESIS AND TECHNIQUE

During the past 10 years, several modifications of Charnley's prosthesis have been introduced throughout the world. Some of these modifications are aimed at reducing load per unit area of the hip joint and, theoretically, maximizing joint stability; other modifications seek to eliminate the necessity of removing the greater trochanter. While in theory these modifications offer improvements on Charnley's technique and prosthesis, the clinical exploration of these other possibilities should be restricted to the original investigators, enabling them to adequately test them and evaluate their long-term results prior to their extensive use.

Bucholz modified Charnley's "St. George Hospital" design by increasing the diameter of the head to 38 mm. and recessing the ventral and medial rim to allow improvement of flexion without subluxation.[5,6] Müller of Switzerland[59,60] increased the femoral head diameter to 32 mm. and advocated not removing the greater trochanter in total hip arthroplasty. This, he said, provides an excellent system of instrumentation for the revised prosthesis. His method is considerably popular both in Europe and the United States and is recommended because of two features: (1) it improves the stability of the hip and (2) it eliminates the need for removal of the greater trochanter. However, there are no clinical studies dealing with this method's long-term performance and only a few dealing with its short-term performance.[23,58]

Lagrange and Letournel[40] reported the early results of 1,355 total hip replacements utilizing a newly designed large femoral head (35 mm.). A similar type of prosthesis with a speccially designed cup and a 35 or 38 mm. head was developed by Aufranc and Turner. Lubinus[49] reported 1,350 total hip arthroplasties in which he used a 35 or 38 mm. head with a "Brunswik" design system. He predicted that the rate of failure in the "foreseeable future" would be between 3% and 4%. Another type of prosthesis that might be mentioned here is Stanmore's prosthesis[24,83]; long-term results are also awaited.

In 1971, Harris reported on a new total hip design, and the clinical results, related in a 1973 study, dealt with 247 total hip operations using this new design with a minimum of 6 months follow-up.[37,38]

Amstutz,[1] following a 2½ year trial of a new type of total hip prosthesis known as Trapezoidal-28, reports that this design provides increased accuracy of "insertion, stability, and versatility," a wide range of motion without neck socket contact, and good stability, but he cautions that additional follow-up is needed to determine the long-term skeletal fixation and the durability of the bearing.

RESULTS IN CONGENITAL DISLOCATION AND DYSPLASIA

Among the first 6,000 low-friction arthroplasties performed at Wrightington Hospital, 96 hips in 81 patients showed evidence of congenital dysplasia, which constitutes about 1.5% of this group. Charnley and Feagan,[19] in reviewing 27 hips in 24 patients with a 1-year follow-up, concluded that the operation was worthwhile because the results were satisfactory. There was one unexplained loosening of the socket in this series, although a much higher incidence of loosening can be expected in this group than in groups with conventional osteoarthritis. Lazansky[47] found that 7.5% (1 of 14 patients) in his series had an unquestionable congenital or childhood disease of the hip joint. He also concluded that when the operation was executed correctly, the results were most gratifying. In a series of 700 total hip replacements (with low-friction arthroplasty performed at our institution)[29] we encountered 30 hips with congenital dysplasia or dislocation; the results obtained remain comparable to those of total hip replacements performed owing to degenerative osteoarthritis. At no time did we feel that equalization of the leg length was a major factor in the decision for or against surgery, or that equalization should be attempted at the risk of ruining an otherwise good arthroplasty. We felt that any leg length discrepancy should be corrected postoperatively with a shoe lift, especially since in most cases of bilateral defect, corrective surgery may become necessary on the opposite side (see Chapter 13).

RESULTS FOLLOWING REVISION OPERATIONS (OTHER THAN THR)

Dupont and Charnley[25] reviewed a series of 217 total hip replacements using low-friction arthroplasty performed at Wrightington Hospital on 203 patients with previous failed operations (with a minimum of a 1-year follow-up).[1] They encountered excellent results in terms of improved walking ability, relief of pain, and gain in function and mobility. Pain was minimal or completely relieved in 96% of the patients, and in no case did it worsen as a result of the revision; a good range of motion (comparable to primary operations) had been achieved, and no hip lost motion after surgery. A high number of positive cultures in 55 hips was of special interest in that

545

study: 13 (23.6%) had a positive culture, but, remarkably, only one of these hips subsequently developed infection (see Chapters 6 and 17).

Of the first 500 low-friction arthroplasty procedures performed between April 1969 and January 1972 at the New York Orthopaedic Hospital, 117 were for failed previous operations. Eftekhar and associates[32,33] recorded the complications in this series but included only 70 of them in the 2-year follow-up (April 1969 to April 1971). The detailed results of these operations were compared with a group of 240 primary procedures performed during the same period, also involving a 2-year follow-up. There were 132 women and 108 men in the primary group, and 40 women and 30 men in the revision group. Bilateral hip disease was present in 178 and unilateral hip disease in 62 of those in the primary group, while 80% of the revision group had bilateral involvement. Twenty-two revisions had been done for failed endoprosthesis, twenty for failed mold arthroplasty, twelve for failed osteotomy, nine for failed fracture fixation, and eight for miscellaneous reasons. The number of previous failed operations varied from one to six prior to total hip replacement. In contrast to the preferred policy in cases of primary intervention, age was not necessarily a factor in selecting these patients, since in most instances a Girdlestone resection would have been indicated if

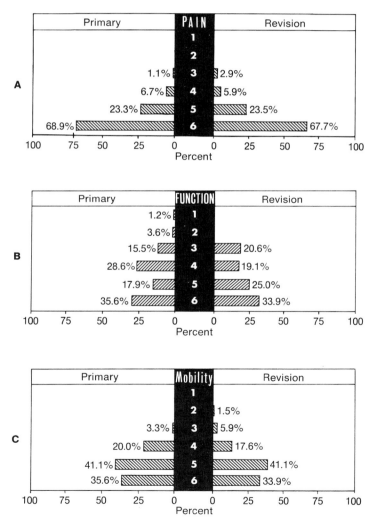

Fig. 15-4. Comparison of primary and revision postoperative results of operations performed during same period. Grading: **A,** pain; **B,** function; and **C,** mobility. (From Eftekhar, N. S., et al.: Clin. Orthop. **95:**48-59, 1973.)

total hip replacement had not been planned. Nevertheless, there were no significant differences in age between the patients in the primary group and those in the revision group. Fig. 15-2 denotes the age distribution in three major categories: primary osteoarthritis, rheumatoid arthritis, and failed surgery. The presence or history of previous infection automatically precluded the use of total hip replacement in these revision procedures. (For the preoperative and postoperative results of these revision operations see Fig. 15-3, which can be compared with the results of the primary operations in Fig. 15-4 performed during the same period.) The specifics of pain, function, and mobility are evaluated pre- and postoperatively according to the D'Aubigne and Postel classification of medical grades. The revision complications compared with the primary operations leads us to the conclusion that low-friction arthroplasty is an excellent salvage procedure, with results comparable to those of primary operations.[32,33] However, we found that there was a greater tendency toward technical and thromboembolic complications in this group; it also became clear that the important task of recognizing a preexisting infection prior to replacement was not easy. The surgeon's awareness of and attention to details of technique were elements of utmost importance in these revisions.

RESULTS IN REVISION OF FAILED TOTAL HIP REPLACEMENTS

Our experience with revision of failed total hip replacements is limited to 60 hips in 56 patients, 30 of which had a minimum of 2 years and a maximum of 6 years follow-up following the revision surgery.[28] Of the 30 patients with failed total hip replacements, 12 were male and 18 were female; age distribution was 52 to 76 years, 1 to 6 years had elapsed since the original procedures, and all patients were followed personally after the revision. The original diagnoses and types of procedures are listed in Table 15-5.

In 21 of these hips the prosthesis had been cemented; in 9 the components were inserted by mechanical interference fit. Loosening was confirmed at surgery, yielding the following outcome: The femoral component was loose in 10 cases, and in one of those the femoral stem also was fractured. The acetabular component was loose in 5 cases, and loosening of both femoral and acetabular components was found in the re-

Table 15-5. Clinical data related to the type of total prosthesis converted to low-friction arthroplasty[28]

	No.	Cemented	Noncemented
Type of prosthesis			
Low-friction arthroplasty	12		
McKee-Farrar	5		
Ring	9		
Other	4		
Total	30		
Diagnosis			
Osteoarthritis	15	10	5
Treated fracture	7	7	
Rheumatoid arthritis	4	1	3
Other	4	3	1
Total	30	21	9

maining 15 cases. Two operations were required for recurrent dislocation of low-friction arthroplasty. Careful preoperative investigation into the cause of the failure ruled out the possibility of infection in all cases. Twenty-eight of these operations were done in one session; in 2 cases, removal of the old prosthesis and implantation of the new device took place at 6- and 8-month intervals.

As expected, increased technical difficulties arose in revision surgery: The mean operative time was 210 minutes compared with 105 minutes in primary intervention, and blood loss averaged 2,000 ml. versus 1,000 ml. Also, during reaming of the cement from the McKee-Farrar–type prosthesis, perforation of the shaft of the femur occurred in three cases. A special guide and reamer were subsequently designed for the removal of the old cement and the rechannelling of the femoral shaft (see Chapter 14).

The clinical results (assessed by the D'Aubigne and Postel method) were favorably comparable to the revision arthroplasties of other conventional operations. Table 15-6 summarizes the preoperative and postoperative grading of the hips in this series for pain, function, and mobility. There was no recurrent infection. Dislocation in one hip required bracing of the patient, which limited excessive flexion and adduction. Because of complicated medical history, no further surgical intervention was attempted. We consider this case to be a failure of revision surgery (see Chapter 17: Fig. 17-2).

Table 15-6. Preoperative and postoperative grading of the hips for pain, function, and mobility in conversion of failed total hip replacements and managed by low-friction arthroplasty[28]

	Preoperative			Postoperative		
Grade	Pain	Function	Mobility	Pain	Function	Mobility
1						
2	12	10	6			
3	14	12	18			1
4	3	8	4		1	5
5		2		12	14	13
6	1		2	18	15	11

SUMMARY OF ESSENTIALS

■ An objective evaluation of the results of clinical studies in a prospective manner is the only way by which the validity of any surgical procedure may be evaluated. During the developmental years of total hip arthroplasty as we know it today, basically two groups of prostheses were used: (1) those having metal-to-metal bearings and (2) those having metal-to-plastic bearings. In the former group, attempts have been made by some surgeons to avoid the use of acrylic cement. Therefore the early reports of total hip arthroplasty in group 1 are considered those of noncemented varieties using metal-against-metal components and those with the use of cement.

■ Early results of noncemented metal-against-metal prostheses, that is, Ring, Tronzo, Sivash, and others, indicated a gradual deterioration in success rates caused by loosening of the component. Although several types of prostheses like these were developed in order to avoid the use of cement, it became apparent that in many instances the use of acrylic cement was essential.

■ McKee and others reported a high degree of early success using chromium-cobalt total hip prostheses in a large series. However, a certain percentage of loosening was subsequently attributed to mechanical failure as the result of high-frictional torque of the prosthesis, low-grade infection, metal sensitivity, and so on. Because of these problems, the trend has now changed to metal-against-plastic prostheses with lower frictional properties.

■ Following early failure of Teflon in a limited clinical trial, high-density polyethylene is now becoming the most common material used in total hip arthroplasties. Charnley and his associates, as well as many other surgeons in centers throughout the world, have reported excellent large-scale results in total hip arthroplasty.

■ The main results of total hip replacement have been total absence of pain, consistent improvement of range of motion, and increased functional activities, often with an excellent gait. Undoubtedly, the state of the art at this point indicates that the operation can be safely applied to older individuals, that is, those who are over 60 years of age, have diminished demand on their joints, and weigh less than 180 pounds. On the other hand, even early results indicate that much longer follow-up results should become available on younger patients prior to its universal application, irrespective of the type of patients selected for total hip arthroplasty.

■ Continuous surveillance of the results of total hip replacement, both in Europe and in the United States, indicates that there is no evidence of deterioration after 9 or 10 years following surgery. However, a number of problems exist both in terms of radiological evidence of loosening of the acetabular component and/or absorption of bone at the region of the calcar femorale, both of which are disturbing, and require further long-term follow-up studies.

■ With the present technique of total hip arthroplasty, the proper indications, and appropriate technique applied, it is safe to assume that after a 10-year follow-up, results of these operations remain satisfactory, that is, without mechanical failure. The stability of the hip joint, the ability to abduct and flex the hip against gravity, and a negative Trendelenburg's test are the most constant and impressive improvements seen following total hip arthroplasty.

■ Postoperative complications after total hip arthroplasty are proportional to the diligence of the surgeon to seek out the potential risks and complications from a medical standpoint and deal with them prior to surgery in addition to excellent postoperative care to diminish or minimize the complications.

■ While the morbidity and mortality of this operation have been considerably lowered by a number of prophylactic measures and early postoperative rehabilitation, a mortality rate of 1% to 2% (mostly owing to pulmonary embolism) and morbidity related to technical failures of 2% to 3% must be considered for a short-term follow-up (up to 5 years).

■ Comparison of the results of different techniques, that is, metal-to-metal components compared with metal-against-plastic components, or surgical technique with or without trochanteric osteotomy is not conclusive because of the selection of the type of patients used in these studies. However, a number of the studies indicate that the result of total hip arthroplasty using a metal-against-metal component with or without cement is inferior to total hip ar-

548

throplasty using a metal-against-plastic bearing. It appears also that the method of evaluation as well as clinical technique reflects the surgeon's experience in presenting these results.

■ Several attempts have been made to show the advantages of performing a total hip replacement using a large femoral head prosthesis without routine trochanteric osteotomy. However, these reports must be considered tentative because of the lack of information regarding the long-range effects of these techniques.

■ A number of modifications of Charnley's prosthesis and technique have been reported in the literature in the past 10 years. These modifications are generally concerned with increasing the ball size of the prosthesis and attempts, in some instances, to perform the operation without removal of the greater trochanter. It is essential that these modifications be tried and tested clinically and only applied preferentially after long-term statistical analyses of the results have been obtained.

■ The results of total hip arthroplasty for congenital dislocation and dysplasia have been reported. Operations for these conditions are technically demanding. However, the results can be most gratifying, and comparable results to those of conventional arthroplasty may be expected providing the acetabulum has partially developed. A completely dislocated (unreduced high dislocation) hip may not lend itself to a satisfactory reconstruction.

■ Results of total hip replacement for failed previous operations have indicated good pain relief and improved functional performance, although the operations are usually more difficult to perform and may be complicated by problems such as heterotopic bone formation, infection, or instability. A higher incidence of wound infection may be anticipated in revision surgery if careful scrutiny in selecting patients for surgery is not considered.

■ There are few reports regarding revision of failed total hip procedures. The technical demands and complications are to be expected in a higher percentage than in routine procedures without prior surgery.

REFERENCES

1. Amstutz, H. C.: Trapezoidal-28 total hip replacement, Clin. Orthop. **95:**158-167, 1973.
2. Bentley, G., and Duthie, R. B.: A comparative review of the McKee-Farrar and Charnley total hip prostheses, Clin. Orthop. **95:**127-142, 1973.
3. Breck, L. W.: Preliminary report on total hip replacement with Urist-Thompson unit without cement, Clin. Orthop. **72:**174-176, 1970.
4. Breck, L. W.: Metal to metal total hip replacement using the Urist socket, Clin. Orthop. **95:**38-42, 1973.
5. Bucholz, H. W.: modification of Charnley artificial hip joint, Clin. Orthop. **72:**69-78, 1970.
6. Bucholz, H. W., and Noack, G.: Results of the total hip prosthesis design, "St. George", Clin. Orthop. **95:**201-210, 1973.
7. Chapchal, G. J., Slooff, T. J. J., and Nollen, A. D.: Results of total hip replacement; a critical follow-up study, Clin. Orthop. **95:**111-117, 1973.
8. Charnley, J.: Arthroplasty of the hip: a new operation, Lancet **1:**1129-1132, 1961.
9. Charnley, J.: The low friction principle in arthroplasty of the hip joint: report of a large scale clinical study (president's guest speaker), American Academy of Orthopaedic Surgeons Meeting, 1963.
10. Charnley, J.: Letter to the editor, J. Bone Joint Surg. **48A:**819, 1966.
11. Charnley, J.: Total prosthetic replacement of the hip. Triangle **8:**211-216, 1968.
12. Charnley, J.: Total prosthetic replacement of the hip, Reconstr. Surg. Traumatol. **11:**9-19, 1969.
13. Charnley, J.: Total hip replacement by low friction arthroplasty, Clin. Orthop. **72:**7-21, 1970.
14. Charnley, J.: Editorial comment, Clin. Orthop. **72:**2, 1970.
15. Charnley, J.: Low friction arthroplasty of the hip joint, J. Bone Joint Surg. **53B:**149, 1971.
16. Charnley, J.: The long-term results of low-friction arthroplasty of the hip performed as a primary intervention, J. Bone Joint Surg. **54B:**61-76, 1972.
17. Charnley, J.: The classic arthroplasty of the hip: a new operation, Clin. Orthop. **95:**4-8, 1973.
18. Charnley, J., and Cupic, Z.: The nine and ten year results of the low-friction arthroplasty of the hip, Clin. Orthop. **95:**9-25, 1973.
19. Charnley, J., and Feagan, J. A.: Low friction arthroplasty in congenital subluxation of the hip, Clin. Orthop. **91:**98-113, 1973.
20. Coventry, M. B.: The surgical technique of total hip arthroplasty, modified from Charnley as done at the Mayo Clinic, Orthop. Clin. North Am. **4:**473-482, 1973.
21. Coventry, M. B., Beckenbaugh, R. D., Nolan, D. R., and Ilstrup, D. M.: 2,012 total hip arthroplasties: a study of postoperative course and early complications, J. Bone Joint Surg. **56A:**273-284, 1974.
22. Debeyre, J., and Goutallier, D.: Urist hip socket and Moore prosthesis without cement for total hip replacement, Clin. Orthop. **72:**169, 1970.
23. DeHaven, K. E., Evarts, C. M., Wilde, A. H., Collins, H. R., Nelson, C., and Razzano, C. D.: Early results of Charnley-Müller total hip reconstruction, Orthop. Clin. North Am. **4:**465-472, 1973.
24. Duff-Barclay, I., Scales, J. T., and Wilson, J. N.: The development of the Stanmore total hip replacement, Proc. R. Soc. Med. **59:**948-951, 1966.
25. Dupont, J. A., and Charnley, J.: Low-friction ar-

throplasty of the hip for the failures of previous operations, J. Bone Joint Surg. **54B:**77-87, 1972.

26. Eftekhar, N. S.: Charnley "low friction torque" arthroplasty, Clin. Orthop. **81:**93-104, 1971.
27. Eftekhar, N. S.: Low friction arthroplasty: indications, contraindications and complications, J.A. M.A. **218:**705-710, 1971.
28. Eftekhar, N. S.: Replacement of failed total hip prostheses in the absence of infection: low friction arthroplasty technique. In The Hip Society: The Hip, proceedings of the fourth open scientific meeting of The Hip Society, 1976, The C. V. Mosby Co., pp. 186.
29. Eftekhar, N. S., and Stinchfield, F. E.: Experience with low friction arthroplasty, a statistical review of early results and complications, Clin. Orthop. **95:**60-68, 1973.
30. Eftekhar, N. S., and Stinchfield, F. E.: total replacement of the hip joint by low friction arthroplasty, Orthop. Clin. North Am. **4:**483-501, 1973.
31. Eftekhar, N. S., Kiernan, H. A., and Stinchfield, F. E.: Systemic and local complications following low-friction arthroplasty of the hip joint: a study of 800 consecutive operations, Arch. Surg. **111:**150-155, 1976.
32. Eftekhar, N. S., Smith, D. M., Henry, J. H., and Stinchfield, F. E.: Revision arthroplasty using Charnley low-friction arthroplasty technique, J. Bone Joint Surg. **54A:**1357-1358, 1972.
33. Eftekhar, N. S., Smith, D. M., Henry, J. H., and Stinchfield, F. E.: Revision arthroplasty using Charnley low-friction arthroplasty technic, with reference to specifics of technic and comparison of results with primary low friction arthroplasty, Clin. Orthop. **95:**48-59, 1973.
34. Evanski, P. M., Waugh, T. R., and Orofino, C. F.: Total hip replacement with the Charnley prosthesis, Clin. Orthop. **95:**69-72, 1973.
35. Freeman, M. A. R., Swasnon, S. A. V., and Heath, J. C.: Biological properties of the wear particles generated by all cobalt-chrome total joint replacement prosthesis. In Chapchal, editor: Arthroplasty of the hip, Stuttgart, 1973, Georg Theime Verlag, pp. 8-10.
36. Freeman, P. A., Lee, P., and Bryson, T. W.: total hip joint replacement in osteoarthrosis and polyarthritis, Clin. Orthop. **95:**224-230, 1973.
37. Harris, W. H.: A new total hip implant, Clin. Orthop. **81:**105-113, 1971.
38. Harris, W. H.: Preliminary report of results of Harris of total hip replacement, Clin. Orthop. **95:**168-173, 1973.
39. Jayson, M.: Total hip replacement, Philadelphia, 1971, J. B. Lippincott Co.
40. Lagrange, J., and Letournel, E.: Lagrange-Letournel hip prosthesis; results of 1355 cases. In The Hip Society: The hip, proceedings of the third open scientific meeting of The Hip Society,

1975, St. Louis, 1975, The C. V. Mosby Co., pp. 278-299.
41. Langenskiöld, A., and Paavilainen, T. M. L.: Total replacement of 116 hips by the McKee-Farrar prosthesis, a preliminary report, Clin. Orthop. **95:**143-150, 1973.
42. Langenskiöld, A., and Salenius, P.: Total hip replacement by the McKee-Farrar prosthesis, a preliminary report of 81 cases, Clin. Orthop. **72:**104-105, 1970.
43. Lazansky, M. G.: A study of bilateral low friction arthroplasty, Internal Publication No. 3, Centre for Hip Surgery, Wrightington Hospital, 1967, England.
44. Lazansky, M. G.: Complications in total hip replacement with the Charnley technic, Clin. Orthop. **72:**40-45, 1970.
45. Lazansky, M. G.: Complications revisited: the debit side of total hip replacement, Clin. Orthop. **95:**96-103, 1973.
46. Lazansky, M. G.: Total hip replacement in patients with bilateral disease. In American Academy of Orthopaedic Surgeons: Instructional course lectures, vol. 23, St. Louis, 1974, The C. V. Mosby Co., pp. 150-153.
47. Lazansky, M. G.: Low friction arthroplasty for sequelae of congenital and developmental hip disease. In American Academy of Orthopaedic Surgeons: Instructional course lectures, vol. 23, St. Louis, 1974, The C. V. Mosby Co., pp. 194-200.
48. Leinbach, I. S., and Barlow, F. A.: 700 total hip replacements, experience with six types, Clin. Orthop. **95:**174-192, 1973.
49. Lubinus, H. H.: Total hip replacement using the "Brunswik system," Clin. Orthop. **95:**211-212, 1973.
50. Lunceford, E. M., Jr.: Total hip replacement using McBride cup and Moore prosthesis, Clin. Orthop. **72:**201-204, 1970.
51. Mallory, T. H.: Total hip replacement with and without trochanteric osteotomy, Clin. Orthop. **103:**133-135, 1974.
52. McKee, G. K.: Artificial hip joint, J. Bone Joint Surg. **33B:**465, 1951.
53. McKee, G. K.: Developments in total hip joint replacement, Proc. Inst. Mech. Engrs. **3F:**85, 1966-1967.
54. McKee, G. K.: Development of total prosthetic replacement of the hip, Clin. Orthop. **72:**85-103, 1970.
55. McKee, G. K., and Chen, S. C.: The statistics of the McKee-Farrar method of total hip replacement, Clin. Orthop. **95:**26-33, 1973.
56. McKee, G. K., and Watson-Farrar, J.: Replacement of arthritic hips by the McKee-Farrar prosthesis, J. Bone Joint Surg. **48B:**245-259, 1966.
57. Moczynski, G., Abraham, E., Barmada, R., and Ray, R. D.: Evaluation of total hip replacement arthroplasties, Clin. Orthop. **95:**213-216, 1973.

550

58. Morris, J. B., and Nicholson, O. R.: Total prosthetic replacement of the hip joint in Auckland, N.Z. Clin. Orthop. **72:**33-35, 1970.
59. Müller, M. E.: Total hip replacement. Paper presented at the Societe Internationale de Chirurgie Orthopedique et Traumatologie Meeting, Mexico City, October, 1969.
60. Müller, M. E.: Total hip prosthesis, Clin. Orthop. **72:**46-68, 1970.
61. Murray, W. R.: Results in patients with total hip replacement arthroplasty, Clin. Orthop. **95:**80-90, 1973.
62. Nicholson, O. R.: Total hip replacement, an evaluation of the results and technics 1967-1972, Clin. Orthop. **95:**217-223, 1973.
63. Owen, R., and Pal, A. K.: The Charnley low friction arthroplasty, J. Bone Joint Surg. **53B:**149, 1971.
64. Patterson, F. P., and Brown, C. S.: The McKee-Farrar total hip replacement: preliminary results and complications of 368 operations performed in five general hospitals, J. Bone Joint Surg. **54A:**257-275, 1972.
65. Ring, P. A.: Complete replacement arthroplasty of the hip by the Ring prosthesis, J. Bone Joint Surg. **50B:**720-731, 1968.
66. Ring, P. A.: Total replacement of the hip, Clin. Orthop. **72:**161-168, 1970.
67. Ring, P. A.: Ring total hip replacement. In Jayson, M., editor: Total hip replacement, Philadelphia, 1971, J. B. Lippincott Co., pp. 26-46.
68. Ring, P. A.: Replacement of the hip joint, Ann. R. Coll. Surg. Engl. **48:**344-355, 1971.
69. Ring, P. A.: problems of the uncemented total hip replacement, J. Bone Joint Surg. **55B:**209, 1973.
70. Ring, P. A.: Total replacement of the hip joint—a review of a thousand operations, J. Bone Joint Surg. **56B:**44-58, 1974.
71. Russin, L. A., and Russin, M. A.: Modified Sivash total hip prosthesis Orthop. Rev. **4:**41, 1975.
72. Shorbe, H. B.: Total hip replacement without cement. McBride acetabular component and Moore femoral prosthesis, Clin. Orthop. **72:**186-200, 1970.
73. Sivash, K. M.: The development of a total metal prosthesis for the hip joint from a partial joint replacement, Reconstr. Surg. Traumatol. **11:**53-62, 1969.
74. Sledge, C. B.: Discussion—osteotomy of the greater trochanter. In The Hip Society: The hip, proceeding of the second open scientific meeting of The Hip Society, 1974, St. Louis, 1974, The C. V. Mosby Co., pp. 247-250.
75. Smith, R. D.: Total hip replacement, Clin. Orthop. **72:**177-185, 1970.
76. Smith, R. D.: Total hip replacement—metal against metal—review and analysis of cases, 1961-1972, Clin. Orthop. **95:**43-47, 1973.
77. Smith, R. E., and Turner, R. J.: Total hip replacement using methyl methacrylate cement, Clin. Orthop. **95:**231-238, 1973.
78. Stinchfield, F. E., and White, E. S.: Total hip replacement, Ann. Surg. **174:**655-662, 1971.
79. Stinchfield, F. E., White, E. S., Eftekhar, N. S., and Kurokawa, K. M.: Low friction arthroplasty, Surg. Gynecol. Obstet. **135:**1-10, 1972.
80. Torgerson, W. R.: Three years of experience with total hip replacement, Clin. Orthop. **95:**151-157, 1973.
81. Urist, M., guest editor: Current problems in surgery; acrylic cement stabilized joint replacements (monograph), Chicago, 1975, Year Book Medical Publishers.
82. Welch, R. B., and Charnley, J.: Low friction arthroplasty of the hip in rheumatoid arthritis and ankylosing spondylitis, Clin. Orthop. **72:**22-31, 1972.
83. Wilson, J. N., and Scales, J. T.: Loosening of total hip replacements with cement fixation: clinical findings and laboratory studies, Clin. Orthop. **72:**145-160, 1970.
84. Wilson, P. D., Jr., Amstutz, H. C., Czerniecki, A., Salvati, E. A., and Mendes, D. G.: Total hip replacement with fixation by acrylic cement, J. Bone Joint Surg. **54A:**207-236, 1972.
85. Wolkow, M. W.: Alloplastik von metallgelenken, Acta. Orthop. Scand. **40:**571-576, 1969.

CHAPTER 16

Local complications

The story of the complications of total hip replacement is just beginning. It is to be hoped that it will be short and conclusive.

J. G. BONNIN

In this chapter, two biological phenomena complicating total hip arthroplasty will be discussed: wound infection complicating total hip arthroplasty and heterotopic ossification following total hip arthroplasty.

Wound infection complicating total hip arthroplasty

In Chapter 6 ("Prevention of Infection") the pathophysiology of infection and prophylaxis was discussed. In this section the following will be discussed: (1) the scope of the problem, (2) diagnosis of infection, (3) definitions and differential diagnosis, (4) limitations of bacteriology, and (5) management of the infected total hip replacement.

SCOPE OF THE PROBLEM

The general pattern of the actual incidence of infected total hip replacements as it appears in the practices of orthopaedic surgeons remains unknown. However, documents are increasingly available from centers where large numbers of these operations are performed annually.[8] Early studies of wound infection by Charnley and Eftekhar[9] indicated a high rate of infection following total hip replacement when no special precautions were exercised in terms of the operative environment or handling of the surgical wound. Similar experiences were encountered by Wilson and associates.[41] In previous chapters, the results of a survey of 17 major institutions evaluating the state of wound infection in the United States were analyzed and discussed (see Chapter 6). It became apparent that if surgeons performing these operations exercised special precautions in the operating room (including the use of prophylactic antibiotics systemically and/or locally as well as the use of a clean-air operating room), the rate of infection remained relatively low (providing there were more than 500 cases), that is, infection within the vicinity of 1%. It was also concluded that the rate of late infection in these centers could not be determined based on the multifactorial origin of wound infection. Likewise, the role played by antibiotic prophylaxis could not be fully evaluated. While the relative rates of infection in major centers were reported to be low, this may not apply to the statistics of orthopaedic surgeons in private practice performing occasional total hip replacement operations in smaller communities.

Because infected total hip replacements are not frequently seen, treatment experiences are limited, and thus an orthopaedic surgeon taking up the technique of total hip replacement may have to face the problem of handling an infected hip when it develops for the first time (despite a larger experience in total hip replacement procedures). For patients, of course, this problem is grave—since the surgeons with greater experience at medical centers may not be able to accommodate them because of the lack of manpower, facilities, and great financial support needed in handling large numbers of these cases.

Because of the seriousness of the complications of infection, a high standard of practice related to prevention must be exercised in performing a major surgical procedure such as a total hip replacement.

We believe that a surgeon performing this type of operation must have a written and an unwritten contract with his patient (a moral contract) to provide him with the highest standard of care and facilities as well as an excellent surgical technique to protect him from infection. He should be prepared to follow the patient (with re-

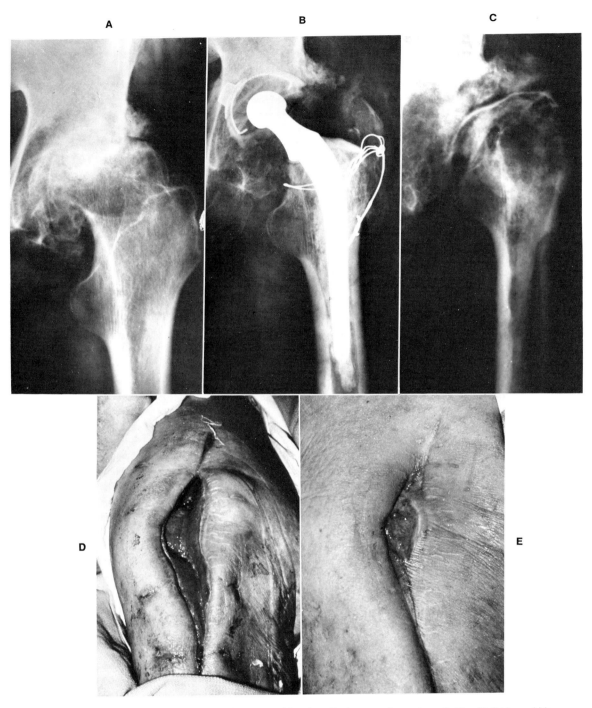

Fig. 16-1. **A,** Preoperative radiograph of 62-year-old male with degenerative osteoarthritis of left hip and history of gout. **B,** Three-month postoperative radiograph of same patient showing early evidence of ectopic bone formation in area of greater trochanter and abductors. This radiograph was taken just prior to removal of total hip replacement device because of lack of response to treatment for infection and systemic signs of toxemia related to multiple abscess formation. **C,** One year following Girdlestone pseudarthrosis and 6 months following resumption of walking with assistance of cane. NOTE: hypertrophic changes of superior acetabular lip and attempt for formation of pseudarthrosis. Patient had only minimal discomfort but could not walk for any distance without cane. Opposite hip was normal. **D,** Eight weeks following removal of artificial hip joint and packing of wound. Packing of wound was selected in this case because of gram-negative organisms (*Escherichia coli*) and subsequently mixed organisms.**E,** State of wound that had nicely granulated by 3 months following Girdlestone pseudarthrosis. Wound ultimately closed by 4½ months following surgery.

553

gard to infection and other complications) as long as both live and be able to consult other physicians as necessary. It is also mandatory that all rational preventive measures (special environment at surgery, extreme aseptic technique, and prophylactic antibiotics) be used—because of the seriousness of the problem should it arise—despite the fact that some of these measures have, as yet, not been scientifically fully proven effective. Finally, the surgeon must be prepared to treat an infected total hip replacement.

Misery of patient vs. cost

The infected total hip replacement is a grave complication, and, next to fatal pulmonary embolism or fatal coronary occlusion, it is the most serious complication of this operation. When considering the cost of special facilities for this type of surgery, the patient's misery and loss must be weighed against the cost of prevention. When a new hospital is designed, surgeons must demand allocation of space and special facilities to perform this type of operation in order to reduce the ultimate price to society and suffering of the patient. A recent study by Nelson[30] estimated the average annual cost to treat an infected total hip replacement in 1974 at $16,000 per case. In a 5-year period the cost to society of treating an infected total hip replacement is approximately $117,000. The following two case histories from our own series best exemplify the economic implications of the infected hip replacement.

CASE 1: *Acute appearance*. H. H., a 62-year-old male, developed an early and acute *Escherichia coli* infection 3 weeks following a total hip replacement; four attempts were made to retain the artificial joint by incision, drainage, and débridement. Ultimately—3 months later—because of persistence of the infection, lack of response to treatment, and systemic signs of toxemia related to abscess formation, the artificial joint and cement were removed; the wound was packed open and the patient was placed in skeletal traction. He was discharged 3½ months following a Girdlestone pseudarthrosis, which was performed for persistence of drainage and pain. At discharge, he had an open-draining wound and a moderate amount of pain with 2½ inches shortening of the extremity. During hospitalization, he was put under general anesthesia five times, 36 units of blood were transfused, and the

total cost of his hospitalization exceeded $82,000—not including nurses' and physicians' fees (Fig. 16-1).

CASE 2: *Chronic appearance*. W. S., a 68-year-old man, developed a febrile illness, presumably pneumonia, 4½ years following a successful total hip replacement. He subsequently developed pain in the hip and shortly thereafter an abscess developed in the hip that required drainage. Mixed organisms were recovered, including *Proteus mirabilis*. The hip was converted to a pseudarthrosis. Following 6 weeks in traction and on removal of the Steinmann's nail in the tibia, he sustained a fracture through the weakened area of the bone following removal of the prosthesis. A total of 6 months hospitalization and immobilization was necessary before healing of the fracture was completed. (He had had 18 operations to promote healing of the wound and to control infection; he had received 60 units of blood and was extremely mentally disabled and depressed.) The cost of treatment was estimated at over $140,000, excluding doctors' and nurses' fees; he had 3½ inches actual shortening of the limb and still had considerable pain on any attempt at weight bearing (Fig. 16-2).

• • •

These 2 case histories exemplify the dramatic impact of the complications of infection from the personal and economic standpoint of the patient and society. Even when infection is more easily controlled and rehabilitation obtained earlier than in the cases cited, from the patient's and surgeon's stance the operation is a failure and only little hope can be given to the patient for further reimplantation of a second artificial hip joint.

DIAGNOSIS OF INFECTION IN TOTAL HIP REPLACEMENT

In every case of a defective result, that is, pain, antalgic gait and so on following total hip replacement, the diagnosis of infection must be suspected unless proved otherwise. It is on the combined clinical, laboratory, radiological, histological, and bacteriological findings (in decreasing order of significance) that a definitive diagnosis is made.

Mode of clinical appearance

Early infection. Early infection is arbitrarily defined as that appearing within the first 12

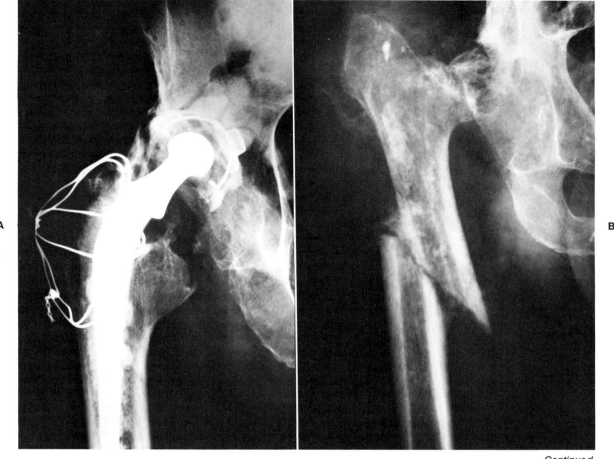

Continued.

Fig. 16-2. A, Note proximal migration of socket as result of loosening. **B,** Six weeks following traction by skeletal Steinmann's nail of tibia following resection pseudarthrosis. Patient sustained fracture through weakened area of old prosthesis site on first attempt out of bed. **C,** Four months later fracture healed despite presence of infection but resulted in considerable shortening in extremity, which was already shortened as result of pseudarthrosis.

weeks after surgery—usually while the patient is in the hospital. There is no special feature in this type of acute infection; it is most likely the result of bacterial contamination in the operating room, although the possibility of hematogenous seeding cannot be entirely dismissed and is recognized by the local and systemic reactions known to most surgeons. It appears in the following manner:

1. Full-blown acute abscess accompanied by elevation of temperature, sedimentation rate, white blood cell differential, and so on
2. A leaking hematoma leading to infection (Cultures initially negative are subsequently positive.)
3. A deep hematoma leading to infection without skin breakage or leaking
4. Defective skin healing leading to infection (This usually is the result of poor skin closure and poor handling of the wound.)

In most early infections the infective organism may be identified by smear or culture, unless systemic prophylactic antibiotics have been given preoperatively. At times, certain organisms may need a lengthy incubation period before they are cultured. Indeed, this is true when the patient has received perioperative antibiotics.

Delayed infection. A delayed infection usually is preceded by perfect wound healing; the delayed signs may occur up to 1 year after surgery.

555

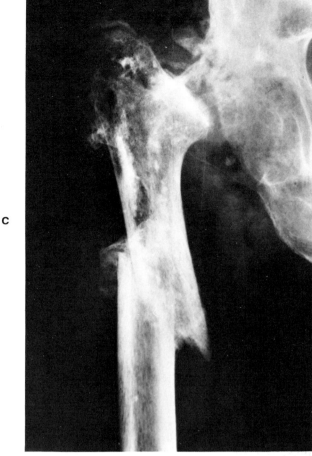

C

Fig. 16-2, cont'd. For legend see p. 555.

Review of the patient's record may or may not uncover the fact that postoperatively the patient was febrile or the sedimentation rate remained elevated, and, at times, the results of arthroplasty were not fully satisfactory but not attributed to infection. This form of infection may be considered "subacute," since it is possible that the low virulence of the organism or the bacteria-host response was such as to delay manifestation.

Early delayed infection. At times we have encountered infections that have appeared many months or years following surgery—yet during the postoperative course there was an indication of delayed healing of the wound or a painful hip following arthroplasty for which a cause was not verified. The patient could tolerate the situation for months or years until the radiological changes of infection or an abscess developed; we have labelled this type of delayed infection "early delayed infection." Although defective wound

healing and poor clinical results of arthroplasty originate in the early postoperative days, the wound remains well healed for many months or years until a diagnosis of infection can be proved. It is in this type of infection that most surgeons consider the theory of a hematogenous origin; on the contrary, we feel that perhaps these are early exogenous infections of a mildly pathogenic nature related to early bacterial seeding.

Late infection. Infections following 1 year are considered late, and these constitute approximately 50% of all infections. True late infections are those that appear after a perfect healing of the wound and a successful arthroplasty. The first signs of infection—such as pain or radiological change—appear 1 or more years after surgery. Generally, patients in this category enjoy a period of pain-free excellent results of the total hip replacement—then there is a sudden onset of pain. It is this mode of appearance that suggests a possible hematogenous route of infection.

Late late infection (hematogenous). Sporadically, yet in increasing numbers, we see patients appearing with infections for which a hematogenous source is suggested. These patients have been limited in our series—perhaps because of the relatively short time that has elapsed since their surgery. The incidence of infection (appearing at particular times) for the entire series of 2,000 low-friction arthroplasties is listed in Table 16-3. There are only a few bona fide, well-documented cases of hematogenous infection of total hip replacements in the literature, but clinical experiences suggest that their occurrence is more common than once supposed.[11,12]

Predicting delayed and late infection and sepsis rate. With the continuance of late-appearing infections, the true incidence of an institution sample is not possible without several years of follow-up. In one series, only 40% of the infections were manifested within 3 months after operation, and 60% of all infections were manifested within 18 months.[8] As a working rule, it appears that an additional 25% increase in the incidence of infection may be expected after 18 months (up to 3 or 4 years), with a chance of an occasional infection occurring later from a possible hematogenous source. General signs of chronic osteomyelitis, such as periosteal elevation, density of cortex, and radiolucencies, in patients who have no other evidence of defective

556

results from their operations might remain obscure unless a routine radiographic examination of all patients is done following total hip replacement. Therefore the true incidence of late, late-appearing infection may never be accurately determined. This is especially true where late infected cases may have been treated in another city or institution.

DIFFERENTIAL DIAGNOSIS
Deep vs. superficial infections

The cardinal sign of infection is pain. One does not expect a painful joint from a superficial wound infection; joint tenderness is almost non-existent but may be present in deep infection. Local inflammation usually is present in superficial infections, whereas in deep infections the skin usually remains intact unless a late sinus has developed. In deep infections generally the wound is indurated and drainage is copious as opposed to superficial infection, where the skin is mobile and drainage is minimal. As a general rule, duration of drainage may itself lead to the differentiation. A superficial infection is a self-limiting process, and within a short period of time the wound will be healed, whereas a continuance of drainage might suggest the possibility of deep infection. A probing of the wound may differentiate between a superficial and deep infection, but a sinogram may be most helpful. Obviously there is no radiological change of the bone in either superficial or deep infection early in the postoperative course (other than incidental findings related to total hip replacement). Later radiological changes such as periosteal reaction and punched-out lesions confirm a deep infection. Undoubtedly the prognoses of the two conditions are entirely different—in the former, improvement is spontaneous; in the latter, the progression of pain and disability leads to the removal of the artificial joint.

Obviously, it is essential to distinguish between the two as early as possible so that appropriate management can be rendered. In a doubtful situation, surgical exploration is the only way by which a correct diagnosis may be established. In a superficial infection with fascial involvement, a thorough débridement and irrigation is carried out. Following exploration and excision of the wound edges, the wound is closed using Hemovac suctions; caution must be exercised not to interfere with deep fascia if the infection is limited to the fat layer (Table 16-1).

Table 16-1. Summary of differential diagnosis between deep and superficial infection

	Wound infection	
	Superficial	**Deep**
Joint tenderness	–	+
Local inflammation	+	–
Wound induration	–	+
Wound drainage	–	+
Wound probe	–	+
Sinogram	–	+
X-ray changes	–	+
Duration	–	+
Prognosis	Good	Poor

+, Yes; –, no.

Deep infection vs. mechanical loosening

One of the most difficult aspects of the diagnosis in a suspected infection of a total hip replacement is in differentiating between deep infection and mechanical loosening; several factors may be of help in this differential diagnosis.

An accurate history may differentiate between deep infection and mechanical loosening; in general, the onset of deep infection is insidious and gradual. The patient reveals a stormy postoperative course, including elevation of temperature, or a defective result, such as pain in the hip, groin, or limbs. Additionally, the history of wound healing might reveal some fact about early trouble within the wound that usually coincides with deep infection. In mechanical loosening the patient generally has a totally pain-free period followed by a sudden onset of pain suggesting a mechanical defect; this may coincide with certain activities that the patient may describe, such as lifting a heavy object, falling, and misstepping. In most instances of mechanical loosening there is no history of defective wound healing.

Pain (definitive characteristics) is the most helpful feature in differentiating between mechanical loosening and deep infection. In a deep infection, pain is generally dull and present at night as well as in the daytime; it is usually deep-seated and may be throbbing or gnawing and constant. This pain may improve with the use of antibiotics and may have no connection with weight bearing, motion, or sharp movements of the hip. On the other hand, with loosening, pain is related to motion as well as weight bearing; antibiotics do not improve it, and any sharp

Table 16-2. Summary of differential diagnosis between mechanical loosening and deep infection

	Mechanical loosening	Deep infection
History		
Onset	−	+
Postoperative course	−	+
Wound healing	−	+
Pain		
With motion	+	−
With weight bearing	+	−
At night	−	+
Dull	−	+
Sharp motion	+	−
Antibiotics	+	−
Non-weight bearing	−	+
Deep	−	+
Throbbing	−	+
Other		
Fever	−	+
Tenderness	−	+
Warmth and fullness	−	+
Sedimentation rate	−	+
Radiographs	+	−
Ectopic bone	−	+

+, Yes; −, no.

movement by the patient (or during examination) brings on pain.

With deep infection, usually a low-grade elevation of temperature is present. The patient will have tenderness during the examination about the hip, particularly with deep palpation of the groin and upper thigh; there is an increased warmth of the skin and, occasionally, increased fullness about the hip (as compared with the opposite side), and slight dilation of the superficial veins. In the majority of cases, an elevated sedimentation rate and slight shift to the left of the white blood cells may suggest infection; additionally, there may be ectopic bone about the hip joint. On the other hand, in loosening, none of the above are present and radiographs are usually suggestive of loosening or defective mechanical fixation by cement. However, radiological changes of the two may be the same if loosening is of a long-standing nature (Table 16-2).

Deep infection vs. nonsuppurative lesions

In a few cases, radiological changes are consistent with signs of osteitis, that is, osteomyelitis of Garré—but the patient remains totally asymptomatic and these changes do not appear to progress to abscess formation (see Fig. 16-4, *C* and *D*). The erythrocyte sedimentation rate remains within the normal range, and the patient remains asymptomatic. Conceivably, slight motion at the time of x-ray examination may be responsible for the alleged radiological changes, but the real cause remains unknown, as most of these patients are asymptomatic and there is no justification for exploration of these cases. (Some of these were explored without any evidence of pus or growth of organisms.) Obviously, antibiotics are not helpful in these situations. A fusiform but symmetrical thickening of the cortex at the junction of the tip of the stem and the remainder of the bone must also be differentiated from this condition; the latter often denotes a good and "athletic performance" following total hip replacement.

Deep infection vs. hematoma

At times the presence of a large, deep hematoma must be distinguished from an acute infection. Patients with a hematoma generally develop acute and sudden onset of severe pain, usually coincidental with an elevated anticoagulation prophylaxis regimen. Severe pain and tenseness is experienced in the wound itself, usually after activity. Examination at an early stage may reveal a tense swelling and perhaps evidence of ecchymoses around the edge of the wound. The patient may have a slight elevation of temperature and even a slight shift in the cell differential. There is usually a drop in the hematocrit. If the patient is put on bedrest (with ice applied to the area of the wound), the pain generally should partly resolve within a few hours. Most importantly, anticoagulation treatment must be reversed. However, in a doubtful situation, a conservative attitude may be dangerous. We prefer in most instances to have the patient in the operating room (after reversing the coagulation profile), where—under aseptic conditions—the wound is opened and the hematoma explored. This mode of action is preferable to aspiration, which risks infection or development of a leaking hematoma. Exploration is especially indicated only when infection is highly suspected.

A draining hematoma (one that has already opened to the surface) is a potential risk for deep wound infection. Many of the infections that result from anticoagulation therapy start with a draining hematoma (in which case the surgeon elects a conservative course). With or without positive culture, the patient with such a hematoma must also be taken to the operating room immediately. Following evacuation and complete irrigation and débridement of the wound, a secondary closure is attempted. Only suction tubes are used for a period of 24 to 48 hours. There should be no "suction irrigation" tubes left in this type of wound. If bacterial contamination of the hematoma is suspected, an irrigation with appropriate antibiotics is used. In any case, once the skin is interrupted, the patient should receive intravenous antibiotics immediately during and after surgery, based on the results of cultures obtained at surgery.

Deep infection vs. ruptured fascia

At times, herniation of the greater trochanter through a defect in the fascia may resemble an infection or hematoma, especially in a slim person with minimum fat coverage over the trochanteric region; this is especially true where the closure of the fascia was inadequately performed, or a hematoma has erupted through the fascia. Nonabsorbable suture material should be routinely used when closing the fascia to prevent premature rupturing.

Deep infection and laboratory data

Of all laboratory parameters, *persistent* elevation of the sedimentation rate is the most reliable single suggestion of chronic infection. Approximately three fourths of patients with infection in the hip will show evidence of an elevated erythrocyte sedimentation rate. However, it must be noted that in the early postoperative course the sedimentation rate is almost always elevated. A rate lingering above 40 mm./hr. late in the postoperative period should be suspected as an indication of infection unless proved otherwise, but at least three values of the sedimentation rate must be determined prior to making a diagnostic decision. Other sources of infection must also be sought when there is a persistently elevated sedimentation rate. A urinary tract infection is a common source of low-grade infection without clinical evidence, especially in patients who have had a postoperative indwelling catheter.

A white blood count and differential might be of some value in determining acute infection, whereas in subacute and chronic infections there is usually no alteration of the white blood count and differential cells.

ASPIRATION OF THE JOINT

When infection is highly suspected and identification of organisms is essential in order to institute appropriate antibiotic treatment, or when the diagnosis of infection cannot be ascertained based on clinical and radiographic appearances, then an aspiration might be indicated. We do not favor routine and multiple aspirations; it is not an innocuous procedure and may itself contaminate the hip joint and lead to infection. Therefore this must be considered a serious procedure. The patient must be hospitalized and the joint aspirated under absolute aseptic conditions; it is not to be regarded as a casual routine office procedure for all symptomatic hips. Aspiration must be done under fluoroscopy (image intensifier) to assure the exact location of the needle. The anterior thigh and groin are properly prepared and draped using a surgical prep technique, that is, ether, alcohol, and tincture of iodine, 2%. Local anesthesia usually suffices, but occasionally a general anesthesia may be considered; preferably the procedure is done in the operating room. A 3-inch spinal needle attached to a glass syringe containing 1 to 2 ml. of normal saline solution is used. The femoral artery is palpated. The point of entry of the needle is approximately 2 inches distal to the mid-Poupart's ligament, just lateral to the femoral artery. If the patient feels radiating pain into the thigh, the needle is directed slightly lateral to the point of entry to the capsule to avoid the femoral nerve.

Attempts at aspiration are done only when it is certain under fluoroscopy that the tip of the needle is within the capsule of the joint next to the artificial joint space. If the attempt at aspiration reveals no fluid, then the normal saline solution is injected into the space and the attempt is repeated. Generally, the entrance of the needle beyond the capsule will be verified by the feeling of the needle passing through a rather dense layer of tissue. However, if in doubt, approximately 2 ml. of radiopaque material can be injected in order to verify that the joint space has been entered. At times, aspiration of the cement-bone junction may be indicated where bone involvement is suspected. An arthrogram may be obtained by injecting radiopaque (Radiographine) solution into the joint cavity through the same needle.

It should be emphasized that the material obtained from the hip joint must be transferred to the culture media immediately; if possible, the

Clinical results and complications

laboratory technician should be present at the time of aspiration and the smears obtained at once. It is of utmost importance that the significance of careful handling and organism identification is emphasized to the laboratory personnel and that they are informed of the implications of the smear and cultures in these patients. Aerobic and anaerobic cultures must be made and a search for L-forms included when the patient has received antibiotics. The laboratory search for L-forms requires great effort in producing an osmotically stable media and the investment of time in identifying the organism. It is essential to have cultures carefully handled—especially in subcultures—and specific reports so that contamination does not cast doubt on the

results. This delayed growth, often found only in subcultures, may be related to (1) prior antibiotic therapy, (2) low-virulence organisms, or (3) even laboratory contamination. Therefore an incubation period of longer than the conventional 24 hours must be allowed and special attention to specimens during the transfer of cultures must be urged.

GRAM'S STAIN AND CELLULAR MORPHOLOGY

Search for bacteria in the smear requires experienced laboratory personnel so that necrotic debris is not mistaken for bacteria. Occasionally, if the patient has had a metallic prosthetic device inserted previously, minute particles of

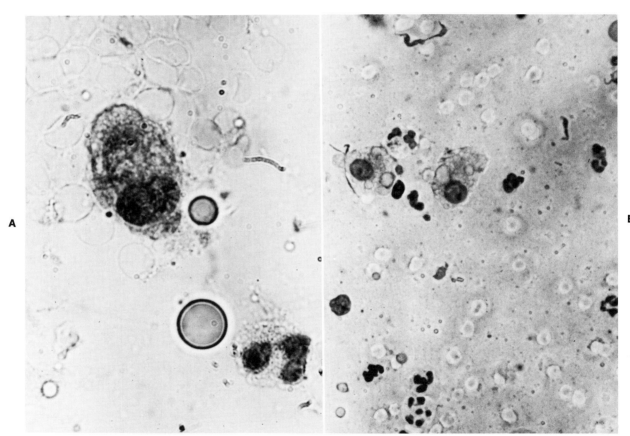

Fig. 16-3. A, High magnification of smear obtained at surgery from revision operation. NOTE: polymorphonuclear cells and red blood cells found in smear. Details of cytoplasmic granules and cytoplasmic membrane are important in assessing presence or absence of infection. Size of red blood cells may differentiate debris and artifacts from organisms in smear. **B,** Note frequency of neutrophils in this field and clear cytoplasm and ruptured cytoplasmic membrane of several neutrophils shown. Also note multiple small fragments of metallic particles in background that must be differentiated from organisms. This smear was obtained at surgery and subsequently revealed *Staphylococcus aureus,* coagulase positive by culture. Nevertheless, no organisms were found in field by Gram's stain. Specimen **A** was considered an infection; **B** was not.

A   B   C   D

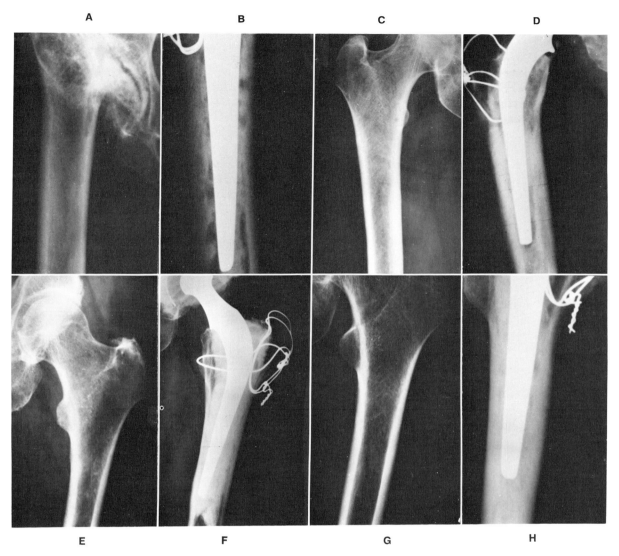

E   F   G   H

Fig. 16-4. Radiological changes of infection must be differentiated from other types of changes including physiological hypertrophy of cortex. **A,** Preoperative radiograph of shaft of right femur in 54-year-old woman prior to total hip replacement. **B,** Radiolucencies appearing at interface between cement and bone "punched-out lesion." These changes are usually signs of infection when they appear at interface. **C,** Preoperative radiograph of 62-year-old female with osteoarthritis of hip joint. **D,** Four years following hip replacement incidental findings of cortical thickening, which is somewhat irregular and extends over two thirds of distal segment of femoral stem. Patient's hip grading at this point was A-6,6,6. Because of excellent clinical results, no surgical intervention was attempted. These radiological changes are compatible with findings of osteitis, but minor loosening cannot be ruled out. No surgical intervention is indicated as long as patient is asymptomatic. Sedimentation rate in this patient was 3 mm./hr. She demonstrated negative Trendelenburg's sign. **E,** Preoperative radiograph of 63-year-old female with degenerative osteoarthritis and avascular necrosis of femoral head. **F,** Postoperative radiograph of **E.** NOTE: prosthesis is inserted in marked valgus orientation. Note also unicortical hypertrophy of cortex of femur on medial side. This is not compatible with infection and probably represents alterations in pattern of forces transmitted via femoral stem to cortex of femur. **G,** Preoperative radiograph of femoral shaft of 56-year-old female with bilateral degenerative osteoarthritis. **H,** Six years' postoperative radiographs of same femur as **G** following low-friction arthroplasty. Patient who was extremely disabled preoperatively graded 6,6,6, bilaterally postoperatively, walked approximately 2 miles/day, and engaged in many physical activities despite surgeon's advice. She enjoyed dancing as hobby. NOTE: fusiform hypertrophy of cortex at lower portion of stem. This marked hypertrophy should be differentiated from osteosclerosis shown in **D.** Physiological hypertrophy of cortex is seen frequently in extremely active individuals following total hip replacement. (See also Fig. 16-8.)

metal may be present in the tissue (the stain resembling that of micrococci). As a general rule, these metal particles are larger than bacteria and can be identified against the background of red cells in the tissue fluid (Fig. 16-3). Yet, more important than the search for bacteria is the search for inflammatory cells in the fluid. An increased number of polymorphonuclear cells, especially neutrophils, is evidence of suppurative infection, and their numbers must be counted within the field of the aspirate material. However, the quality of these neutrophils is more important than their number per se. When lysosomal activity is present within the cytoplasm, that is, bacterial infection, the neutrophils are depleted of cytoplasmic granules, and degrading neutrophils are prevalent in large numbers in the microscopic field (Fig. 16-3, *B*). Prevalence of plasma cells, however, might indicate the presence of chronic infection.

DEEP WOUND INFECTION AND RADIOLOGICAL APPEARANCE

No information is obtainable by radiographs prior to 6 weeks. In previous studies of radiographs of infected total hip replacements, approximately 3 to 6 months lapsed before radiological signs of infection appeared.[9] Common changes include a radiolucent zone at the bone-cement interface, scalloping effect at the cortex, periosteal reaction resembling lamination, or evidence of osteitis represented by radiodensity or radiolucency such as found in osteomyelitis (Fig. 16-4). The most reliable interpretation of radiographs is based on examination of periodic routine films; the standard view must include the upper third of the femur and the hip joint. Early and minor changes are not recognized without previous films for comparison. The use of laminagrams may be indicated in certain situations; they will detect any interruption of the

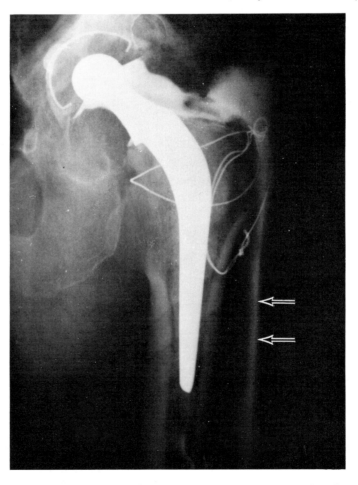

Fig. 16-5. Arrows indicate distal extension of dye into thigh and in posterior region of trochanter following arthrogram obtained in patient with acute infection following total hip arthroplasty.

cement column, that is, mechanical loosening, or show evidence of punched-out lesions in the cortex common in osteitis. Magnification views of the cortex of the femur or acetabulum may verify the details of bone trabeculae that might not otherwise be seen on routine films. These signs are magnified by increasing the tube-plate distance and increasing the intensity of kilovoltage and the use of spot cassettes. Special x-ray machines are required to produce these films.

ARTHROGRAM, SINOGRAM, AND BONE SCAN

Arthrograms are not helpful in the diagnosis of infection per se and could be misleading when they are positive with regard to the presence or absence of loosening. However, when there is soft tissue involvement, arthrograms might be helpful in detecting the extent and location of soft tissue involvement about the artificial hip joint (which can be helpful in surgical management). Subtraction technique is essential to verify the details when radiopaque cement is used.

Sinograms are of extreme help in verifying the extent of involvement of the soft tissue—whether or not the soft tissue infection extends to the deeper structures and down to the artificial joint. All patients undergoing surgery for removal of the artificial joint (following infected total hip replacement with existing sinus) should have a sinogram to verify the extent of involvement of the hip joint itself (Figs. 10-4 and 16-5).

Bone scanning is suggested to be of value in differentiating between mechanical loosening and infection. Our limited experience with this method does not allow us to make a definitive judgment on its diagnostic value at this time.

BACTERIOLOGY OF INFECTION AFTER TOTAL HIP REPLACEMENT

Any opinion regarding prevalence of organisms and their types can be formulated only from a large series of infections. Between 1960 and 1970, following 5,800 total hip replacements, 85 infections developed at Wrightington Hospital (representing a rate of 1.6%). In that series, *Staphylococcus aureus* could be incriminated in 33 cases (or 39.5%). In 23 cases of infection, bacteriology of the wound could not be evaluated and was not considered valid (27.5%), since a late sinus had developed at the time cultures were obtained.[8] An additional problem is the interpretation of cultures from which no organism can be grown despite presence of clinical infection. This occurred in 10 patients (12% of all cases). Coliform bacilli were present in 5, *Proteus* in 6, coagulase-negative staphylococcus in 4, *Pseudomonas* in 1, hemolytic streptococcus in 1, *Streptococcus agalactiae* in 2. Delayed positive cultures (after several days) and chances of laboratory contamination create difficulty in interpreting the results in subcultures.[8]

Seven infections occurred in the first 1,500 cases at New York Orthopaedic Hospital; the types of organism recovered and the time of appearance of the infections are presented in Table 16-3.

The types of organism related to early and late infections have been studied. In Charnley's series 34 infections were considered early and 51 late. In 17 of 34 early infections *Staphylococcus aureus* was the cause, and in 16 late infections (31%) the same organism could be identified. Therefore *Staphylococcus aureus*, coagulase positive, remains the major cause of both early and late infections after total hip replacement. There was a greater number of sterile infections in the early group (6 or 18%) than in the delayed group (4 or 8%). All 4 infections by coliforms (12%) were in the early group, and there were 6 infections with mixed organisms—namely mixed coliforms with coagulase-negative organisms.[8]

Over the period of study, a progressive reduction of both absolute and relative numbers of "sterile" infections exonerates the possibility that these sterile infections were caused by chemical irritation from implanted plastics.[8,9]

It is of considerable interest that if one considers the susceptibility to infection in an individual, one might expect a similar outcome following surgery of the opposite hip (after the first hip becomes infected). However, it is generally considered safe to proceed with the operation on the second hip (following infection in the first hip) without fear of infection in the second side. This usually should be planned, of course, in the absence of acute exacerbation of infection or presence of copious drainage from the infected hip. (See Chapter 8.)

LIMITATIONS OF THE GERM THEORY IN TOTAL HIP REPLACEMENT

A real dilemma arises when interpreting negative cultures from a wound where there is gross

Table 16-3. Correlation of intracapsular cultures with organism recovered from operative wounds following infection (New York Orthopaedic Hospital)

Primary arthroplasty	Diagnosis	Intracapsular culture	Months to infection	Infection culture
C. J.	OA	No growth	46*	Mixed
H. H.	OA	No growth	1	*Staphylococcus aureus Enterococcus*
R. S.	CDH	No growth	20	*Staphylococcus aureus Pseudomonas*
D. D.	AN	No growth	11	Not available
A. G.	OA	No growth	12	Not available
Revision arthroplasty				
W. S.	OA	No growth	39*	*Proteus*
P. L.	OA	Beta hemolytic streptococcus	21	*Staphylococcus aureus*

*Hematogenous infection. OA, osteoarthritis; CDH, congenital dislocation of hip; AN, avascular necrosis.

Table 16-4. Total hip replacement intraoperative wound cultures (New York Orthopaedic Hospital)[38]

	Primary	Revision
Staphylococcus epidermidis	9	6
Staphylococcus aureus	5	2
Streptococcus viridans	4	2
Clostridium perfringens	3	1
Enterococcus	2	1
Diphtheroid	2	
Enterobacter	1	
Bacteroides	1	1
Peptococcus	1	
Mixed (*Escherichia coli,* *Clostridium perfringens*)	1	
Serratia		1
Bacillus		1
Total	29	15
Incidence	2.3%	6.4%

A routine culture was obtained in the first 1,500 total hip replacements performed at our hospital[38] (1,421 cultures became available for study). In 1,187 primary operations included in this series, 29 (2.3%) revealed a positive culture from the wound; of 234 revision operations performed for failed previous operations, 15 also revealed positive cultures (6.4%). Table 16-4 shows the type and frequency of organisms recovered in these two groups (a higher incidence of positive cultures have been reported by others; see Table 16-5). (It must be noted that routine preoperative antibiotics had been instituted in all these cases.) All these patients received prophylactic antibiotics perioperatively. Furthermore, it must be noted that in none of the primary or revision patients with a positive intraoperative culture has infection developed with the same organism (Table 16-3). It is most remarkable that none of these patients (primary or revision groups) today have shown evidence of clinical infection or a defective result following their operation. It is of further special interest that at surgery Gram's stains of the joint fluids obtained in the revision group were negative in all hips. During the period between April 1969 and August 1974 (which was selected for this study) seven deep wound infections developed (Table 16-3). As one can see, the infective organisms in these cases did not correlate with the types of organisms recovered at surgery. Possible explanations for positive cultures from "virgin hips" are: (1) laboratory contamination;

evidence of clinical and radiological infection (without previous antibiotic therapy), and no other explanation can be offered. Even more disturbing is the unexplained and provocative presence of organisms in the "virgin" hip where no previous operation was performed; this unexplained finding has been reported by others* (Tables 16-4 and 16-5) and has also been studied at the New York Orthopaedic Hospital.

*See references 7, 16, 17, 19-21, 36, and 40.

Table 16-5. Correlation of "positive cultures" in primary and revision surgery with deep wound infections in different institutions

Primary operations	New York Orthopaedic Hospital[38]	Charnley[7]	Murray[29]	Dupont[16]	Mayo Clinic[19]
Cultured cases	1,187		511		437
Number positive cultures	29		160		111
Percent positive cultures	2.3		31.3		25.4
Deep infections	5		4		2
Revision operations					
Revision cases	234	217	229	168	221
Cultured cases	234	59	229	168	221
Percent positive cultures	6.4	29	32	24	38
Deep infections	1	8	8	7	5
Positive cultures in clinical infected cases	0 (+1 with different organism)	4 of 5	2 of 8 (+2 with different organisms)	3 of 6	1 of 5 (+3 with different organisms)

(2) repeated transfer of the original culture specimens to new media (subcultures) caused accidental contamination to take place; (3) the operative wound was already inoculated at the time the acetabular culture was obtained; (4) transient bacteremia resulted in hematologic seeding of the diseased hip joint with the organism. Paradoxically, all wounds healed per primam without subsequent development of infection.

While it is difficult to explain a positive culture from a "virgin hip," a positive culture following previous surgery is of more concern and requires treatment; we recommend a period of 6 weeks of antibiotic therapy for both groups. If the types of organisms recovered from the wound are gram negative or highly virulent, a longer period of antibiotic therapy may be indicated.

MANAGEMENT OF THE INFECTED TOTAL HIP

Treatment will be considered in situations where infection is: (1) acute, (2) low grade without osteitis, and (3) chronic with osteitis, sinus formation, and the like.

Acute infection

The principles of treatment of acute surgical infection apply to the infected total hip where there is swelling, redness, toxemia, and other systemic and local evidence of infection. As soon as the diagnosis is made, a differential between "deep" and "superficial" must be established. The entire wound is opened, and the deep fascia and artificial joint are fully exposed only if infection is deep to the fascia. At the discretion of the surgeon, the greater trochanteric fixation may be left undisturbed. Following complete débridement and removal of necrotized and devitalized tissue, copious irrigation of the wound is performed. Loculations of soft-tissue abscesses about the joint are thoroughly opened and the infective tissue is excised by sharp dissection. Supportive therapy—including blood transfusions and intravenous fluids—must be administered as necessary. Antibiotics specific to the organism must be given intravenously in large doses. The appropriate antibiotic is determined by serum bactericidal level against the organism recovered from the hip.

The method of treatment of the wound following surgery (based on our present policy) depends on the type of organism, that is, for a gram-negative sepsis—wound packed open; for a gram-positive sepsis—insertion of suction irrigation tubes. The suction irrigation must not be left in place more than 3 to 5 days (at the discretion of the surgeon) since oftentimes a secondary contamination is unavoidable. Primary wound closure must be done *only* if the surgeon feels that the débridement has been

565

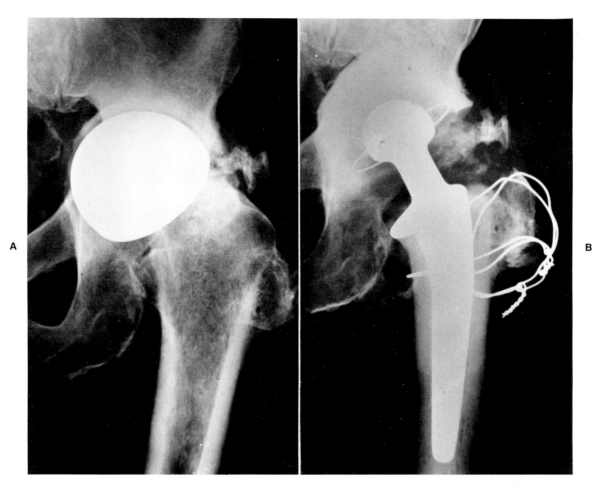

Fig. 16-6. A, Radiograph 12 years following cup arthroplasty in 72-year-old man who originally had osteoarthritis for which mold arthroplasty had been performed. Three months following mold arthroplasty abscess was present in area of incision for which incision and drainage were performed, irrigation-suction system was installed, and oxacillin was administered both intravenously as well as locally to control infection. Infection had been controlled successfully for 12 years. **B,** Two years following conversion of previously infected cup arthroplasty to total hip replacement. At surgery the patient's sedimentation rate was 15 mm./hr., and there was no evidence of induration, tenderness, heat, and so on. Multiple aspiration of joint was also negative. Tissue obtained at surgery revealed no evidence of infection and was compatible with chronic inflammatory process similar to tissue adjacent to implant (cup). Patient's hip assessment was 6,6,6 and arthroplasty was considered successful.

complete and antibiotic sensitivity has revealed a highly susceptible organism (such as streptococcus). Intravenous antibiotics must be extended for 4 to 6 weeks postoperatively in large doses and continued orally for at least 6 months or more. Control of infection is determined by periodic examination of the wound and sedimentation rate, as well as other parameters such as white blood count. Experience suggests that approximately 50% of all infections appearing in acute form following a total hip replacement may be treated successfully in this manner. The remainder will gradually be converted to a subacute or chronic form requiring further treatment as indicated at a later date.

Low-grade infection without osteitis

Treatment of this type of infected total hip replacement is quite controversial at the present time; there are no adequate statistics to support the most suitable treatment in this type of infection. DuPont and Charnley[15] reported positive

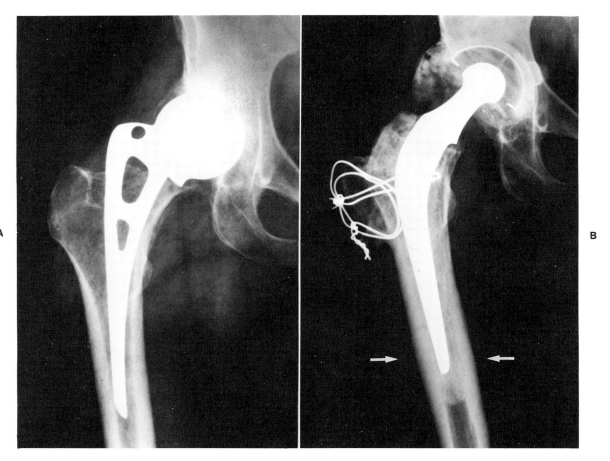

Fig. 16-8. A, Fifty-four-year-old female with failed Moore self-locking prosthesis, which had been inserted for fracture of neck of femur. Patient had no history of drainage from wound following insertion of prosthesis. Sedimentation rate was 13 mm./hr., and at surgery there was no suspicion for infection when hip was explored for attempt at replacement. **B,** Eight years following conversion of Moore self-locking prosthesis to low-friction arthroplasty. Multiple specimens obtained at surgery from medullary canal and acetabulum all revealed heavy growth of *Staphylococcus aureus,* coagulase positive. Patient was started on intravenous oxacillin for period of 2 weeks and continued on antibiotics postoperatively for 6 weeks. When last seen 8 years following arthroplasty, hip grades were 6,6,6, sedimentation rate was 15 mm./hr., and there is no evidence of any sign of "mischief" in hip. Cortical hypertrophy indicates good function (arrow).

cultures from operative specimens in 13 hips following revision for a failed previous operation; nine of these cultures showed evidence of growth of *Staphylococcus albus,* coagulase negative, and one showed growth of *Staphylococcus aureus,* coagulase positive. They reported successful treatment in 8 of these 10 staphylococcal infections, with a definite deep infection in one patient and a suspected deep infection in another—but follow-up was encouraging regarding the mode of treatment in a subacute infection in these cases. Since Wilson's original report,[39] we have occasionally accepted a patient with a low-grade infection for total hip arthro-

plasty (Fig. 16-6 to 16-8). It is still difficult to formulate an opinion regarding the type of infection that may be successfully treated by this method, but the following details appear to be essential in overall success.

1. Select only healthy patients with very disabled (painful) hips who can tolerate a major ordeal.
2. If the bacteria involved is of low virulence, that is, *Staphylococcus epidermidis,* sensitive *Staphylococcus aureus,* streptococcus, sterile wounds, and so on, be cautious in the selection of patients with gram-negative and mixed organisms.

569

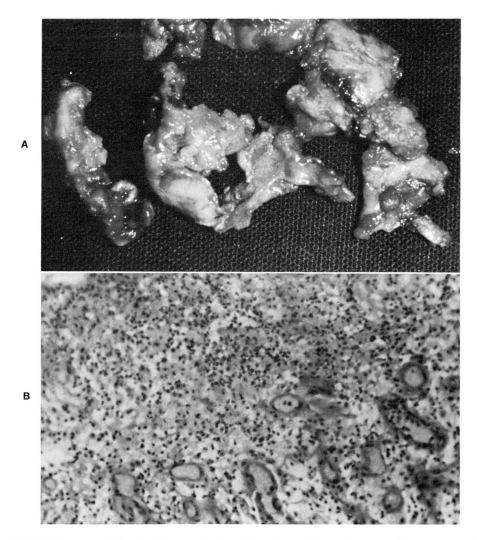

Fig. 16-9. A, Presence of abundant "granulation-type tissue" found at surgery may only suggest possibility of infection. **B,** Real confirmation of pyogenic nature of material is by histological evidence of suppurative elements, that is, fibrinoid necrosis, infiltrative polymorphs, hypervascularity, and so on. NOTE: material shown here relates to Fig. 16-10.

Fig. 16-10. A, Preoperative radiograph of hip in 54-year-old baker with severe and advanced degenerative osteoarthritis. **B,** Six months following total hip replacement by low-friction arthroplasty in another institution. NOTE: radiological changes of femur at level of tip of prosthesis and slight subsidence of prosthesis (arrows). On admission to our hospital sedimentation rate was 35 mm./hr. There was no history of infection following operation. **C,** At surgery Gram's stain obtained from tissue revealed no organism, but granulation tissue was abundant and microscopically suggestive of infection (Fig. 16-9). Therefore operation was terminated following débridement, but acetabular cup was left in place and reoperation following cultures and sensitivity of organisms was considered. Six months following removal of femoral component in second attempt for replacement, abundant amount of granulation tissue and purulent material was observed. Purulent material was definitely suggestive of infection although no organism was present on smear. **D,** After multiple biopsies were obtained, suction-irrigation system was instituted and operation was terminated following removal of cup. Radiographs shown here are 1 year following conversion of hip to pseudarthrosis. Patient has good functional results, thus decision regarding reoperation has been indefinitely postponed. This hip never grew any organism. Patient had not received preoperative antibiotics. Sedimentation rate always remained below 40 mm./hr. However, histologically and clinically hip was considered infected.

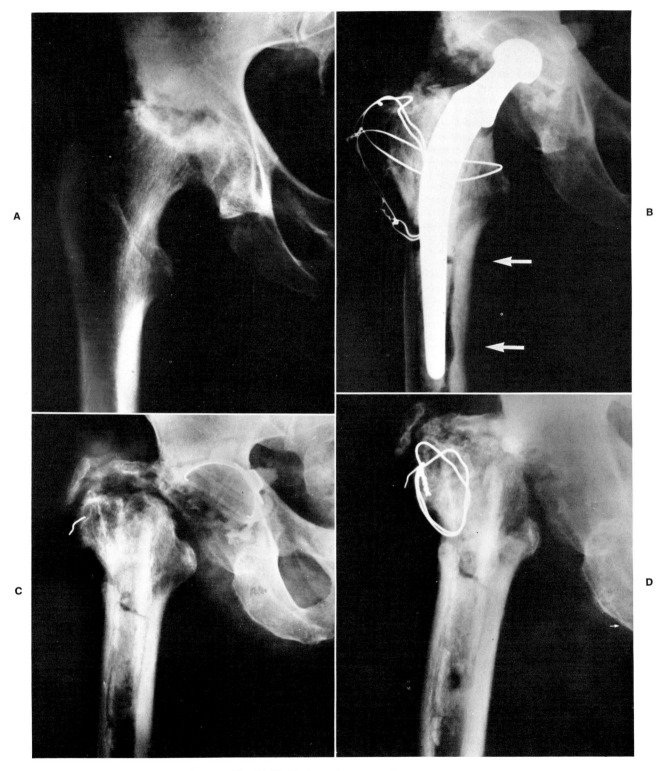

A

B

C

D

Fig. 16-10. For legend see opposite page.

3. If the wound is not indurated, warm, or showing evidence of drainage (closed sub-clinical infection) the chances for success are good.

4. The operation must be staged whenever there is doubt about the activity of infection or invasiveness of organisms.

5. The first responsibility is to perform adequate surgical débridement, and secondly, to suppress the organism with a large dose of effective antibiotics.

6. No revision should be undertaken in open wounds, in the presence of extensive osteomyelitis, mixed organisms, and gram-negative infections.

7. The entire plan must be based on (and is dependent on) the patient's understanding of the magnitude of the surgery, the risks involved, and the chances for failure. (Patients must realize beforehand the arduous nature of treatment—especially long-term antibiotic treatment.)

Wilson and associates[39] reported 19 patients suffering from subacute (latent) or recently arrested sepsis of the hip joint treated by massive doses of antibiotics and total prosthetic reconstruction. There was a minimum of 2 years recorded follow-up with failure caused by recurrence of infection in two patients; they attributed this failure to inadequate antibiotic treatment. The authors concluded that the results were superior to those from a simple Girdlestone procedure, and they emphasized the importance of identifying the organism and adequate antibiotic therapy in these patients. They caution against treating gram-negative infections in this manner, however.

Buchholz and Gartmann[3] have expressed similar difficulty in sepsis caused by gram-negative organisms, especially *Pseudomonas* and anaerobic bacteria. In those situations, high doses of intravenous antibiotics are recommended, similar to treatment for bacterial endocarditis after valve replacement surgery.* A minimum of 3 months of antibiotic treatment has been recommended. If the infective organism has not been identified by aspiration, then exploration of the hip joint for a biopsy and débridement of the hip joint are done for cultures from the synovium and capsule. Pulverized specimens are more definitive in producing organisms.

---

*See references 1, 14, 26, 35, and 42.

Finally, it must be recognized that recovery of the organism is fundamental to appropriate management of these cases and that all organisms are potential "pathogens" when recovered from a previously infected hip. For example, as in general surgery, coagulase-negative Staphylococcus is a common organism found in postoperative infections in total hip replacement.

Staging of surgery in subacute infections without osteitis. In deciding whether or not to proceed with replacement of an infected hip without osteitis, the criteria of the histology, cellular morphology, and the state of the wound at surgery must be considered (Fig. 16-9). This information is evaluated along with x-ray changes and the nature and virulence of the bacteria and its sensitivity to antibiotics. When a two-stage operation is planned, the interval between the two operations must be decided on the basis of all available criteria, such as the virulence of organisms, the nature of bone changes on radiographs, and the state of the wound at surgery. Ideally, the operations should be staged with an interval of 6 months or longer to allow the wound to become quiescent and for adequate antibiotic administration. Obviously, there is no comprehensive data to indicate the optimum time period before the second operation can safely be performed. The disadvantages of proceeding too early would seem to outweigh those of waiting too long. During this interval, patients can be protected by crutch walking and, perhaps, partial weight bearing. Prolonged and continuous skeletal traction during the interphase is not indicated (except for the early postoperative course of immobilization to overcome excessive shortening of the extremity) (Fig. 16-10).

It must be recognized that in both Charnley's and Wilson's series the most frequently offending organisms were *Staphylococcus albus* and other mild pathogens (Table 16-6). It is further noted that in both series (all 13 of Charnley's cases and in 16 of Wilson's 19 cases) no cement had been used. Histologically, direct contact of cement with bone makes it impossible for bone to escape contamination when an organism reaches the interface. On the other hand, in an uncemented intramedullary stem, for example, in a Thompson prosthesis, because of motion a fibrous layer develops, forming a sleeve about the stem of the prosthesis that may protect the bone from developing osteomyelitis (Fig. 16-11). At revision surgery this entire fibrous sleeve can

Table 16-6. Type of organism recovered in cases of low-grade infection prior to total hip replacement

	DuPont and Charnley[15] 13 hips*	Wilson et al.[39] 19 hips†
Staphylococcus albus	9	9
Staphylococcus aureus	1	2
Pseudomonas		1
Diphtheroids		1
Gram-positive cocci		1
Mixed	1	
Other	2	5
Total	13	19

*All noncemented.
†Three cemented.

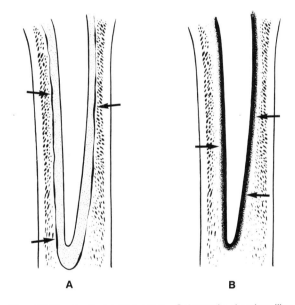

Fig. 16-11. A, Cemented stem. Schematic drawing illustrating that cement is in direct contact with bone with only occasional thin layer of fibrous tissue (arrows) present at interface. **B,** Noncemented stem. Thick layer of fibrous tissue (arrows) forms at interface between metal and bone as result of motion.

usually be removed from the medullary canal without extensive contamination of bone. Therefore, at least in theory, a better opportunity exists for removing infective material in a noncemented situation than with a cemented prosthesis.

Chronic infection with osteitis

Indications for surgery are pain and systemic manifestations of infection. While the patient obviously shows evidence of osteomyelitis, some patients have little discomfort in the hip—and at times, no pain whatsoever. There are occasional patients who can tolerate the presence of infection and go on walking for some years before surgical intervention becomes necessary (Fig. 16-6). On the average, the time lapse from the original diagnosis to removal of the artificial joint varies from 3 to 4 years, with a maximum of 8 to 9 years in some instances.

Obviously a conservative attitude is justified. Not all infected hips require an immediate decision for removal of the artificial device. Further, radiological evidence of osteitis alone never is an indication to remove the total hip device.

REMOVAL OF THE TOTAL HIP PROSTHESIS AND CEMENT

Like Charnley, we believe that once it has been clinically and radiologically established that the total hip replacement is infected and the patient is sufficiently symptomatic, the entire implant (including the methyl methacrylate cement) will have to be removed. From the patient's standpoint, this is no more drastic than if a femoral head prosthesis without cement became infected and would have to be removed. The task for the surgeon, however, is somewhat more difficult. We believe that under no circumstances is a second replacement justified when there has been evidence of osteomyelitis of the upper femur. This is in contrast to the opinion rendered in the recent experiences of Buchholz and others[3,4] that an infected hip with osteomyelitis can be saved by reoperation and reinsertion of a total hip prosthesis.

The timing for the removal of the total hip prosthesis depends on the severity of the infection and the patient's symptoms. If pain develops early, early removal of the prosthesis is advisable since bone will be less involved and there will be a better chance for a primary wound closure after removal of the entire implant. On the other hand, if the infection is long-standing, removal is often easy since the cement will be sequestrated. But the treatment of the osteomyelitis is more involved (Fig. 16-12). If symptoms are minimal but the erythrocyte sedimentation rate is elevated and radiological changes are present, biopsy is not indicated because it may precipitate

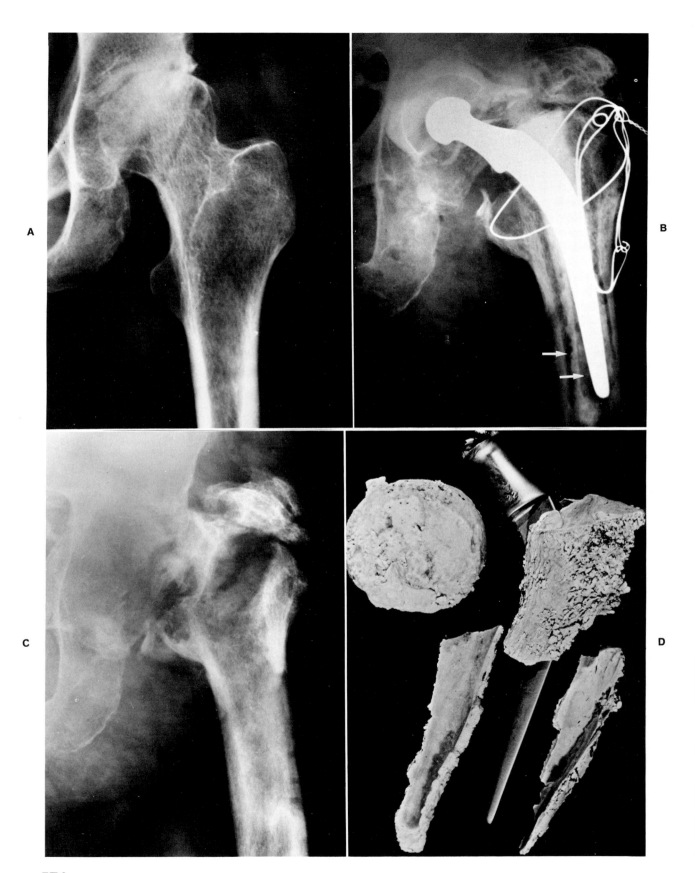

a sinus or flare-up of the infection, leading to an early need for pseudarthrosis, despite the patient's satisfaction with the arthroplasty. In contrast, early removal must be considered for the patient with long-standing pain who has not been advised to have the artificial joint removed and who has had only minor surgical procedures done, such as repeated abscess drainage.

PSYCHOLOGICAL PREPARATION OF THE PATIENT FOR SURGERY

The patient who is undergoing removal of his total hip prosthesis must be psychologically prepared and supported to accept a Girdlestone pseudarthrosis, which frequently results in a relatively good functional hip after an infected total hip replacement. It must be recognized that most patients are mystified by the fact that they are going to have no hip joint at all, and they compare their status with amputation or total invalidism; it must be stressed that a Girdlestone operation was once an accepted method for treatment of primary hip disorders. The greatest disadvantages of a Girdlestone operation most often are instability and shortening of the limb, thus necessitating the use of a cane and lift in the shoe in most instances. The pain, many times, will be less than with the infected total hip. Therefore the patient who has considerable pain should be encouraged to accept the Girdlestone resection. (Visiting another patient with such a procedure often is helpful and supportive.) In preparation for a good result, the patient must be told that 6 weeks' traction will provide him with better stability in the hip as well as good alignment for the lower extremity once rehabilitation begins. This is an extremely important detail since most patients have the notion that following removal of the artificial joint the course will follow one similar to that of the original replacement operation. If there is any evidence of systemic sepsis—such as elevation of temperature, lack of appetite, or signs of chronic toxemia (such as anemia)—there will

be very little persuasion necessary for acceptance of the removal of the artificial device.

PATIENT'S FITNESS AND SURGICAL PREPARATION

Removal of the artificial hip joint and conversion of an infected total hip replacement to a pseudarthrosis is a procedure of greater magnitude than a total hip replacement; much greater care must be paid to the patient's physiological status—particularly to kidney function, pulmonary status, and hemodynamics. The patient's skin is of further consideration. The skin must be protected because of the long stay in traction; if the patient has sensitive skin, special precautions such as an air or water mattress may be useful. Because of possible reactivation of infection, isolation may be necessary during the early postoperative course. Hospitalization costs and other monetary aspects must be considered because of the long hospital stay. A consultation with the Social Services Department of the hospital is often helpful. The patient's blood type (as well as proper antibiotics) must have been determined and appraised, and cooperation with an infectious disease expert is invaluable in prescribing antibiotics.

SURGICAL TECHNIQUE AND POSTOPERATIVE MANAGEMENT

A conventional lateral approach with the incision centered over the greater trochanter is used (Fig. 16-13). If necessary, the proximal end of the incision may be fashioned in a T shape or a "goblet" shape to allow complete access to the top of the femur and the pelvic region. The abductor muscles are elevated from the greater trochanter by an electric knife to minimize bleeding (Fig. 16-13) and wires are removed. After dislocation of the prosthesis, the femoral component is knocked out with a blunt chisel. It is most important to mobilize the upper femur from the scar tissue and perform an iliopsoas tenotomy to obtain access to the neck of the femur and shaft. Approximately 1 inch of the ce-

Fig. 16-12. A, Preoperative radiograph of degenerative osteoarthritis of hip in 73-year-old ex–tennis coach and instructor. **B,** Two years following total hip replacement performed in another institution patient had developed early infection for which multiple surgical procedures had been performed to eradicate infection. Patient was referred to us for definitive treatment. **C,** Immediate postoperative radiograph following removal of total hip device and cement. Radiograph shows osteomyelitic sequestra about hip, necessitating removal of entire cement. **D,** On exploration, cup literally fell out of acetabulum and entire cement mass was extracted with ease in three pieces. In this situation, because of chronic osteomyelitis of bone, anterolateral trough was made to remove all pieces of sequestra, although cement removal did not require windowing of cortex.

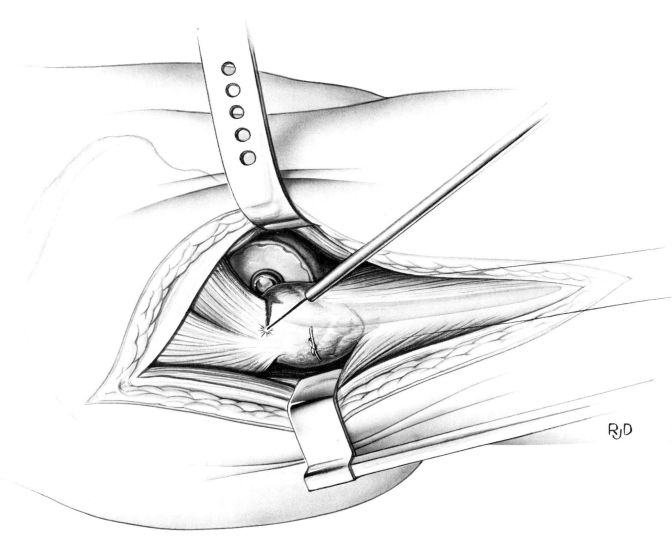

Fig. 16-13. Surgical technique involved in removal of infected total hip includes conventional lateral approach with incision centered over greater trochanter. Abductor muscles are elevated from greater trochanter by electric knife to minimize bleeding. Wires are removed, making sure surgeon will not puncture his gloves thus contaminating himself with infected material. Upper femur must be mobilized prior to removal of prosthesis and cement from shaft of femur.

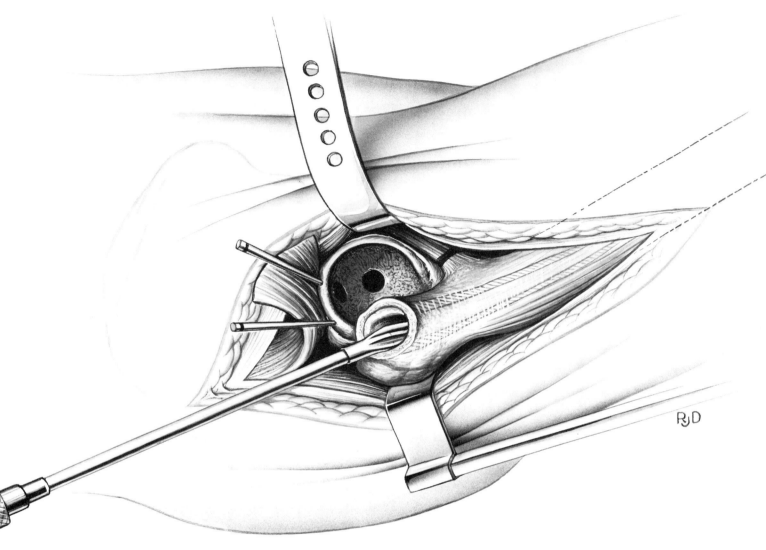

Fig. 16-14. Low-speed, high-torque drill is being used to remove cement from the upper femur. NOTE: acetabulum has been fully exposed by insertion of pin retractors to superior acetabular area and by retracting abductor muscles. Total exposure must be greater than incision and exposure used in performing conventional total hip operation.

ment can be easily removed through the neck; removal of the remainder of the cement is facilitated by a low-speed, high-torque drill, using graded Küntscher reamers or similar reamers (Fig. 16-14). Nevertheless, if the infection is not of long-standing duration and the cement is rigidly fixed to the bone, then guttering approximately one third of the circumference of the anterolateral aspect of the shaft of the femur is necessary (Fig. 16-15). The guttering of the shaft (which automatically eliminates the pos-sibility of future replacement) must be carefully done to avoid pathological fracture of the upper end of the femur. It must be realized that *all* cement must be removed or a sinus will persist (Fig. 16-16). The use of a tapered corkscrew-like instrument or a special hook may remove large fragments of cement. The use of fiberoptic light may facilitate visualization of unrecognized pieces in the shaft.

Removal of the acetabular component is generally easier than the femoral component. The

577

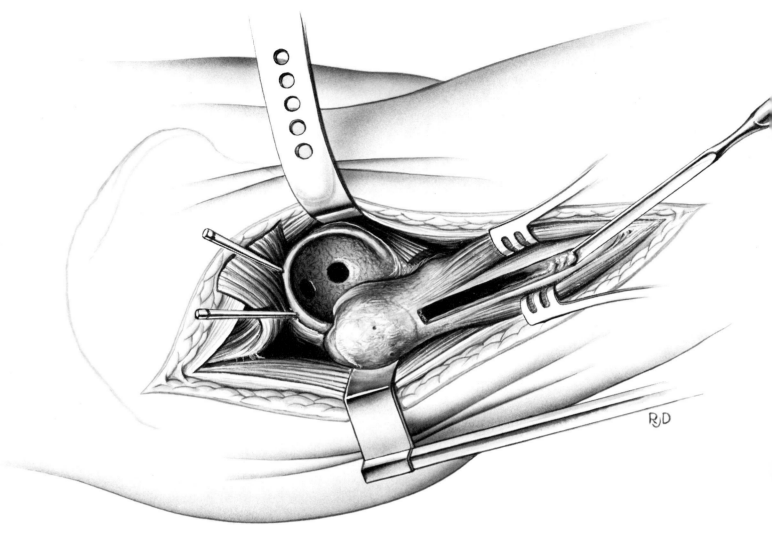

Fig. 16-15. When infection is not long-standing and cement is rigidly fixed to bone, guttering of proximal end (one third of circumference) of shaft of femur at anterolateral aspect is necessary. Four small drill holes should be used to map out size of window. Use of sharp gouge connecting four holes is encouraged. Width of trough must not exceed one third of circumference of femur.

cephalad periphery of the acetabulum must be identified by insertion of one or two (or more) pin retractors (Fig. 16-17); a Smith-Petersen curved arthroplasty gouge and a Watson-Jones gouge facilitate entering at the junction of cement and bone, using heavy hammer blows. With progressive blows, a curved gouge will fall into the space between the cement and the acetabulum, and the entire implant can be removed in toto. If anchorage columns of cement (anchor holes) penetrating into the pelvis are fractured, they are then removed separately.

As a practical point, at the end of surgical removal a radiograph must be obtained in the operating room to verify entire cement removal (Fig. 16-18). If the postoperative radiograph reveals the presence of sequestrum or cement, at the second operation (first repacking of the wound), an opportunity exists to remove the remainder of the cement and necrotic bone.

The abductors are sutured as distally as possible over the lateral aspect of the shaft. Wires or catgut are used for this purpose. Two pairs of suction tubes are placed deep into the wound

578

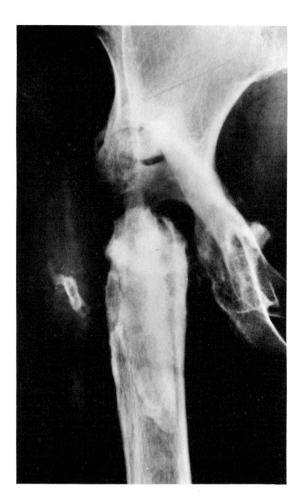

Fig. 16-16. Radiograph of 36-year-old female who had total hip arthroplasty performed in another institution. She was sent to us for definitive treatment of "stubborn" infection. She had had 18 major procedures to eradicate infection from hip joint. Organisms were mixed gram-negative and gram-positive bacteria. Three sinuses were present anteriorly and two laterally in hip region. The anteroposterior view of hip illustrates problem: unremoved cement from shaft. Despite multiple surgical procedures in this patient, cement and sequestrated bone had not been removed even though approximately 3 inches of upper femur and acetabular region had been extensively excised.

adjacent to the shaft of the femur and acetabulum, then primary closure of the wound is performed.

When irrigation is planned, two additional tubes are used and suction irrigation with appropriate antibiotics is instituted immediately. While suction irrigation may selectively be chosen in some instances, in most cases where osteomyelitis is present we prefer packing of the wound instead; it is done with a 5-yard roll soaked in povidone-iodine (Betadine) solution. However, large suctions may be placed deep to the wound and deep to the packing. The packing is then held in place by four or five through-and-through retention sutures applied through the fascia, fat, and skin. These suction tubes remain undisturbed until the first dressing is done 5 days later under general anesthesia, at which time they may be replaced or may be kept for

further packing. Infrequent packing is recommended; the first packing after the original operation must again be done under general anesthesia in order to evaluate the wound and debride further if necessary.

It is preferable to place the extremity in balanced suspension traction (Fig. 16-18) for comfort after the insertion of a Steinmann's nail into the upper tibia. A period of 6 weeks of uninterrupted traction is followed by a crutch-walking, non-weight-bearing period of an additional 6 weeks, following which gradual weight bearing is resumed. The use of a cane is encouraged only after the patient is able to bear weight more than 50% of the time on the affected side without pain.

This program provides maximum length of the extremity and a more stable hip than a treatment program that encourages the patient to

579

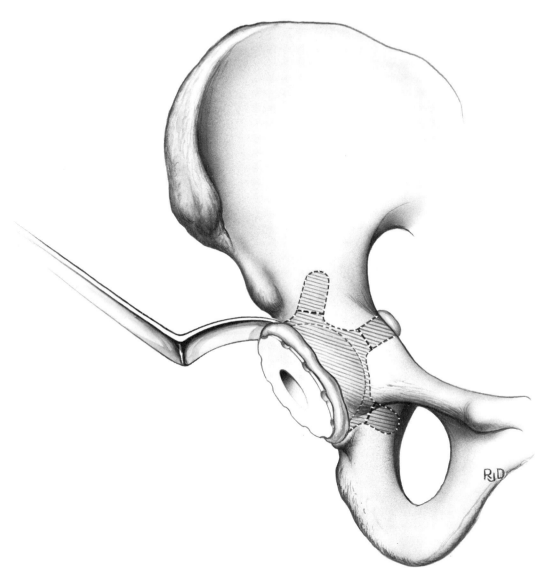

Fig. 16-17. Removal of acetabular component is generally easy, but prior to attempt at removal, periphery of acetabulum must be well identified by insertion of pin retractors (Figs. 16-14 and 16-15). Conventional acetabular gouge, that is, Smith-Petersen curved arthroplasty gouge or Watson-Jones gouge, facilitates entering junction of cement and bone using heavy hammer blows. With progressive blows curved gouge will fall into space between cement and acetabulum and entire implant can be removed in toto. Remainder of cement at site of anchor holes may be removed separately following removal of major components.

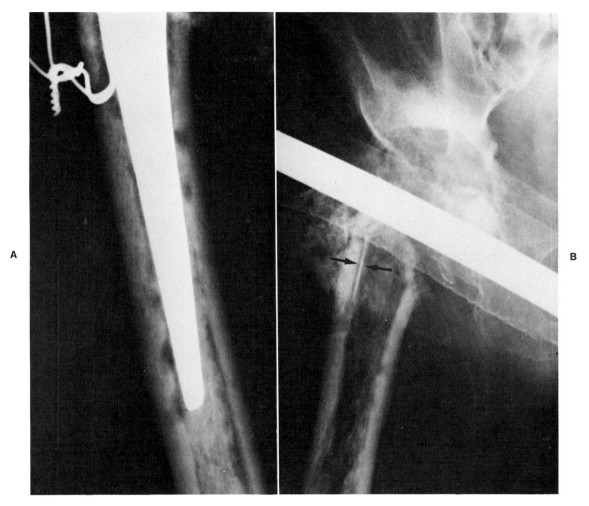

Fig. 16-18. A, "Punched-out" lesions of cortex at interface between cement and bone indicate mild osteosclerosis of outer cortex. Patient's pain and elevation of sedimentation rate developed 6 months following low-friction arthroplasty. Immediately during postoperative course hematoma had spontaneously evacuated into dressing and cultures from hematoma had grown staphylococcus coagulase-negative organisms but wound had healed uneventfully. **B,** Following Girdlestone pseudarthrosis patient is placed in balanced suspension traction. Good and detailed radiograph postoperatively is essential to assure that all cement and "dead bone" have been removed. Arrow shows flake of cement within lateral aspect of shaft (see text).

assume activities and range of motion early in the postoperative course. An attempt at fusion is not recommended after the removal of the total hip replacement. Fusion is obviously difficult to obtain, and under these conditions an older patient generally may not tolerate the lengthy and complicated postoperative course of the fusion procedure. Instead, it is extremely important to transfer cheerful confidence to the patient during rehabilitation. Patients are always worried that they may never walk again. It is important that they understand the mechanics of

the hip joint and how a pseudarthrosis can become functional. It is quite gratifying to see that a well-planned, well-executed program of resection pseudarthrosis may be functional indeed. A joint space is created some months after surgery and the patient may walk with only minor discomfort (Fig. 16-1).

POSTOPERATIVE ANTIBIOTICS FOLLOWING REMOVAL OF THE PROSTHESIS

Antibiotics must be based on bacterial sensitivity. Specific antibiotics should be determined

581

by tube dilution technique, and a broad-spectrum antibiotic should *never* be used in treating an infected total hip replacement. Newer broad-spectrum antibiotics must only be used when specific and time-tested antibiotics are not suitable for treatment. Antibiotics must be given in high doses to maximize the serum bactericidal level, which must be controlled throughout the treatment. At least 4 weeks of intravenous antibiotics must be instituted following removal of the artificial hip. Further antibiotic administration may be justified after 3 to 6 months following removal if the sedimentation rate is not within the normal range and if the wound shows evidence of suppuration.

OPPOSITE HIP REPLACEMENT FOLLOWING INFECTION

Experience indicates that the opposite hip may be operated on despite the presence of infection in the side requiring removal. It is necessary to provide the patient with one stable, pain-free hip because of the pseudarthrosis of the opposite side. A combination of a painful hip and a Girdlestone operation in one patient is extremely disabling. The patient's fear of the second hip becoming infected is a real one; however, based on the available statistics he should be encouraged to accept the second hip surgery. If other joints (such as the knees) are involved and surgery is necessary, it may be done as long as the infected hip wound is completely closed and there is no evidence of drainage from the hip area. In these complicated situations it would be better to have a second opinion (for the patient's psychological support and comfort) when the decision is reached to proceed with the second hip surgery. In Charnley's cases, 11 out of 14 infected hips had been converted to a pseudarthrosis by the time the opposite side was operated on.[5] However, three patients were operated on the second side while an infected arthroplasty was still present. In all 14 examples the dictum of performing the operation on the opposite hip with a history of infection on the other side was supported by the fact that none of the operations on the second side became infected. This problem, of course, is much more than a question of scientific interest—since most of these patients are seriously disabled in view of a Girdlestone pseudarthrosis and a painful hip for which treatment must be rendered. This also casts doubt on the possibility of generally lowered resistance of patients to a hematogenous source of infection that might cause infection in the second hip as well. It further exonerates bloodborne infection as a cause of deep infection, which has so often been suggested. In three hips in which a total hip replacement was performed with infection present in the other hip (but with the implants in place), the patient responded to rehabilitation well after the second operation prior to converting the first hip to a pseudarthrosis. This has been a helpful situation because rehabilitation on the side with the new implant was accomplished before the artificial joint was removed from the infected hip.[5] (See Chapter 8.)

Heterotopic ossification following total hip arthroplasty

Although bone formation following hip surgery has long been recognized as a complication, its cause remains unknown. Appearance of myositis ossificans following cup arthroplasty or other surgical intervention has been reported in the past. The role of this complication in reducing range of motion (thus failure of total hip arthroplasty) does not appear to be as serious a problem as in cup arthroplasty.

Obviously the main concern with regard to this complication is its limiting effect on the range of motion produced as a result of heterotopic ossification following total hip arthroplasty. This is especially significant in bilateral arthroplasties because generally both hips are subjected to this complication. While insignificant in most cases, it can become a great handicap where the principal aim of surgery is to promote mobility. This is particularly true in cases of bilateral degenerative osteoarthritis requiring correction to increase mobility. It is further disturbing to recognize a systemic cause for heterotopic bone formation, which, in most instances, leads to a similar consequence following surgery of the second hip. Surgical experience indicates that removal of heterotopic bone is often complicated by a high rate of recurrence following its removal. Our limited experience suggests that heterotopic ossification following total hip replacement may be successfully removed, a procedure that is helpful in some selected cases.

582

The role of diphosphonates and irradiation is under clinical investigation. Early reports and experiences with the use of both reveal their modest usefulness in prevention of this complication.

ETIOLOGY

The many causes listed in the etiology of myositis ossificans include metaplasia of primitive connective tissue, migrating bone marrow cells, interstitial hemorrhage and muscle necrosis, trauma to the soft tissue or periosteal lesions, presence of bone dust, motion between the implant and bone, and last but not least, infection. But the true cause of heterotopic ossification following surgery remains unknown; consequently, no method to prevent this condition has evolved. However, from a clinical standpoint and our own observations there seems to be a definite possibility of undetected low-grade inflammatory process, especially in bilateral operations with unilateral bone formation. It may also be concluded that patients with peripheral nerve or cord injury (especially sciatic nerve palsy and traumatic fracture dislocations about the hip) are particularly predisposed to bone formation. If a patient has formed bone following surgery of one hip, it is highly likely that bone will form on the second side postoperatively. We have also observed that stiffness may result from diminished "clearance" between the upper femur and the acetabulum as the result of excessive deepening of the socket or unremoved peripheral osteophytes and bridging of the hip joint by new bone formation. However, our experiences suggest that immobilization following surgery does not promote or prevent formation of heterotopic bone. In general, formation of bone occurs within the first year after total hip arthroplasty, and it appears that the bone is completely matured and bone formation ceases by the end of the first year. In over 90% the first radiological sign of heterotopic ossification may become evident within the first 3 months—and in 10%, within the first 6 months. Most early evidence of radiological changes may first appear within 6 weeks or slightly thereafter. By 6 months the major portion of heterotopic bone is clearly evident on radiographs—pain is the prodromal symptom and usually may precede the x-ray changes.

A preponderance of male patients forming heterotopic bone has been noted by Lazansky, Delee, and associates, and in our own series.[*] The condition appears to involve stiffer hips and those with pronounced marginal osteophyte formation, particularly in heavy, bony male patients. There appears to be no recurrence of an osteophyte per se following removal at surgery; however, these individuals are more prone to form bone than other groups of patients. In our experiences there have been no female patients under 65 years of age forming severe heterotopic bone. This may suggest a hormonal basis for the prevention of bone formation following surgery. It is of special interest that patients who have had previous hip surgery are not particularly prone to forming heterotopic bone; nevertheless, those patients who had formed bone following their previous operation are likely to form heterotopic bone following the total hip arthroplasty. We have concluded that if a patient has developed heterotopic bone following one total hip arthroplasty, there is a better than 90% chance that heterotopic bone will develop on the second side. Although exceptions are also observed (Fig. 16-20) in bilateral total hip arthroplasty, there appears to be no correlation between bone formation in the second hip and the interval between the two operations. We have encountered individuals who have had an interval of 4 or 5 years between surgeries, and the second hip operation had an identical outcome with regard to bone formation. This *phenomenon* suggests, perhaps, that a systemic factor may play a role in the development of heterotopic bone.[24] When heterotopic bone is formed unilaterally in a patient with bilateral hip surgery, infection should be considered as a contributing factor. When the result of total hip arthroplasty is defective and the patient has pain, loosening of the components should also be considered as an etiological factor as well as low-grade infection. In our experience, removal of an osteophyte has not necessarily provoked bone formation about the hip; in fact, there is greater proclivity toward bone formation about the hip when the osteophytes are left alone, since there is less clearance between the proximal femur and acetabular margin. It has been suggested that nonunion of the greater trochanter or routine osteotomy of the greater trochanter has contributed to a

---

[*]See references 13, 17, and 32.

greater number of patients developing heterotopic ossification following total hip arthroplasty.[33] But the fact that capsulectomy performed in operations without removal of the trochanter prevents heterotopic ossification has not been clinically proved. We have not encountered a greater, or significant, formation of bone following trochanteric osteotomy, nor have we been able to relate the higher incidence of heterotopic ossification to the removal of the greater trochanter than those with uneventful healing of the trochanter. It is of considerable interest to note that patients developing the greatest amount of heterotopic ossification are among those patients who have had the greatest restriction of range of motion preoperatively.

The type of original disease does not appear to relate to the formation of heterotopic bone,[13] nor does there seem to be any correlation between patients receiving steroid therapy before or after total hip arthroplasty. There is no correlation between the patient's activities and formation of bone. In our experience the first evidence of heterotopic ossification was noted at about 3 months following surgery, and in a much smaller number of patients it was first seen 6 months after surgery. In most cases the mass of heterotopic bone was fully matured at about 6 months (as evidenced by radiodensity). We have not encountered heterotopic ossification after 1 year following total hip arthroplasty. We agree with Delee and his associates that osteoarthritic patients are the most likely to form heterotopic bone. In their studies, patients with congenital dislocation or subluxation constituted the second most likely group, and patients with rheumatoid arthritis constituted the third. Ankylosing spondylitis formed bone only in a small percentage of the cases.[13]

INCIDENCE

The amount of bone formation reported by different series, manifested by serial radiography, varies from 3% to 30%.[13,27,31,33,34] This, of course, is contingent on the degree of search and the method of classification of those reports (Table 16-7). Traces of minor bone islands may be found in postsurgical radiographs of many patients, which could substantially increase the incidence. However, these bony islands are clinically insignificant and only a small percentage actually restrict range of motion[6,7,23,25] following total hip arthroplasty (Fig. 16-19).

Table 16-7. Incidence of heterotopic ossification

Source	No. of cases	Incidence (%)	Type of operation
Wilson et al.[41]	100	30	McKee-Farrar
Lazansky[25]	501	8.1	LFA
Brooker et al.[2]	100	21	Müller type
Parker et al.[33]	100	12	With trochanteric osteotomy
Parker et al.[33]	100	5	Without trochanteric osteotomy
Eftekhar et al.[17]	800	10	LFA
DeLee et al.[13]	2,173	14.6	LFA

Brooker and associates,[2] in an evaluation of 100 consecutive patients treated by total hip arthroplasty, found a 21% incidence of heterotopic ossification (Table 16-7). The degree of ossification was classified as follows: class 1, islands of bone within the soft tissue about the hip; class 2, bone spurs from the pelvis or proximal end of the femur leaving at least 1 cm. between opposing bone surfaces; class 3, bone spurs from the pelvis or proximal end of the femur reducing the space between opposing bone surfaces to less than 1 cm.; class 4, apparent bony ankylosis as the result of heterotopic ossification. There were seven patients in class 1, five in class 2, seven in class 3, and two in class 4. It is of interest that although most of the patients did not have a trochanteric osteotomy for total hip arthroplasty, a high rate of heterotopic ossification nevertheless was observed in this series.

In the study of complications in our own series,[17] and in comparison with conventional techniques such as mold arthroplasty or Moore self-locking prosthesis, there seems to be a similar incidence of heterotopic bone formation. However, the restricting effects characteristic of heterotopic ossification following total hip arthroplasty have been less significant than in other types of arthroplasty. With our series, the stiffer the hip preoperatively, the more likelihood that it would become stiff from heterotopic bone formation following surgery. Approximately 10% of our hip arthroplasties developed a significant amount of bone as noted on radiographs (Table 16-7). Of these, 2% had significant reduction in their range of motion and, similar to other experiences of heterotopic ossification, it occurred more commonly in men than in women (ratio of 3 to 1). We also observed on radiographs

Text continued on p. 590.

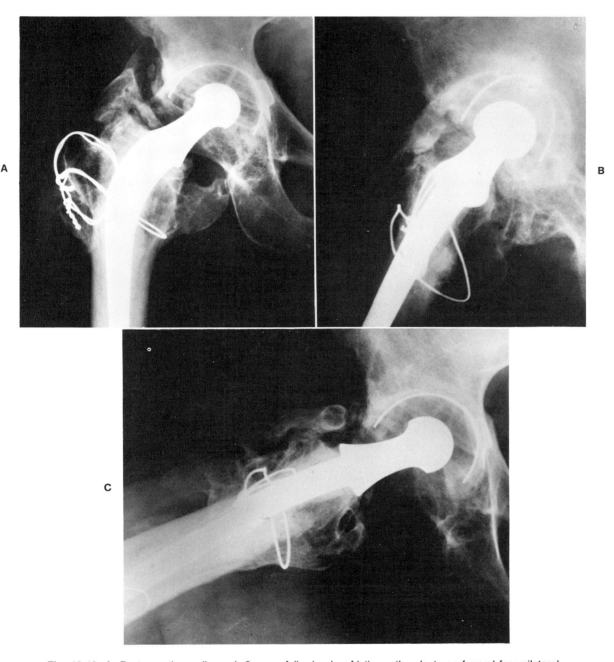

Fig. 16-19. A, Postoperative radiograph 2 years following low-friction arthroplasty performed for unilateral degenerative osteoarthrosis of hip in 64-year-old female. NOTE: extent of bone formation in area of abductors and on medial aspect along insertion of iliopsoas tendon. Hip grading is A-6,6,6, despite heterotopic bone formation. **B,** Hip is flexed to 90 degrees of flexion and 20 degrees of abduction. Anteroposterior radiograph was taken in conventional manner. **C,** Hip abducted to approximately 45 degrees and again anteroposterior view is obtained. This case illustrates clearly that despite heterotopic bone formation good range of motion of hip may persist. Bone has formed in areas that do not cause impingement.

585

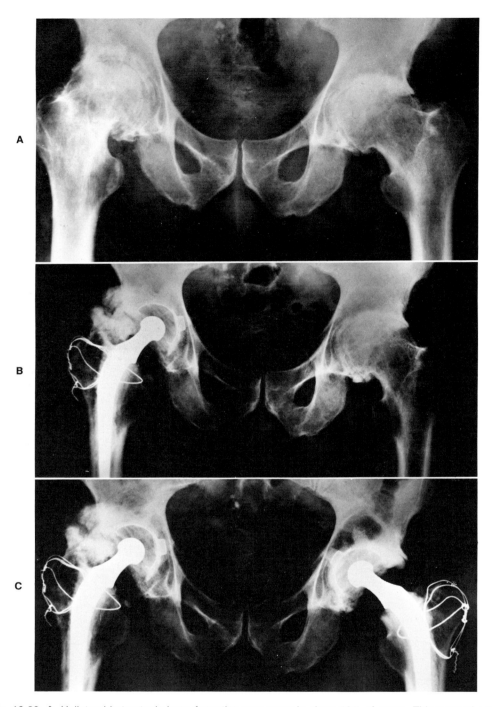

Fig. 16-20. A, Unilateral heterotopic bone formation may occur in about 10% of cases. This unusual complication (unilateral extensive heterotopic bone formation) is illustrated in this 73-year-old man with bilateral hyperproductive degenerative osteoarthrosis. Right hip was ankylosed in 30 degrees of external rotation, 20 degrees of flexion, and 5 degrees of adduction. **B,** Following surgery, right hip developed extensive ectopic bone, by 1 year bridging across hip joint leading to complete ankylosis but hip ankylosed in neutral rotation no more than 10 degrees of flexion and neutral abduction-adduction. Although discouraged by this complication, patient's grading of hip was 6,3,1. At patient's request left hip was operated on 2 years later. **C,** Radiograph 5 years following surgery on right and 3 years on left. No heterotopic bone formation was observed up to 3 years of follow-up on left side. Patient's grading of hips is B-right, 6,5,1; left, 6,5,4.

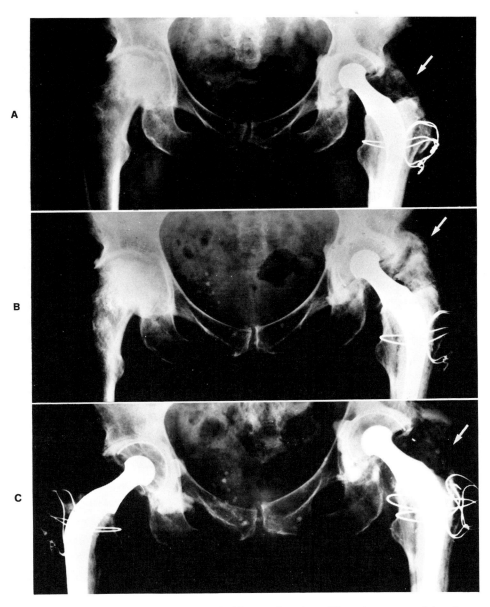

Fig. 16-21. Resection of heterotopic bone is worthwhile exercise when stiffness is severe or deformity present. Fifty-five-year-old female with bilateral avascular necrosis of femoral head owing to alcohol abuse required surgical intervention. **A,** Three month postoperative radiograph of left hip indicating appearance of heterotopic bone (arrow) in region of abductors and superior capsular region. **B,** At 18 months bone has bridged across completely (arrow) and hip is completely ankylosed. **C,** Right hip was operated on because of pain and within 2 weeks left hip was revised. Two years following surgery of left hip only traces of bone have formed (arrow). Patient is pleased with results. Grading of hip is as follows: B, right- 6,6,6; left- 5,6,5. Patient did not receive either EHDP or irradiation prior to or after surgery as adjunctive measure to surgical resection of bone.

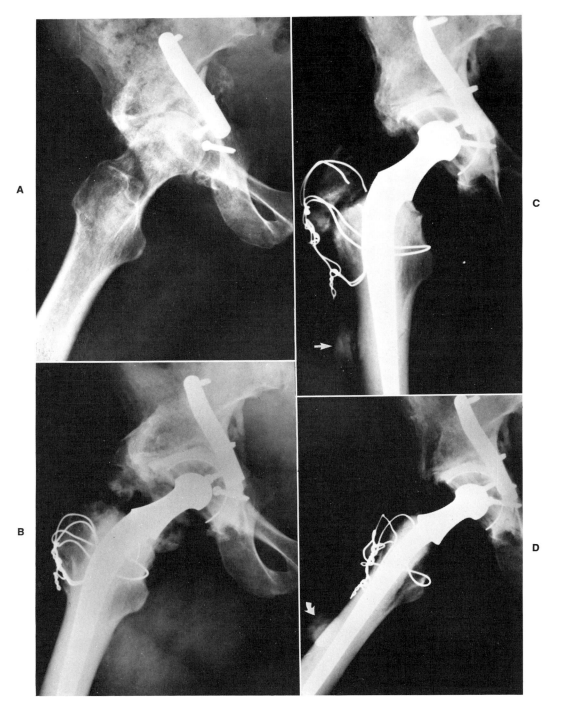

Fig. 16-22. A, Fifty-one-year-old female sustained severe fracture dislocation of right hip, following which open reduction had been performed. She had also sustained complete right sciatic nerve palsy. Hip was fixed in abduction position 1 year following surgery, grade, C-4,3,1. **B,** Following low-friction arthroplasty. NOTE: bone formation on medial and superior portion of hip joint. At 1 year following surgery hip assumed position of abduction and flexion with unsightly gait and marked stiffness. There was only jog of motion present in hip. **C,** Two years following resection of heterotopic bone and revision of low-friction arthroplasty. Only femoral component was exchanged. Wires are fractured and greater trochanter developed fibrous union but remained asymptomatic. NOTE: cement extrusion at junction of lower third and distal third of prosthesis through "vent hole" made to allow new cement to reach this point (arrow). **D,** Lateral view of same hip shows absence of bone formation in hip area 2 years following surgery. Preoperative grading of hip prior to revision was 5,2,1. Postoperative improvement following resection of heterotopic bone was 5,4,4. Patient remained somewhat restricted because of other injuries including ankle and spine. This patient received EHDP pre-operatively and for 1 year following surgery. **C** and **D** were taken 1 year following cessation of EHDP.

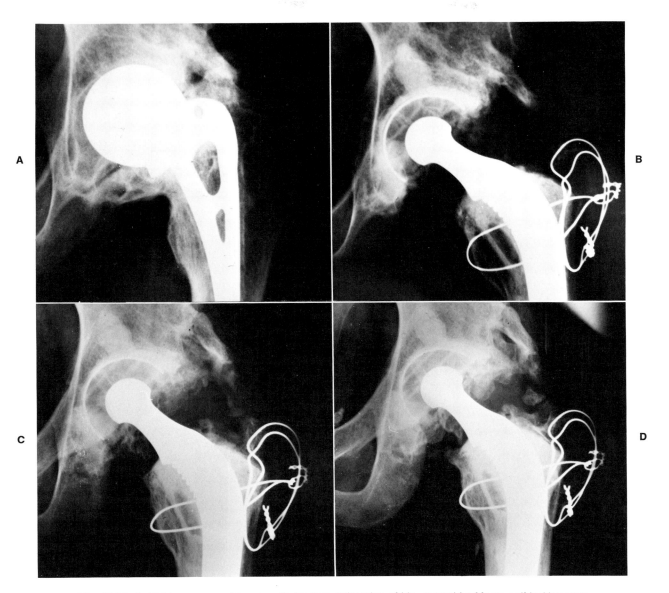

Fig. 16-23. A, Thirty-one-year-old male with fracture dislocation of hip, treated by Moore self-locking prosthesis following which severe ectopic bone formed encapsulating prosthesis. Patient literally had osseous union of upper femur to pelvis. Grading of hip prior to surgery was A-6,3,1 postoperatively is 6,5,6. Indication for surgery was progressive pain in knee, which caused patient to be unable to work. **B,** Radiograph 6 months following surgery by revision. **C,** Radiograph of hip at 12 months following surgery. **D,** Radiograph 2 years following surgery. NOTE: moderate amount of bone is formed but patient's flexion is to 90 degrees, abduction to 40 degrees, and adduction to 30 degrees, with 10 degrees of external and 10 degrees of internal rotation. Patient demonstrates no limp. This patient was on double-blind study and received EHDP (see text).

that those patients who had extra-articular ossification demonstrating hypertrophic osteoarthritis prior to surgery were prone to formation of bone postoperatively. As stated before, we also conclude that the type of prosthesis and the type of surgical approach (with or without trochanteric osteotomy) had no correlation with the amount of bone formed following total hip arthroplasty. We had, for example, observed several cases of arthroplasty utilizing a Müller prosthesis without removal of the trochanter inserted on one side and a Charnley prosthesis with removal of the trochanter on the opposite side without any significant difference in the amount of bone formation or the range of motion. There was no difference in the incidence of bone formation after instituting copious irrigation of the wound to remove bone dust at surgery. The presence of bone dust has been suggested by some surgeons as being an etiological factor in the formation of heterotopic bone. Approximately 10% of patients with bilateral hip arthroplasties have formed bone only on one side. To date, we have not been able to document evidence that infection is a causative agent in the formation of bone in these patients (Fig. 16-20). However, if a patient with a bilateral total hip replacement develops heterotopic bone in one hip, he has better than a 90% chance to develop it in the opposite hip as well.

PREVENTION AND MANAGEMENT OF HETEROTOPIC OSSIFICATION FOLLOWING TOTAL HIP ARTHROPLASTY

An attempt has been made to prevent heterotopic ossification following total hip arthroplasty by the administration of EHDP.* Because the incidence of significant heterotopic bone formation in limiting the range of motion is relatively low, and because the beneficial effects of EHDP are still under controlled clinical studies, routine administration of these drugs to prevent heterotopic ossification does not seem advisable.

Recent studies have hinted that there may be beneficial effects from the use of EHDP, both in reducing the incidence and the severity (extent) of this complication.[18] Coventry[10] and associates found that irradiation of 2,000 rads in the course of 10 treatments starting early in the

postoperative course decreased the formation of ectopic bone. It is true, however, that when bilateral hip disease is present and the patient has already developed heterotopic ossification following one arthroplasty, administration of these agents might be of help in preventing heterotopic ossification on the opposite side.

Resection of heterotopic bone following surgery has been discouraged in the past because of a high incidence of recurrence. In a recent collaborative study of surgical removal of heterotopic bone, we found relief from ankylosis and gain in mobility have been impressive. While it is too early to judge the effect of EHDP used in conjunction with the removal of heterotopic bone, clinical results and radiological findings are encouraging* (Figs. 16-21 to 16-23). Recommending surgical removal of heterotopic bone in bilateral hip disease where arthroplasty has been complicated by excessive bone formation and complete ankylosis of the hip seems to be justified. We have elected to remove the greater trochanter and femoral components for free access to the front and the back of the hip joint as well as into the superior capsular region and abductor region where most often a large amount of bone is present, and its removal is difficult without osteotomy of the greater trochanter (see Chapter 14).

SUMMARY OF ESSENTIALS

- Early experiences with total hip replacements suggested a high incidence of infection following this procedure. However, awareness and prophylactic measures against infection appear to have reduced the rate of infection, and in most centers the incidence is approximately 1% early and no more than 3% late.
- Second only to fatal pulmonary embolism, infection following total hip replacement is the most serious complication of this operation because of the difficulty in treating this condition successfully in addition to the cost and misery to the patient.
- Diagnosis of infection based on the mode of clinical appearance is either early or late. The early infection appears as an acute abscess, a leaking hematoma leading to infection, a deep hematoma (without breakage of skin), or a defective skin healing leading to infection. A late infection, on the other

---

*Ethane hydroxy diphosphonate (etidronate disodium [generic name], Didronel [trade name]).

*Under present protocol 20 mg./kg. EHDP is given 4 weeks prior to surgery and 10 mg./kg. for 52 weeks after surgery. Generous support of Procter & Gamble Co. is acknowledged for conducting this study.

hand, is usually the result of perfect healing of the wound but a delayed appearance of a sinus or an abscess several months or years following surgery. Late infections (appearing after 1 year) constitute between 40% to 50% of all infections. "Late late" infection sporadically seen after several years of surgery may be attributed to the focus of infection elsewhere in the body and seeding of the organism via the bloodstream.

- With the continuance of late-appearing infections the true incidence is not possible. As a working rule, 40% of infections appear within 3 months after operation and 60% of all infections within 18 months following surgery, with additional appearance of isolated cases up to several years following surgery.

- A differential diagnosis of deep infection must be made with superficial infection, mechanical loosening of the prosthesis, a deep-seated hematoma, or a ruptured fascia. The most significant laboratory data in making a diagnosis of infection is a persistently elevated sedimentation rate, which is present within three fourths of the patients with deep wound infection following total hip arthroplasty. Only when infection is established and of long duration are radiological changes typical.

- Aspiration of the joint, Gram's stain, and cultures may not be of value (when negative), especially if the patient has received antibiotics postoperatively or the organism is of low virulence. Arthrograms are of no value in diagnosing the presence or absence of infection. However, they may be of assistance in determining the extent of soft tissue involvement.

- In addition to a Gram's stain, the cellular morphology of the aspirated joint or bone is of great assistance in identifying the presence of infection based on the type and frequency of inflammatory cells in the fluid.

- The most prevalent organism in infected total hip replacements is *Staphylococcus aureus*, comprising approximately one half of the infections in most series.

- It should be recognized that the diagnosis of infection is a combined clinical, radiological, and bacteriological endeavor and that a negative culture from the hip would not necessarily by itself rule out the infection.

- Treatment must be separately considered for acute, low-grade infection, without and with chronic osteitis. The principal treatment of acute infection is incision and drainage of the abscess, complete débridement, and removal of devitalized tissue, accompanied by copious irrigation of the wound. A primary closure of the wound utilizing a suction-irrigation system or packing of the wound is done based on the nature of the organism and the status of the wound.

- Low-grade infection without osteitis may be considered for reimplantation of a total hip prosthesis. The issue, which is controversial at the present time, is considered experimental until more experience becomes available. The operation may be staged, including treatment of infection in the first stage and definitive replacement as the second stage. The treatment must be carefully planned and coupled with intensive antibiotic therapy. The role of antibiotic-impregnated cement in treating bone infection awaits clinical studies.

- Chronic infections with osteitis are best treated by removal of the prosthesis and cement, converting the hip to a pseudarthrosis.

- In performing a pseudarthrosis following an infected total hip replacement, patients must be psychologically prepared and physically strengthened to undergo a major procedure, including a lengthy rehabilitation. All the foreign material as well as necrotic bone must be removed. The patient is placed in skeletal traction for 6 weeks, followed by a gradual weight-bearing program.

- The treatment of the wound following a resection pseudarthrosis is based on the nature of the wound and the offending organism. Gram-negative organisms are treated by packing the wound, and gram-positive organisms are treated by primary closure with suction.

- The surgical technique to remove an artificial hip joint is demanding, and the magnitude of surgery is considerably greater than insertion of a total hip prosthesis. The surgical technique should be directed toward removal of all of the cement as well as necrotic debris from the acetabulum, femur, and soft tissue. An intensive program of antibiotic treatment is essential in most instances.

- The opposite hip, if it requires replacement, may be considered for replacement. Experiences suggest that if a low-grade infection is recognized and removal of the total hip prosthesis is contemplated, the opposite hip must be seriously considered for surgery because of the disabling nature of the pseudarthrosis and opposite hip involvement.

- Heterotopic ossification is a recognized complication of all hip surgery, including total hip arthroplasty. This complication occurs in approximately 10% of hips following total hip arthroplasty. Of these, 2% to 3% are severe enough to cause restriction of motion and/or ankylosis of the hip.

- The true cause of heterotopic ossification following total hip arthroplasty remains unknown; however, heterotopic bone formation occurs nearly three times as often in males as in females. The heavy, bony-skeletal male with large marginal osteophytes and marked stiffness preoperatively is particularly prone to postoperative formation of heterotopic bone.

- Osteoarthritis seems to be more complicated by

591

this condition than rheumatoid arthritis. However, the more limited the range of motion preoperatively, the more severe the degree of bone formation postoperatively, thus there is a more limited range of motion postoperatively.

■ Since there appears to be a systemic factor that plays an important role in the formation of heterotopic bone, it may be concluded that 90% or more of the patients developing heterotopic bone in one arthroplasty will develop a similar complication on the opposite side. While removal of osteophytes or the greater trochanter during total hip arthroplasty does not promote heterotopic bone formation, formation of heterotopic bone as a coincidental finding following infection is a documented fact.

■ When extreme stiffness is present following bilateral total hip arthroplasty, resection of heterotopic bone is justifiable. It is also indicated if a unilateral total hip arthroplasty is complicated by heterotopic ossification in addition to severe flexion and adduction deformity.

REFERENCES

1. Beeson, P. B.: Bacterial endocarditis. In Beeson, P. B., and McDermott, W., editors: Cecil-Loeb textbook of medicine, ed. 13, Philadelphia, 1971, W. B. Saunders Co., pp. 1098-1106.
2. Brooker, A. F., Bowerman, J. W., Robinson, R. A., and Riley, L. H.: Ectopic ossification following total hip replacement, J. Bone Joint Surg. **55A**(8): 1629-1632, 1973.
3. Buchholz, H. W., and Gartmann, H. D.: Infektions prophylaxe and operative Behandling der schleichenden tiefen Infektion bei der totalen Endoprothese, Chirurg **43**:446-453, 1972.
4. Buchholz, H. W., and Siefel, A.: Erfahrungen mit refobacin palacos in der prosthesenchirurgi, Acta Traumatol. **3**:233, 1973.
5. Charnley, J.: Total hip replacement following infection in the opposite hip. Internal publication No. 48, Centre for Hip Surgery, Wrightington Hospital, England, 1974.
6. Charnley, J.: Total hip replacement by low-friction arthroplasty, Clin. Orthop. **72**:7-21, 1970.
7. Charnley, J.: The long-term results of low-friction arthroplasty of the hip performed as primary intervention, J. Bone Joint Surg. **54B**:61-76, 1972.
8. Charnley, J.: Postoperative infection after total hip replacement with special reference to air contamination in the operating room, Clin. Orthop. **87**:167-187, 1972.
9. Charnley, J., and Eftekhar, N.: Postoperative infection in total prosthetic replacement arthroplasty of the hip joint, Br. J. Surg. **56**(9):641-649, 1969.
10. Coventry, M. B.: Personal communications.
11. Cruess, R. L., Bickel, W. S., and VonKessler, K.

L. C.: Infections in total hips secondary to a primary source elsewhere, Clin. Orthop. **106**:99-101, 1975.
12. D'Ambrosia, R. D., Shoji, H., and Heater, R.: Secondarily infected total joint replacements by hematogenous spread, J. Bone Joint Surg. **58A**: 450-453, 1976.
13. DeLee, J., Ferrari, A., and Charnley, J.: Ectopic bone formation following low friction arthroplasty of the hip. Internal Publication No. 59, Wrightington Hospital, England, November, 1975.
14. Dismukes, W. E., Karchmer, A. W., Buckley, M. J., Austen, W. G., and Swartz, M. N.: Prosthetic valve endocarditis: analysis of 38 cases, Circulation **48**:365-377, 1973.
15. Dupont, J. A., and Charnley, J.: Low-friction arthroplasty of the hip for the failures of previous operations, J. Bone Joint Surg. **54B**:77-87, 1972.
16. Dupont, J. A., and Lumsden, R. M.: Significance of operative cultures in total joint replacements, J. Bone Joint Surg. **57A**:138, 1975.
17. Eftekhar, N. S., Kiernan, H. A., and Stinchfield, F. E.: Systemic and local complications following low-friction arthroplasty of the hip joint, Arch. Surg. **111**:150-155, 1976.
18. Finerman, G. A. M., Krengel, W. F., Jr., Lowell, J. D., Murray, W. R., Volz, R. G., Gold, R. H., and Bowerman, J.: The role and use of diphosphonate (EHDP) in prevention of heterotopic ossification following total hip arthroplasty, Orthop. Trans. **1**(1):69-70, 1977.
19. Fitzgerald, R. H., Jr., Washington, J. A., II, Coventry, M. B., and Peterson, L. F. A.: Contamination of the surgical wound in the operating room, J. Bone Joint Surg. **56A**:849, 1974.
20. Fitzgerald, R. H., Jr., Peterson, L. F. A., Washington, J. A. II, Von Scoy, R. E., and Coventry, M. D.: Bacterial colonization of wound and sepsis in total hip arthroplasty, J. Bone Joint Surg. **55A**:1242-1250, 1973.
21. Forsgren, A., and Forsum, U.: Agglutination of *Staphylococcus aureus* by sera, Infect. Immun. **5**:524-530, 1972.
22. Forsgren, A., Nordstrom, K., Philipson, L., et al.: Protein A mutants of *Staphylococcus aureus,* J. Bacteriol. **107**:245-250, 1971.
23. Harris, W. H.: Clinical results using Müller-Charnley total hip prosthesis, Clin. Orthop. **86**: 95-101, 1972.
24. Jowsey, J., and Coventry, M. B.: Heterotopic ossification: theoretical consideration, possible etiologic factors and a clinical review of total hip arthroplasty patients exhibiting this phenomenon, Orthop. Trans. **1**(1):69, 1977.
25. Lazansky, M. G.: Complications revisited: the debit side of total hip replacement, Clin. Orthop. **95**:96-103, 1973.
26. Lerner, P. I., and Weinstein, L.: Infective en-

docarditis in the antibiotic era, N. Engl. J. Med. **274:**323-331; 388-393, 1966.

27. McKee, G., and Chen, S.: The statistics of Mc-Kee-Farrar method of total hip replacement, Clin. Orthop. **95:**26-33, 1973.

28. Mitchell, R. C.: Classification of *Staphylococcus albus* strains isolated from the urinary tract, J. Clin. Pathol. **21:**93-96, 1968.

29. Murray, W. R.: Results in patients with total hip replacement arthroplasty, Clin. Orthop. **95:**80-90, 1973.

30. Nelson, P. J.: Personal communications.

31. Nollen, A. J., and Slooff, T. J.: Para-articular ossifications after total hip replacement, Acta. Orthop. Scand. **44:**230-241, 1973.

32. Owen, R.: The Charnley arthroplasty. In Jayson, M., editor: total hip replacement, Philadelphia, 1971, J. B. Lippincott, pp. 68-85.

33. Parker, H. G., Wiesman, H. S., Edward, F. C., Thomas, W. H., and Sledge, C. B.: Comparison of immediate and late results of total hip replacement with and without trochanteric osteotomy (Proceedings), J. Bone Joint Surg. **56A:**1537, 1974.

34. Patterson, F. P., and Brown, C. S.: The McKee-Farrar total hip replacement, J. Bone Joint Surg. **54A:**257-275, 1972.

35. Perrin, J. C. S., and McLaurin, R. L.: Infected ventriculoatrial shunts: a method of treatment, J. Neurosurg. **27:**21-26, 1976.

36. Salvati, E. A., and Wilson, P. D., Jr.: Long-term results of femoral-head replacement, J. Bone Joint Surg. **55A:**516-524, 1973.

37. Salvati, E. A., Freiberger, R. H., and Wilson, P. D.: Arthrography for complications of total hip replacement, a review of thirty-one arthrograms, J. Bone Joint Surg. **53A:**701-709, 1971.

38. Tietjen, R., Stinchfield, F. E., and Michelsen, C.: The significance of intracapsular cultures in total hip operations, Surg. Gynecol. Obstet. **144:**699-702, 1977.

39. Wilson, P. D., Jr., Aglietti, P., and Salvati, E. A.: Subacute sepsis of the hip treated by antibiotics and cemented prosthesis, J. Bone Joint Surg. **56A:**879-989, 1974.

40. Wilson, P. D., Salvati, E. A., Aglietti, P., and Kutner, L. J.: The problem of infection in endoprosthetic surgery of the hip joint, Clin. Orthop. **96:**213-221, 1973.

41. Wilson, P. D., Jr., Amstutz, H. C., Czerniecki, A., Salvati, E. A., and Mendes, D. G.: Total hip replacement with fixation by acrylic cement, J. Bone Joint Surg. **54A:**207-236, 1972.

42. Wilson, T. S., and Stuart, R. D.: *Staphylococcus albus* in wound infections and in septicemia, Can. Med. Assoc. J. **93:**8-16, 1965.

CHAPTER 17

Technical complications

The responsibilities of those performing this type of surgery are immense, and nobody is encouraged to adopt this technique without very careful training in the new technologies involved.

SIR JOHN CHARNLEY

No one is encouraged to perform this type of operation unless he is prepared and willing to treat his complications when they arise.

FRANK E. STINCHFIELD

Some major technical complications are discussed in earlier chapters: (1) loss of fixation (see Chapter 3); (2) failure of prosthesis and cement (see Chapters 3 and 4); and (3) infection, heterotopic ossification, and hematoma (see Chapter 16).

In this chapter the following complications will be discussed: dislocation and instability, fracture of the femur complicating total hip replacement, trochanteric complications, and other technical complications.

DISLOCATION AND INSTABILITY

Dislocation following total hip replacement is a complication that is usually related to surgical technique. Without attention to the technical details that will ensure a "stable" hip at surgery, this complication may seriously jeopardize the outcome of the surgery. A longer hospital stay, traction, cast immobilization, or reoperation are often required to rectify this situation, the sum of which may carry added morbidity for the patient.

Some reports in the recent literature suggest a direct but inverse relationship between the size of the femoral head component of the total hip prosthesis and the rate of dislocation following anthroplasty of the hip.* On that basis, it has been suggested that a 22-mm. head prosthesis of the Charnley type is more prone to instability and dislocation than a prosthesis with a larger, that is, 32-mm. diameter head (such as the Mül-

ler modification of the Charnley prosthesis). Indeed, some authors have actually referred to the 22-mm. prosthetic head as an "inherently unstable prosthesis." Also, it has been suggested that a small head makes critical alignment of the components imperative; thus there would be less allowance for error at the time of surgery with a smaller head.[2,53] Development of the so-called second generation of total hip replacements as well as the introduction of single-unit prostheses is aimed at "improved stability" of the hip by increasing the diameter of the head and increasing the ball-neck diameter ratio.[30,31] Preferentially, an anterior approach without removal of the greater trochanter has also been recommended by some surgeons to avoid dislocation and to enhance the stability of the hip joint.[27,28,43,44]

Terminology

Dislocation is defined as displacement of the head of the femoral prosthesis out of the prosthetic socket and completely out of the bony acetabulum. Terms such as "anterior," "posterior," "superior," and "inferior" are applied to designate the direction of the prosthetic femoral component in relation to the bony acetabulum. Arbitrarily, dislocations occurring during the first 3 weeks following surgery (while the patient, usually, is in the hospital) are considered "immediate"; between 3 weeks and 3 months they are considered "early"; and after 3 months postoperatively, they are considered "late." "Traumatic

---

*See references 1, 2, 27, 28, 30, 41, 44, and 53.

594

dislocation" is referred to as dislocation following a severe trauma or a severe fall. "Static subluxation" is defined as displacement of the head of the femoral prosthesis out of the acetabular socket but still in some contact with the rim and completely confined within the bony socket (this is best illustrated by interposition of a fragment of cement or soft tissue between the two components of the prosthesis). Subluxation may be "functional" or "dynamic" and only felt by the patient as a palpable or audible click in certain ranges in motion of the hip or seen in radiographs—as evidenced by an increased distance between the femoral head component of the prosthesis and the socket, which may be related to a lack of tissue tension or severe scarring. The term "operative instability" is applied when prior to reattachment of the greater trochanter, the femoral prosthesis can be pulled more than 1 cm. out of the socket by longitudinal traction. In such cases the hip usually dislocates during "rehearsal" for stability by flexion, adduction, with or without internal or external rotation.

Experiences with instability and dislocation

A special review, with the aim of identifying the incidence and the scope of this problem, was undertaken.[21] Between April 1969 and April 1975, 1,550 total hip replacements were performed at The New York Orthopaedic Hospital. The first 1,400 consecutive low-friction arthroplasty procedures were performed using exclusively the Charnley technique and prosthesis. The operative proforma provided a space for degrees of instability of the hip as tested at surgery as well as the quality of trochanteric fixation prior to wound closure. An anteroposterior radiograph of the hip taken in the operating room or in the recovery room was seen routinely by the surgical team prior to discharge of the patient from the recovery room (see Chapters 9 and 11).

All operations were performed under general anesthesia, and the greater trochanter was routinely osteotomized. Most of the patients without previous surgery were allowed out of bed and permitted full weight bearing on the sixth or seventh postoperative day. Only those with excessive osteoporosis, those who underwent revision of previous surgery, depending upon the quality of the trochanteric fixation, or patients who developed a complication were retained in bed until the fourteenth to twenty-first postoperative day. Fifteen patients were placed in a hip spica

plaster cast immediately following surgery—either for intraoperative fractures of the femur or inadequate fixation of the trochanter; 12 additional patients were treated similarly because of instability encountered at the time of operation. Postoperatively, the hips were maintained in abduction by a special abduction splint,[20] and, in addition to immediate postoperative radiographs, all hips were radiographed at 1 week and 12 days postoperatively. Only nine patients were treated with balanced suspension apparatus to maintain the position of abduction postoperatively. Surgical technique was uniformly adopted from Charnley—using a straight lateral approach to the hip with routine detachment of the greater trochanter and the utilization of a 22-mm. Charnley prosthesis. Only in the last 650 hips included in this series was the acetabular cup with a posterior extended wall used (when necessary, a small Charnley cup or a straight-stem femoral prosthesis was used).

Eight dislocations and three cases of severe instability were recognized (eight in 1,400 operations; incidence 0.5%). All dislocations were posterior. Three of the eight dislocations were traumatic and caused by severe automobile accidents in two patients, and a severe fall in the other. There were two "immediate," three "early," and three "late" dislocations. Four subluxations were also recognized (0.25%) by radiograph. The rate of functional subluxation was approximately 2% in the first 700 hips included (only the first 700 cases were studied for subluxation). Because the detailed case histories reflect the pathomechanics of dislocation in total hip arthroplasty, most of the representative case histories are presented. Table 17-1 presents the details of the entire series, demonstrating that in most cases more than one factor contributes to dislocation.

CASE 1. W. S., a 64-year-old white male, was admitted in December 1971 with an 18-year history of left hip pain. In 1969, 2 years prior to admission, he had a Moore self-locking prosthesis inserted for the diagnosis of degenerative osteoarthritis of the hip. Because of persistent pain, a conversion of the painful Moore self-locking prosthesis to a low-friction arthroplasty was done in December 1971. Moderate instability of the hip was observed at surgery. The hip could be pulled apart approximately 1 cm.; however, following a firm reattachment of the greater trochanter, the hip was stable on testing at the final stage of the operation.

595

Table 17-1. Contributing factors in eight cases of postoperative dislocation

Case history	B. J.	D. M.	M. L.	G. E.	D. B.	F. O.	F. C.	W. S.
Original diagnosis	Osteoarthritis	Fracture: neck of femur	Fracture: neck of femur	Osteoarthritis	Osteoarthritis	Fracture: neck of acetabulum	Fracture: neck of femur	Osteoarthritis
Sex	F	F	F	M	M	M	F	M
No. of operations prior to LFA	0	2	3	0	0	3	2	1
Type of operation prior to LFA		Girdlestone pseudarthrosis	Girdlestone pseudarthrosis			Charnley LFA	Moore self-locking prosthesis	Moore self-locking prosthesis
Age at LFA	54	34	68	61	67	72	67	64
Malposition, cup						X	X	
High position, cup						X		X
Malposition, femur						X		
Instability at surgery						X		
Poor muscle or extensive scarring		X	X				X	X
Severe trauma	X	X	X					
Early extensive range of motion				X	X			
No. of dislocations	1	2	2	4	1	8	20	2
No. of closed reductions	1	2	2	4	1	8	20	2
No. of open reductions						*	1†	
Trochanteric nonunion and wire breakage		X	X					
No. of factors contributing to dislocations	1	3	3	1	1	3	3	3

*Only femoral component of arthroplasty was revised.
†Hip arthroplasty was revised.
From Eftekhar, N. S.: Clin. Orthop. **121:**120-125, 1976.

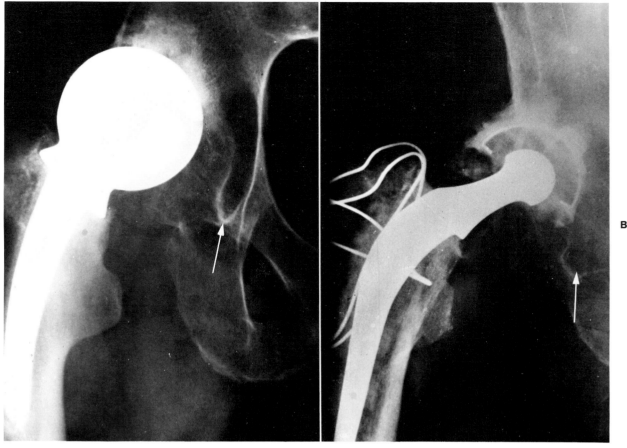

Continued.

Fig. 17-1. A, W. S. 2 years following insertion of Moore self-locking prosthesis. Evidence of marked proximal migration of prosthesis in relation to acetabulum and sclerosis of acetabulum. Arrow indicates original site of acetabulum (teardrop), **A** to **C. B,** Immediate postoperative radiograph of hip following low-friction arthroplasty. NOTE: high position of socket at migrated site of original prosthesis. **C,** Posterior and superior dislocation of low-friction arthroplasty. NOTE: high position of socket and greater trochanteric fixation, which has remained undisturbed following dislocation. Relationship of cemented socket to teardrop indicates reduction in effective neck length (see text).

In the recovery room 2 hours after surgery the patient became restless and sat up in bed. A deformity of the lower extremity was subsequently noted, and a posterior dislocation of the prosthesis was confirmed by radiography. With intravenous injection of meperidine (Demerol), the hip was easily reduced with traction and maintained in the position of abduction by an abduction splint. A second dislocation was observed on the fourth postoperative day when the patient flexed the hip in bed; the second dislocation was reduced under general anesthesia by manipulation, and the patient was placed in a 1½ hip spica cast for 6 weeks. The greater trochanter remained undisturbed, and the hip has remained

located for 4 years following surgery (Fig. 17-1).

CASE 2. F. C., a 67-year-old female schoolteacher, sustained a subcapital fracture of the right hip in 1968 for which a Moore self-locking prosthesis was inserted. Pain persisted postoperatively and, in June 1969, a revision of the prosthesis was done with a long-stem Moore self-locking prosthesis. Because of the persistent pain, a right low-friction arthroplasty was performed in July 1971. Two months following surgery the hip dislocated. Reduction was accomplished under general anesthesia, followed by application of a hip spica cast and immobilization for 3 weeks. Subsequently, 20 dislocations occurred, most of which the patient was able to

597

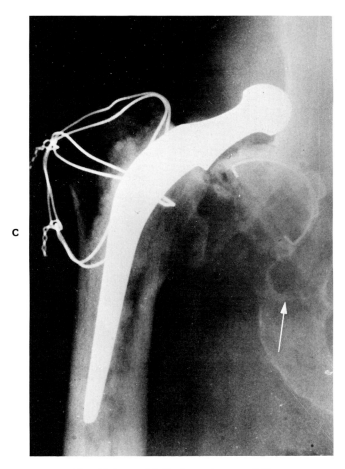

Fig. 17-1, cont'd. For legend see p. 597.

The low-friction arthroplasty had been performed for a central fracture dislocation of the hip 1 year prior to his admission here. He had experienced four postoperative dislocations; the first at 3 weeks, the second at 9 weeks, the third at 12 weeks, and the fourth at 16 weeks. Two closed reductions and two open reductions had been performed prior to his transfer. Attempts at closed reduction by means of skeletal traction through a tibial pin were unsuccessful, therefore the patient was taken to the operating room and open reduction was performed. At surgery, the acetabular component was found to be excessively vertical (approximately 30 degrees to the axis of the body), the femoral component excessively retroverted, and a large lump of cement was present inferior to the socket, facilitating the dislocation (Fig. 17-2, *A* to *C*). A revision of the femoral component of the prosthesis and removal of the cement was done; however, because of the defective floor owing to previous fracture, the vertical orientation of the acetabular cup was accepted and the acetabular portion of the prosthesis was left undisturbed. Eight weeks following the revision a recurrent dislocation took place while the patient was sitting in a chair. A closed reduction was done and the hip remained located for approximately 1 year, at which time the patient fell and recurrent dislocation took place. Six dislocations subsequent to this were reduced by closed methods. The patient was finally fitted into an abduction brace (Fig. 17-2, *D*) and no further surgery was contemplated in view of the patient's arteriosclerotic heart disease and intercurrent episode of cerebrovascular disease. Severe instability and recurrent dislocations in this case were related to the residual defect of the orientation of the acetabular cup and extensive scarring of the hip as a result of previous surgery.

Traumatic dislocations. There were three traumatic dislocations in this series.

CASE 1. M. L., a 68-year-old woman with multiple failed surgical procedures including hip nailing, removal of the nail, insertion of a Moore self-locking prosthesis, and removal of the prosthesis, underwent low-friction arthroplasty in 1972. Following revision surgery, the patient did well with the exception of a nonunion of the greater trochanter. Two years postoperatively, she was completely symptom free and extremely pleased with the results of arthroplasty, although radiographs revealed breakage of wires used

reduce at home; only three necessitated manipulation by the treating surgeon under general anesthesia. At this point, the patient was apprehensive about the dislocation and refused to walk on the extremity even when the joint was relocated. Radiographs revealed a vertical orientation of the acetabular prosthesis (30 degrees to the axis of the body and 15 degrees retroversion, which was confirmed at surgery). Approximately 1 year following low-friction arthroplasty, revision of the entire arthroplasty was done using a long-neck Charnley-Müller total prosthesis. Following this operation the patient was placed in a unilateral hip spica cast for 6 weeks. The hip has remained located for over 5 years following revision arthroplasty.

CASE 3. F. O., a 72-year-old man, was referred here from another institution following recurrent dislocations of a low-friction arthroplasty.

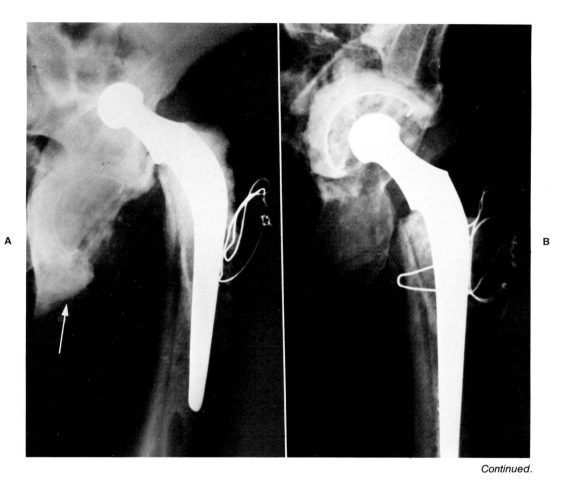

Continued.

Fig. 17-2. A, F. O. Radiograph shows posterior and superior dislocation of left low-friction arthroplasty. Evidence of only slight vertical orientation of acetabular component (30 degrees to longitudinal axis of body) is seen. Femoral component was found retroverted at surgery. NOTE: large lump of cement facilitating dislocation (arrow) inferior to socket. **B,** Postoperative revision of femoral component and removal of excess cement. Acetabular component was not revised because of defective floor and good fixation as tested at surgery. **C,** Recurrence of dislocation following revision owing to uncorrected malposition of acetabular component and marked atrophy and scars about hip joint. **D,** Abduction brace such as this one may be worn where recurrent dislocation is complicated by patient's general health and contraindications for further surgical intervention. Brace is securely fastened to thigh via leather thigh cuff, *3,* and pelvic band, *2.* Hinge is located at level of hip joint, *1,* which only allows flexion to about 60 to 70 degrees and maintains hip joint in neutral or slight abduction. Brace is worn at all times but especially when patient is out of bed or sitting in chair. Brace also may be used for postoperative treatment of revised hip replacements following dislocations.

599

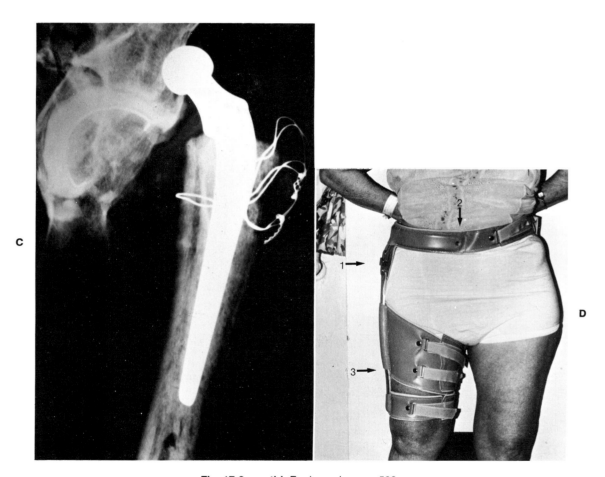

Fig. 17-2, cont'd. For legend see p. 599.

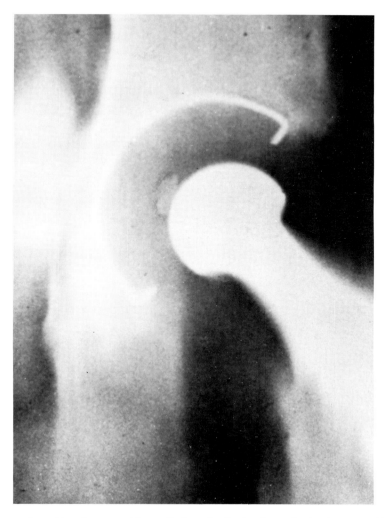

Fig. 17-3. If cause for subluxation cannot be verified on standard radiographs, laminagram of hip may clearly visualize a cement fragment. Cut is at 11.5 cm. and only level to show fragment.

for trochanteric fixation. Following a fall 2 years postoperatively, a posterior dislocation occurred, which was reduced easily by manipulation. A second dislocation was also experienced some 3 weeks following sitting on a low chair. At the time of examination it was possible to demonstrate by flexion, adduction, and internal rotation, a momentary subluxation that made the patient apprehensive. Two weeks following the second dislocation, the patient was placed in an abduction splint for a total of 3 weeks and further immobilization in a walking brace, which the patient wore for approximately 3 months following traumatic dislocation. No further recurrence of dislocation has been reported.

CASE 2. D. M., a 34-year-old female, had sustained an intracapsular fracture of the hip (for which a Ring prosthesis had been inserted) complicated by a femoral shaft fracture in another institution. This hip was first converted to a pseudarthrosis and followed by a low-friction arthroplasty. She had a pain-free hip but was left with approximately 1½ inches of shortening in the affected extremity. She could move about well and achieved approximately 90 degrees flexion and 30 degrees abduction and adduction, with 20 degrees external and internal rotation. Three years after surgery, the patient was involved in a severe automobile accident and sustained a fracture at the base of the skull, as well as traumatic

601

dislocation of the hip with disruption of the greater trochanter wires and separation of the fibrous union of the trochanter, which had been diagnosed previously. At this point it was reduced but dislocated once again. She was placed in a hip spica plaster cast for a period of 6 weeks following which the hip has remained located.

Static subluxation. Occasionally, the hip may appear "subluxed" on routine postoperative x-ray examination. A persistent subluxation may indicate the presence of interpositional soft tissue, bone, or cement fragments within the joint. Clinically, there is no evidence of pain or "click," but the fragment may alter the wear pattern in the joint. At times, routine radiographs may not reveal such a fragment of bone or cement, but a laminagram may show the interpositioning fragment (Fig. 17-3).

Instability without dislocations. There have been seven cases of severe instability noted at the time of operation, but only one dislocated postoperatively. The following cases of subluxation (demonstrated by radiographs postoperatively) deserve special comment.

CASE 1. I. S., a 68-year-old man, had been treated for a failed fracture fixation by a Moore self-locking prosthesis, which was converted to a low-friction arthroplasty in 1970. At the time of surgery, it was noted that the abductor mechanism had been partially destroyed and the greater trochanter was absent. The scarified abductor mechanism had been reattached at the time of insertion of the Moore self-locking prosthesis to the tensor fascia femoris. Because of instability at the time of surgery (low-friction arthroplasty), the patient was placed in a bilateral hip spica

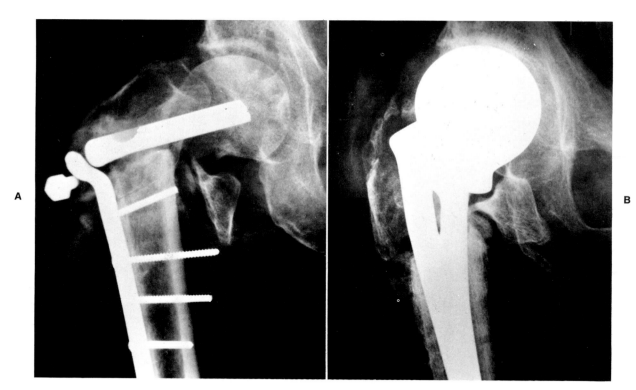

Fig. 17-4. A, Established nonunion of intertrochanteric fracture of right hip in 68-year-old man was treated by hemiarthroplasty (Moore self-locking prosthesis) in another institution. **B,** Two years following insertion of Moore self-locking prosthesis, radiograph shows evidence of proximal migration of prosthesis. Further surgical intervention became necessary. **C,** At revision surgery bone on lateral aspect of shaft of femur (which was thought to be greater trochanter) proved to be only heterotopic ossification. There was no trace of abductor muscles or tendon, which presumably had been removed at time of insertion of Moore self-locking prosthesis. Following resection of loose bone fragment, revision of prosthesis, and low-friction arthroplasty, hip was unstable. Despite application of hip spica cast, head dislocated inferiorly out of socket (arrows). **D,** Following removal of hip spica cast and vigorous generalized exercise program (isometric), hip joint tightened up, thus centering head within socket. **E,** Four years after replacement head has remained in socket and hip remains stable.

602

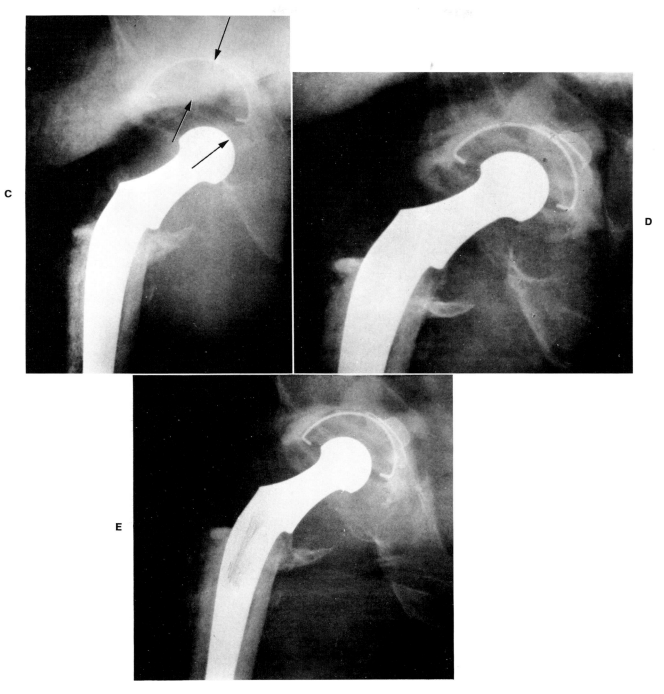

Fig. 17-4, cont'd. For legend see opposite page.

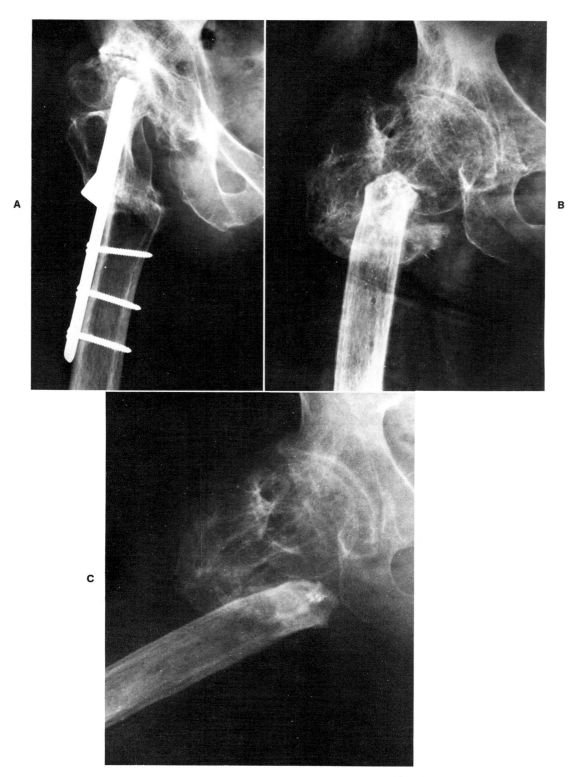

Fig. 17-5. **A,** Status postvalgus osteotomy in 69-year-old female. **B** and **C,** Established nonunion at subtrochanteric level following removal of internal fixation device. **D,** Because of instability noted at surgery following removal of proximal fragment of nonunited upper femur, hip spica cast was applied. Distal migration (subluxation) was observed on sixth postoperative day while patient was still in hip spica cast. **E,** Following institution of isometric exercises without removal of cast, reduction of hip occurred and hip remained stable thereafter (see text).

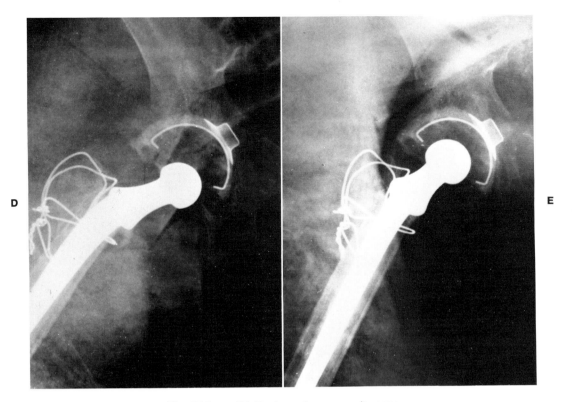

Fig. 17-5, cont'd. For legend see opposite page.

cast immediately upon completion of surgery. The neck of the femur was excessively short, since it had been removed during the insertion of the Moore self-locking prosthesis. Extreme fibrotic and scarified abductor mechanism and soft tissue were encountered about the hip. Despite proper orientation of the components and the application of a hip spica cast, an outward migration of the femoral component was observed on the sixth postoperative day. Following isometric exercises, the hip, which had remained concentrically within the mouth of the cup, reduced itself and there was no further instability or dislocation in this case (Fig. 17-4). A long-neck prosthesis probably would have obviated this complication.

CASE 2. G. H., a 69-year-old woman, had remained chairbound because of bilateral degenerative osteoarthritis secondary to congenital dysplasia of the hip. She had previously undergone bilateral valgus displaced osteotomies of the hip with nonunion of the right osteotomy. Because of instability as the result of the removal of the proximal fragment of the nonunited upper fe-

mur at the time of operation and scars of previous surgery, severe instability was observed at surgery for which a hip spica cast was applied at the end of the operation. Although the hip remained located, separation of the components was observed on the sixth postoperative day while still in the hip spica cast (Fig. 17-5). Following institution of isometric exercises, spontaneous reduction of the hip occurred, and the hip has remained located 4 years following surgery. A long-neck prosthesis probably would have obviated this problem.

CASE 3. L. M., a 58-year-old man with degenerative osteoarthritis of the hip and a severe external rotation deformity, underwent a low-friction arthroplasty. Following a successful arthroplasty, subluxation of the hip was observed and a fragment of cement was detected interposed between the two components of the prosthesis, although there had been no intraoperative detection of the cement fragment. No surgical intervention was contemplated because of absence of pain and otherwise satisfactory results from the arthroplasty (Fig. 17-6).

605

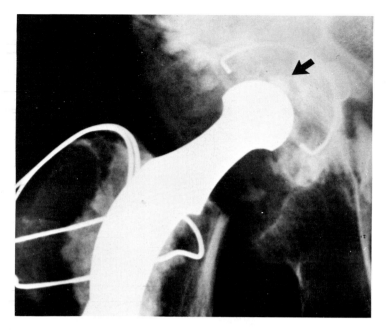

Fig. 17-6. Persistent subluxation noted in postoperative radiograph in this 58-year-old man is due to interposing fragment of cement. NOTE: margin of head out of periphery of acetabulum. Arrow indicates fragment of cement.

Table 17-2. Incidence of dislocation related to different techniques and use of different types of prostheses

Author	Period of operations	No. cases reported	No. dislocations	Percent dislocations	Type prosthesis
McKee[41]	1965-1967	100	3	3	MF
McKee and Chen[42]	1965-1969	300	6	2	MF
McKee and Chen[42]	1971-	100	2	2	MF
Ring[48,49]	1964-1973	1,045	3	0.2	R
Welch and Charnley[57]	1963-1967	307	4	1.3	C
Charnley and Cupic[12]	1962-1963	185	6	3.2	C
Charnley and Cupic[13]	1966-1971	5,000	30	0.6	C
Charnley and Cupic[13]	1971-1972	1,200	3	0.16	C
Eftekhar and Stinchfield[24]	1969-1972	700	4	0.5	C
Murray[45]	1968-1972	808	32	3.9	MF, M, C, etc.
Bergstrom et al.[3]	1970-1972	283	13	4.5	C
Lazansky[36]	1966-1972	501	7	1.3	C
Chapchal et al.[4]	1968-1972	340	11	3.2	MF, M
Johnston[33]	1970-1972	326	3	0.9	C
Amstutz[1]	1970-1972	175	2	1.1	T
Leinbach and Barlow[37]	1968-1972	700	6	0.8	MF, M, etc.
Nicholson[46]	1967-1972	939	26	2.15	C
Freeman et al.[29]	1967-1972	360	14	3.8	H
Coventry et al.[16]	1969-	2.012	60	2.9	C

McKee-Farrar, MF; Charnley, C; Müller, M; Ring, R; Trapezoidal, T; Howse, H.
From Eftekhar, N. S.: Clin. Orthop. **121:**120-125, 1976.

Pathomechanics of dislocation and instability

Regardless of the type of prosthesis used in their early experiences with total hip replacement, most authors reported a higher incidence of dislocation than in their subsequent hip replacement reports (Table 17-2). Information was imparted in Charnley's early teaching that a high rate of dislocation may be experienced when using a 22-mm. femoral head prosthesis.[17,19,35,36] Basically, this idea was generated to emphasize the importance of the greater trochanter detachment and its subsequent transplantation to provide stability for the hip in Charnley's low-friction arthroplasty procedure.[23] As further experience was gained, the mechanism of stability following total hip replacement was better understood; dislocation now is considered to be a rare complication in institutions where large numbers of operations are performed.[7,12] The incidence of dislocation in our series compares favorably with its occurrence following prosthetic replacement of the femoral head for fractures.[19] This suggests the possibility of the lack of relationship between the size of the femoral head and incidence of dislocation. It appears that the range of motion following total hip arthroplasty is more dependent upon the soft tissue to produce stability than on the size of the head and the geometry of the ball and socket. Quite frequently, a range of motion of 110 degrees or 120 degrees flexion is obtained irrespective of the type of prosthesis used (see Chapter 3). Undoubtedly, scarred tissue and lack of elasticity play an important role in instability and dislocation; it is of special interest in our series that five of eight cases of dislocation and six of seven hips with severe postoperative instability were in patients who had undergone more than one previous operation prior to low-friction arthroplasty.

Greater trochanteric reattachment technique requires special emphasis and detailed consideration. Walking with crutches for 6 weeks—and then using a cane to protect the trochanter—ensures postoperative union. A relatively large number of dislocations reported in some series incriminating the removal of the trochanter must be attributed to the faulty technique of individual surgeons, because we consider the trochanteric reattachment an aid in establishing the stability of the joint following replacement. It may also be that separation of the trochanter

occurs following the dislocation itself and not the cause of the dislocation.

A factor that allows a large range of angulatory motion without dislocation is related to the ratio between the diameter of the head and the thickness of the femoral neck. It must be noted that with the Charnley 22-mm. head prosthesis, the center of the head is 2 mm. deep within the diameter of the socket. This feature, while reducing the angle of dislocation, increases the resistance against dislocation. The posterior extended wall of the Charnley prosthesis is an additional deterrent to posterior dislocation (see Chapter 3).

A higher rate of dislocation following low-friction arthroplasty has also been reported by surgeons who have performed the operation with the patient in a lateral decubitus rather than supine position[15,16]—or those who attempted to perform the operation without detachment of the greater trochanter. It is felt that dislocation of either the large- or small-diameter head is less likely if the acetabular component is slightly horizontally oriented, that is, closer to a 45-degree angle (rather than 30 degrees) to the long axis of the body. With more than 15 degrees antever-

Table 17-3. Dimensional characteristics of three types of total hip prostheses

Type prosthesis	Charnley*	Charnley-Müller†	McKee-Farrar‡
Ball diameter (mm.)	22	32	41
Cup inner diameter (mm.)	22	32	41
Neck-shaft angle (degrees)	128	135	128
Collar-shaft angle (degrees)	38	45	30
Neck cross-section area (mm.²)	133	201	415
Socket dimension outer diameter (mm.)	40-44	49-56	41
Neck-socket contact flexion§	91	106	119

*Thackray Ltd., England.
†Protek Ltd., Switzerland.
‡Howmedica, Inc., United States.
§At 0 degrees with 0 degrees external rotation. With any abduction and external rotation, flexion increases without neck-socket contact.

Three interrelated factors contributing to instability and dislocation following total arthroplasty of the hip

I. Mechanical factors
  A. Geometry and design
    1. Ball
    2. Socket
    3. Neck
  B. Attitude of components
    1. Anteversion
    2. Retroversion
    3. Vertical
  C. Clearance between components
    1. Osteophyte
    2. Projected neck osteophyte
    3. Deep placement
    4. Ectopic bone
    5. Unremoved excess cement
II. Anatomical factors
  A. Socket level
    1. High position
    2. Shallow position
    3. Deep position
  B. Effective neck length
    1. Capsule
    2. Ligaments
    3. Muscles
    4. Fascial septa
  C. Femoral neck length
  D. Tissue elasticity (tension)
    1. Scar
    2. Atrophy
    3. Paralysis

III. Technical factors
  A. Orientation
    1. Anteversion
    2. Retroversion
    3. Position on table
  B. Preservation of soft tissue
    1. Abductors (trochanter fixation)
    2. Nerve (tensor fascia femoris)
    3. Capsule
  C. Rehearsal for stability
    1. Stable prior to cement
    2. Stable after cement
    3. Stable prior to reattachment of greater trochanter
  D. Firm reattachment of greater trochanter
    1. Mechanical locking double-wire fixation
    2. Distal position (revision)
    3. Simultaneous tightening of wires—heavy wire
  E. Rehabilitation
    1. Crutch walking, 6 weeks
    2. Cane walking, 6 weeks
    3. Walking in abduction
    4. *Avoid* early flexion/adduction

---

sion or retroversion (with the extended posterior wall cup), one is risking anterior or posterior dislocations, respectively (Fig. 12-37).

There are several interrelated principles involving instability of the hip joint following total hip replacement (see boxed material). These factors include:

1. The mechanical features of the prosthesis
2. Anatomical factors related to the soft tissue and femur or acetabulum
3. Technical handling at surgery and postoperative management

Mechanical factors

Stability as related to the design features of the prostheses has been discussed elsewhere (Chapter 3). While the stability of a total hip joint after arthroplasty is unrelated to the size of the femoral head, stability per se may be affected by the design of the neck and the head-neck diameter ratio and the location of the center of the ball in relation to the center of the socket, therefore the depth of the socket.

A prosthesis with a greater neck recession allows greater freedom from inpingement (Table 17-3). Simulated range of motion of the total hip device indicates that the impingement of the neck against the socket takes place at 91 degrees with the Charnley prosthesis. However, these figures are measured at 0 degrees of abduction and 0 degrees of external rotation. In a normal functional situation, attempt at flexion of the hip often accompanies a position of abduction and external rotation facilitating relief of the impingement at the neck socket angle (see Chapter 3).

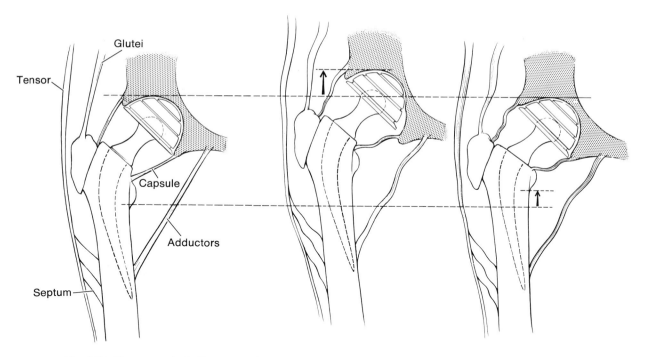

Fig. 17-7. Diagrammatically illustrates "effective-neck length." **A,** Reveals taut musculoseptal fascia as well as muscular tension when appropriate length of femur in relation to acetabulum is preserved by correct position of both components. **B,** High position of socket leading to instability as result of soft tissue laxity. Similar situation can be created if acetabulum is placed excessively deep. **C,** Similar situation to that of **B** as result of excessive shortening of neck of femur despite correct positioning of acetabular component. Similar situation can be created if prosthesis is placed in excess varus position in shaft of femur or excessively short-neck prosthesis is used.

Anatomical factors

The structures contributing to the stability of the hip following total arthroplasty include tensor fascia femoris, gluteus medius and minimus, capsule of the joint, and its reinforcing ligaments. Obviously, scarified structures, calcification and heterotopic bone about the hip, or paralysis of the muscles will lead to obvious inelasticity (or laxity), which explains the frequent incidence of dislocations in revision operations in our series. In a normal hip joint, the amount of separation of the femoral head from the depth of the acetabulum is governed by muscular resistance to force, capsule and capsular ligaments, and ligamentum teres. Under anesthesia and after resection of the capsule and ligamentum teres, forceful elongation of the limb is limited by fascial structures of the thigh, predominantly the iliotibial tract and muscular septa. The iliotibial tract contributes to the stability of the hip by its strong abduction power, and any exposure of the hip joint that might damage the nerve supply to the tensor fascia femoris—either by cutting or stretching beyond repair—would deprive the hip joint of this stabilizing mechanism. Likewise, the resection of the inferior capsule must be avoided (unless necessary to gain exposure), since it also becomes taut after reduction of the prosthesis.

Undoubtedly, preservation of the anterior capsule and the Y-shaped ligament of Bigelow prevents anterior dislocation by external rotation of the hip. This structure must also be preserved at the time of arthroplasty unless its removal is required to overcome a fixed deformity.

Most important of all, the length of the neck of the femur contributes to the tightening of these structures following reduction of the prosthesis. Proximal placement of the socket at surgery, excessive shortening of the limb by removing too much neck, excessive deepening of the acetabulum without compensation by neck length, and positioning of the femoral prosthesis in varus all predispose the hip to excessive laxity, thus inviting dislocation (Figs. 17-7 and 17-8).

609

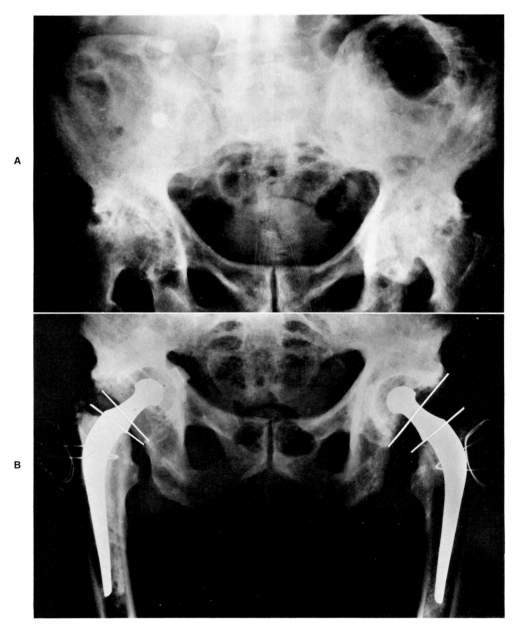

Fig. 17-8. A, Advanced degenerative osteoarthritis of hips and Paget's disease in 74-year-old priest. NOTE: thickness of floor of acetabulum on both sides and available bone stock for seating of acetabular components. **B,** Maximum deepening of hip on right, thus loss of clearance between upper femur and acetabulum (maximum medialization) but only optimal deepening on left side. Patient developed sensation of click in right hip while walking downstairs and definite subluxation in certain degrees of range of motion. It is believed that combination of excessive medialization and lack of clearance on right side is responsible for this phenomena. Standard neck length prosthesis was used in both hips. Patient was large-boned man. It is now preferable not to do extreme medialization in these situations (see Chapter 13). Preoperative grading of hip, right, 2,2,1 and left, 2,2,1; postoperative grading right, 6,6,6 and left, 6,6,6.

Technical factors

Because of the importance of soft tissue in contributing to the stability of the hip after total replacement, it is essential to preserve the iliotibial tract and its function by careful suturing of the tensor fascia femoris at the termination of the operation. This must be done with the hip in the position of abduction using nonabsorptive suture materials. If a transverse incision of this structure is done in order to obtain exposure during the operation, this also must be carefully repaired. Gentle retraction of the anterior fibers of the gluteus medius and tensor fascia femoris and preservation of the nerve to the tensor fascia femoris are essential. Detachment of the gluteus medius and minimus by removal of the greater trochanter facilitates the exposure—thus minimizing trauma to the anterior fibers of this muscle, which contributes to the stability of the hip joint. A firm distal and lateral reattachment of the greater trochanter will subsequently augment stability when surgery has been performed for revision of a failed previous operation. However, it must be emphasized that the hip joint (at the time of arthroplasty) must be stable prior to the reattachment of the greater trochanter. An excessively shortened neck of the femur can be compensated for by the use of a long-neck prosthesis. Orientation of the Charnley prosthesis must be carefully determined at surgery, and there should be no anteversion or retroversion of either component. Femoral components should not be subjected to more than 5 degrees of anteversion; the axis of the cup should be 45 degrees to the longitudinal axis of the body, and certainly reduction of this angle toward the longitudinal axis of the body predisposes the hip to dislocation. (See Chapter 12 and Figs. 17-2 and 17-9.) Orientation of other types of prostheses must be done strictly according to the designer's instruction.

Since high positioning of the socket is a major contributory factor in instability (caused by relaxation of the soft tissue and ligaments), it is essential to place the socket at the level of the triradiate cartilage (true acetabulum) (Fig. 17-3). When the acetabulum is located high (cephalad migration), it is recommended that the marking of the floor and its preparation be done in a transverse plane to the axis of the pelvis in order to locate the socket low. This can be assessed by a radiographic template preoperatively (see Chapters 10 and 12).

Rehearsal and testing for stability during surgery is essential and must be done prior to the cementing of the femoral component after completion of the fixation of the acetabular prosthesis. Tests for stability include over 90 degrees flexion in neutral adduction to over 20 degrees with neutral rotation. The hip must also be stable both in external and internal rotation; ideally, one must not be able to separate the two components more than 5 mm. by longitudinal traction at the time of operation. It is essential to transfer the greater trochanter as distally as possible in revision operations (especially when, at surgery, a marked degree of instability is observed).

In addition to proper orientation of the components, mechanical clearance of the implanted prosthesis must be assured prior to closure (Fig. 17-8). It is often necessary to palpate for impingement anteriorly (Fig. 17-9), while flexing or adducting the hip joint. If dislocation takes place posteriorly, common offenders are an anterior or medial osteophyte of the acetabulum or a cement lump (Fig. 17-9). (See also Fig. 17-2.) Likewise, an osteophyte over the anterior neck of the femur could be responsible. Clearance may be reduced if: (1) excessive deepening of the acetabulum is done without removal of the marginal osteophyte; (2) a projecting anterior neck or anterior and inferior acetabular osteophytes are present; or (3) cement is not removed from the periphery of the acetabulum or the neck of the femur, acting as a fulcrum.

Twenty-five percent of 32 dislocations following 5,000 low-friction arthroplasties studied by Charnley and Cupic[13] were related to separation of the greater trochanter. In none of the early dislocations in our series was greater trochanter detachment the responsible cause. In two nonunions of the greater trochanter following a severe trauma, further separation of the trochanter was observed and both were treated successfully by nonoperative means.[21] In the Charnley series, only 15% of those hips that dislocated had previous surgery. In five of eight hips in our series, one or more previous operations had been performed. In the Charnley series, three late dislocations occurred at 5, 6, and 8 years following surgery. Late dislocations in these cases occurred in patients who did not have early postoperative dislocations. Those who had early postoperative dislocations were not followed by recurrent problems; postoperative subluxation did not

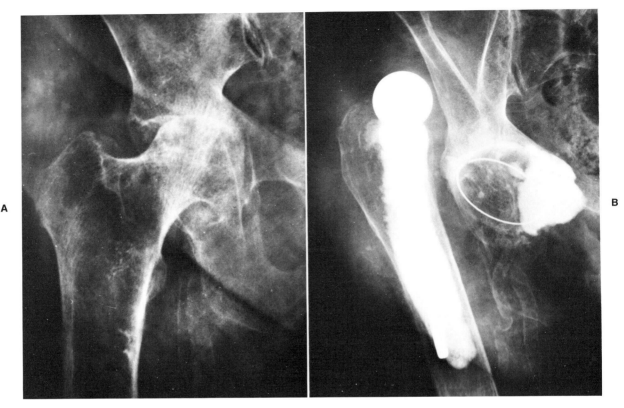

Fig. 17-9. Advanced degenerative osteoarthritis of right hip in 81-year-old woman. **A,** Preoperative radiograph shows medial migration of head present as well as large medullary canal and severe osteoporosis. Proper orientation of components becomes critical. Because of patient's age, surgeon decided to do total hip replacement using larger head prosthesis and without removal of greater trochanter for "quick" surgery to obviate complication of more involved techniques! Operation is said to have been free of complications and performed in less than 60 minutes. Dislocation was observed in recovery room. **B,** Note large lump of cement unremoved from anteroinferior aspects of prosthesis and severe retroversion of cup facilitating dislocation (see text).

cause a dislocation in that series.[13] In our series (with a minimum of 3 years' follow-up), there has been no dislocation occurring after 1 year; two dislocations occurred approximately 6 months following original surgery in a man with a subluxating hip. We have encountered no late spontaneous dislocations in our series.[21,25] Based on the limited number of surgeons performing in our series (two surgeons responsible for more than 85% of all cases), we believe late dislocations have come to our attention through referred patients. Recent dislocations must be treated by skin or skeletal traction for the first 24 hours, which often successfully reduces the hip joint. Radiographs are taken as weight is added to the traction. If reduction attempts are not successful within the first 24 hours following dislocation, the hip must then be reduced under gen-

eral anesthesia. Failure to reduce the hip under general anesthesia requires an open reduction and search for the cause of dislocation. Following reduction, the hip is immobilized for a period of 6 weeks in a hip spica cast, or bedrest with the hips abducted is employed.

FRACTURE OF FEMUR COMPLICATING TOTAL HIP REPLACEMENT

Total hip replacement complicated by fracture of the femur is unusual; however, it can seriously jeopardize the surgical outcome when it does occur. These fractures may be classified as:

- preoperative
- intraoperative
- postoperative

Each of these categories have specific problems deserving care and management. Preoperative fracture for which total hip replacement becomes necessary has been dealt with in Chapters 8 and 14; therefore only intraoperative fractures and postoperative fractures are discussed here.

Incidence and location

The true incidence of intraoperative fracture is impossible to determine; some of these fractures go unrecognized because postoperative radiographs do not reveal all of the details when cement has been used. Obviously, more fractures occur in patients with osteoporosis. Therefore the clinical material (both operative records and radiographs) must be considered when discussing the incidence. For example, Welch and Charnley[57]—in a series of 307 patients with rheumatoid arthritis—treated eight fractures (an incidence of 2.6%). In a series by Scott and associates,[52] their experiences with 5,000 operations (combined osteoarthritis, rheumatoid arthritis, and other conditions) yielded 18 recognized fractures (an incidence of about 0.4%). Paterson and Brown[47] reported three fractures in 369 patients (0.8%), and Arden and Ansel[2a] reported six fractures in 189 patients with rheumatoid arthritis (3%). With recent advances in surgical technology, the low incidence of infection, and minimum complications, this technical failing is serious. Intraoperative fractures can be disastrous if they are not recognized and properly treated during the operation.

The true incidence of fractures occurring during or after total hip replacement surgery is not clearly known. Scott and associates[52] analyzed intraoperative and postoperative fractures of the femur in 25 hips, 18 of which were of the former type, and 7 the latter. One patient had a preoperative as well as an intraoperative fracture, and another patient had a fracture intraoperatively as well as postoperatively. These intraoperative fractures occurred while the surgeon was reaming the canal, seating the femoral components, or manipulating the femur in patients who were predisposed to fractures. In their experiences, most postoperative fractures occurred through a cortical defect near the tip of the femoral component. A long-stem femoral component was helpful in treating such fractures once the cortical defect was recognized.[51] Sixteen of the fractures in this group were sustained in the proximal third of the femur, and two were in the middle and distal thirds. Of the proximally located frac-

tures, seven occurred during reaming of the canal, four during the final seating of the femoral components, and two when the surgeon was attempting to dislocate the hip after capsulectomy. One fracture occurred during the removal of a failed Moore self-locking prosthesis; another occurred during an attempt to drive the fractured stem of a Thompson prosthesis down the femoral canal; and a third occurred during osteotomy of the neck of the femur.

McElfresh and associates[40] reported on the incidence of postoperative fractures in 5,400 cases of total hip arthroplasty performed at the Mayo Clinic. Six occurred in the proximal third of the femur, and one was combined with acetabular fracture. Neither in the studies of McElfresh nor of Scott and associates did fracture healing appear to be adversely affected by the presence of the prosthesis or cement.

Experiences with fractures

In a special review of our own cases at the New York Orthopaedic Hospital, the first 1,200 total hip replacements were subjects of this study (between April 1969 and December 1973).[34] In subsequent experience[18] the rate of fractures is reduced to approximately 1 in 500 cases. We define intraoperative fractures as any evidence and/or recognition of injury to the femur at surgery or proof of such an injury by postoperative radiograph. We were able to collect data on and analyze 32 intraoperative fractures. This study was possible because of special operative records (see Chapter 9) indicating several references to this complication when it occurred. Twenty-six patients were female and six were male (in other series also the prevalence of fractures during the operation was higher in females than males). The youngest patient was 40 years old, and the oldest was 79 years old—mean age was 62 years. Preoperative diagnoses were: osteoarthritis (11 patients), congenital dysplasia (2 patients), the largest group (18 patients) was for revision of failed previous operations, and one patient had Paget's disease in the hip joint.

Overall average anesthesia time was 252 minutes; average blood loss was 3,125 ml.; and average hospital stay was 35 days. Charnley's technique was used in all cases, including routine trochanteric osteotomy. In these 32 intraoperative fractures, dislocation of the hip caused two fractures; removal of the femoral head prosthe-

Table 17-4. Comparison of intraoperative fractures in primary and revision surgery (major fractures only)

Fracture type	Revision	Primary
Fracture (upper)	4.3%	0.9%
Shaft perforation	2.9%	0.4%

Mechanism of 32 fractures in 1,200 total hip replacements	
At dislocation	2
Broaching canal	13
Removal of previous prosthesis	9
Removal cement	4
Previous shaft defect	2
Insertion of prosthesis	2
Total	32

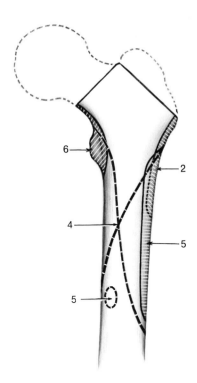

Fig. 17-10. Pattern of major fractures as occurred in our series. Most serious fractures are considered to be those extending to shaft of femur and beyond level of tip of stem of prosthesis.[34] Numbers indicate the number of fractures in each category (see text).

sis produced nine fractures; broaching of the femoral canal caused thirteen fractures; insertion of a femoral prosthesis produced two fractures; removal of the cement was responsible for four fractures; and two fractures resulted from a previous surgical defect (see boxed material above). The fractures in our series could be divided into two categories—major and minor.

Minor fractures. Minor fractures were defined as those including only a small fragment of the neck or calcar region and not affecting the stability of the femoral component or in any way altering postoperative management; the long-term follow-up results were similar to those of other uncomplicated cases. There were 10 fractures so classified (see boxed material on p. 624).

Major fractures. Major fractures, however, did affect the immediate stability of the femoral component, and postoperative management was altered to include further immobilization of the hip following total hip replacement.

The 22 major fractures consisted of two high-lateral cortex fractures, five low-lateral cortex fractures, five perforations of the shaft, six fractures of the calcar, and four fractures of the shaft at the junction of the middle and upper third (see box on p. 624). Fig. 17-10 illustrates the pattern of fractures and their frequency in our series.

Predisposing factors and prevention

A review of our operative record revealed that one or more mechanisms or conditions contributed to the intraoperative fractures (see boxed material on p. 624 and above).

Narrow canal. Congenital dysplasia, rheumatoid arthritis, and in one case, the characteristic abnormal bone of Paget's disease were the principal causes of fracture in 16 cases (Figs. 17-11 and 17-12). Increased femoral neck anteversion was an additional factor in dysplastic femurs. In attempts to broach the femoral canal in "neutroversion," the axis of the broach jammed so often with the axis of a dysplastic canal that it exploded the shaft. The narrow canal, with increased femoral neck anteversion, must be carefully approached by using a narrow, straight-stem prosthesis and broach, and attempts to force through a curved-stem broach must be avoided. In a very small canal, serial graded Küntscher reamers are useful before the straight-stem broach is used (Fig. 17-13). The site of entry by reamers to the femoral canal in

Text continued on p. 619.

614

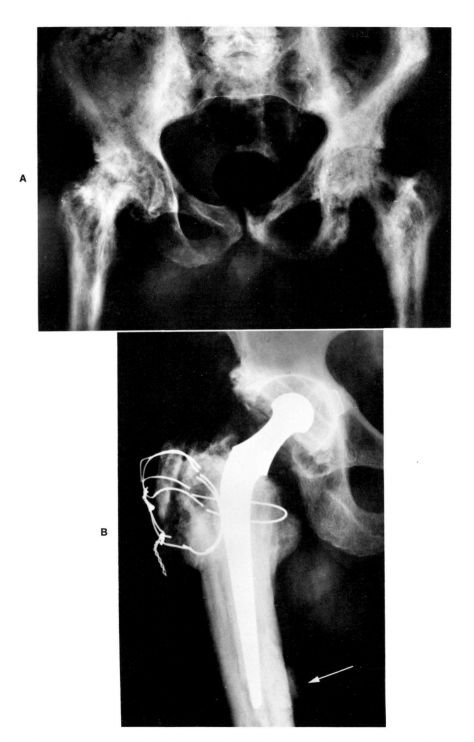

Fig. 17-11. Pathological condition of bone must be carefully handled during hip replacement because of abnormal mechanical strength of bone. **A,** Preoperative radiograph of 63-year-old man with Paget's disease and osteoarthritis. **B,** During preparation of left hip medial perforation of shaft was sustained (arrow). NOTE: medullary canal on both sides is extremely narrow and despite large size of bone only straight, narrow-stem prosthesis could be utilized.

615

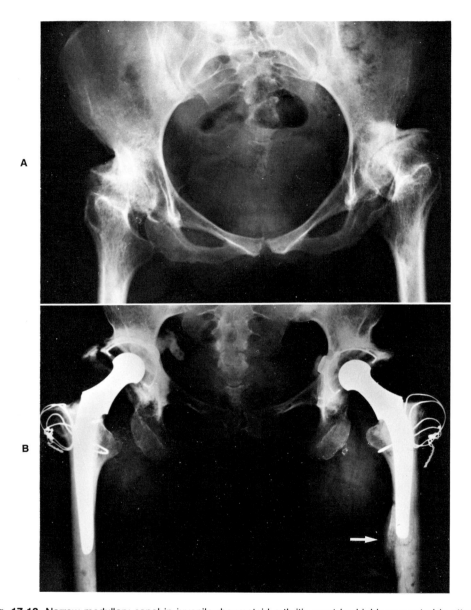

Fig. 17-12. Narrow medullary canal in juvenile rheumatoid arthritis must be highly respected in attempt to accommodate prosthesis. Medullary canal is dysplastic and does not possess natural neck-shaft angle. Graded Küntscher reamers are used to expand medullary canal. However, oversized reaming may result in perforation. **A,** Bilateral juvenile rheumatoid arthritis in 36-year-old woman. NOTE: marked dysplasia of femurs. **B,** Postoperative appearance of hips following bilateral low-friction arthroplasty. NOTE: it was necessary to use shortened and narrowed-down prosthesis in both hips (custom-made). Despite attention to extreme dysplasia of bone and preparation for this case by special prostheses, left hip preparation was complicated by perforation of shaft on medial side by thinning of cortex during use of graded reamers (arrow). Also note that cortex similarly has been markedly thinned down on right side.

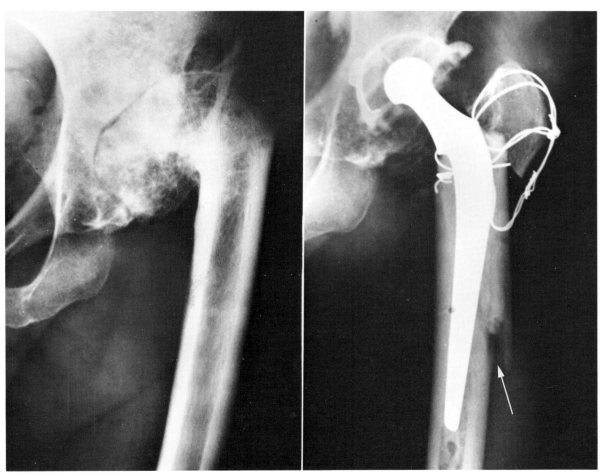

A   B

Fig. 17-13. Straight and narrow shaft will not accommodate curved broach. **A,** Advanced degenerative osteoarthritis superimposed in coxa vara in 63-year-old female. **B,** Low lateral cortical fracture (arrow) observed on immediate postoperative radiograph and unrecognized by surgeon at time of surgery. During surgery standard broaches had been used with aim to accommodate larger prosthesis because of patient's age and vigor, but finally straight, narrow stem was all that was possible for insertion. This complication could have been avoided if graded reamers had been used and straight, narrow stem had been accepted as first choice.

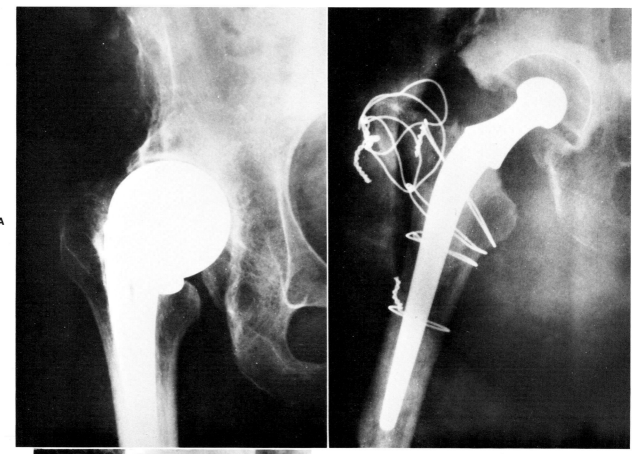

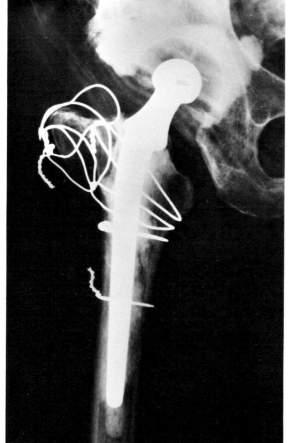

Fig. 17-14. Removal and dislocation of Moore self-locking prosthesis has been most common cause of serious fractures of proximal femur. **A,** Sunk-in femoral prosthesis in 62-year-old female. NOTE: fixed external rotation deformity as well as subsidence of prosthesis into medullary canal. **B,** During dislodgment of prosthesis by heavy hammer blows entire upper femur "exploded" and long spiral fracture was sustained. Fracture was fixed with circlage wires and operation was supplemented by use of hip spica cast. **C,** One year following surgery, fracture is well healed and patient has full weight bearing without any further problem.

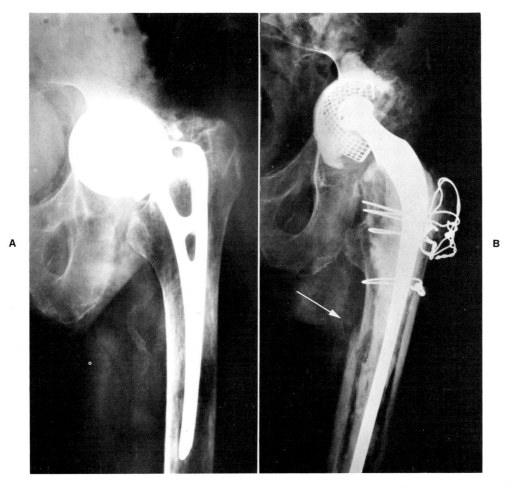

Fig. 17-15. A, Proximal and distal migration of Moore self-locking prosthesis in 71-year-old patient with rheumatoid arthritis and severe osteoporosis. Patient was chairbound prior to surgery. **B,** During dislocation of femoral head from depth of acetabulum only minor external rotation caused severe fracture extending from trochanteric area to midshaft region. Use of circlage wires and long-stem prosthesis was employed to rectify this complication. After 2 months supplementary cast immobilization, rehabilitation began protected weight bearing. Radiograph at 6 months revealed complete healing of fracture. Step-off of medial cortex is related to "less-than-perfect" reduction of fracture achieved at surgery. Additional circlage wire distal to arrow would have rectified this step-off.

dysplasia is often located posteriorly, which must be kept in mind (see Chapter 13, Fig. 13-19).

Removal of femoral head prosthesis. Removal of the femoral head prosthesis has been the most common cause of serious fractures of the proximal femur (Figs. 17-14 and 17-15), especially when a self-locking device was used, and proximal fenestration of the prosthesis filled with bone and fibrous tissue prevented dislodgment of the prosthesis. Fractures were produced with heavy hammer blows at the time of dislodgment in attempts to unseat the bone from the fenes-

tration. External rotation of the femur at the time of dislocation of the prosthesis out of the acetabulum also caused serious fractures (Fig. 17-14). The oscillating power-driven saw that is used to remove the fenestration bone should obviate this complication (see Fig. 14-8, Chapter 14). It is essential to remove all soft tissue and ectopic bone around the neck prior to making attempts at dislodging the prosthesis from the canal (Fig. 17-15).

Dislocation of the hip. In primary arthroplasties, dislocation of the hip has caused only one

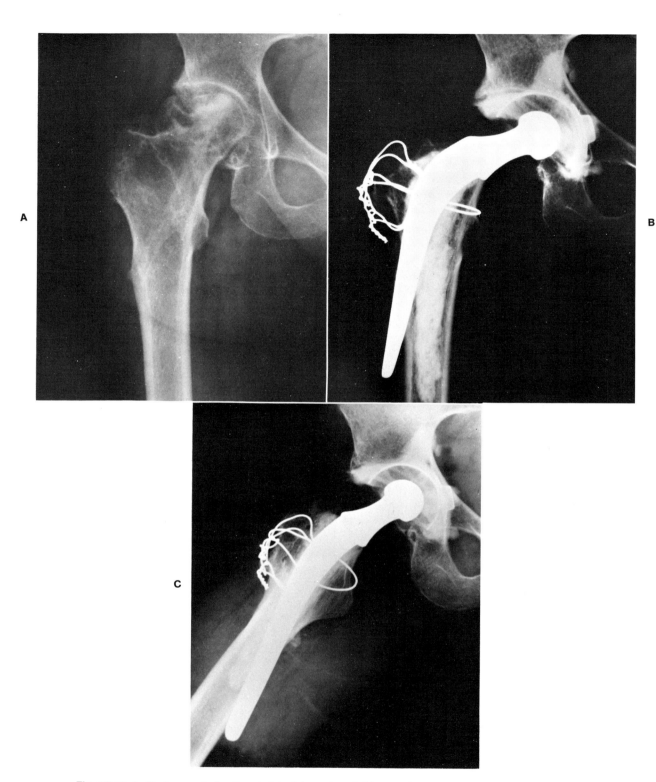

Fig. 17-16. A, Postremoval of nail and plate fixing subcapital fracture in 61-year-old female. **B,** Preparation had been conducted through medullary canal, but unfortunately prosthesis had been inserted through defect, which was posterolateral. **C,** When leg is in external rotation, tip of stem appears as if it has penetrated medially. **D,** "Shoot through" lateral view illustrates exact location of tip of stem to be posterior. **E,** With internal rotation of hip, tip of stem appears to be lateral. **F,** With leg in neutral rotation stem appears as if it is lying side by side with shaft. This series of radiographs illustrates importance of biplane x-ray examination of shaft searching for possible perforations.

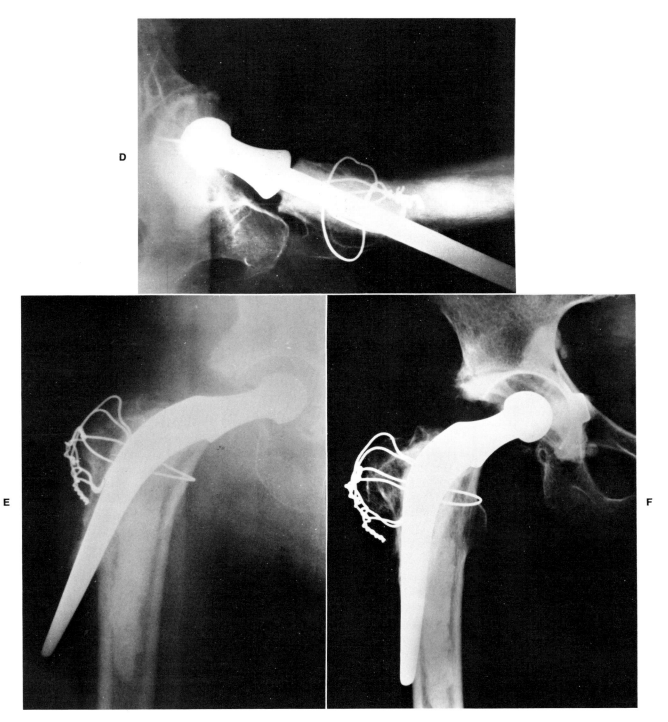

Fig. 17-16, cont'd. For legend see opposite page.

fracture of the femur—when an external rotation maneuver was executed in an effort to dislocate the head. If the hip is extremely stiff, the interpositioning of a Watson-Jones gouge between the head of the femur and the acetabulum, accompanied by adduction of the femur, often facilitates dislocation. External rotation must be avoided prior to disengagement of the head from the depth of the acetabulum (Fig. 17-15). *In situ* osteotomy of the neck when the hip is ankylosed may be necessary to avoid this complication (see Chapter 13). If osteotomy is performed, an oscillating saw should be used (Fig. 2-4). Scar tissue about the hip from previous operations must be completely excised before any attempt is made to dislocate the femoral head; likewise, peripheral ectopic bone, when present, must also be removed (see Chapter 14) prior to attempting dislocation of the head. In the revision of a failed total hip replacement the entire anterior and posterior capsule (1 to 2 cm. thick fibrotic tissue) must be completely excised.

Fracture through a femoral defect. A cortical defect (previous fixation site) of the lateral aspect of the shaft may serve as a weak point and cause fracture during the attempt to dislocate the hip joint. This occurred in four cases. In another two cases the broach had taken a path through an old nail track that was not recognized at surgery. Preferably the hardware will be left *in situ* prior to dislocation of the hip and then removed afterward. This minor detail is important, since removal often weakens the bone at the nail site. Additionally, considerable effort to remove screws may damage the shaft, and it will not tolerate the added stresses during the attempt at dislocation.

During reaming of the canal, special attention must be directed to avoiding entry at the previous defect. One should undertake a deliberate exploration of the site where the prosthesis or nail had previously penetrated the cortex. By direct palpation and placing a finger (first assistant) at the entry site of the broaches, penetration of cement or the prosthesis can be prevented (Fig. 17-16). Perforation of the shaft is likely when the upper femur has not been adequately mobilized and the surgeon is forced to ream the femur without directly being able to assess the alignment. The degree of anteversion of the neck of the femur or previous displaced osteotomy must also be carefully evaluated before surgery (see Chapter 14). Observing the anterior

bowing of the femur and the appropriate selection of the site of entry to the shaft will prevent posterior perforation of the shaft.

Broaching and removal of cement. In broaching the femoral canal the concave side of the broach must never reach the calcar region, since attempts to force the reamers in this area lead to a low calcar fracture. Broaches should never fit too snugly; slight rotation of the broaches during insertion and extraction prevents jamming. The use of graded tapered reamers is to be encouraged in extremely narrow canals. Perforations usually occur when a curved-stem prosthesis (such as a Müller or McKee-Farrar) had been previously cemented into place, and reaming is done with a straight drill or reamer (Fig. 17-17). The technique of rechannelization (see Chapter 14) can now facilitate removal of the cement. But again, unless a genuine effort is made in careful removal of the cement, perforations are likely to occur. The use of long-handled gouges and fiberoptic light are also invaluable in the removal of cement from the shaft under direct vision.

Intraoperative fractures of the femur during hip replacement are associated with revision surgery, old congenital deformity, or severe osteoporosis (see box on p. 624). Lack of familiarity on the part of the surgeon concerning unforseen problems (based on the examination of radiographs) often leads to this mishap. Often more than one factor predisposes the hip to these types of fractures. For example, in revision surgery a hip is usually stiffer, hardware is difficult to remove, and extreme osteoporosis is present (Fig. 17-15). Disregard concerning such situations by the surgeon or assistant who vigorously manipulates the femur will lead to fracture. Pre-existing bony defects in the shaft (from previous surgery) must also be carefully considered when revising a failed prosthesis.

Management of intraoperative fractures

Intraoperative fractures of the femur are better prevented than treated. These complications can be anticipated and prevented by a careful preoperative review of the radiographs. A good quality lateral view of the upper third of the femur is essential and prerequisite for revision surgery. However, the surgeon must be fully equipped to deal with a fracture when, and if, it does occur during surgery.

When a fracture occurs during an operation,

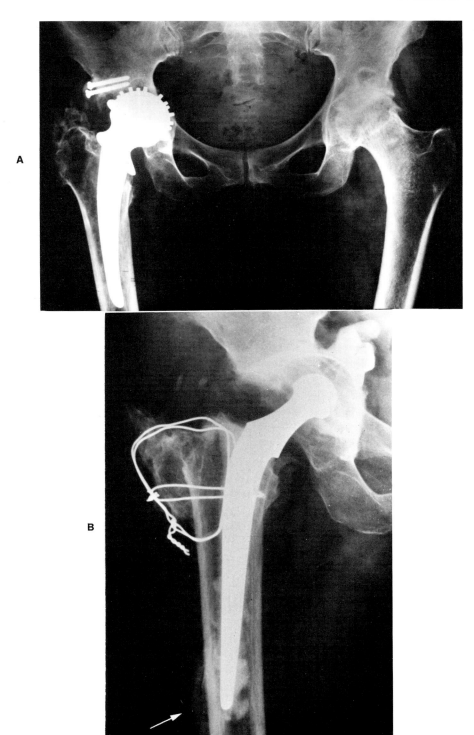

Fig. 17-17. Removal of cement at revision of failed cemented prosthesis may complicate surgery by perforation. This is especially true when previously inserted cement is nonradiopaque. **A,** Postoperative hip replacement in 55-year-old female with rheumatoid arthritis by McKee-Farrar prosthesis. NOTE: absence of radiographical evidence of cement. **B,** Preparation of femur was complicated by perforation of shaft at distal end (arrow), in addition to varus orientation of prosthesis. Large defect of acetabular floor also had not been appraised, thus leading to escape of cement restrictor into lesser pelvis.

623

Classification of 32 fractures in 1,200 total hip replacements

Major	
High lateral cortex	2
Low lateral cortex	5
Perforations	5
Calcar	6
Shaft (spiral)	4
Minor cortex	10
Total	32

Etiology of intraoperative fractures (1,200 total hip replacements with 32 fractures)

Osteoarthritis	11
Previous surgery	18
Congenital dysplasia	2
Paget's disease	1
Total	32

it must be carefully and completely evaluated. Immediate access to intraoperative radiographs provides an indispensable tool in evaluating these fractures, since the femoral shaft may often be fractured extensively in a spiral manner extending from the calcar, or a displacement might be present that cannot be appreciated without a radiograph. It is essential to repair an intraoperative fracture of the femur with care and patience; the goal is to fix the fracture and to perform the total hip procedure.

Following a two-plane x-ray evaluation, the fracture site should be exposed and the cortices opposed. One or more circlage wires are used to secure and maintain the position prior to insertion of the femoral component (Fig. 17-18) or the fracture may be fixed by a small plate and unicortical screws and the use of a long-stem prosthesis. If a fracture has occurred during dislocation, it is advisable to leave it alone until

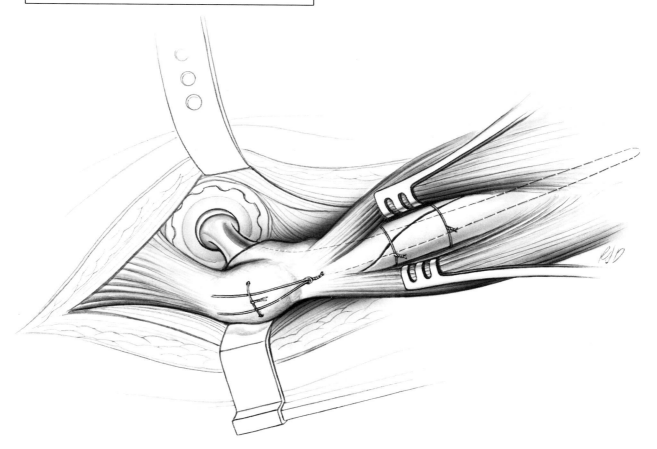

Fig. 17-18. Lateral view of hip following insertion of long-stem prosthesis and fixation of fracture by two circlage wires. NOTE: oblique (spiral) line extending throughout upper third of femur. Muscle split approach through vastus lateralis allows good exposure of shaft. Circlage wires need not be removed following insertion of cement and prosthesis.

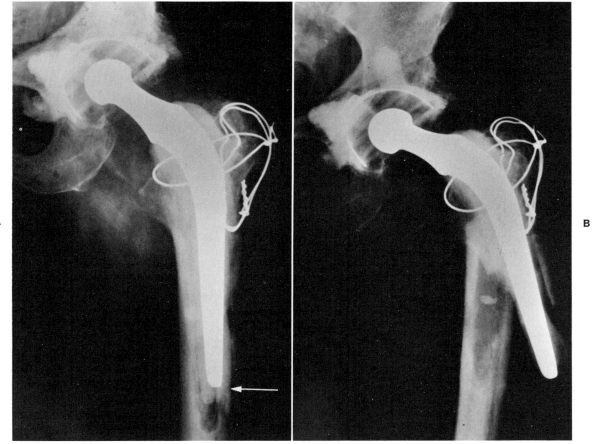

Fig. 17-19. A, Total hip replacement in this 63-year-old female was complicated by obvious penetration of cement through lateral cortex of femur (tension side of femur, arrow). No modification of postoperative rehabilitation was instituted in relation to protecting femur. **B,** Approximately 4 months following surgery patient sustained fracture through defective lateral cortex. **C,** Following skeletal traction and cast immobilization, fracture is united in this precarious position; however, 2 years following fracture patient is free of pain and no further surgical intervention has become necessary. Perhaps this complication could have been avoided by protective weight bearing during postoperative course and by period of non-weight bearing postoperatively.

the acetabular component is cemented in place because manipulation of the shaft during work on the acetabulum may jeopardize the fixation of the femur. The surgeon must alert the anesthetist to an extended need for anesthesia (often twice the normal operative time) and extra blood transfusions. The vastus lateralis muscle may be split to expose the fracture site when the fracture extends to the lateral cortex; similarly, by splitting the vastus lateralis and with subperiosteal retraction with a Bennett-type retractor, the medial aspect of the shaft may be adequately exposed. To avoid comminution of the fracture, the bone must be handled gently, avoiding the use of bone clamps. To maintain alignment,

a Lowman-type bone-holding forceps is often necessary. The presence of cement does not inhibit the healing of a fracture, but any amount of interpositioning cement between the fracture fragments may invite delayed union or nonunion. It is essential to obtain maximum apposition of the ends of the bones at the time of reduction with minimum stripping of the soft tissue. The femur is stabilized (by the second assistant) firmly and steadily, while further preparation of the femoral canal is completed. The surgeon must have available two long-stem prostheses (one with a regular neck length and one with a long neck) to be sure of obtaining satisfactory fixation and reduction. The length of the

625

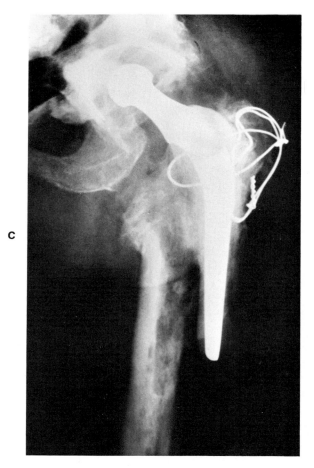

c

Fig. 17-19, cont'd. For legend see p. 625.

stem to be used must be carefully evaluated, as excess narrowing of the canal or bowing of the shaft may necessitate the use of a shorter one (a stem may be too long and pierce the cortex of the femur). Prostheses made of stainless steel may be shortened at surgery, if necessary. Osteotomy of the greater trochanter is indispensable in these operations. After fixation of the fracture and insertion of the prosthesis at the trial stage, a radiograph (anteroposterior and lateral) of the femur may be useful in confirming the position and accuracy of the fracture fixation. Refrigeration of the methyl methacrylate cement prior to use in the operating room may subsequently provide added working time (see Chapter 4). The stem length must pass the fracture site and be fixed with proper alignment and rotation. The circlage wires, preferably, should not be removed until after the fracture has healed or they may be left in place indefinitely. Re-

gardless of the efficacy of fixation by internal means, the fracture must be protected until osseous union occurs; for a fractured femur, this period ranges from 6 months to 1 year (this must be clearly discussed with the patient and his cooperation requested). A careful follow-up with regard to healing must be conducted.

Immediately (postoperatively), internal fixation may be supplemented by a balanced suspension apparatus; alternatively, a hip spica cast may be used as a supplement to internal fixation. Based on the extent of the fracture and the degree of internal fixation, the supplemental cast may be discontinued within 2 to 3 months after surgery. It should be emphasized, in the case of a femoral shaft fracture accompanied by total hip replacement, that we must concern ourselves with proper healing of the fracture if successful results of arthroplasty are to be expected. Thus prolonged and protected weight bearing is fundamentally essential to ensure bony union and to prevent late loosening of the component. Inadequate fixation, as well as inadequate postoperative management, may lead to a painful nonunion or malunion of the femur, which can be a very difficult technical problem to rectify (Fig. 17-19).

Postoperative fractures

A severe fall (or other accident) may cause a patient to suffer a fractured femur, usually occurring at the junction between the flexible segment (distal to the tip of the stem) and the rigid segment (the stem and cement). These fractures usually are amenable to treatment by nonoperative means and should be treated as such (Fig. 17-20); rarely should they be treated by open methods and surgical intervention. The difficulty in achieving perfect fixation is enormous, and it does not necessarily reduce the postoperative recovery period or lessen morbidity. The patient must be placed in skeletal traction (using a tibial Steinmann's pin) for a period of 6 to 8 weeks, at which time the fracture site may show signs of callous formation as evidenced by diminished pain. In the first weeks of traction, repeated roentgenograms must reveal good apposition of the fracture fragment as well as proper alignment and rotation (Figs. 17-20 and 17-21). The hip must also be radiographed to be sure that traction has not caused dislocation of the hip. After approximately 6 to 8 weeks of traction, the patient may be placed in a single-leg hip spica

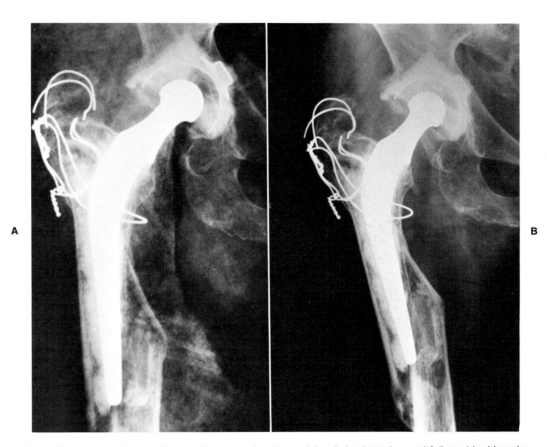

Fig. 17-20. Postoperative fractures of femur are best treated by skeletal traction and followed by hip spica cast until fracture is healed. **A,** Six weeks following skeletal traction using tibial pin, hip of this 62-year-old female was placed in unilateral hip spica cast. **B,** At 3½ months following fracture, good union of fracture is present. *Continued.*

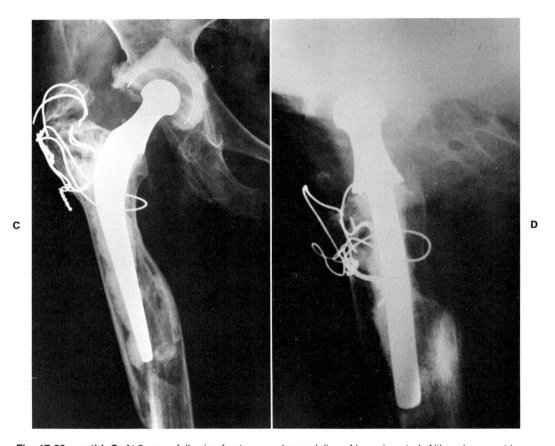

C

D

Fig. 17-20, cont'd. C, At 2 years following fracture good remodeling of bone is noted. Although cement has been disrupted at distal portion of prosthesis, patient in completely asymptomatic. **D,** Lateral view of the same as shown in **C.**

Fig. 17-21. A, Failed Moore self-locking prosthesis used for fracture sustained by this 73-year-old female was converted to low-friction arthroplasty, **B.** NOTE: tip of prosthesis is in contact with medial cortex. **C,** Three months following surgery patient sustained fall, following which oblique fracture at level of tip of prosthesis was sustained. It is possible that at original surgery medial cortex had been damaged. **D,** Rather than traction patient had been placed in hip spica cast. NOTE: angulatory deformity of femur at tip of stem; complete union had occurred with approximately 40 degrees of malalignment. Although hip has remained located, patient now has very disturbing gait because of valgus strain of knee. **E,** One year postunion fracture. Patient now has knee pain due to angulatory deformity of femur.

A B C

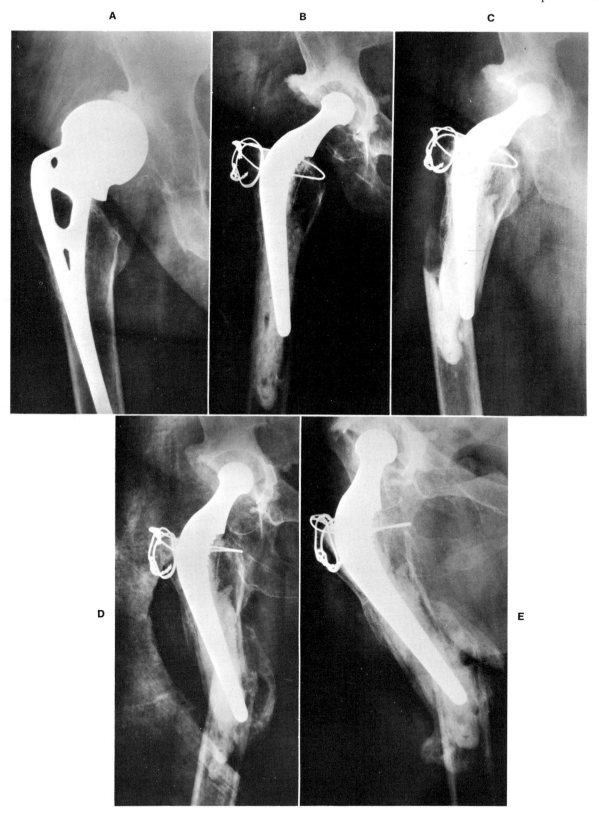

D E

Fig. 17-21. For legend see opposite page.

cast, providing that clinically and radiologically there is evidence of callous at the fracture site. Ambulation begins with non-weight bearing, but progresses to weight bearing within the first 6 or 8 weeks with the hip spica cast. The minimum required amount of immobilization by cast is evaluated clinically and radiologically. Preferably, the knee should be thoroughly mobilized from 6 to 8 weeks following application of the cast, by shortening the cast at knee level. Weight bearing must be accomplished on a graduated schedule, and based on the speed of the fracture's healing and callous formation.

In summary, the ideal treatment of intraoperative fractures includes immediate operative evaluation by radiographs, immediate fixation of the fracture by circlage wires (or plate and screws), and insertion of the total hip prosthesis (with a long stem); ideal postoperative care includes that for total hip replacement plus postoperative care for a fracture of the femur. When the femur is fractured after surgery, a nonoperative method is the treatment of choice.

TROCHANTERIC COMPLICATIONS

A discussion of the rationale for the use of the transtrochanteric approach in total hip arthroplasty has been advanced in Chapters 2, 3, 12, 13, and 14. A consistently better exposure, less damage to the abductor mechanism, and restoration of biomechanical equilibrium contribute to the more satisfactory performance of hips replaced with trochanteric osteotomy. The advantages of trochanteric osteotomy can be offset if a high rate of complications results from this technique, but without trochanteric osteotomy in certain situations such as obese or muscular patients, revision surgery, stiff hips, osteoporotic patients, and protrusio acetabuli, a higher rate of complications may result. Factors that decidedly influence the rate of union without loss of fixation of the trochanter include: (1) a detailed and precise technique used in detachment and reattachment; (2) the quality of bone of the trochanter; (3) repeated surgery and the pathological condition of the bone; and (4) the patient's postoperative cooperation and the use of crutches during the first 6 weeks postoperatively. It must be emphasized that an improved method of fixation directly reduces the complications of the greater trochanter; in most instances, however, the complications of trochanteric fixation are technical and preventable, re-

flecting the surgeon's expertise with trochanteric detachment and subsequent reattachment. Trochanteric complications have been further reported in several series and are serious enough to dissuade some surgeons from performing "routine" trochanteric osteotomies in total hip replacement cases. Continuous efforts are being made by surgeons to overcome these problems by either insisting on using surgical approaches that circumvent the need for trochanteric osteotomy* or finding new methods for better fixation of the greater trochanter.[1,26,54,55]

Despite a high percentage of nonunion (averaging 7%), detachment and reattachment of the greater trochanter seemed an indispensable part of the operation.[5-9,12-14]

Early reports indicated that a two-plane fixation (that is, horizontal and coronal) of the greater trochanter augmented union better than a single horizontal loop wire.[14] Modifications in the procedure have been continually directed toward an improvement of fixation of the trochanter,[9,11] principally to prevent forward and backward motion of the trochanter, which may prevent union or cause fixation failure. In this context the use of a trochanteric staple clamp.† has been recently introduced by Charnley.[10] We recognized that the conventional double-cross-wire technique of fixation does not prevent forward and backward movements of the trochanter unless the trochanter is interlocked into the prominence of the vastus lateralis ridge (Figs. 12-49 and 17-22). (See Chapter 12.) With this modification, in addition to the use of 16-gauge wire employing the "alternate" tightening technique, our results have been most encouraging (see box on p. 632). It must be noted that the interlocking technique may not be feasible in the revision of failed previous surgery, especially in the presence of abnormal bone of the trochanter and the femur in addition to the ectopic bone that is often present, which prevents satisfactory distal advancement of the trochanter. The rate of trochanteric complications has been three times greater in revision groups than in primary operations. It is a fact that in revision surgery and in "large-boned" men a supplemental fixation by trochanteric staple-clamp or cancellous bone screws will result in better fixation.

---

*See references 31, 38, 39, 43, and 50.
†This method[10] has been in use for 1 year, and early experiences are extremely encouraging.

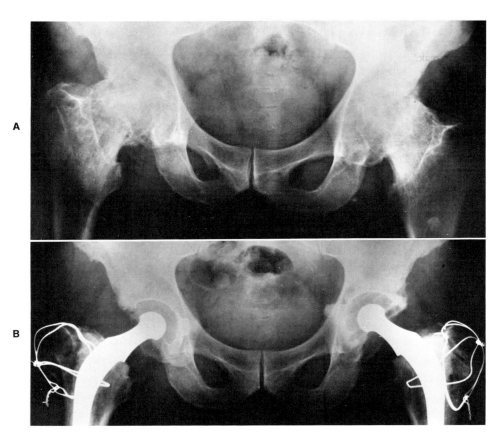

Fig. 17-22. A, Bilateral degenerative osteoarthritis of hips in 63-year-old man weighing 200 pounds. **B,** Post-operative low-friction arthroplasties within 1 week apart. Left hip was done first. Trochanter was fixed to its original site, (position 3) and on left fixed onto vastus lateralis ridge by interlocking technique in position 2. Ambulation began 1 week following second operation and 2 weeks following first operation. NOTE: early wire ruptures noted at 6 weeks postoperatively on left side. Same surgeon performed both operations. Pathology of hip was symmetrical and similar wire technique had been used on both sides with exception of interlocking of trochanter on right side (see text).

631

Clinical and radiological evaluation of trochanteric complications of 100 consecutive low-friction arthroplasties performed as a primary intervention

Painless union	95
Delayed union (6 months)	3
Nonunion (painless)	2
Local tenderness (bursitis)	3*
Wire breakage (late)	4
Wire breakage (early)	1†

*Only in one case did the wire break; none required treatment.

†A proximal migration (1 cm.) of the trochanter, but trochanter united at 6 months.

From Eftekhar, N. S.: Trochanter on or off? Paper presented before First Open Scientific Meeting of International Hip Society, Berne, Switzerland, April, 1977.

Specific problems and their solutions

The problems of trochanteric transfer include asymptomatic nonunion (radiographic), painful nonunion without displacement, painful nonunion with migration, delayed union (radiological), painful bursitis (union), early avulsion with or without dislocation of the hip, nonunion and late dislocation, or heterotopic ossification.

Radiographic evidence of nonunion may be underestimated (and/or miscalculated) if the evaluation is done from a single anteroposterior view of the radiographs, since the position of the extremity, that is, external rotation, may cause overlapping of the trochanter onto the shaft. On the other hand, the rate of union may be overestimated if delayed union is not considered, since in some instances union of the trochanter may occur several months or even years after surgery. The incidence of fibrous union of the trochanter in total hip replacement has been reported to be as high as 10% to 15%, but these figures reflect early experiences of individuals, with a limited number of cases studied. The true incidence of trochanteric nonunion is somewhere between 2% and 3%: Charnley and Cupic,[12] 2.7%; Lazansky,[36] 1.8%; Eftekhar, et al.,[25] 3%; Eftekhar,[22] 1%. An additional rate of 2% to 3% delayed union is to be expected.[36] (Admittedly these figures may be unrealistic to the surgeons who only occasionally remove the trochanter or make no special effort to develop a "meticulous technique" in reattaching the trochanter.) An additional 5% to 10% breakage of

wires may be anticipated—some occurring quite late and completely unrelated to nonunion (Figs. 17-22 and 17-23). In a personal series of 100 consecutive operations (including only primary operations) only a small percentage of trochanteric complications was observed[22] (see boxed material on this page).

Nonunion of the greater trochanter is often asymptomatic and manifested on radiographic examination alone, usually it is recognized within 3 to 6 months following surgery. There would be no point in mentioning this to the patient if the result of arthroplasty is satisfactory; on the other hand, a small number of nonunions might be painful, especially if there is gross motion between the greater trochanter and the bone of the femur, or marked separation and proximal displacement of the greater trochanter makes the abductor power weak, resulting in a severe gluteus medius gait. As a rule, conservative non-operative treatment is the method of choice if the patient can tolerate it; however, with pain or a severe limp (or with accompanied recurrent dislocation) reoperation may be necessary. A successful union by surgery may be difficult since the local tissue blood supply is poor, and the bone of the trochanter is osteoporotic. Excision of a trochanteric fragment is to be discouraged as an alternative to a bone graft or modified techniques to achieve union. The precise method of fixation of the trochanter undoubtedly plays an important role in prevention of trochanteric nonunion and/or migration. A completely complication-free method has not yet been devised, but of the number of methods available, one that is simple and produces maximum fixation (both craniad and forward and backward directions) is a cruciate double- or triple-strand wire technique with or without supplemental transfixation screws or staple-clamp.

The most common causes of early loss of fixation may be faulty technique—usually resulting from the inadequate size of the greater trochanter such as fragmentation, severe osteoporosis leading to a poor fixation. The surgeon's experience plays an important role in this context. One of the important factors in trochanteric fixation is good coaptation and surface contact between the bone of the trochanter and the lateral aspect of the femur; insufficient bony surface contact or trochanteric fragment contact with cement may result in nonunion, so special care must be taken at surgery to pro-

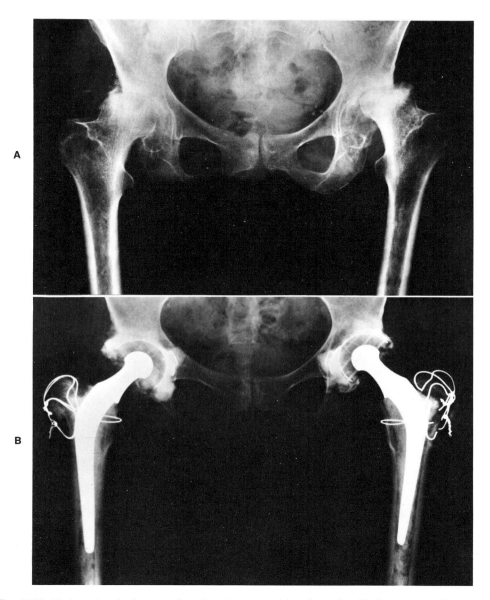

Fig. 17-23. Early ruptured wires may be related to overactivity when other hip is symptomatic and patient enthusiastically discards her support and/or upper extremities are involved with arthritis and patient is unable to use cane or crutches. **A,** Bilateral advanced degenerative changes of hips in rheumatoid arthritis in 34-year-old woman. **B,** Bilateral low-friction arthroplasties performed within 6 weeks apart. Left hip was done first; broken wires were noted by radiographs 6 weeks following hip replacement. It is believed that rupture of wire was sustained on left because of inability of patient to use cane or crutches (owing to advanced rheumatoid arthritis of upper extremities) and the fact that opposite hip (right) was involved and patient's weight bearing was principally supported by left hip (see text).

vide adequate surface contact for the greater trochanter. Wire fixation must be done with heavy wire (16 gauge) if a cruciate fixation method is used. Wires must be handled carefully (to avoid kinks or scratching) with wire-holding forceps in order to prevent early rupture. A short or contracted abductor muscle is especially prone to detachment and nonunion (this is common in cases of revision surgery). Mobilization of abductors from their origin (wing of ilium) or distal advancement by Z-plasty of the tendon is less satisfactory than simple shortening of the neck of the femur or the use of a short-neck prosthesis to allow good fixation of the trochanter. Protected weight bearing with crutches for 6 weeks may improve the rate of union.

As stated, the majority of nonunions occur in patients who have already had previous surgery with inadequate trochanteric fixation caused by a contracted, shortened, scarified, or ossified abductor mechanism with increased tension on the wires. Because short abductors generate significant tension, mobilization of the abductor muscle and a careful preparation of the site on which the trochanter is fixed are necessary (see Chapter 14) (Fig. 12-47). Interlocking of the greater trochanter (Fig. 12-49, see Chapter 12) is most effective in order to minimize nonunion. All soft tissue interpositioning at the site of the trochanter must be carefully removed to allow osseous union. Extreme stripping of the vastus lateralis and periosteum from the lateral aspect of the trochanter is unwise, as this usually reduces the local blood supply and encourages myositis with ossification. As stated, additionally, the use of crutches for 6 weeks enhances union by sparing the forceful use of the abductor muscles. It should be emphasized that the cooperation of the patient during the immediate postoperative course is essential (Fig. 17-23); because of their enthusiasm, many patients (despite forewarnings) overdo their exercises, cross their legs, or sit early and flex their hip in excess. These individuals need special instructions and are to be discouraged from "overdoing." When delayed union is noted, the patient must be advised to protect the hip by using a cane or crutches until union takes place (Fig. 17-23) to avoid separation.

Likewise, following lengthening of the extremity by a new position of the socket, the abductors may become relatively "short" in reaching the site of fixation onto the shaft of the femur

or may only reach the outer aspect of the cement or prosthesis without good bony contact.

We have found no correlation between the healing (union) of the trochanter and postoperative immobilization. We originally allowed patients out of bed only after 7 to 10 days postoperatively (to prevent nonunion). The present policy allowing ambulation within 72 hours has not changed the rate of success regarding union; however, postoperative protection using an abduction splint to alleviate tension on the wires and avoidance of early sitting continues to be a part of the routine postoperative course (see Chapter 11). Volz and Turner,[55] English,[26] Coventry,[15] and others have used a modification of the technique of trochanteric fixation. The first two have used a special bolt and assembly device to increase the rate of union.

Coventry, on the other hand, found no problem with a double-loop technique originally used by Aufranc for trochanteric fixation. Our main experience has been based on a double (horizontal and vertical) wire technique (see Chapter 12), interlocking the trochanter and using a conventional osteotome and gouge for improved interlocking (Fig. 12-49); wires are tightened alternately and simultaneously. A three-wire loop fixation (a cruciform system and a vertical double) recently introduced by Charnley has improved the quality of fixation by wires alone or with the supplemental use of the staple-clamp. (See Chapter 12 and Fig. 12-53.)

Significance of wire breakage

Wire breakage may take place early or late. Early wire breakage is usually the result of a poor fixation at surgery or mishandling of the wires, especially if they are exposed to acute bending or twisting at the points of ties; they may break during surgery if overtightening by the wire tightener creates too much tension. At times, a noncooperative patient who becomes too active early during the postoperative course may cause early wire breakage. Delayed rupture is the result of cyclic bending of the wire between the rigidly fixed portion in the bone and the mobile segment in the soft tissue and may take place months or years after surgery. Fracture of the wire may also occur following union of the greater trochanter; it is usually inconsequential, and the patient is unaware of it (Fig. 17-24, *A*). Overly tightened wires, excess osteoporosis, or poorly placed wires may result in loss of fixation of the

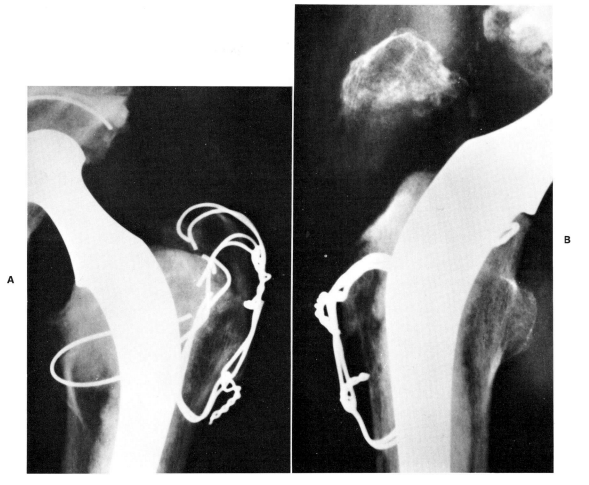

Fig. 17-24. A, Late wire rupture despite union of trochanter was observed 3 years following surgery in this 39-year-old female with rheumatoid arthritis. **B,** "Complete escape" of trochanter through wire loops two weeks following total hip replacement in 56-year-old man, without wire breakage (see text).

trochanter without wire breakage (Fig. 17-24, *B*). Early rupture of wires may be painful; it may be the result of trauma and usually accompanies trochanteric displacement, separation, or fragmentation. A loosely applied wire in fixation may also lead to early wire fractures (Fig. 17-25). Broken wires that are asymptomatic should not be a source of concern to the surgeon or to the patient. Many patients who were completely satisfied with their arthroplasties became worried or anxious when the surgeon told them their "wires were broken"! On the other hand, when bursitis is present and the wires are palpable under the skin, as in a thin person, they may be removed (following adequate conservatism) to alleviate pain at the area of the greater trochanter. If the wiring has been done properly

and the vastus lateralis muscle tendinous cuff has covered the wires, this type of bursitis and pain is extremely rare (see Chapter 12). In my own experience to date, I have not removed a wire from the trochanter because of bursitis, nor have I injected steroids into the area to alleviate pain. If a patient is concerned about broken wires, he must be assured that despite the removal of the wires, pain over the trochanteric bursa may persist; it should be remembered that trochanteric bursitis is often a self-limiting process, providing patients avoid sleeping or lying on the affected side temporarily. The removal of wires may be encouraged only when fractured fragments of wires are within the joint (Fig. 17-26). This disturbing complication should be rectified because of its potential for

635

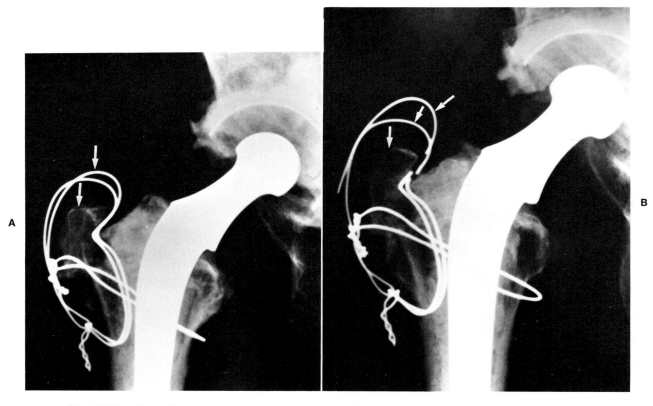

Fig. 17-25. A, Immediate postoperative radiograph following low-friction arthroplasty. NOTE: technical error of inadequate tightening of both loops of wires (or soft tissue entrapment), especially vertical double wire as indicated by arrow to show distance between wires and cortex of trochanter. Trochanter has not migrated proximally in this case. **B,** Same hip as **A** 1 year later. Fractured wires are results of cyclic and repetitive bending at bone–soft tissue level.

damage to the cup and the femoral prosthesis. However, even in this situation, if the patient refuses surgery because of the absence of symptoms, his decision must be respected. Nevertheless, the joint should still be observed closely for signs of accelerated socket wear.

Painful bursitis

Trochanteric bursitis may be present following hip surgery regardless of the type of surgical approach used. This is especially true where the incision is located over the trochanteric region and in thin patients (or those with a thin layer of fat over the trochanteric area). The true incidence of this complication is not known because this is of relative concern to the patients and often is spontaneously resolved after avoidance of the cause of irritation, that is, lying on the side. If a patient has genuine pain, the cause of the pain must be sought elsewhere as well. By conventional orthopaedic ideas, patients

with bursitis can be treated by local injections of steroids, and often removal of the wires (partially or in toto) is advised. However, local injections are to be discouraged for fear of superimposing infection (wires are in continuity with the prosthesis). It is very important for patients to be psychologically supported and advised against lying on the operated side. Anything other than mild analgesics (such as aspirin) should not be needed. Patients are often relieved by knowing that this is only a local phenomenon, unrelated to the function of their arthroplasty, and that the condition is self-limiting; that is, avoidance of the irritation will lead to subsidence of the symptoms. When the patient complains of pain about the trochanteric region, deep bursitis in the hip or "sciatica" must be considered in the differential diagnosis. Occasional pains from the low back area—present in or radiating to the trochanteric region—should also be differentiated. It is of special interest that most patients com-

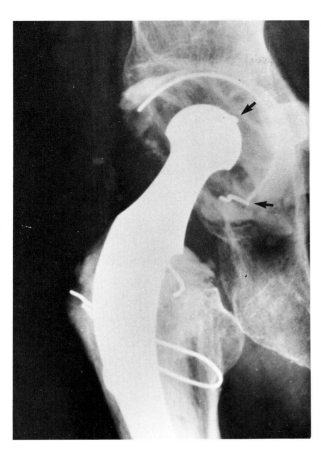

Fig. 17-26. Postoperative radiograph of 48-year-old female following excision of greater trochanter for established nonunion (performed in another hospital). This patient developed instability and had severe limp owing to weakness of abductors. NOTE: inclusion of wire fragment (arrow).

plaining of trochanteric pain either have a low threshold for pain or preoperatively did not grade "severe" for their pain on the evaluation sheet, and consequently were considered borderline candidates for total hip replacement surgery selection. They are often borderline neurotics or miracle seekers!

At times, wire migration into the soft tissue of the hip following fracture is seen. If revision surgery becomes necessary, the migrated wire pieces often may be lost, and it is futile to waste time trying to find all the pieces.

Nonunion of trochanter and dislocation

A relatively high rate of nonunion of the trochanter accompanying dislocation of the hip has been reported (see "Instability and Disloca-

tions"). As stated previously, nonunion of the trochanter was accompanied by dislocations only twice in our series. In both cases, severe trauma with further separation of the trochanter was sustained by the patient (leading to the dislocation). It may then be stated that if the trochanter is not united, there is an increased risk of its separation as the result of trauma, leading to dislocation. Undoubtedly, early separation of the greater trochanter is accompanied by an increased risk of dislocation.

Avulsion and painful migrated trochanter

Early loss of the trochanter (that is, its fixation or fragmentation) can usually be traced to the surgical technique. Fragmentation of the trochanter can occur often in severe osteoporosis or revision of failed previous operations. At surgery fragmentation and fracture may occur from careless handling of the trochanteric clamp or forceful retraction of the trochanter (see Chapter 12). On occasion, however, despite good and careful wiring, an extremely osteoporotic trochanter may escape through the wires (if they have cut through the bone) (Fig. 17-24, *B*). An osteoporotic trochanter is usually recognized at the time of its removal; the lack of bony trabeculae within the trochanter (revealed by radiography) testifies to this and mandates careful handling during surgery. Further postoperative bedrest or immobilization may be justified if fixation is not optimum at surgery. As a solution to handling an osteoporotic trochanter, the use of wire mesh has been advocated.[32] We have no experience with this method.

The painful migrated trochanter should be treated as follows.

1. The nonunion site should be exposed and the fibrous union should be excised.
2. As much cancellous bone as possible should be preserved with the trochanter.
3. The short abductors should be advanced distally but rarely proximally (through separate incision and by subperiosteal release of abductor origin from iliac bone).
4. Wires supplemented by two screws or trochanteric staple-clamps should be used or the technique of Volz should be employed.
5. If cancellous bone of the trochanter is insufficient, a bone graft taken from the ilium may serve as an interposition graft.
6. The cement should not be in contact with the newly reattached trochanter.

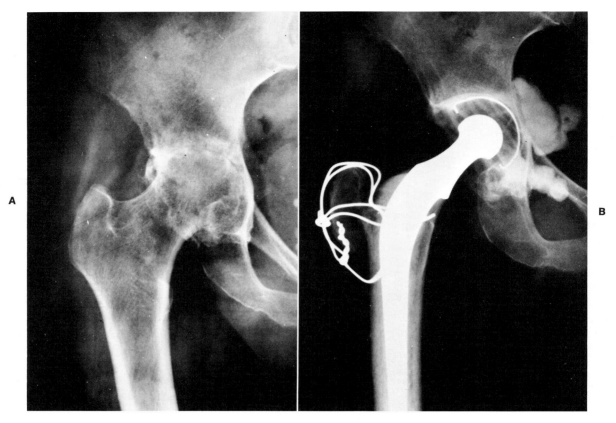

Fig. 17-27. A, Preoperative radiograph of 53-year-old woman with rheumatoid arthritis. Concentric involvement and minimal progression are noted. **B,** Excess damage to floor and ischiopubic region. Postoperatively patient had complete femoral and obturator nerve palsy, presumably from damage by trauma or heat of polymerization of cement. Femoral nerve partially recovered 1 year following surgery.

Ectopic bone formation in trochanteric region

It is often said that the bone dust from the removal of the trochanter will cause ectopic bone formation; our experience does not support this view. We have seen an equal amount of ectopic bone in the same individual who underwent bilateral total hip arthroplasty involving unilateral trochanteric osteotomy. As indicated earlier in this chapter, excess stripping of the vastus lateralis muscle below the vastus lateralis ridge may encourage myositic ossifications in this region.

NEUROVASCULAR COMPLICATIONS

Vascular damage including rupture of the major vessels such as the internal iliac artery or vein, femoral artery or vein, and circumflex vessels may lead to excessive bleeding during or immediately after total hip replacement. Immediate recognition of this complication by arteriography and management by surgical correction immediately or at reoperation may be lifesaving. Sporadic reports of isolated cases have appeared in the literature with the emphasis on avoidance of these unfortunate complications. Embolization of smaller vessels following detection by arteriography has also been suggested.

Peripheral neuropathies associated with total hip arthroplasty have been reported in many clinical series in the past. The most vulnerable nerves are the sciatic, femoral, and obturator nerves, in order of their frequency. Posterior dislocation of the hip, direct contact of methyl methacrylate cement with the nerve, and excessive stretching at the time of surgery by lengthening the extremity may be considered etiological factors.

The most common cause of sciatic nerve palsy in our series during the first 2,000 total hip arthroplasties has been postoperative hemorrhage, as the result of anticoagulation treatment. Six sciatic and two femoral nerve palsies were encountered. In all, a hematoma was demonstrated to be the responsible cause, and in five out of six sciatic palsies in which hematoma was evacuated recovery of the sciatic nerve was prompt and complete. The obturator and femoral nerves are more prone to damage by the flow of cement (Fig. 17-27) into the region of the pubis and anterior aspect of the acetabulum. Additionally, the femoral nerve may be overly stretched or permanently damaged by injudicious use of Hohmann-type retractors applied within the pelvis. Nerve palsies resulting from overstretching in lengthening the extremity must be extremely rare. No correlations are found between the amount of lengthening gained at surgery and femoral nerve palsy.[56] In fact, in our experience this has not been the cause of any nerve palsies. This is presumably because of fixed length of the fascia and septal layer of the thigh, which does not allow "overstretching" by elongation. It is of special interest that female patients have been more prone to nerve palsy than male patients.[56] One must consider patients with previous surgery or difficult technical problems more prone to develop this complication.

Another type of nerve palsy is caused by external rotation and direct pressure on the nerve postoperatively. If fixed external rotation deformity is not corrected by surgery or develops postoperatively, direct pressure on the peroneal nerve at the level of the neck of the fibula may result.

To prevent peripheral neuropathy the surgeon must constantly remind himself of the anatomical relationship of the sciatic nerve and its intimacy to the posterior acetabulum. The possibility of polymerizing cement through defective areas, that is, anchor holes, acetabular floor, and so on, to produce nerve damage must also be kept in mind. It is also essential to create anchoring holes without excessive damage to the bone. During rehearsal for the stability of the hip, one must protect the sciatic nerve from being stretched over the dislocating head posteriorly (see Chapter 12). Additionally, placement of the Hohmann retractors, if used, must be carefully verified in relationship to the nerves about the hip.

Every patient following total hip replacement must be tested for nerve function immediately on recovery from the anesthesia. Repeated examination of the patient for possible nerve palsy during the daily follow-up course is also equally essential, since pressure-induced nerve palsies such as those from hematomas induced by anticoagulation or other hemorrhagic conditions can be detected and treated immediately. If anticoagulation and hemorrhage are the causes of nerve palsy developing postoperatively, it should be treated by immediate decompression of the nerve by reoperation. The fascia is opened, and nerve is freed up to the sciatic notch at reexploration. In general the recovery following nerve palsy is good unless the nerve has been completely destroyed, either by the heat of polymerization of the cement or by transection at surgery. The prognosis is excellent when decompression of the hematoma has been done by evacuation immediately after detection. An immediate peroneal nerve palsy associated with total hip arthroplasty is the result of sciatic nerve damage at the level of the arthroplasty. On the other hand, when peroneal palsy (footdrop) develops following surgery, it is either the result of direct pressure from contact over the neck of the fibula or a progressive hematoma causing pressure on the sciatic nerve.

SUMMARY OF ESSENTIALS

- Dislocation following total hip replacement is a complication of surgical technique that is usually avoidable if the details of technique are observed.
- Some reports in recent literature suggest a direct but inverse relationship between the size of the femoral head (component of the total hip prosthesis) and the rate of dislocation following total hip arthroplasty. On this ground a small femoral head prosthesis has been incriminated for being inherently "unstable."
- It is our conclusion that the rate of dislocation following total hip replacement is not related to the size of the femoral head component of the prosthesis.
- Dislocations may be classified as anterior, posterior, superior, and inferior; and immediate, early, and late. Subluxations may be static or dynamic (functional). In subluxation the head has escaped from the acetabular cup but is still in contact with its rim and remains within the confinement of the bony socket.
- Operative instability is created by the ability of the surgeon to pull the femoral prosthesis out of the

Clinical results and complications

socket more than 1 cm., by longitudinal traction on the limb, or by certain ranges of motion (without the use of traction) to produce dislocation with ease.

■ A review of dislocations in 1,400 low-friction arthroplasties (using a 22-mm. diameter ball) performed revealed eight dislocations, resulting in an incidence of 0.5%. All dislocations were posterior, three of the eight dislocations were traumatic. Two dislocations were immediate, three were early, and three were late. Four subluxations were also recognized (an incidence of 0.25% by radiography). The rate of functional subluxation (dynamic) was approximately 2%. None of the subluxations required any specific treatment, and none were complicated by subsequent dislocations.

■ Understanding the pathomechanics of dislocation is important in order to avoid this complication. There are several interrelated principles involving instability of the hip joint following total hip replacement. These factors include mechanical features of the prosthesis, anatomical factors related to the soft tissue and femur or acetabulum, technical handling at surgery, and postoperative management.

■ Of the mechanical factors of the prosthesis contributing to dislocation, the head-neck ratio diameter, the neck length, the depth of the socket, the recession of the neck, and orientation of the components within the bony acetabulum and femur should be considered. Of the anatomical factors the key stabilizing muscles include the tensor fascia femoris, gluteus medius and minimus, and the capsule of the joint and its reinforcing ligaments. Obviously, damage to the nerves to these muscles as well as scarified structures, calcifications, and heterotopic bone about the hip may prejudice their function in producing stability.

■ Because of the importance of soft tissue in contributing to the stability of the hip after replacement, preservation of the iliotibial tract and repair of this structure at the end of operation and gentle retraction of the glutei and tensor fascia femoris muscle and preservation of their nerves are essential. Reattachment of the greater trochanter must be done with care to augment stability of the joint. A high positioning of the socket or extreme shortening of the neck reduces the effective neck length of the femur, thus reducing the tension of the musculofascial septa inviting dislocation.

■ At surgery the hip joint must be stable prior to the reattachment of the greater trochanter. An excessively shortened neck of the femur can be compensated for by the use of a long-neck prosthesis.

■ Orientation of the prosthesis is most crucial in avoiding dislocations. Preoperative planning for locating the "acetabular site" and preparation at the appropriate level (by the use of a radiographic template) should reduce the chance for dislocation.

■ Mechanical clearance between the femur and acetabulum must be assured prior to closure. Often marginal osteophytes or unremoved cement may lever the femoral head out of the socket similar to excessive deepening of the acetabulum.

■ Recent dislocations must be treated by skin or skeletal traction for the first 24 hours; often this may successfully reduce the hip joint. When reduction is not successful within the first 24 to 48 hours following dislocation, the hip must be reduced under general anesthesia. Failure to reduce the hip under general anesthesia necessitates an open reduction to search for the cause(s) of dislocation.

■ When the hip is reduced (by closed or open methods), it should be immobilized for a period of 6 weeks in a hip spica cast or in bed with the hip in an abducted position.

■ Fractures of the femur complicating total hip replacement may be divided into preoperative, intraoperative, and postoperative fractures. A true incidence of intraoperative fracture is only possible if surgeon's records accurately document these complications and/or postoperative radiographs are carefully scrutinized for these complications.

■ Factors predisposing to fracture include anatomical pathology of the bone or joint, previous surgery, osteoporosis, and careless handling at surgery. The study of our first 1,200 consecutive total hip replacements revealed 32 intraoperative fractures; 10 were considered minor fractures, which in no way affected the stability of the femoral component or postoperative management of the patient; 22 were considered major, requiring treatment or careful observation.

■ Specifically, predisposing factors in fractures in our series were narrow medullary canal, rheumatoid arthritis, and increased anteversion of the femoral neck.

■ Revision surgery also carried considerable risk in producing these fractures including removal of the femoral head prosthesis, such as the Moore self-locking prosthesis, removal of the nail and plate, and dislocating the hip at surgery. Broaching of the femur or removal of the cement from canals was an added etiological factor in producing these fractures.

■ The best methods of preventing fractures are careful planning; careful examination of radiographs preoperatively, that is, narrow medullary canal, previous hardware, previous damage to the shaft of the femur, and so on; and careful preparation of the femur using graded reamers prior to the use

640

of broaches. The previous defects of the shaft or severe osteoporosis are alarming enough to proceed at a slower pace with added caution to avoid penetration by broaches.

■ Intraoperative fractures of the femur must be treated immediately on their recognition and evaluated fully by two perpendicular-plane radiographs. In our experiences a circlage-wire technique and the use of a long-stem prosthesis have been best suited for major shaft fractures. Proximal cortical fractures also are best treated by circlage wire and the use of conventional hip replacement prostheses.

■ Immediately following surgery, a supplemental balanced suspension apparatus or a hip spica cast may be used in addition to the internal fixation. Full weight bearing must be avoided until complete healing of the fracture.

■ Postoperative fractures resulting from trauma are best treated by nonoperative means using skeletal traction and application of a hip spica cast as indicated. The rate of a successful union following this method indicates that operative intervention is rarely indicated for this type of fracture.

■ The advantages of trochanteric osteotomy may be offset if a high rate of complication results from this technique. Factors that decidedly influence the rate of union of the trochanter are related to detailed and precise technique used in detachment and subsequent reattachment of the trochanter.

■ The quality of the bone of the trochanter, repeated surgery and pathological conditions of the bone of the femur, and the patient's lack of cooperation postoperatively contribute to trochanteric complications.

■ The problems of trochanteric osteotomy include asymptomatic nonunion (radiographic), painful nonunion without displacement, painful nonunion with migration, delayed union (radiological), painful bursitis (union), early avulsion with or without dislocation of the hip, nonunion and late dislocation, and heterotopic ossification in the trochanteric region.

■ Nonunion of the greater trochanter is often asymptomatic and manifests itself on radiographic examinations alone within 3 to 6 months following surgery. A small number of nonunions eventually unite even after many months or years following surgery.

■ Because most nonunions are asymptomatic and since a successful union by reoperation may be difficult, no further surgical intervention is justifiable unless the patient develops pain or a severe limp.

■ The technique of fixation of the trochanter plays an important part in preventing dislocation. Good contact between the bone of the trochanter and the outer aspect of the femur and maintenance of the fixation during the early postoperative phase is essential to ensure union.

■ A completely "complication-free" method has yet to be developed, but any method used should include a two-plane fixation of the trochanter, longitudinally and horizontally.

■ While the rate of nonunion of the trochanter in primary interventions is low, nonunion and proximal migration are most frequently encountered in revision of previously failed operations, where the bone is osteoporotic and the abductor mechanism is scarified and shortened. In addition to mobilization of the abductors, additional fixation elements such as screws, bolts, and staple-clamps may be used to overcome the difficulties encountered in obtaining union in these cases.

■ The breakage of wires may be early or late. The late breakage of wire following union of the trochanter is inconsequential and to avoid anxiety should not be mentioned to the patient. However, the early rupture of wires may risk migration of the trochanter and the possibility of an unstable hip. Broken wires that are asymptomatic should not be a source of concern to the surgeon or the patient.

■ Repeated local steroid injections for painful bursitis over the trochanter should be discouraged. The wires from the trochanter rarely require removal; only when the fractured fragments of wires are lodged within the joint is removal encouraged. Removal of the ununited trochanteric fragment is not indicated.

■ A painful proximally migrated trochanter with severe limp must be rectified by reoperation, which includes exposure of the nonunion site, excision of the fibrous union, distal advancement of the short abductors, and a rigid fixation of the ununited trochanter. Trochanteric avulsion complicated by dislocation usually requires rewiring especially when dislocation is recurrent or displacement is severe.

REFERENCES

1. Amstutz, H. C.: Trapezoidal-28 total hip replacement, Clin. Orthop. **95:**158-167, 1973.
2. Amstutz, H. C., and Markoff, K. L.: Design features in total hip replacement. In The Hip Society: Proceedings of the second open scientific meeting of The Hip Society, 1974, St. Louis, 1974, The C. V. Mosby Co., pp. 111-122.
2a. Arden, G. P., and Ansel, B. M.: Total hip replacement in inflammatory arthritis. In Jason, M., editor: Total hip replacement, Philadelphia, 1971, J. B. Lippincott Co., pp. 86-102.
3. Bergström, B., Lindberg, L., Persson, B., and Önnerfält, R.: Complications after total hip arthroplasty according to Charnley in a Swedish series of cases, Clin. Orthop. **95:**91-95, 1973.

4. Chapchal, G. J., Slooff, T. J. J. H., and Nollen, A. D.: Results of total hip replacement: a critical follow-up study, Clin. Orthop. **95:**111-117, 1973.

5. Charnley, J.: The healing of human fractures in contact with self-curing acrylic cement, Clin. Orthop. **47:**157-163, 1966.

6. Charnley, J.: Total hip replacement by low-friction arthroplasty, Clin. Orthop. **72:**7-21, 1970.

7. Charnley, J.: The rationale of low-friction arthroplasty. In The Hip Society: Proceedings of the first open scientific meeting of The Hip Society, 1973, St. Louis, 1973, The C. V. Mosby Co., pp. 92-100.

8. Charnley, J.: Biomechanical considerations in total prosthetic design. In The Hip Society: Proceedings of the first open scientific meeting of The Hip Society, 1973, St. Louis, 1973, The C. V. Mosby Co., pp. 101-117.

9. Charnley, J.: Elevation of the greater trochanter in total hip replacement, J. Bone Joint Surg. **57B:** 395, 1975.

10. Charnley, J.: Instructions for the use of the trochanter staple-clamp. Internal Publication No. 65, Centre for Hip Surgery, Wrightington Hospital, England, September, 1976.

11. Charnley, J.: Scientific exhibit (combined meeting of the English speaking world) London, September, 1976.

12. Charnley, J., and Cupic, Z.: The nine and ten year results of the low-friction arthroplasty of the hip, Clin. Orthop. **95:**9-25, 1973.

13. Charnley, J., and Cupic, Z.: Etiology and incidence of dislocation in Charnley low-friction arthroplasty. Internal Publication No. 46, Centre for Hip Surgery, Wrightington Hospital, England, January, 1974.

14. Charnley, J., and Ferrera, A.: Transplantation of the greater trochanter in arthroplasty of the hip, J. Bone Joint Surg. **46B:**191-197, 1964.

15. Coventry, M. B.: The surgical technique of total hip arthroplasty, modified from Charnley as done at the Mayo Clinic, Orthop. Clin. North Am. **4:** 473-482, 1973.

16. Coventry, M. B., Beckenbaugh, R. D., Nolan, D. R., and Ilstrup, D. M.: 2012 total hip arthroplasties: a study of postoperative course and early complications, J. Bone Joint Surg. **56A:**273-284, 1974.

17. Eftekhar, N. S.: Low-friction arthroplasty: indications, contraindications and complications, J.A.M.A. **28:**705-710, 1971.

18. Eftekhar, N. S.: Intraoperative fractures of the femur. Paper presented at the American Academy of Orthopaedic Surgeons meeting, Miami, 1974.

19. Eftekhar, N. S.: Mechanical failure in low-friction arthroplasty. In American Academy of Orthopaedic Surgeons: Instructional course lectures, vol. 23, St. Louis, 1974, The C. V. Mosby Co., pp. 230-242.

20. Eftekhar, N. S.: Abduction splint for hip surgery, a new device, Orthop. Rev. **3:**51-52, 1974.

21. Eftekhar, N. S.: Dislocation and instability complicating low-friction arthroplasty of the hip joint, Clin. Orthop. **121:**120-125, 1976.

22. Eftekhar, N. S.: Trochanter on or off? Paper presented before first Open Scientific Meeting of International Hip Society, Berne, Switzerland, April, 1977.

23. Eftekhar, N. S.: Charnley "low–friction torque" arthroplasty, a study of long-term results, Clin. Orthop. **81:**93-104, 1971.

24. Eftekhar, N. S., and Stinchfield, F. E.: Experience with low-friction arthroplasty, a statistical review of early results and complications, Clin. Orthop. **95:**60-68, 1973.

25. Eftekhar, N. S., Kiernan, H. A., and Stinchfield, F. E.: Systemic and local complications following low-friction arthroplasty of the hip joint, a study of 800 consecutive operations, Arch. Surg. **111:**150-155, 1976.

26. English, T. A.: The trochanteric approach to the hip for prosthetic replacement, J. Bone Joint Surg. **57B:**395, 1975.

27. Evanski, P. M., Waugh, T. R., and Orofino, C. F.: Total hip replacement with the Charnley prosthesis, Clin. Orthop. **95:**69-72, 1973.

28. Evarts, C. M., Wilde, A. H., DeHaven, K. E., Nelson, C. L., and Collins, H. R.: Total hip joint arthroplasty, J. Bone Joint Surg. **54A:**1562, 1972.

29. Freeman, P. A., Lee, P., and Bryson, W. T.: Total hip joint replacement in osteoarthrosis and polyarthritis, a statistical study of the results, Clin. Orthop. **95:**224-230, 1973.

30. Harris, W. H.: A new total hip implant, Clin. Orthop. **81:**105-113, 1971.

31. Harris, W. H.: A new approach to total hip replacement without osteotomy of the greater trochanter, Clin. Orthop. **106:**19-26, 1975.

32. Harris, W. H., and Jones, W. N.: The use of wire mesh in total hip replacement surgery, Clin. Orthop. **106:**117-121, 1975.

33. Johnston, R. C.: Clinical follow-up of total hip replacement, Clin. Orthop. **95:**118-126, 1973.

34. Kiernan, H., Bush, D., Eftekhar, N., and Stinchfield, F.: Fractures of the upper femur during total hip replacement, Unpublished data.

35. Lazansky, M. G.: Complications in total hip replacement with the Charnley technic, Clin. Orthop. **72:**40-45, 1970.

36. Lazansky, M. G.: Complications revisited: the debit side of total hip replacement, Clin. Orthop. **95:**96-103, 1973.

37. Leinbach, I. S., and Barlow, F. A.: 700 total hip replacements, experience with six types, Clin. Orthop. **95:**174-192, 1973.

38. Luck, J. V.: An approach for hip construction: broad visualization without osteotomy of the greater trochanter, Clin. Orthop. **91**:70-85, 1973.

39. Luck, J. V., Brannon, E. W., and Luck, J. V., Jr.: Total hip replacement arthroplasty; causes, orthopaedic management, and prevention of selected problems, J. Bone Joint Surg. **54A**:1569-1571, 1972.

40. McElfresh, E. C., and Coventry, M. B.: Femoral and pelvic fractures after total hip arthroplasty, J. Bone Joint Surg. **56A**:483, 1974.

41. McKee, G. K.: Development of total prosthetic replacement of the hip, Clin. Orthop. **72**:85-103, 1970.

42. McKee, G. K., and Chen, S. C.: The statistics of the McKee-Farrar method of total hip replacement, Clin. Orthop. **95**:26-33, 1973.

43. Müller, M. E.: Total hip prosthesis, Clin. Orthop. **72**:46-68, 1970.

44. Müller, M. E.: Total hip replacement without trochanter osteotomy. In The Hip Society: Proceedings of the second open scientific meeting of The Hip Society, 1974, St. Louis, 1974, The C. V. Mosby Co., pp. 231-237.

45. Murray, W. R.: Results in patients with total hip replacement arthroplasty, Clin. Orthop. **95**:80-90, 1973.

46. Nicholson, O. R.: Total hip replacement, an evaluation of the results and technics, 1967-1972, Clin. Orthop. **95**:217-233, 1973.

47. Patterson, F. P., and Brown, C. S.: The McKee-Farrar total hip replacement—preliminary results and complications of 368 operations performed in five general hospitals, J. Bone Joint Surg. **54A:** 257-275, 1972.

48. Ring, P. A.: Total replacement of the hip, Clin. Orthop. **72**:161-168, 1970.

49. Ring, P. A.: Total replacement of the hip joint, Clin. Orthop. **95**:34-37, 1973.

50. Sarmiento, A.: Personal communications.

51. Scott, R. D., and Turner, R. H.: Avoiding complications with long-stem total hip-replacement arthroplasty, J. Bone Joint Surg. **57A**:722, 1975.

52. Scott, R. D., Turner, R. H., Leitzes, S. M., and Aufranc, O. E.: Femoral fractures in conjunction with total hip replacement, J. Bone Joint Surg. **57A**:494-501, 1975.

53. Sledge, C. B.: Discussion on osteotomy of the greater trochanter. In The Hip Society: Proceedings of the second open scientific meeting of The Hip Society, 1974, St. Louis, 1974, The C. V. Mosby Co., pp. 247-250.

54. Volz, R. G., and Mayer, D. M.: The predictive factors necessitating trochanteric osteotomy in total hip replacement, Orthop. Rev. **5**:23-25, 1976.

55. Volz, R. G., and Turner, R. H.: Reattachment of the greater trochanter in total hip arthroplasty by use of a bolt, J. Bone Joint Surg. **57A**:129-131, 1975.

56. Weber, E. R., Daube, J. R., and Coventry, M. B.: Peripheral neuropathies associated with total hip arthroplasty, J. Bone Joint Surg. **58A**:66-69, 1976.

57. Welch, R. B., and Charnley, J.: Low-friction arthroplasty of the hip in rheumatoid arthritis and ankylosing spondylitis, Clin. Orthop. **72**:22-32, 1970.

643

Index

Index

Index